E

E

(

ATLAS OF CLINICAL
RHEUMATOLOGY

Project Editor:	**David Bennett**
Art Director:	**Mehmet Hussein**
Design:	Mick Brennan
	David Buss
	Julian Dorr
Illustration:	Pam Corfield
(Artwork)	Max Dyson
	Edwina Hannam
	Lydia Malim
Illustration:	Jeremy Cort
(Linework)	Maurizia Merati
	Andrew Park
	Gill Short
Index:	Dr. John Gibson

ATLAS OF CLINICAL RHEUMATOLOGY

Paul A Dieppe
BSc MB BS MRCP
Consultant Rheumatologist and
Senior Lecturer in Medicine
Bristol Royal Infirmary Bristol UK

Paul A Bacon
MB BCHIR FRCP
Professor of Rheumatology
University of Birmingham
Birmingham UK

Andrew N Bamji
MB BS MRCP
Consultant Rheumatologist
Brook General Hospital London &
Queen Mary's Hospital Sidcup UK

Iain Watt
MB BS MRCP FRCR
Consultant Radiologist
Bristol Royal Infirmary Bristol UK

Editorial Advisors
Barbara Ansell   Harrow UK
Paul Byers   London UK
Joseph D Croft Jr   Washington DC USA
Ian Haslock   Middlesbrough UK
Marcel Kahn   Paris France
Thomas Scott   London UK
Colin Tribe   Bristol UK
Thomas Vischer   Geneva Switzerland

Gower Medical Publishing · London · New York 1986

Brought to You as a Medical Service by G. D. Searle & Co.

Distributors of English Editions
USA and Canada
Lea and Febiger
600 Washington Square
Philadelphia 19106, USA.

ISBN 0-906923-75-1 (Gower)

Library of Congress Cataloging in Publication Data:
Main entry under title

Atlas of Clinical Rheumatology.
    Includes bibliographies and index.
    1. Rheumatism–Diagnosis–Atlases. I. Dieppe, Paul.
[DNLM: 1. Rheumatology–atlases. WE 17 A879]
RC927,A85 1985   616.7'23   85-23129

Originated by Mandarin Offset.
Reprinted in Hong Kong in 1988.

Preface

Rheumatic diseases account for a major proportion of those who suffer chronic pain and disability. These diseases range from rare, severe, systemic diseases such as polyarteritis nodosa to common self-limiting, localized disorders like tennis elbow. The majority of these conditions can be diagnosed and assessed with a simple clinical, radiographic and pathological examination without employing complex technology. It is most appropriate therefore, that the rheumatic diseases be presented in a clinically orientated atlas.

The Atlas of Clinical Rheumatology comprises a selection of clinical and radiological appearances, pathological specimens and histological sections illustrating common and important features of the rheumatic diseases. Diagrams, operative views and some tables and lists have also been included where it was felt that they would enhance understanding. All illustrations are accompanied by a detailed descriptive caption and, where appropriate, an explanatory diagram. The text is intended to complement the illustrations rather than to be a comprehensive treatise on rheumatology. The aim is to help the reader place the pictures in the context of the overall disease process. The chapters are divided according to current concepts of disease processes rather than by anatomical region. Where possible, an attempt has been made to illustrate modern concepts regarding the pathology of the disease process and to explain the clinical and radiological changes shown. Our hope was to aid understanding, stimulate thought, and encourage research into these crippling diseases. The Atlas should also provide useful teaching material for both undergraduate and postgraduate education. We hope teachers will find it helpful and that it may make some contribution to increasing rheumatology in medical curriculae.

The field of rheumatology is a very broad one. Had we attempted a complete and comprehensive coverage, the result would have been an atlas much too large to be genuinely useful. Instead, our aim has been to include top quality examples of important aspects of the rheumatic diseases. The text and captions explain each choice and how it illustrates a particular aspect of clinical rheumatology.

The concept of the Atlas started in the Bath/Bristol area and much of the material originated locally. We are deeply indebted to our many colleagues and friends who contributed items from personal slide collections. We would particularly like to acknowledge the work of the late Colin Tribe, whose untimely death came during the production of this Atlas, to which he made a major contribution.

We would also like to thank Mrs. Margaret Clarke for invaluable secretarial help, and David Bennett of Gower Medical Publishing Ltd. for continued care of the project through its long gestation.

PAD
PAB
ANB
IW

CONTRIBUTORS

Dr Carol Black, West Middlesex University Hospital, Isleworth, UK.

Dr Joseph Croft Jr., Arthritis Rehabilitation Center, P.C., Washington, D.C., USA

Dr W. Carson Dick, The Royal Victoria Infirmary, Newcastle-Upon-Tyne, UK.

Dr Ian Haslock, Middlesbrough General Hospital, Middlesbrough, UK.

Professor Malcolm Jayson, Hope Hospital, Salford, UK.

Dr John Kanis, The Medical School, The University of Sheffield, Sheffield, UK.

Dr John Klippel, National Institutes of Health, Bethesda, Maryland, USA.

Dr Peter Maddison, Royal National Hospital for Rheumatic Diseases, Bath, UK.

Dr Philip Platt, The Royal Victoria Infirmary, Newcastle-Upon-Tyne, UK.

Dr David G.I. Scott, The Medical School, The University of Birmingham, Birmingham, UK.

Professor Thomas Vischer, Hôpital Cantonal, Universitaire de Genève, Geneva, Switzerland.

Dr Rodney Waterworth, Napier Hospital, Hawkes Bay, New Zealand.

Contents

1

The Clinical Evaluation of Rheumatic Diseases

Rheumatology involves the study of diseases affecting joints and periarticular structures. In spite of recent advances in sophisticated diagnostic techniques such as joint imaging and clinical immunology, rheumatology remains an essentially clinical discipline. The majority of rheumatic diseases can be diagnosed from a careful clinical history and examination of the patient. Furthermore, the precise anatomical site of the pathology, and the functional problems caused by the disease, can be assessed accurately during the clinical examination. A number of numerical measurements are also available to the clinician which further aid his ability to follow the course of rheumatic diseases and chart the effect of various treatments used. It is therefore appropriate to begin this survey of rheumatic diseases with the clinical evaluation of joints and periarticular structures. No attempt has been made to cover all aspects of this vast subject, but a selection of illustrations is presented depicting various examinations and measurements in joint diseases.

The Symptoms and Signs of Joint Disease

A diagrammatic cross-section of a synovial joint and its periarticular structures is shown in figure 1.1. Any pathological condition affecting the bone ends, articular cartilage, synovium or capsule can result in joint disease. In addition, abnormalities of the surrounding soft tissue, including muscles, ligaments, tendons and bursae may give rise to similar signs and symptoms, and are included in the category of rheumatic diseases.

Musculoskeletal symptoms include pain, stiffness, deformity and loss of function (Fig. 1.2). Pain is the major symptom of most rheumatic diseases, but its pattern and its relationship to activity varies considerably; for example, pain usually gets worse on use in osteoarthritis, and tends to be severe at the beginning of the day in rheumatoid disease. Joint stiffness is another important symptom, and again its pattern, severity and duration may help to discriminate between different diseases: stiffness in the morning is a feature of all inflammatory diseases of the synovium, whereas short lasting but severe stiffness after inactivity is a prominent feature of osteoarthritis. Patients may also complain of deformity and loss of motion in individual joints or limbs, or of increasing functional disability. A careful history of the patient's ability to carry out the normal everyday tasks of daily living is therefore an important part of the history. Many rheumatic diseases also result in generalized systemic illness and symptoms arising from many other organs.

Joints are examined by inspection, palpation and movement. After careful inspection of the whole limb, and comparison of the two sides of the body, individual joint and periarticular structures should be palpated. Increased vascularity may result in heat and redness of the joints, with inflammation causing tenderness. The exact point of tenderness is important in locating the site of the pathology (Figs. 1.3 & 1.4). Swelling may be bony, due to soft tissue hypertrophy, or result from fluid exudation into the area (Figs. 1.5 & 1.6). Subluxation, dislocation, or angulation deformities can be palpated and measured (Fig. 1.7), and joint motion should be examined by both active and passive movement (Fig. 1.8). Restriction of movement, instability, and joint crepitus should be recorded. Finally, the patient should be asked to carry out some simple everyday tasks involving the joint in question.

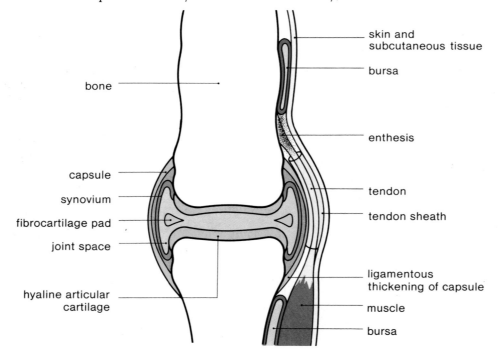

SYMPTOMS AND SIGNS OF JOINT DISEASES
Symptoms
Pain
Stiffness
Deformity
Loss of Function
Systemic Illness
Signs
Heat
Redness
Swelling
Loss of Movement
Deformity
Tenderness
Abnormal Movement
Crepitus
Functional Abnormality

Fig. 1.1 Diagrammatic cross-section of synovial joint and its periarticular structures, illustrating some of the structures which give rise to pain and inflammation in rheumatic diseases. Note the synovial lining of the joint, bursae and tendon sheaths.

Fig. 1.2 The major symptoms and signs of joint diseases.

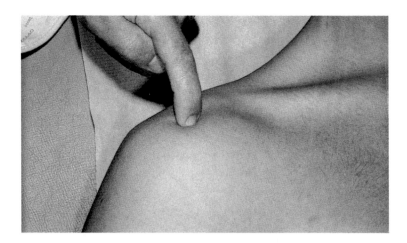

Fig. 1.3 Tenderness over the joint line indicates articular disease. The acromio-clavicular joint line is being palpated by the examiner's index finger to see if pain is arising from this joint or from a nearby related structure.

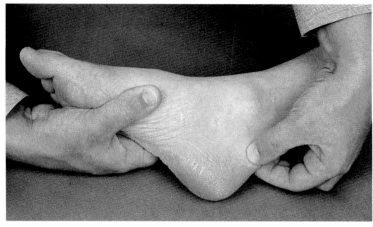

Fig. 1.4 Testing for tenderness over the insertion of the achilles tendon. This is an example of a periarticular site causing 'joint' pain.

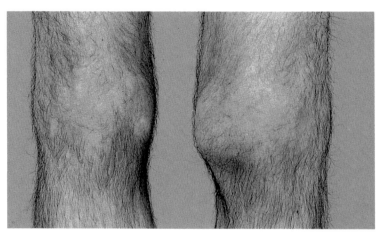

Fig. 1.5 Bony swelling of a joint; in this case due to bony overgrowth at the knee in hemophiliac arthropathy.

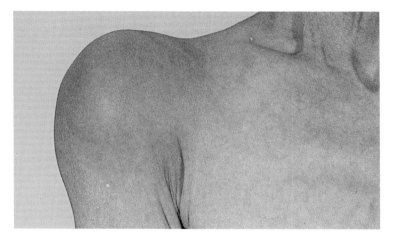

Fig. 1.6 Soft tissue swelling; a large swollen shoulder joint due to 'pseudogout'. About 150 mls. of synovial fluid was aspirated from this joint.

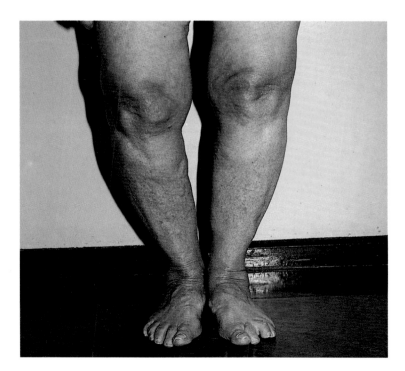

Fig. 1.7 Varus deformity of the knee joint due to osteoarthritis.

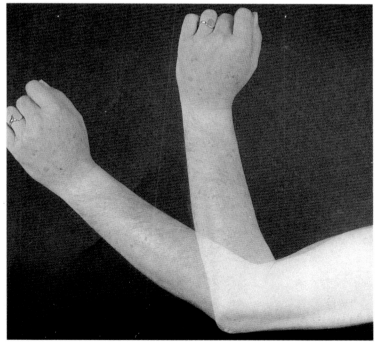

Fig. 1.8 Restricted range of joint motion due to arthritis of the elbow; the patient has flexed and extended the joint as far as she can.

Inflammation of Joints and Periarticular Structures
Inflammation is a major component of many rheumatic diseases. The classical features of inflammation described by Galen include heat, redness, swelling, pain and loss of function (Fig. 1.9). Stiffness in the morning can be added to the list as it is a particularly common feature of rheumatic diseases and its duration and severity reflect the amount of inflammation present. Swelling in or around the joint may have a variety of causes and a careful palpation of the area is necessary to distinguish bone, cartilage and periarticular soft tissue changes, from inflammatory fluid exudates or hypertrophy of the synovium (Fig. 1.10). Although any swollen inflamed joint may be warm to touch, redness of the overlying skin implies involvement of periarticular tissue as well as of the synovium. This occurs in a limited number of rheumatic diseases including gout, septic arthritis, inflamed Heberden's nodes, rheumatic fever and palindromic rheumatism (Fig. 1.11). Heat can often be fairly accurately assessed by running the back of the hand over the area; differences of about one degree centigrade can be detected in this way after exposure of the limb.

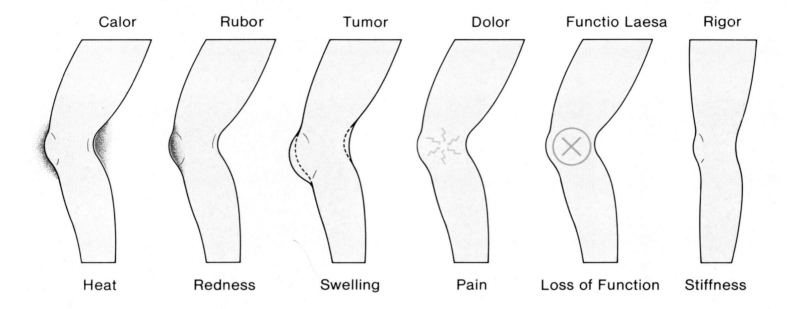

Calor	Rubor	Tumor	Dolor	Functio Laesa	Rigor
Heat	Redness	Swelling	Pain	Loss of Function	Stiffness

Fig. 1.9 The cardinal signs of inflammation as described by Celsus, Galen and others.

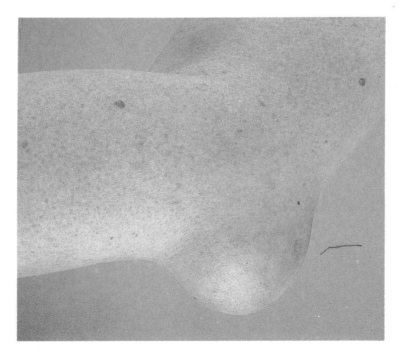

Fig. 1.10 Inflammation of the olecranon bursa in rheumatoid arthritis causing a large swelling. Extra-articular bursae and tendon sheaths may cause confusion with intra-articular swellings.

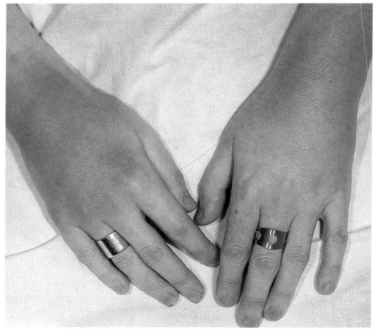

Fig. 1.11 Redness of the skin overlying inflamed joints, in this case due to rheumatic fever.

Inflammation of the joints may also result in systemic symptoms such as fever, malaise and weight loss.

Regional Examination of Joints

Good examination techniques cannot be conveyed adequately by a small number of illustrations. A small number are included here to show some aspects of the regional examination of the musculoskeletal system; many other examples can be found in other chapters.

The Upper Limbs. Hand, wrist, elbow and shoulder function can be assessed by observing the patient carrying out a few simple tasks, for example picking up objects on the bedside, trying to write, putting their hands together as if praying, or combing their hair. The functional limitations and site of the problem usually become immediately obvious. Full regional examination should then include careful palpation of the joints and periarticular structures, as well as assessment of neurological deficits and muscle power. Some examples of the techniques used are shown in figures 1.12 – 1.19.

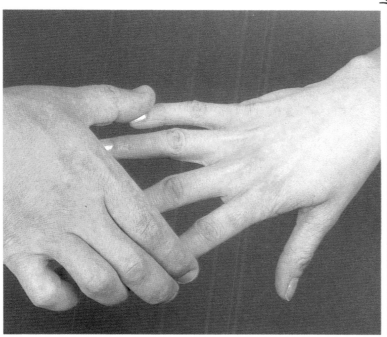

Fig. 1.12 Examination of the hands. The patient's index finger is being flexed and extended while the examiner's fingers are palpating the flexor tendons to detect crepitus or restriction of movement from tenosynovitis.

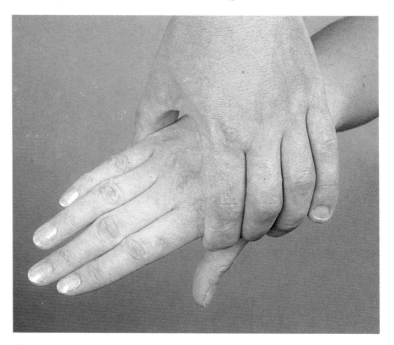

Fig. 1.13 Lateral pressure over the metacarpophalangeal joints to elicit tenderness, an early sign of inflammatory disease of the MCPs.

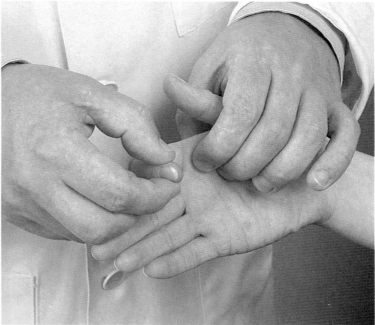

Fig. 1.14 Testing for power of the interossei muscles of the fingers. The patient is trying to keep her fingers spread apart against the examiner's pressure (left). Testing for power of the muscles of the thenar eminence (right). The patient is trying to oppose the thumb against resistance.

The Spine. Palpation of the spine and assessment of movement in each region should be performed. Limitation of lumbar spine movement, due to ankylosing spondylitis for example, can be missed unless the patient is asked to take his clothes off and examined leaning forward (Figs. 1.20 & 1.21). Further illustrations of techniques used to examine the back and sacroiliac joints are covered under 'Spinal Diseases and Back Pain' and 'Ankylosing Spondylitis'.

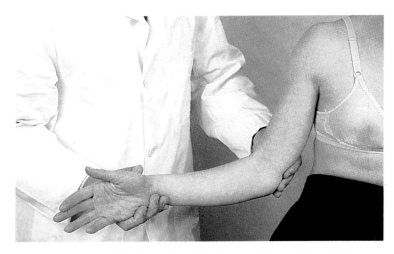

Fig. 1.15 Examination of supination and pronation of the forearm. This is a function of both wrist and elbow movement.

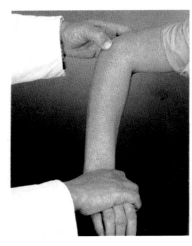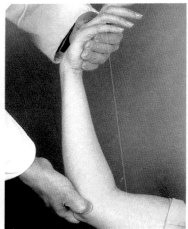

Fig. 1.16 Eliciting tenderness over the lateral epicondyle of the elbow. This is the site of origin of the long extensors of the forearm. The patient is tensing these muscles by trying to extend the wrist against the examiner; pain is felt at the origin in lateral epicondylitis ('tennis elbow') (left). Pain over the medial epicondyle occurs in 'golfer's elbow' (medial epicondylitis) (right) and can be elicited by palpation or by resisted flexion of the wrist which tenses the long flexor origin at the epicondyle.

Fig. 1.17 Palpating for tenderness of the subacromial bursa (left) and long head of biceps (right).

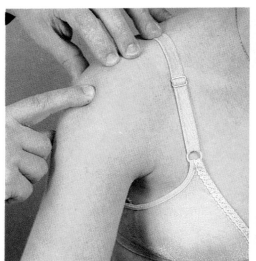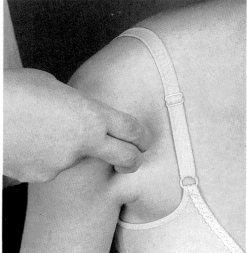

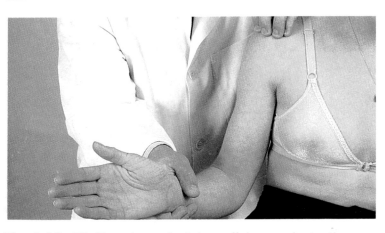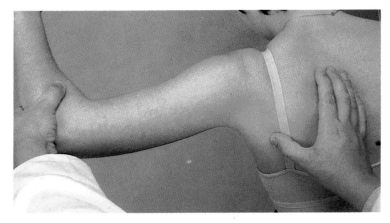

Fig. 1.18 Eliciting signs of rotator cuff damage by testing resisted external rotation of the shoulder. The patient is pushing against the examiner's hand, thus stretching the infraspinatus tendon.

Fig. 1.19 Examining movements of the shoulder joint. scapula is fixed with one hand so that gleno-humeral movement can be assessed.

The Lower Limb. Examination of the lower limb is incomplete unless the patient is asked to stand and observed walking. As in the upper limb, this overall functional assessment is important in revealing the major site and type of problem. Thereafter, the hip, knee, hindfoot and forefoot can be assessed separately and again a limited number of techniques used have been illustrated (Figs. 1.22 – 1.30).

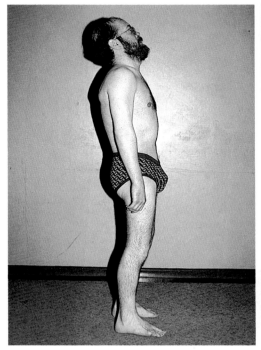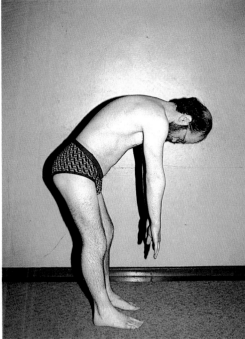

Fig. 1.20 Spinal movement in ankylosing spondylitis. A patient is trying to extend (left) and flex (right) the spine – movement of the lumbar spine itself is minimal. Flexion is entirely at the hips and the patient has also flexed the left knee in order to bend this far.

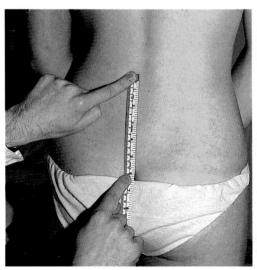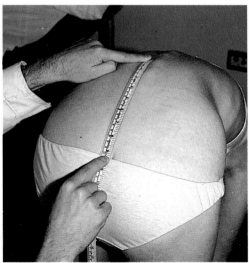

Fig. 1.21 Measurement of lumbar spine flexion. With the patient erect the tape measure is held along the lumbar spine; a point is marked 15cm from the natal cleft (left). When the patient bends forward the distance from the top point to the natal cleft increases, in this case to 22cm (right).

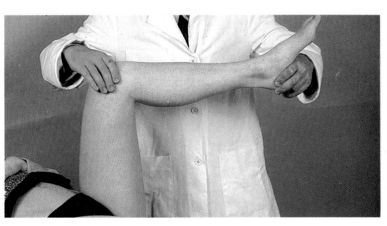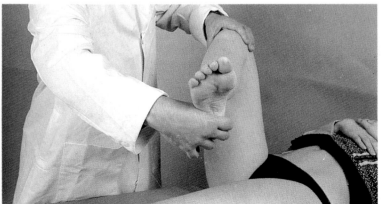

Fig. 1.22 Assessing internal (upper) (left) and external (lower) (right) rotation of the hip joint with the knee flexed at 90°. The leg acts as a pointer which shows the angle of rotation.

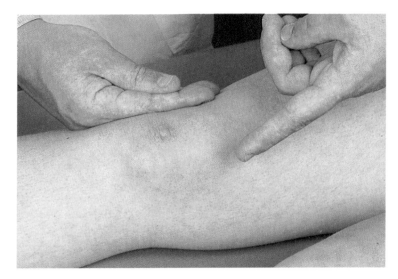

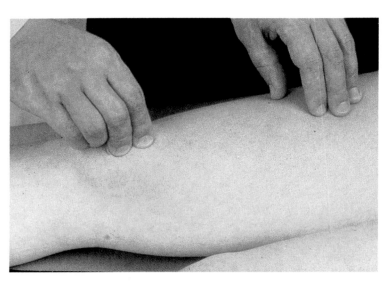

Fig. 1.23 The bulge sign for small effusions of the knee joint. Pressure is being applied to the lateral side of the knee and the examiner is looking on the medial side for evidence of movement of the fluid: a bulge appears on the medial side as the fluid flows across the joint.

Fig. 1.24 Examination for patello-femoral disease. Pressure is being applied to the patella while the patient contracts the quadriceps muscle. The examiner may feel patello-femoral crepitus, and the patient feels pain.

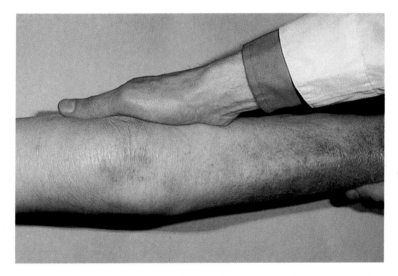

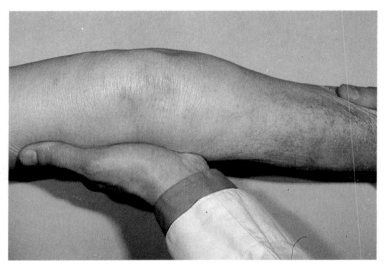

Fig. 1.25 Testing the stability of the collateral ligaments of the knee joint. With the knee slightly flexed to avoid normal 'locking' lateral pressure is applied to see if the knee will rock from side to side.

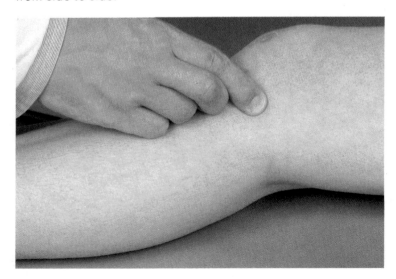

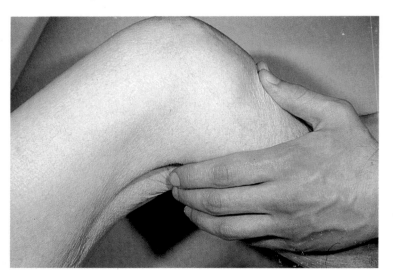

Fig. 1.26 Palpating the insertion of the medial collateral ligament of the knee joint, a common site of 'joint' tenderness, particularly in association with osteoarthritis.

Fig. 1.27 Testing the integrity of the cruciate ligaments of the knee. The examiner flexes the knee, immobilizes the patient's foot, and grasps the upper end of the tibia to see if it will move (rock) forwards and backwards on the femur.

Functional Assessment

Testing the patient's ability to carry out normal functional tasks is an essential part of a rheumatological examination and allows one to detect possible ways of reducing disability. The occupational therapist and physiotherapist play a major role in this part of the clinical examination. Hand function is particularly important and can be assessed in a variety of ways. Different grips should be tested individually (Figs. 1.31 – 1.33).

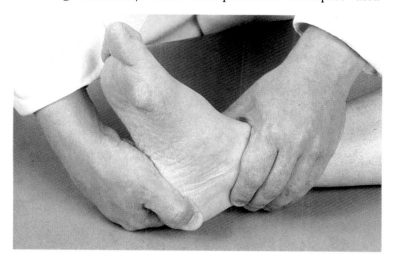

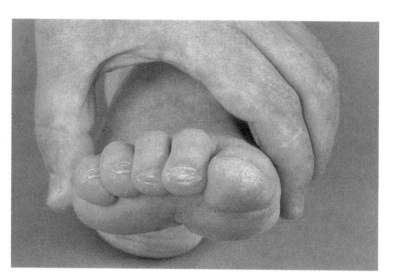

Fig. 1.28 Examining the subtalar joint. The ankle joint is firmly fixed with one hand while the calcaneus is rocked from side to side.

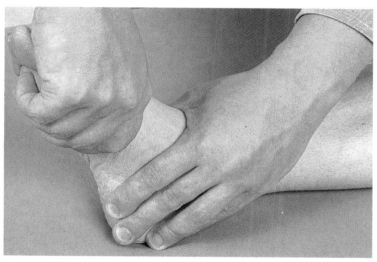

Fig. 1.29 Examining the midtarsal joints. The hindfoot is firmly grasped in one hand and forefoot rotated with the other.

Fig. 1.30 Applying pressure across the heads of the metatarsals for evidence of tenderness. This is an early sign of inflammation in the MTPs or associated bursae.

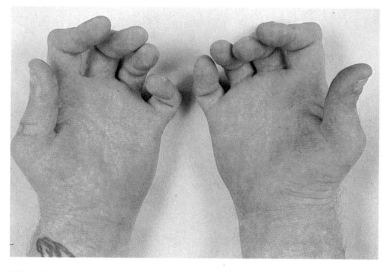

Fig. 1.31 A patient with rheumatoid arthritis who has been asked to make a fist – this reveals marked restriction of finger flexion.

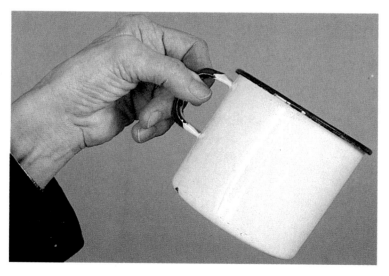

Fig. 1.32 A patient with rheumatoid arthritis who has difficulty holding a cup.

The patient's ability to dress, wash, eat, and cook can also be examined by the occupational therapist (Figs. 1.34 & 1.35). Function does not always bear any relation to the apparent deformity and disability that is observed.

Patients with severe advanced rheumatic diseases are often able to carry out surprisingly dextrous tasks with their hands (Fig. 1.36). The physiotherapist can often help in the examination of function of the lower limbs.

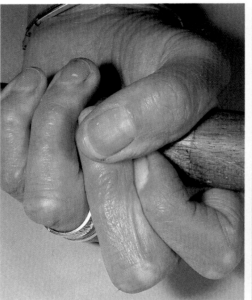 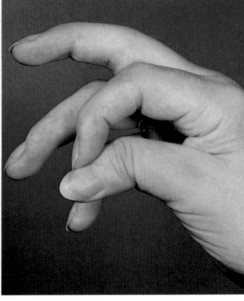

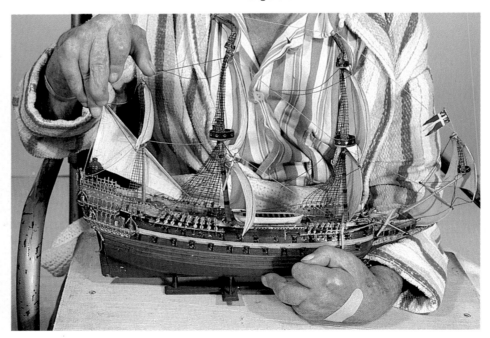

Fig. 1.33 Testing the power grip (left): the index and middle fingers will not close around the bar properly. Testing the pinch grip (lower): in this case instability of the interphalangeal joint of the thumb is interfering with function.

Fig. 1.34 An occupational therapist assessing the use of various cutlery grips to aid eating in a patient with impaired hand function. Restricted finger flexion from rheumatoid arthritis means that the patient can only grasp large diameter handles.

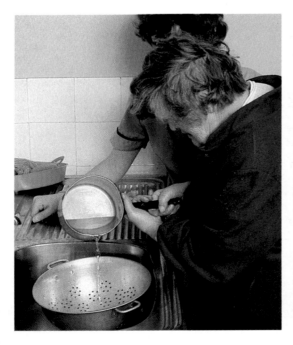

Fig. 1.35 An occupation therapist assessing the patient's ability to carry out kitchen tasks. Various aids are available to improve function.

Fig. 1.36 This patient who has built a model boat despite severe rheumatoid changes of the hands demonstrates that function is not necessarily related to joint deformity.

Walking time can be measured and the patient should be observed climbing steps and stairs (Figs. 1.37 & 1.38). The quadriceps is an example of a muscle which often becomes wasted in rheumatic diseases and the physio-therapist's assessment of power and help in restoring normal function can be of major importance (Fig. 1.39). Examining the patient's shoes also gives useful clues to the joint problems they are experiencing (Fig. 1.40).

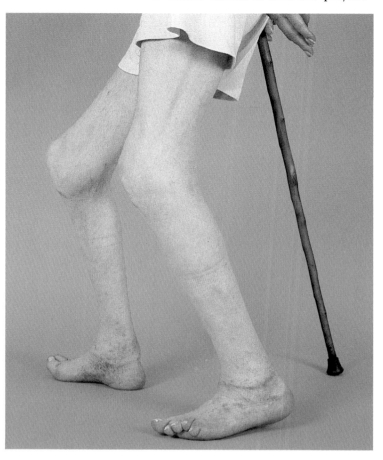

Fig. 1.37 Examination of gait is an essential part of a rheumatological examination. Walking time can also be measured; for example, the time taken to walk 20 metres may be assessed before and after treatment.

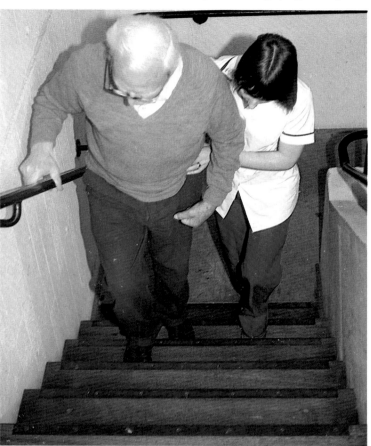

Fig. 1.38 A physiotherapist assessing the ability of a patient to manage stairs.

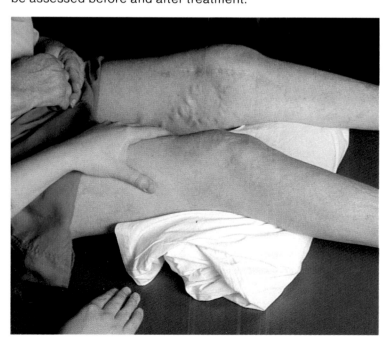

Fig. 1.39 A physiotherapist assessing the power of the quadriceps muscle. The patient is trying to extend the knee and the physiotherapist is feeling the bulk of the muscle. Thigh diameter at a set point above the knee is sometimes also measured.

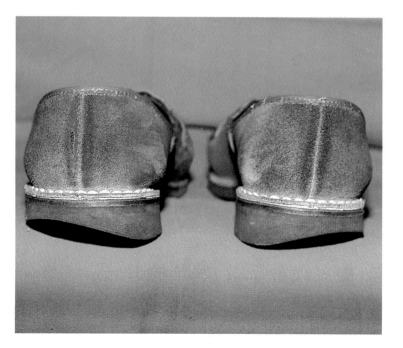

Fig. 1.40 Examination of the patient's shoes. This pair shows very uneven heel wear and the inner aspects of the heels are scuffed where they rub against each other. Their owner had bilateral varus deformities of the knees.

1.11

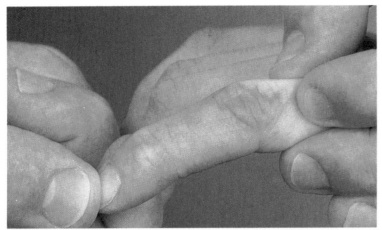

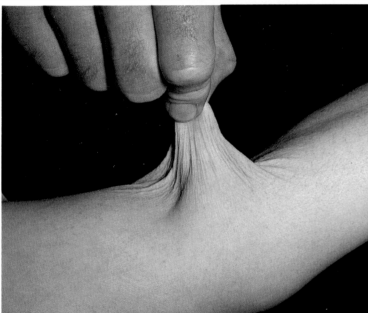

The Periarticular Tissues

The multiple abnormalities of skin and periarticular tissues that occur in different rheumatic diseases are included elsewhere in this collection of illustrations. Figures 1.41 – 1.45 show one or two examples of involvement of these structures. Muscle wasting and bursitis or tendinitis are common features of many rheumatic diseases, and alteration of skin texture or elasticity can occur. A variety of nodules, lumps and bumps may or may not be related to rheumatic diseases and the nails, finger pulps, ears, eyes and numerous other sites are often worthy of examination revealing important clues to the nature of the underlying condition.

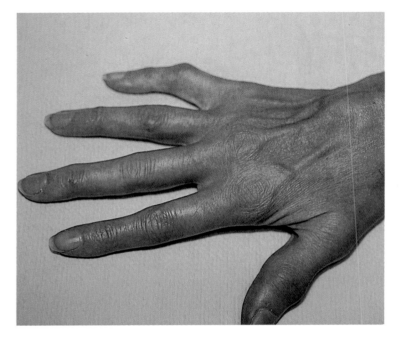

Fig. 1.41 Skin tethering in systemic sclerosis (upper). The examiner is pinching up the skin over the phalanges to test its tethering and extensibility. Excess mobility of the skin in Ehlers Danlos syndrome (lower). The skin can be pulled right away from the subcutaneous tissue, and will snap back like rubber. Courtesy of Dr. H. Bird.

Fig. 1.42 The hand in early rheumatoid arthritis. The most striking feature is the swelling of the extensor tendon sheath over the wrist. The metacarpophalangeal joints are swollen and there is early spindling of the proximal interphalangeal joints. Courtesy of Dr. J.D. Croft.

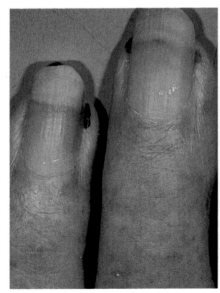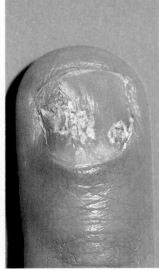

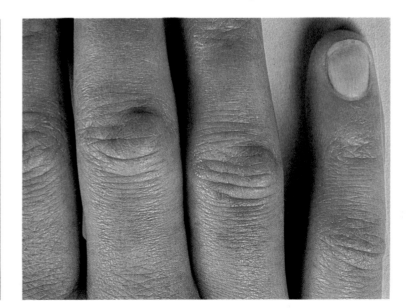

Fig. 1.43 Examination of the finger-nails in RA. Nail fold lesions representing small infarcts due to vasculitis (left). Nail pitting and onycholysis are characteristic of psoriasis, the PIP joint underlying such a nail is often affected by arthritis (right).

Fig 1.44 Garrod's fatty pads over the proximal interphalangeal joints of the hand. These are subcutaneous fibro-fatty pads of no significance, often misdiagnosed as indicating joint disease.

1.12

Many diseases, including rheumatoid arthritis, the connective tissue diseases and the seronegative spondarthritides, are generalized systemic conditions which happen to affect the joints more obviously than other organs. The general examination of the patient, and assessment of all symptoms, is therefore important if the correct diagnosis is to be made and if the extra-articular manifestations of these diseases are not to be missed.

Clinical Measurements in Rheumatology

The techniques of examination illustrated and mentioned so far are entirely subjective. For many years, rheumatologists have tried to produce accurate ways of numerically measuring joint disease and function, in particular to aid assessment of the efficacy of treatment. Simple subjective scores made by the patients such as their own feeling of change for better or worse and their measurement of pain can provide useful and important information. The remaining figures illustrate one or two ways in which the physician or clinical metrologist may further numerically score aspects of joint disease (Fig. 1.46). The Ritchie index is a widely used assessment of joint tenderness which allows one to record the degree and distribution of joint line tenderness and is therefore an index of the activity of synovitis (Fig. 1.47).

Fig. 1.45 Hands of a patient with rheumatoid arthritis showing a nail fold lesion and a nodule over the fifth metacarpophalangeal joint.

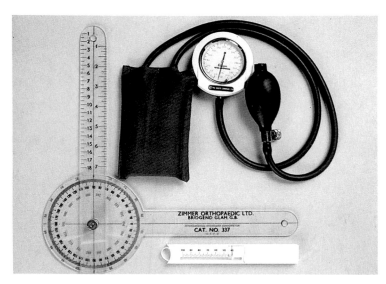

Fig. 1.46 A goniometer, grip strength recorder and ring size assessor used by the clinical metrologist in therapeutic trials.

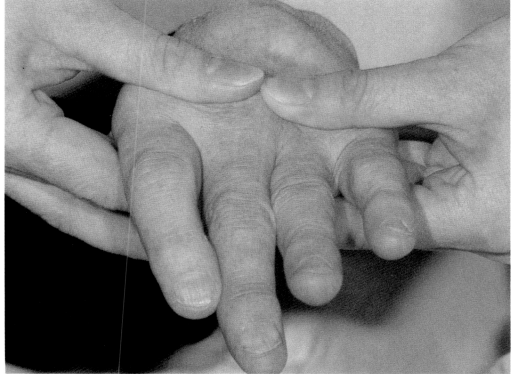

Fig. 1.47 Ritchie index assessment of synovitis. Joint tenderness is elicited by firm pressure over the joint line or by movement (left). Tenderness is scored as 0, 1 (pain), 2 (pain and wince), or 3 (pain and withdrawal). The score at each of the standard sites is filled in on a form and the total score recorded (right).

RITCHIE INDEX

JOINTS EXAMINED	LEFT	RIGHT
Temporomandibular		
Cervical Spine *		
Sternoclavicular		
Acromioclavicular		
Shoulders		
Elbows		
Wrists		
M.C.P.		
P.I.P.		
Hips *		
Knees		
Ankles		
Talocalcaneal *		
Midtarsal *		
Metatarsals		
TOTAL :		

KEY: 0 · not tender   +3 · tender, winced and withdrew
      +1 · tender   * · move: others press!
      +2 · tender and winced

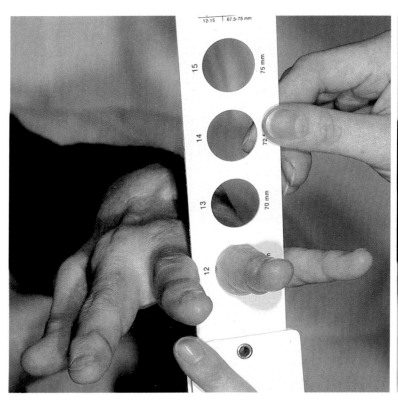
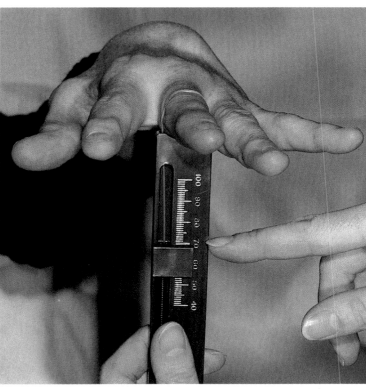

Fig. 1.48 Two methods used to measure the diameter of the proximal interphalangeal joints. Rings of varying diameter can be used to find the smallest one that will pass over the joint (left), or a flexible band is used to measure joint size (right).

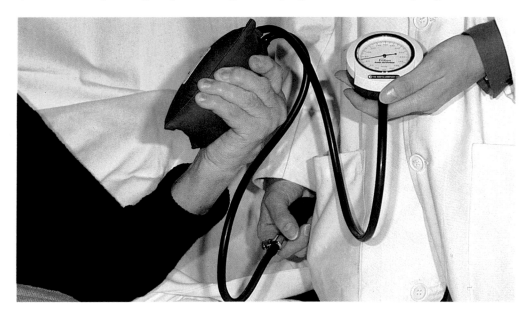

Fig. 1.49 Testing grip strength in a patient with rheumatoid arthritis. A standard bag is attached to a sphygmomanometer and inflated to 30 mmHg. The patient grips the bag as hard as possible and the rise in pressure on the manometer recorded.

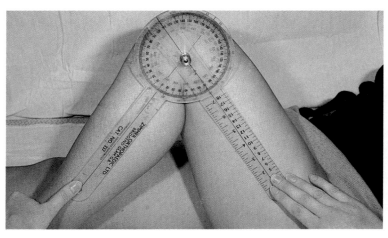
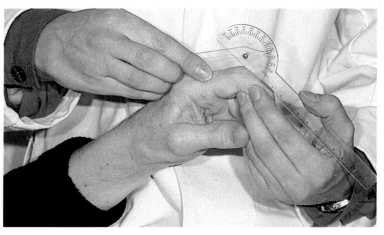

1.14

Fig. 1.50 Precise measurement of the angle of knee joint flexion using a large goniometer (left). Measuring flexion of the proximal interphalangeal joint using a small goniometer (right).

Other techniques used to assess inflammatory diseases, and rheumatoid arthritis in particular, include measuring the diameter of the proximal interphalangeal joints by a ring size gauge or by other instruments (Fig. 1.48), and assessing the grip strength by using a modified sphygmomanometer (Fig. 1.49). Grip strength may be reduced for a variety of reasons one of which is inflammatory synovitis, and quite a marked improvement can be achieved with anti-inflammatory therapy alone.

The Range of Motion of Joints

Joint motion can be measured accurately with a goniometer (Fig. 1.50). Movements must be measured from a defined zero starting position, and the 'extended anatomical position' of the limb is usually accepted as zero degrees. Limb movements should be compared on opposite sides of the body, and can be expressed as a percentage loss on the affected side, or as total movement in degrees. Extension is the natural motion opposite to flexion at the zero position; hyperextension means abnormal movement opposite to flexion. Flexion deformities can be expressed by recording knee joint motion for example as +10° to +130° instead of the normal 0° to +130° flexion. Ankylosis produces complete loss of movement. The normal range of joint motion varies with age (decreasing with age), race, and disease. Some conditions, such as Marfan's syndrome or the Ehlers-Danlos syndrome, result in increased motion (Fig. 1.51); most rheumatic diseases cause loss of movement. Approximate ranges of normal motion in the upper and lower limbs are shown in figures 1.52–1.56. Back movement is illustrated separately under 'Spinal Diseases and Back Pain'.

This brief introduction to the clinical evaluation of rheumatic diseases should help to stress the importance of the initial examination, and the strong clinical basis of all rheumatology. Numerous further examples are to be found in subsequent chapters.

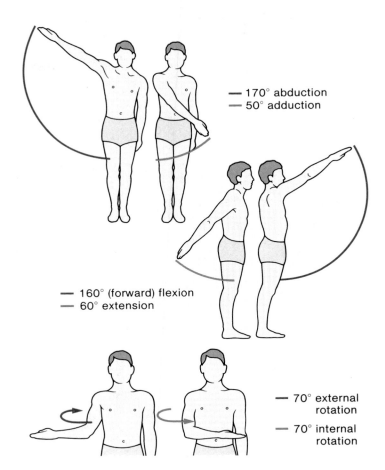

— 170° abduction
— 50° adduction

— 160° (forward) flexion
— 60° extension

— 70° external rotation
— 70° internal rotation

Fig. 1.52 Normal movements of the shoulder joint.

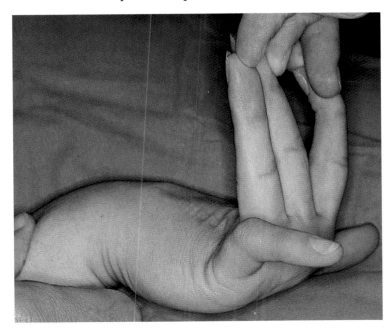

Fig. 1.51 Joint hypermobility producing an increased range of finger movement. Courtesy of Dr. H. Bird.

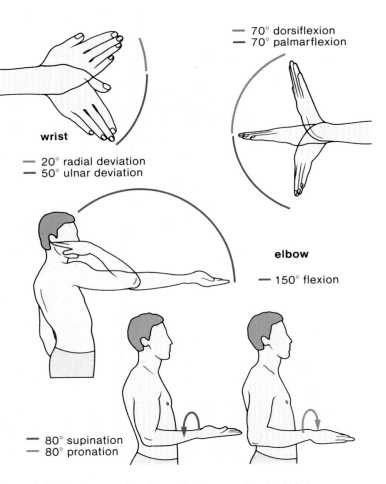

— 70° dorsiflexion
— 70° palmarflexion

wrist

— 20° radial deviation
— 50° ulnar deviation

elbow

— 150° flexion

— 80° supination
— 80° pronation

Fig. 1.53 Range of motion of elbow and wrist joints.

1.15

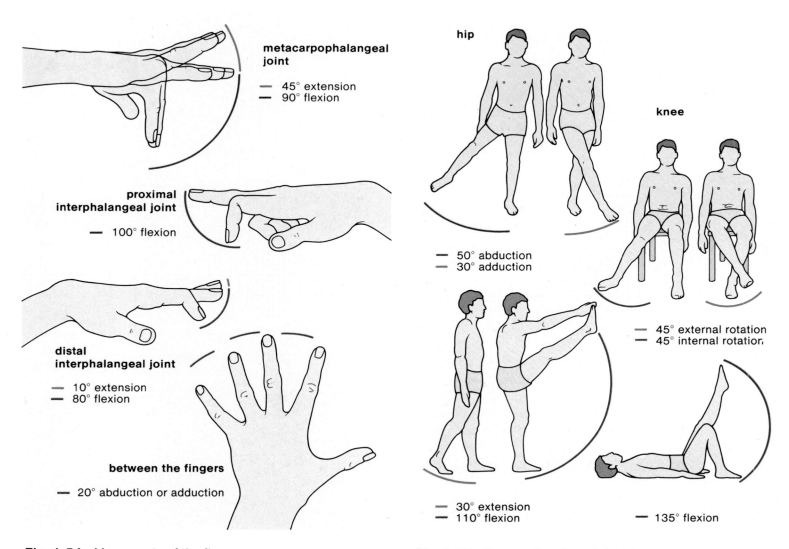

metacarpophalangeal joint

— 45° extension
— 90° flexion

proximal interphalangeal joint

— 100° flexion

distal interphalangeal joint

— 10° extension
— 80° flexion

between the fingers

— 20° abduction or adduction

hip

— 50° abduction
— 30° adduction

— 30° extension
— 110° flexion

knee

— 45° external rotation
— 45° internal rotation

— 135° flexion

Fig. 1.54 Movements of the fingers.

Fig. 1.55 Range of motion of the hip and knee joint.

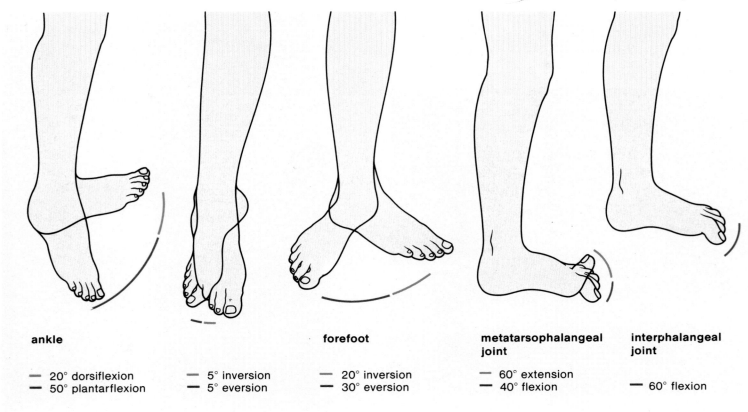

ankle

— 20° dorsiflexion
— 50° plantarflexion

— 5° inversion
— 5° eversion

forefoot

— 20° inversion
— 30° eversion

metatarsophalangeal joint

— 60° extension
— 40° flexion

interphalangeal joint

— 60° flexion

1.16   **Fig. 1.56**   Movements of the ankle, foot and great toe.

2

The Investigation of Rheumatic Diseases

A wide spectrum of different investigative techniques is available in rheumatological practice. Some tests assist the clinician in establishing a diagnosis or categorizing a disease. Some demonstrate the extent and nature of any pathological changes in or around joints and other tissues. Others are necessary to monitor the activity of an inflammatory condition and help assessment of treatment responses (Fig. 2.1). A few examples of some of the established methods of investigation will be illustrated (Fig. 2.2).

Non-Specific Markers of Systemic Disease

Inflammation in a systemic disease such as rheumatoid arthritis (RA) results in several different hematological and biochemical responses. A normocytic normochromic anemia is usual (the 'anemia of chronic disease') and may be accompanied by a mild leucocytosis or thrombocytosis. The liver increases output of several different proteins including fibrinogen, C-reactive protein (CRP), some complement components, enzyme inhibitors and carriage proteins (the acute phase proteins). These proteins contribute to the elevated erythrocyte sedimentation rate (ESR) and high blood viscosity.

A full blood count and ESR (or viscosity) are used routinely to screen patients who may have an inflammatory disorder. They also help exclude primary or secondary hematological abnormalities such as anemia of chronic disease or aplastic anemia. The hemoglobin, ESR, CRP, and other acute phase proteins can also be used in the clinical assessment of disease activity and treatment responses. Typical changes in a patient with active RA who responded to suppressive therapy with D-penicillamine are shown in figure 2.3.

Immunological Markers of Systemic Disease

Many of the chronic rheumatic diseases are associated

USE OF INVESTIGATIVE TECHNIQUES

Establish diagnosis

Monitor disease activity

Demonstrate anatomical and pathological changes

Follow disease progression and response to treatment

Fig. 2.1 Table of some of the main uses of investigative techniques in rheumatology.

INVESTIGATIVE TECHNIQUES IN RHEUMATOLOGY

Hematology and biochemistry

Immunological markers of disease

Synovial fluid analysis

Imaging techniques:
    plain radiograph
    contrast studies
    scintigraphy
    C.T. scanning
    thermography

Arthroscopy

Biopsy and histology

Neurophysiology

Fig. 2.2 Investigative techniques in rheumatology. This list summarizes the primary techniques available to the clinical rheumatologist.

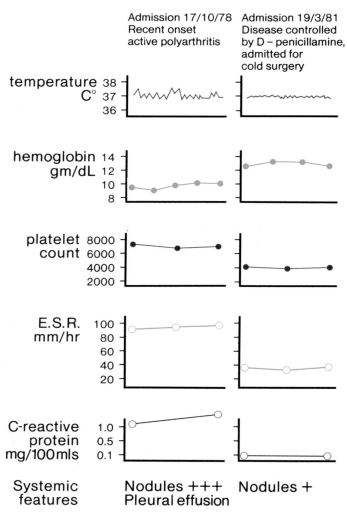

Mr C.C./Age 34/Rheumatoid arthritis

Fig. 2.3 Systemic, biochemical and hematological responses to active rheumatoid arthritis. The temperature, hemoglobin, ESR, platelet count and C-reactive protein have been plotted in a patient with rheumatoid disease during two separate hospital admissions. At the onset, the disease was extremely active. Following treatment with D-penicillamine the condition improved and the indices had returned to more normal levels by the time of the second admission.

with immunological abnormalities. Immunological investigations include:

AUTOANTIBODIES Rheumatoid factors (RF) are immunoglobulins of the IgG or IgM class which react with the Fc portion of the IgG molecule. They are prevalent in patients with rheumatoid arthritis. The commonly used latex and sheep cell agglutination tests detect and quantify IgM rheumatoid factor (Fig. 2.4). High RF titers indicate a poor prognosis and are associated with the development of erosive disease and nodules. RF is sometimes found in other connective tissue diseases and in other disorders such as fibrosing alveolitis.

Autoantibodies directed against nuclear proteins (antinuclear factors -ANF) are also common in the connective tissue diseases. Antibody to native double-stranded DNA is relatively specific for systemic lupus erythematosus (Fig. 2.5).

The continued refining of techniques has revealed numerous subclasses of antibodies with more highly defined specificities. Disease classification by antibody is being attempted (eg. the diagnosis of mixed connective tissue disease by the presence of antinuclear antibody of the speckled type directed against an extractable nuclear antigen of ribonuclear protein). However there is overlap of antibodies in apparently different diseases which may cause confusion clinically. The occurrence of these various antinuclear and other antibodies in many different connective tissue diseases may be indicative of common underlying disease mechanisms.

IMMUNE COMPLEXES The detection of circulating complexes containing immunoglobulin and complement, and the demonstration of tissue deposits, may assist in the diagnosis of disease. Complexes have been demonstrated in RA synovium and are deposited in many sites in SLE (Fig. 2.6).

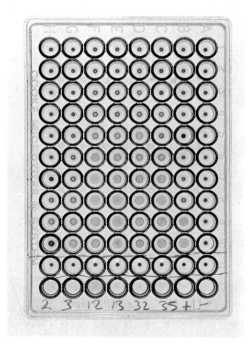

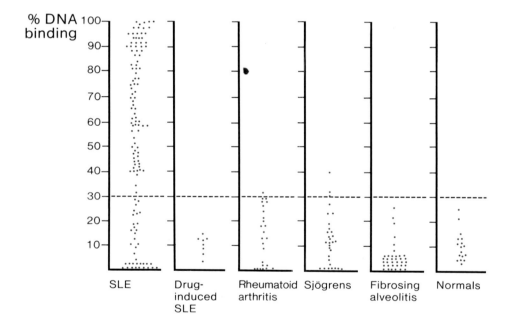

Fig. 2.4 Rheumatoid arthritis hemagglutination (RAHA) test for rheumatoid factor. Each well of the microtiter plate contains sheep red cells coated with rabbit IgG; if added serum contains anti-IgG then the cells will agglutinate; if not, the cells settle as a 'button'. To each vertical column is added a serial dilution of each serum – on this plate the bottom well is empty and the next a control without serum. The two columns on the extreme right are a positive and negative control. The 'titer' for each serum is taken as the point before the negative button reappears. For serum no. 2 this is 1/8, for serum no. 32 it is 1/640. Courtesy of Dr. W. Irving.

Fig. 2.5 DNA binding in the positive antinuclear factor (ANF) test. A positive test is common in many diseases and occasionally occurs in normal people. The diagram shows the activity of ANF positive sera against DNA, assessed by the Farr technique. High levels of antibody to DNA are often found in SLE, but are rare in other conditions. The normal level is less than 30%.

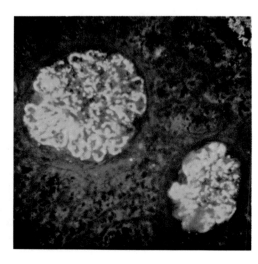

Fig. 2.6 The kidney in SLE: immunofluorescent staining for IgG and complement revealing a diffuse pattern of deposition in the glomeruli. Courtesy of Professor D. Doniach.

Many different techniques have been used to detect complexes in the serum (Fig. 2.7); high levels are often found in active SLE and rheumatoid vasculitis, but may occur in many other disorders.

HISTOCOMPATIBILITY ANTIGENS A number of different diseases have been found to be associated to a variable degree with particular histocompatibility antigens. The archetype of such associations is that of ankylosing spondylitis with the B27 allele where individuals positive for this tissue type are nearly 100 times more likely to develop the disease than B27 negative subjects. There is an association of severe erosive RA with HLA DR4, although in this case the relative risk is much lower (Fig. 2.8).

As yet tissue typing has a limited role in diagnosis especially where disease and HLA concordance is not high. However, the absence of a particular antigenic type may provide useful contributory evidence in a case where the diagnosis is in doubt on clinical grounds.

Synovial Fluid Analysis

Examination of the joint fluid is essential and specific for the diagnosis of septic arthritis or crystal-induced synovitis. The findings are non-specific in other conditions, but may give some guide to the likely diagnosis or the activity of a disease.

Joint aspiration is a simple technique. The procedure can be carried out in a clinic room with no special precautions except careful skin cleansing and a scrupulous non-touch technique to minimize the risk of introducing infection (Fig. 2.9). Some common puncture sites for different joints are shown (Figs. 2.10-2.13).

The fluid should be examined in several different ways (Fig. 2.14). The viscosity and turbidity respectively reflect the amount of hyaluronic acid and cells in the fluid. Active synovial inflammation results in a thin turbid fluid with a predominance of polymorphonuclear leucocytes (Fig. 2.15).

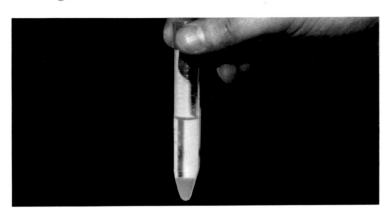

Fig. 2.7 Cryoglobulinemia. This test tube contains serum from a patient with circulating immune complexes. The serum has been stored overnight at 4°C and some of the complex has precipitated (a cryoprecipitate). This is one of several different indirect tests used to detect the presence of circulating immune complexes in patients with SLE, rheumatoid arthritis and other connective tissue diseases.

ASSOCIATIONS OF SOME RHEUMATIC DISEASES WITH THE HLA SYSTEM

Disease	Associated allele	Increased risk of disease conferred by presence of allele
Ankylosing spondylitis	B27	x 91
Reiter's disease	B27	x 37
Rheumatoid arthritis	DR4	x 6
Behçet's disease	B5	x 7

Fig. 2.8 HLA associations of rheumatic diseases. This table shows some of the rheumatic diseases in which an increased risk is conferred by possession of a particular HLA antigen.

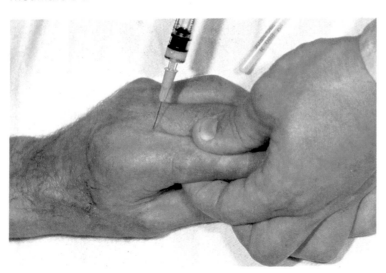

Fig. 2.9 Joint aspiration and injection. In this instance the index finger metacarpophalangeal joint (MCP) is being injected with steroid. The finger is being distracted to open the joint line, the skin has been cleaned, and the needle is passing through the skin and into the joint space from the lateral aspect of the joint line.

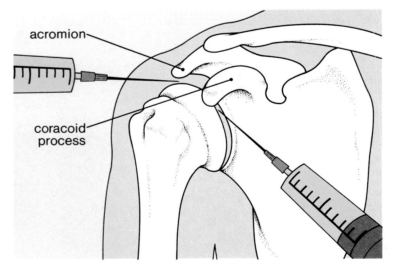

Fig. 2.10 Sites for aspirating the shoulder joint and subacromial bursa. The diagram shows the anterior approach to the shoulder joint. The needle is inserted just below the coracoid process and directed upwards and outwards to enter the joint. Insertion of the needle into the subacromial bursa between the top of the humerus and the acromio-clavicular joint is also shown.

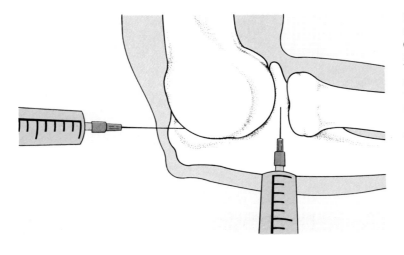

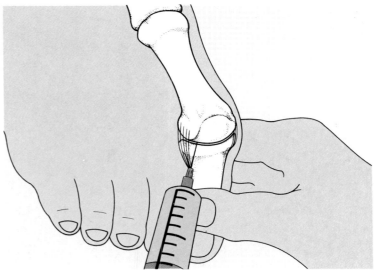

Fig. 2.11 Sites for aspirating the elbow joint. The humero-radial joint can be approached with the forearm flexed to 90 degrees. The head of the radius is palpated and the needle is inserted into the joint line from the lateral aspect. The humero-ulnar joint can be approached from the lateral epicondylar region. The needle is inserted posteriorly below the lateral epicondyle of the humerus so that the line of the needle is parallel to that of the shaft of the radius. Since there is a communication of the radio-ulnar and humero-ulnar joints, aspiration of both is possible from one site.

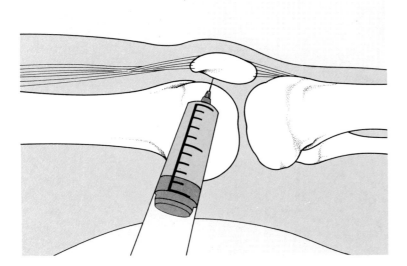

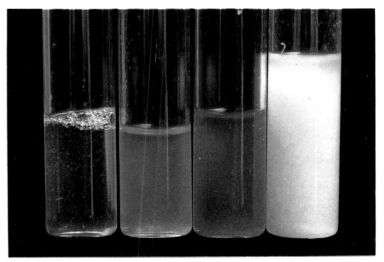

Fig. 2.12 The medial approach to aspirating the knee joint. There are several different possible sites of entry to the knee joint. The diagram shows the medial approach in which the needle is inserted into the knee joint proper. The patella and femur can be palpated and the needle is inserted into the space beneath the patella at its mid-point. The condylar anatomy is such that the space is wider on the medial side.

Fig. 2.13 Aspirating the first metatarsophalangeal joint (MTP). The diagram shows the examiner flexing and distracting the great toe in order to open up the joint space. The needle can then be inserted from the superior surface directly into the joint line. A similar technique can be used for injection of other small joints of the hands and feet.

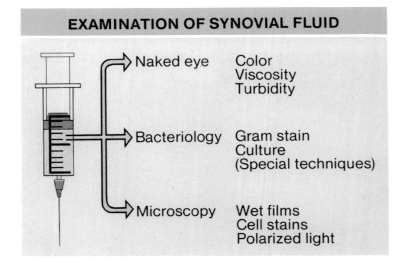

EXAMINATION OF SYNOVIAL FLUID

→	Naked eye	Color Viscosity Turbidity
→	Bacteriology	Gram stain Culture (Special techniques)
→	Microscopy	Wet films Cell stains Polarized light

Fig. 2.14 Techniques used in the examination of synovial fluid. The most important tests are the naked eye examination of colour, viscosity and turbidity of the fluid, the bacteriological examination for the presence of organisms and microscopy to establish the cell and crystal content of the fluid.

Fig. 2.15 The naked eye appearance of synovial fluid in different diseases. The normal synovial fluid in the tube on the left is viscous and clear. The two tubes in the middle contain fluid from joints with mild synovial inflammation. The blood staining of the third tube was caused by trauma. The tube on the right contains fluid from a severely inflamed joint. It is thin and opaque due to a very high polymorph count.

Several different conditions cause bloodstaining of fluid (Fig. 2.16).

'Pus' is usual but not invariable in septic arthritis, and is occasionally aspirated from joints with a crystal synovitis or other inflammatory arthropathy (Fig. 2.17). A thorough bacteriological examination is essential if sepsis is possible. The type of stain, and transport and culture media used, will depend on the the likely diagnoses. If there is suspicion of TB or gonococcal arthritis for example, close cooperation with the bacteriologist is essential.

The viscosity of synovial fluid, and its cell and particle content can be examined from a single drop. The viscosity can be tested between finger and thumb, (Fig. 2.18) and a clean slide can be used for microscopic examination (Fig. 2.19). The differential cell count is often useful, and can be measured on a stained smear of the centrifugal deposit − thus polymorphs dominate in RA, but mononuclear cells are seen in osteoarthritis (OA). If crystal synovitis is a possible diagnosis then a polarized light microscope should be used to try and identify urate or pyrophosphate crystals (Fig. 2.20).

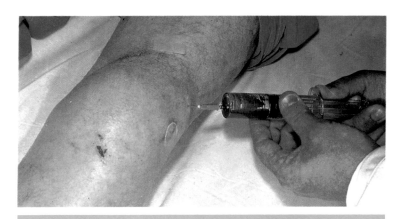

SOME CAUSES OF A HEMARTHROSIS

Trauma
Bleeding disorders
Villonodular synovitis
Pyrophosphate arthropathy
Charcot joint
Resolving infection
Contamination during aspiration

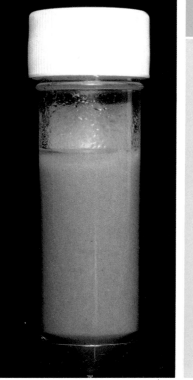
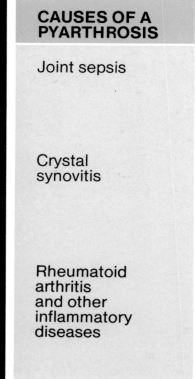

CAUSES OF A PYARTHROSIS

Joint sepsis

Crystal synovitis

Rheumatoid arthritis and other inflammatory diseases

Fig. 2.16 Hemarthrosis. Joint fluid may become contaminated with blood at the time of aspiration. Uniform blood staining of synovial fluid (upper) can also occur as a result of a number of specific rheumatic diseases (lower).

Fig. 2.17 Pyarthrosis. Synovial fluid resembling pus strongly suggests infection (left). However a similar appearance can occur in crystal synovitis and occasionally with severe inflammation in other inflammatory rheumatic disorders (right).

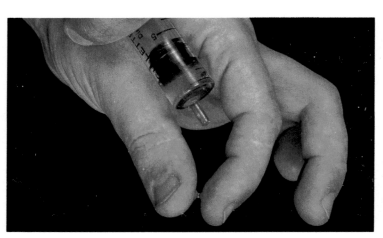

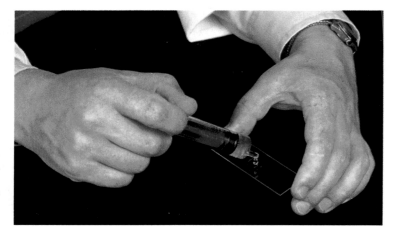

Fig. 2.18 Testing the viscosity of synovial fluid. A small drop of fluid placed between finger and thumb can be used to test viscosity. Hyaluronic acid in the fluid makes normal samples highly viscous and the fluid can be drawn out into a string. With increasing synovial inflammation the hyaluronate is destroyed and the fluid becomes thinner.

Fig. 2.19 A drop of synovial fluid placed on a clean glass microscope slide to examine the cell and particle content. Even if the joint puncture was apparently dry a little fluid can often be expressed from the needle onto the slide and used to help establish a diagnosis.

Imaging Techniques

Various different ways of imaging bones, joints and periarticular tissues are available (Fig. 2.21). They are among the most vital investigative techniques in rheumatology and provide information on diagnosis, disease activity and distribution and the evolution of rheumatic diseases. They also help monitor treatment responses and aid the assessment of complications and extra-articular features of rheumatic diseases. The plain radiograph remains the single most important investigation.

THE PLAIN FILM It is essential to obtain high resolution images with preservation of soft tissue detail because the soft tissue planes give invaluable information on joint swelling and activity (Fig. 2.22). (Both sides should be examined for comparison initially, although this may be unnecessary when assessing disease progression.) A single view will suffice for most joints although views at different angles are sometimes helpful (eg. AP and lateral views of the knee, Fig. 2.23). A single AP view of the pelvis and a lateral view of the lumbar or thoracolumbar spine are sufficient to detect most back disorders.

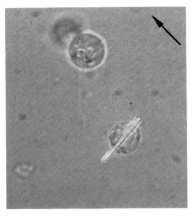
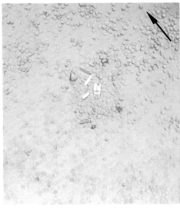

Fig. 2.20   Crystals in synovial fluid. Examination of a drop of fresh synovial fluid or its centrifuged deposit may help identify crystals with the aid of polarized light microscopy. These pictures show the microscope field between crossed polars after insertion of a first order red compensator giving the red background: a typical negatively birefringent urate crystal attached to a cell (left, x 1200) and a cluster of positively birefringent calcium pyrophosphate dihydrate crystals in blood-stained synovial fluid (right, x 600). The direction of the optical axis on the compensator is marked.

IMAGING TECHNIQUES

Plain X-ray	Sialography
Xeroradiograph	Angiography
Scintigraphy	Tenography
Arthrography	Radiculography
Ultrasound	Discography
C.T. scanning	Thermography

Fig. 2.21   Some of the imaging techniques used in rheumatology.

Fig. 2.22   Plain radiograph of the hands in early rheumatoid arthritis. The soft tissue outlines reveal swelling of the MCPs, and proximal interphalangeal joints (PIPs). There is also periarticular osteoporosis of the MCPs and PIPs and erosion of the middle finger MCPS.

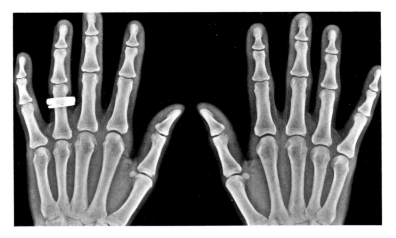
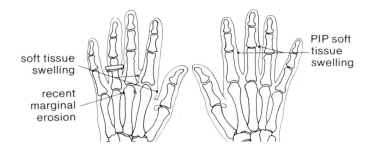

soft tissue swelling

recent marginal erosion

PIP soft tissue swelling

Fig. 2.23   Lateral and anteroposterior radiographs of the knee joint. The lateral view (left) shows an effusion extending into the enlarged suprapatellar pouch. The AP view (right) shows chondrocalcinosis of the meniscus.

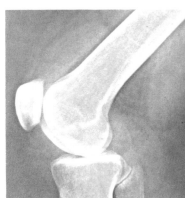
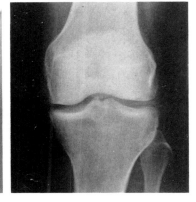
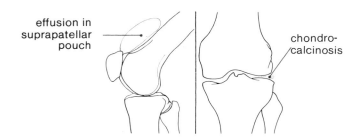

effusion in suprapatellar pouch

chondro-calcinosis

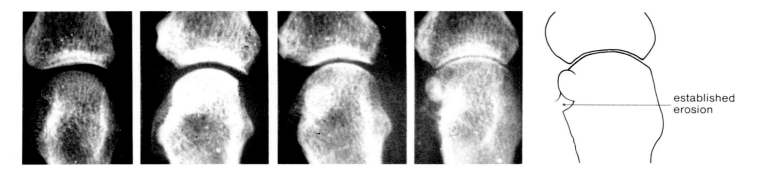

Fig. 2.24 Radiographic progression of rheumatoid changes of an MCP joint over five years. The first radiograph (left) shows a little periarticular osteoporosis but no other changes. With the progress of the disease the joint space can be seen to become narrowed and erosions develop at the joint margin on the head of the metacarpal (right).

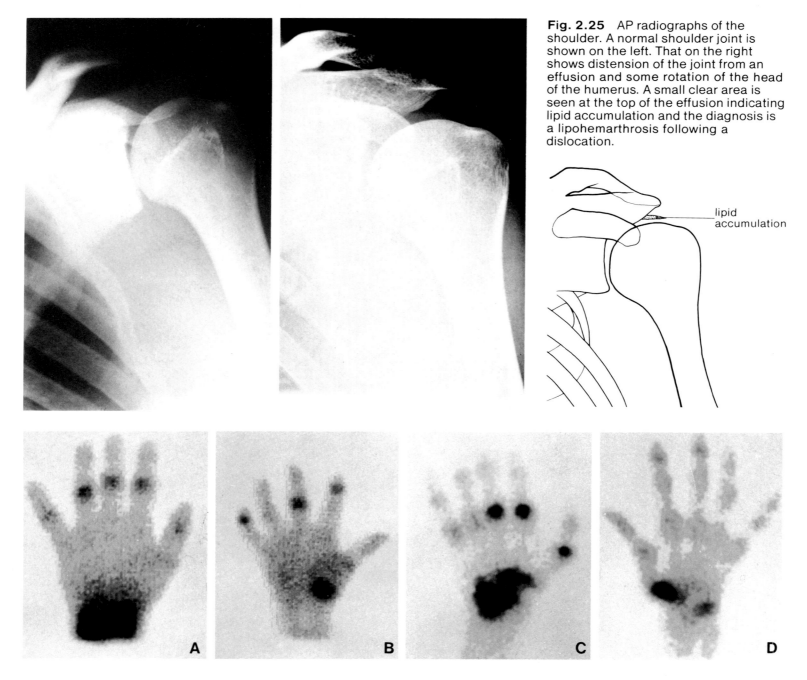

Fig. 2.25 AP radiographs of the shoulder. A normal shoulder joint is shown on the left. That on the right shows distension of the joint from an effusion and some rotation of the head of the humerus. A small clear area is seen at the top of the effusion indicating lipid accumulation and the diagnosis is a lipohemarthrosis following a dislocation.

Fig. 2.26 Perfusion (A, B) and late phase (C, D) technetium-labelled disphosphonate scans of hands in rheumatoid arthritis and osteoarthritis. Scans A and C are of patients with rheumatoid arthritis and scans B and D are of patients with osteoarthritis. Scan A shows increased uptake in the wrist and proximal interphalangeal joints during the perfusion phase in a patient with active rheumatoid arthritis. The perfusion scan B shows the increased uptake at the carpometacarpal joint (CMC) of the thumb and in some interphalangeal joints. Scan C was taken four hours after injection of isotope and during this bone perfusion phase there is increased uptake in the wrist and medial MCPs due to active rheumatoid arthritis. Scan D is a bone phase image from a patient with osteoarthritis of the thumb CMC. In these cases the distribution of joint involvement, and pattern of synovitis in the early phase, allow distinction between RA and OA.

Views of the hands and feet are most helpful for peripheral arthropathies. Close cooperation between clinicians and radiologists is essential to review techniques and results and to help avoid unnecessary and expensive 'joint surveys' or inadequate films.

The plain radiograph provides a current but static view of joint effusions and synovial thickening. It is an historical record of bone and cartilage changes which have to be extensive and relatively longstanding before being apparent on the film. The examination of serial films taken at reasonable time intervals will be helpful in most rheumatic diseases (Fig. 2.24). Soft tissue changes, bone and periosteal reactions and joint space narrowing (cartilage attrition) are documented and often fit a pattern specific for a given diagnosis (Fig. 2.25).

SCINTIGRAPHY This technique offers a simple means of documenting the pattern of joint involvement and current status of disease activity. Scanning with 99m technetium-labelled phosphate compounds permits assessment of abnormal perfusion around a bone or joint when images are made immediately after injection; delayed 'bone scan' images reflect the combination of abnormal perfusion to bone and increased calcium turnover. Discrimination between active synovitis in RA and established bone changes in OA of a single joint is therefore possible (Figs. 2.26-2.28).

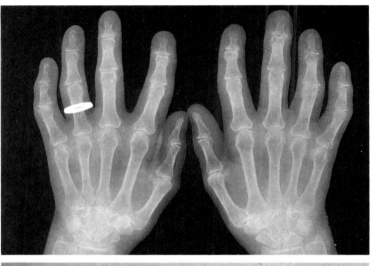

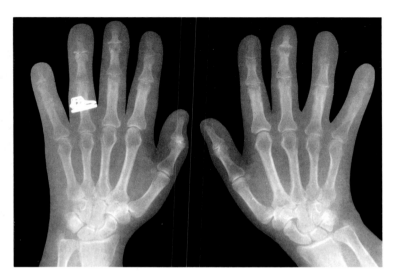

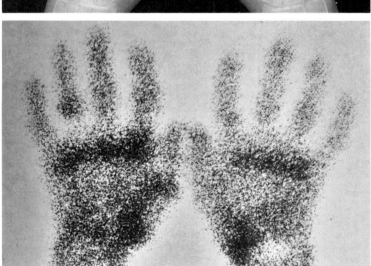

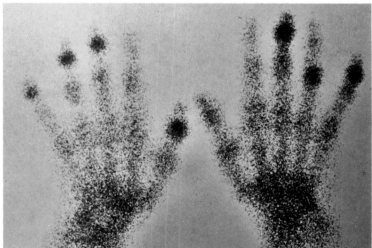

Fig. 2.27 Plain radiograph and perfusion phase diphosphonate scan of the hands in a patient with rheumatoid arthritis. The radiograph shows the soft tissue swelling and periarticular osteoporosis and the scan shows increased perfusion of the same joints.

Fig. 2.28 Plain radiograph and late phase diphosphonate bone scan in a patient with erosive osteoarthritis. The radiograph shows typical osteoarthritic changes in several interphalangeal joints. The diphosphonate scan image taken four hours after injection of isotope shows well-defined areas of increased uptake in the involved interphalangeal joints.

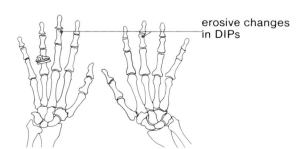

erosive changes in DIPs

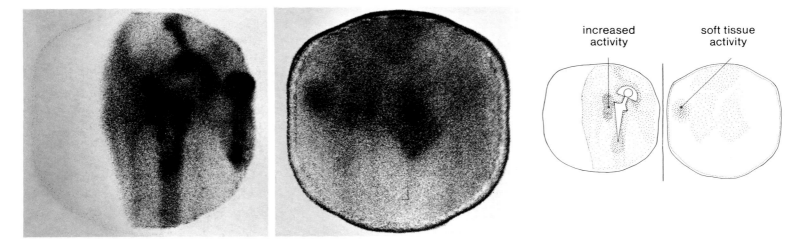

increased
activity

soft tissue
activity

Fig. 2.29 Technetium and gallium scans of an infected total hip replacement. The image on the left shows the delayed phase bone scan following injection of technetium-labelled diphosphonate. There is increased activity around the whole replacement, particularly laterally. The image on the right was taken 24 hours after injection of Gallium 67. The increased uptake arises in part from the isotope entering active polymorphs. The increased uptake is indicative of infection. There is soft tissue activity due to the associated sinuses.

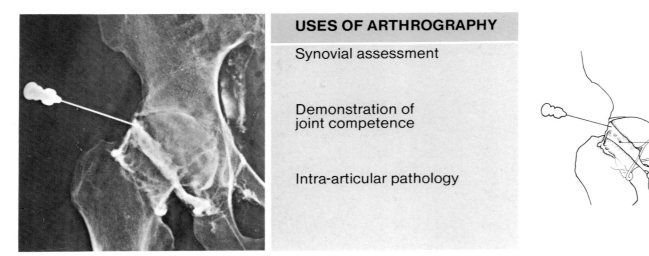

USES OF ARTHROGRAPHY

Synovial assessment

Demonstration of joint competence

Intra-articular pathology

regional lymph node

nodular synovial hypertrophy

lymphatics

Fig. 2.30 Arthrography. Arthrograms are usually performed under screening control (left). A needle can be seen entering the joint space and contrast medium can be injected. In this hip arthrogram in a patient with rheumatoid disease there is synovial hypertrophy with extensive drainage of contrast medium into the regional lymphatics and lymph nodes. This is often seen in joints with active synovitis. Arthrography is used for synovial assessment to demonstrate joint competence and to assess intra-articular pathology (right).

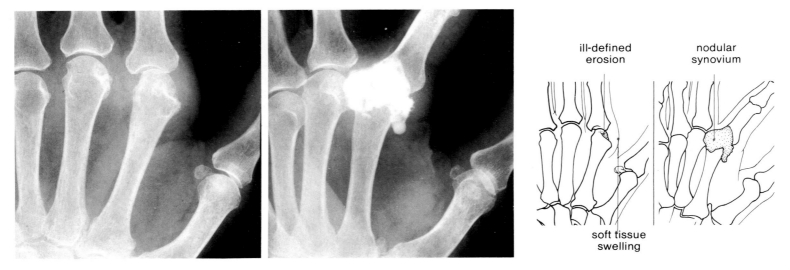

ill-defined
erosion

nodular
synovium

soft tissue
swelling

Fig. 2.31 A plain radiograph and arthrogram of an MCP with villonodular synovitis. The plain film (left) shows soft tissue swelling, loss of joint space and an ill-defined area of bony erosion on the metacarpal. The arthrogram (right) shows an enlarged synovial space with extensive indentation of the contrast medium due to the nodular outgrowths of the synovial tissue.

67 gallium citrate is an expensive agent which highlights active inflammation or infection, and is particularly used for the latter (Fig. 2.29). Numerous other isotope techniques are available including ventilation-perfusion scans for lung involvement and pertechnetate studies of salivary gland disease.

ARTHROGRAPHY This should be performed under screen control and has three major uses (Fig. 2.30):

1. assessment of the synovium may help in the diagnosis of diseases such as villonodular synovitis or synovial chondromatosis (Fig. 2.31),
2. joint competence can be demonstrated, Baker's cysts and joint ruptures being shown and distinguished from deep venous thromboses (Fig. 2.32),

3. demonstration of other intra-articular pathology is especially useful in monoarthritis, for example meniscal injury in the knee or ulno-carpal ligament rupture at the wrist (Fig. 2.33).

Almost any joint can be examined under local anesthesia with minimal complication rates. The joint contents can be aspirated during the prodecure, relieving pressure and providing fluid for analysis.

Other imaging techniques are only used occasionally, but include:-

Ultrasound, which promises to be a simple screening test for joint rupture and detection of Baker's cysts, and may be of value in assessing the size of the lumbar canal (Fig. 2.34).

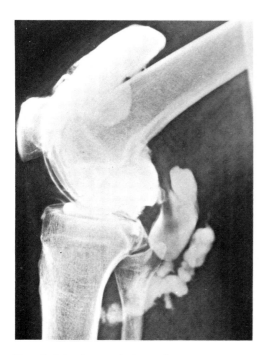
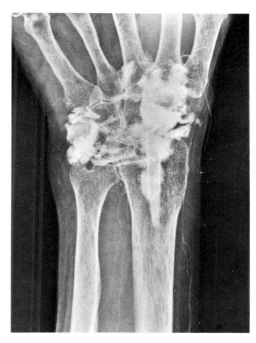
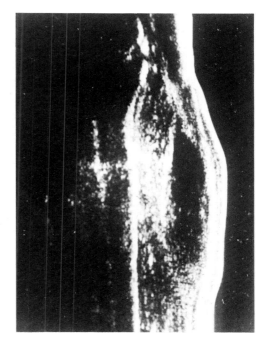

Fig. 2.32 Lateral view of a knee arthrogram showing joint rupture. The contrast medium can be seen extending into the suprapatellar pouch. There is also an extension of the joint space posteriorly (Baker's cyst). Contrast medium has leaked from a rupture of the cyst into the calf.

Fig. 2.33 Arthrogram of the wrist in a patient with rheumatoid arthritis. Contrast medium is outlining a nodular hypertrophied synovial space. There is intercarpal leakage and extensive drainage of the contrast medium into the lymphatics of the forearm. The contrast medium is also extending into a tendon sheath overlying the head of the radius and the ulno-carpal ligament of the wrist has ruptured.

Fig. 2.34 Ultrasound scan showing a popliteal cyst (extending intramuscularly into the calf) which appears as a clear (black) area behind the tibia in this sagittal section. Courtesy of Dr. L.G. Darlington.

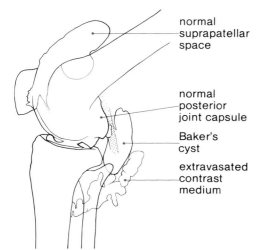

normal suprapatellar space

normal posterior joint capsule

Baker's cyst

extravasated contrast medium

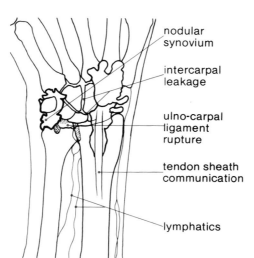

nodular synovium

intercarpal leakage

ulno-carpal ligament rupture

tendon sheath communication

lymphatics

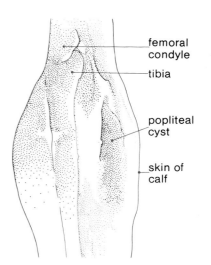

femoral condyle

tibia

popliteal cyst

skin of calf

Computer assisted tomography (CT scans), which may prove useful in assessing areas of anatomy such as the spinal canal and sacroiliac joints that are otherwise difficult to visualize (Fig. 2.35).

Sialography, which may be used to demonstrate the effects of sicca syndrome on the salivary glands and differentiate this from mechanical obstruction due to salivary calculus (Fig. 2.36).

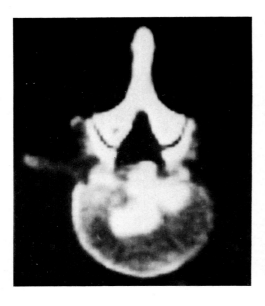

Fig. 2.35 CT scan of the lumbar spine at the level of the disc space and the facet joints. Contrast medium has been previously injected at discography and a posterior protrusion is shown.

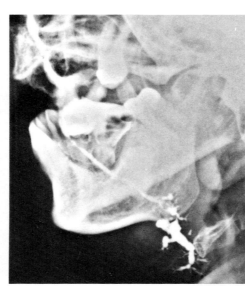

Fig. 2.36 A sialogram showing abnormalities due to the sicca syndrome. There is dilatation of the central ducts of the salivary gland with decreased branching and strictures of the smaller ducts. The main duct is normal.

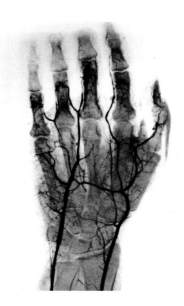

Fig. 2.37 Angiogram in systemic sclerosis. The main vessels are normal but the smaller vessels to the fingers show strictures and occlusions. There is extensive collateral vessel formation but the terminal phalanges of the middle and ring fingers have been lost due to ischemia.

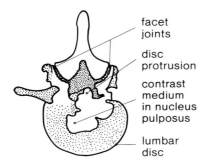

facet joints

disc protrusion

contrast medium in nucleus pulposus

lumbar disc

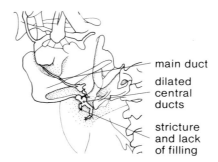

main duct

dilated central ducts

stricture and lack of filling

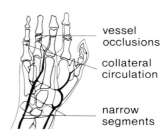

vessel occlusions

collateral circulation

narrow segments

Fig. 2.38 Tenography. The radiograph (left) shows contrast medium outlining the tendon sheath of the tibialis anterior. The normal sheath is expanded due to rheumatoid inflammation. The lateral arthrogram of the wrist (right) shows contrast medium flowing into the flexor tendon sheaths of the forearm. The synovitis has resulted in the development of a communication between joints and tendon sheaths. Extensive lymphatic filling has occurred, consistent with the inflammatory changes.

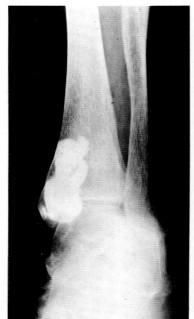

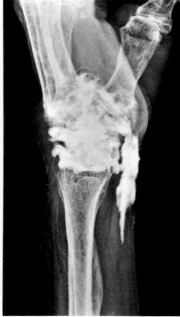

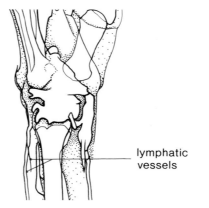

lymphatic vessels

Angiography, which permits assessment of small vessel disease in connective tissue disorders like systemic sclerosis, and differentiation from major vessel disease of alternative etiology (Fig. 2.37). The aneurysms of polyarteritis can also be demonstrated.

Tenography, which may be undertaken to demonstrate either tendon rupture or mass lesions due to synovial hypertrophy (Fig. 2.38).

Myelography, radiculography, ascending lumbar venography and discography are most likely to be used in the assessment of low back pain or rheumatoid disease of the cervical spine (Figs. 2.39-2.41).

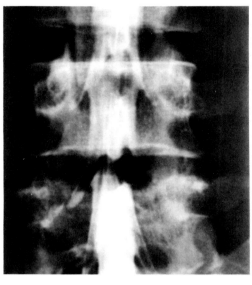

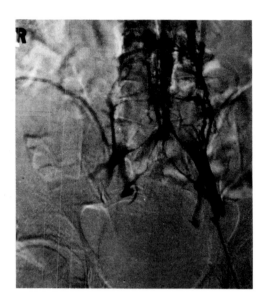

Fig. 2.39 Radiculogram from a patient with a disc protrusion at the L4/5 level. The AP view shows indentation of the column of contrast medium and obliteration of the L5 root sheath on the left (left). The lateral view clearly shows the posterior indentation of the column due to the disc prolapse (right).

Fig. 2.40 Ascending lumbar venography showing L4/5 disc protrusion. There is occlusion of the right pedicular vein at S1 due to disc protrusion. Compare this with the normal vein on the left.

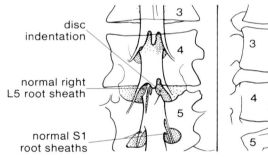

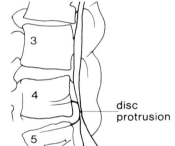

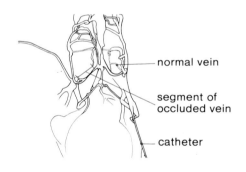

Fig. 2.41 Discogram showing abnormalities at the L3/4 and L4/5 levels. Contrast medium has been injected into the nucleus pulposus of both discs. A posterior leak due to damage to the nucleus pulposus can be seen at the L3/4 level. There is also chronic damage to the L4/5 disc and the abnormal extension of contrast medium anteriorly and posteriorly as well as through fissures in the disc space itself are clearly shown.

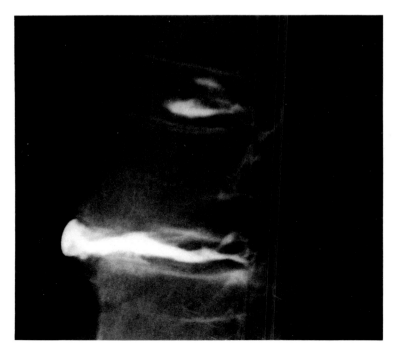

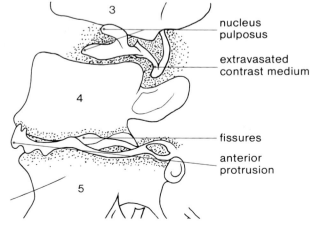

Thermography is an imaging technique based on infra-red heat emission from the skin over bones and joints. Active synovitis can be assessed and quantified with this technique, and the response to treatment measured (Fig. 2.42). Thermography can also be used to investigate reduced peripheral blood flow in disorders such as Raynaud's phenomenon, and increased blood flow in bone as in Paget's disease (Fig. 2.43).

Arthroscopy

Arthroscopy provides a useful technique for the direct examination of a joint cavity. Only certain joints (and principally the knee) can be examined routinely. Sterile conditions are necessary (Fig. 2.44 & 2.45).

The cartilage and synovium of the joint can be visualized, and biopsies taken under direct vision (Figs. 2.46-2.48). The investigation is particularly useful for diagnosis of internal derangements of the knee joint, and for obtaining biopsy material in conditions like tuberculosis, or villonodular synovitis, which can cause patchy synovial changes which may be missed using a 'blind' percutaneous biopsy technique.

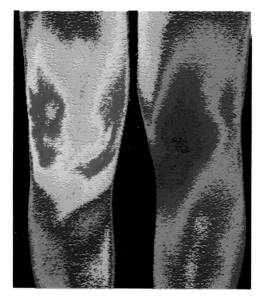 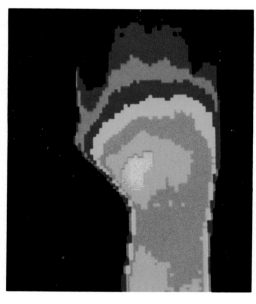 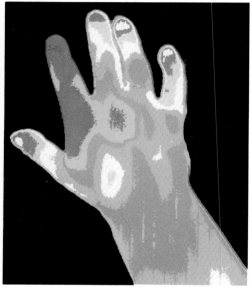

Fig. 2.42 Thermogram of the knee joint in acute monoarthritis. The left knee is normal. The inflamed, right, knee has the V-shaped red area of increased heat emission (anterior view). Temperatures range from 25°C (dark blue) to 35°C (white).

Fig. 2.43 Thermograms of the hands in Raynaud's phenomenon taken before and after cold stress. The cold results in loss of blood flow to the fingers resulting in 'thermal amputation' (left).

Following cold stress some fingers show reactive hyperemia (right).
Figs. 2.42 and 2.43 courtesy of Mr. E.F.J. Ring, Royal National Hospital for Rheumatic Diseases.

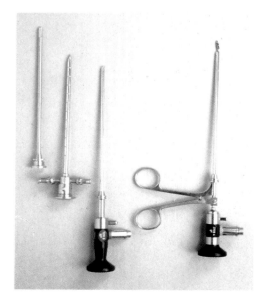 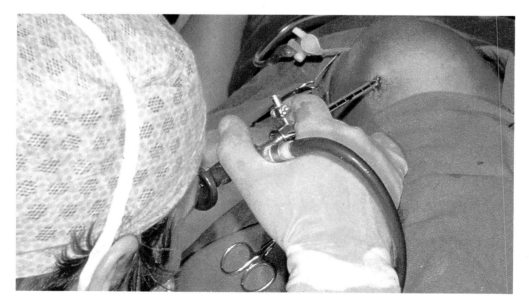

Fig. 2.44 A Stortz arthroscope. The trochar and cannula are shown on the left. In the middle the telescope which produces a magnified image to the observer is seen. To the right of the picture are the biopsy forceps used to take samples of tissue under direct vision.

Fig. 2.45 Arthroscopy of the knee joint. The examination is being carried out with the patient under local anesthetic. The knee is flexed and the arthroscope has been inserted into the intercondylar notch from the lateral aspect. A cannula has been inserted into the infrapatellar space to allow continuous washing of the knee joint with normal saline. Strict aseptic techniques are being observed.

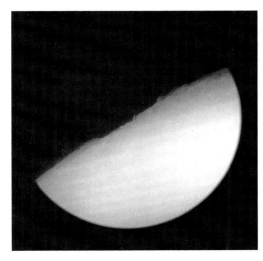
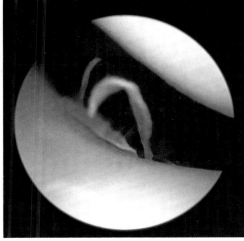
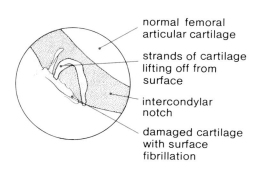

normal femoral articular cartilage

strands of cartilage lifting off from surface

intercondylar notch

damaged cartilage with surface fibrillation

Fig. 2.46 Two views of the articular cartilage through an arthroscope. The view of the back of the patella shows the normal smooth surface and white glistening appearance of normal articular cartilage (left). An area of cartilage ulceration and fibrillation can be seen in the lateral intercondylar area (right). Courtesy of Dr. D. Yates.

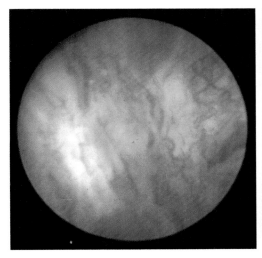
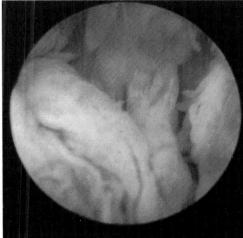
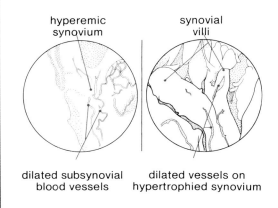

hyperemic synovium

synovial villi

dilated subsynovial blood vessels

dilated vessels on hypertrophied synovium

Fig. 2.47 Synovial abnormalities viewed through an arthroscope. The view on the left shows marked hyperemia of the synovium on the medial wall of the joint space, that on the right shows hypertrophied, inflamed synovial villi in a case of rheumatoid disease. Courtesy of Dr. D. Yates.

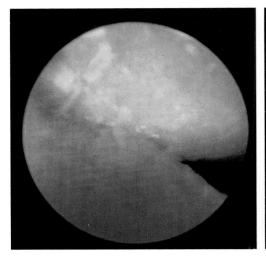
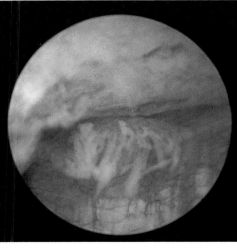
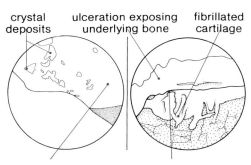

crystal deposits

ulceration exposing underlying bone

fibrillated cartilage

femoral articular cartilage

cartilage segment lifting off articular surface

Fig. 2.48 Cartilage and bone abnormalities viewed through the arthroscope. The picture on the left was taken from a case of gout and shows crystal deposits in the articular cartilage, that on the right shows an area of bony erosion with a segment lifting out from the underlying bone in a case of chronic destructive joint disease. Courtesy of Dr. D. Yates.

Tissue Diagnoses

Several rheumatic diseases are associated with specific histological changes and biopsy material is essential to make the diagnosis of disorders such as giant cell arterius, amyloidosis or a synovioma. Various tissues are useful.

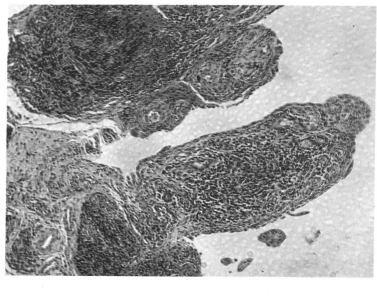

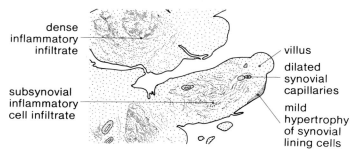

Fig. 2.49 A synovial biopsy showing an inflamed synovial villus with extensive infiltration and inflammatory cells in the subsynovial tissue. However, these changes are non-specific and can be seen in a variety of different inflammatory arthropathies. H & E stain, x 180. Courtesy of Dr. B Ansell.

Fig. 2.50 Synovial pathology in villonodular synovitis. The gross specimen of the synovium (upper, courtesy of Dr. B. Ansell) shows the typical hypertrophied fronds and darkly-stained pigmented synovium due to accummulation of pigments from the blood. The histological sections (lower) show infiltration with macrophages and giant cells (left, H & E stain, x 200) and the interstitial deposits of hemosiderin pigment (right, Perl's stain, x 200).

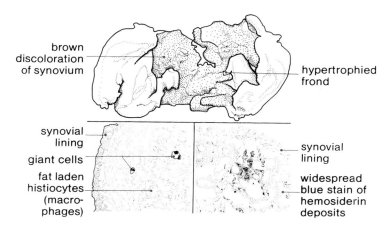

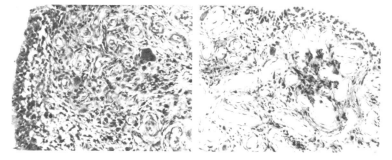

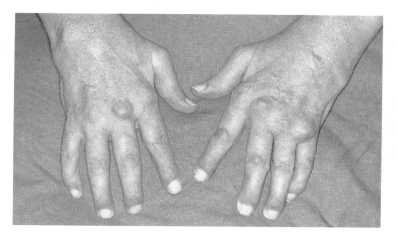

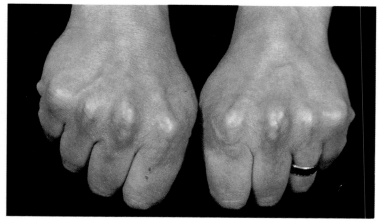

Fig. 2.51 Nodules in rheumatic disease. A variety of rheumatic diseases may give rise to nodules on the hands and elsewhere. The cases shown are of nodules due to rheumatoid disease (left) and hyperlipidemia (right).

Synovial changes, surprisingly, are often unhelpful. The histological appearance of most common rheumatic diseases is similar, showing non-specific inflammatory changes (Fig. 2.49). However, a few uncommon diseases such as villonodular synovitis are diagnosed on synovial biopsy (Fig. 2.50). Skin and subcutaneous tissue may be useful. For example, xanthomas and rheumatoid nodules may look the same to the clinician, but have quite different histological appearances (Fig. 2.51). Those of rheumatoid arthritis are usually associated with high titers of rheumatoid factor. If this is not present a biopsy to establish the diagnosis is indicated. Immunofluorescent staining of the skin may aid the diagnosis of SLE (Fig. 2.52). Muscle biopsy is helpful in diagnosing polymyositis (Fig. 2.53) and vasculitis can be confirmed by skin, vessel, nerve, or rectal biopsy (Fig. 2.54). Temporal artery biopsy may confirm giant cell arteritis, renal or rectal biopsies amyloidosis, and lip gland biopsy the sicca syndrome. Bone may need to be examined for osteomalacia.

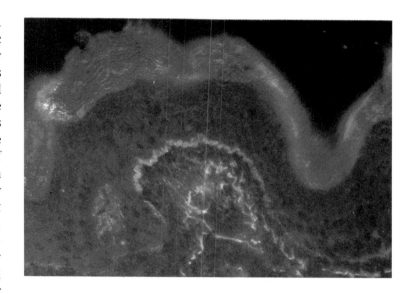

Fig. 2.52 The Lupus Band Test. The skin biopsy taken from the forearm of a patient with SLE shows a green band of immunofluorescent staining with IgG at the dermal-epidermal junction.

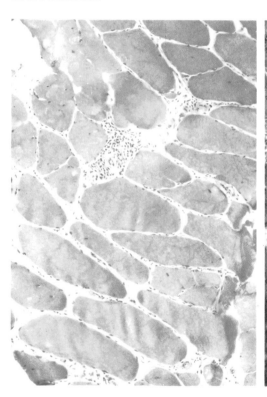
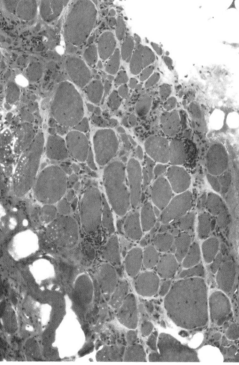
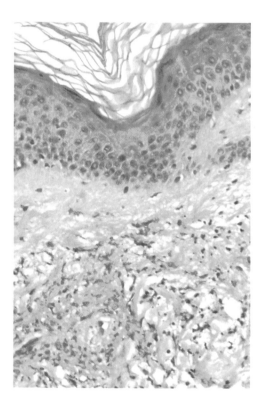

Fig. 2.53 Histological examination of the muscle in a case of polymyositis. The section on the left shows a perivascular inflammatory infiltrate between the muscle fibres (H & E stain, x 300). The section on the right shows variation in the size of the muscle fibers, and interstitial inflammatory infiltrate and increased fibrosis in a patient with chronic polymyositis (H & E stain, x 300). Courtesy of Dr. D. Isenberg.

Fig. 2.54 Skin biopsy showing an area of subepidermal leucocytoclastic vasculitis with an inflammatory cell infiltrate and fragmenting neutrophils around a small arteriole. H & E stain, x 300.

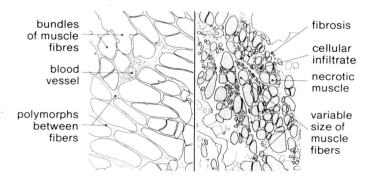

bundles of muscle fibres

blood vessel

polymorphs between fibers

fibrosis

cellular infiltrate

necrotic muscle

variable size of muscle fibers

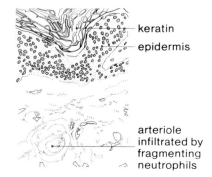

keratin

epidermis

arteriole infiltrated by fragmenting neutrophils

Neurophysiology

Neurophysiological tests are of value in the assessment of peripheral nerve lesions and some muscle disorders. The most common example is the confirmation of a compression or entrapment neuropathy. Diminished conduction in the median nerve across the carpal tunnel, for example, suggests compression (Figs. 2.55). The electrical pattern obtained by needling muscle can help to distinguish between polymyositis and other muscle disorders (Fig. 2.56).

Conclusion

A few of the investigative techniques used in rheumatological practice have been mentioned. Other special tests are sometimes useful in assessing joint diseases and their systemic complications. A wide range of techniques is therefore available to help clinicians investigate the anatomical changes and processes involved in the pathogenesis of rheumatic disorders.

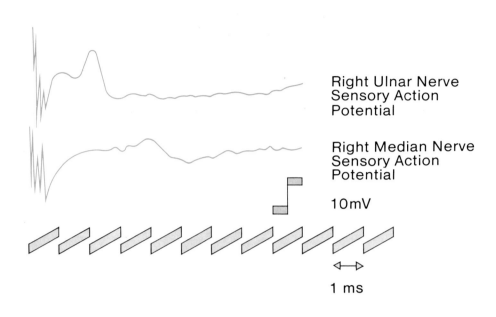

Right Ulnar Nerve
Sensory Action
Potential

Right Median Nerve
Sensory Action
Potential

10mV

1 ms

Fig. 2.55 Nerve conduction studies in a patient with carpal tunnel syndrome. There is delayed conduction in the median nerve with a low-voltage potential. Courtesy of Dr. C. Fowler.

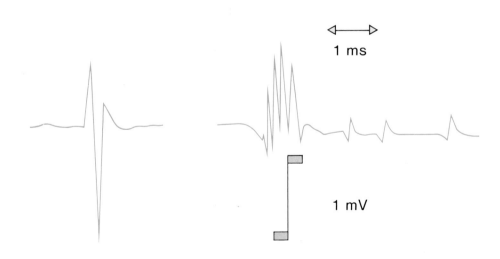

1 ms

1 mV

Fig. 2.56 Electromyography: a single motor unit recorded from normal muscle (left) and the pattern seen in polymyositis, with a polyphasic unit of normal amplitude and several small biphasic fibrillation potentials (right). Courtesy of Dr. M. Harrison.

3

Introduction to Rheumatoid Arthritis

Rheumatoid arthritis (RA) is a chronic, idiopathic, inflammatory disease, which can affect almost any part of the body (synonym: rheumatoid disease). Synovial joints usually bear the brunt of the inflammation, and as the disease progresses, deforming, disabling damage to cartilage and bone often occur.

The prevalence of RA is difficult to estimate, but is probably about 3%; women are more commonly affected than men (F : M ratio 3 : 1). The peak age of onset is 25–50 years, although it can begin at any age. RA is no respector of race or climate, although its severity varies in different countries; severe deforming disease is particularly common in northern Europe for example (Fig. 3.1).

The etiology of RA remains unknown, but is probably multifactorial. Of interest are its relatively recent development as a major disease (the first descriptions only appear in the middle of the nineteenth century), the high risk conferred by HLA D4, and its high prevalence in women. Autoimmunity is a feature of the disease: the inflammatory synovitis contains focal areas of plasma cells and lymphocytes, and the serum usually contains various antibodies to native IgG. There is also circumstantial evidence suggesting that infection may trigger an autoimmune synovitis in susceptible individuals.

The three main pathological features of the disease are serositis, nodules and vasculitis (Fig. 3.2). Clinical and radiological features vary considerably in different patients, and in different stages of the disease; joint inflammation dominates the early picture, whereas joint destruction and systemic complications may be prominent in the chronic phase. There is no known cure for rheumatoid arthritis.

THE CHARACTERISTICS OF RA

Systemic chronic inflammatory disease

Mainly affects synovial joints

Variable expression

Prevalence about 3%

Worldwide distribution

Female : male ratio 3:1

Peak age of onset 25-50 years

Fig. 3.1 The main characteristics of rheumatoid arthritis.

THE PATHOLOGY OF RA

Serositis

1 – Synovitis
Joints
Tendon sheaths
Bursae

2 – Serositis of pleura and pericardium

Nodules

Vasculitis

Fig. 3.2 The main pathological features of rheumatoid arthritis.

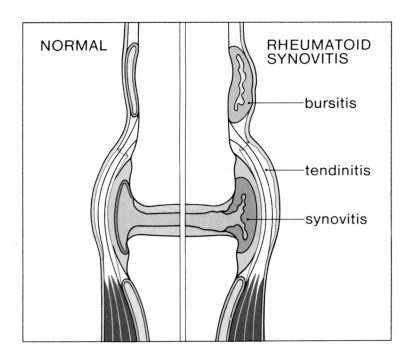

Fig. 3.3 The three major sites of rheumatoid synovitis.

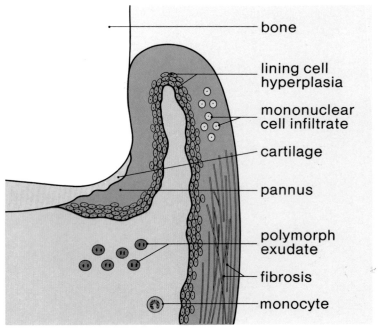

Fig. 3.4 The main features of rheumatoid synovitis.

Serositis

The relentless inflammation of synovial tissue, which is the hallmark of this disease, can affect the lining of any diarthrodial joint in the body, as well as the numerous bursae and tendon sheaths (Fig. 3.3). Serositis in other organs is described in 'Rheumatoid Disease'. Synovitis in RA has features of both acute and chronic inflammation. In the first stages of the disease edema, vascular dilatation and an exudate rich in polymorphs are seen, but as the condition develops the synovial tissue becomes infiltrated with lymphocytes and plasma cells and the lining cells proliferate; fibrosis and the development of granulation tissue occur. In active RA it is common to see a mononuclear cell infiltrate in the synovium, a polymorph cell exudate in the fluid, and at the synovium-cartilage junction, proliferative granulation tissue (the pannus) which appears to erode the cartilage (Fig. 3.4).

The clinical features of RA are most varied, but usually it first appears in peripheral joints and tendon sheaths, and then spreads to involve more central articulations, sparing the back but not the cervical spine. It is usually fairly symmetrical. The frequencies of involvement of different joint sites at presentation, and in established RA are given in figures 3.5 & 3.6. Early synovitis of joints may cause swelling of proximal interphalangeal (PIP) joints, or tenderness of metacarpophalangeal (MCP) or metatarsophalangeal (MTP) joints (Fig. 3.7). Tendinitis or bursal inflammation can also be early features.

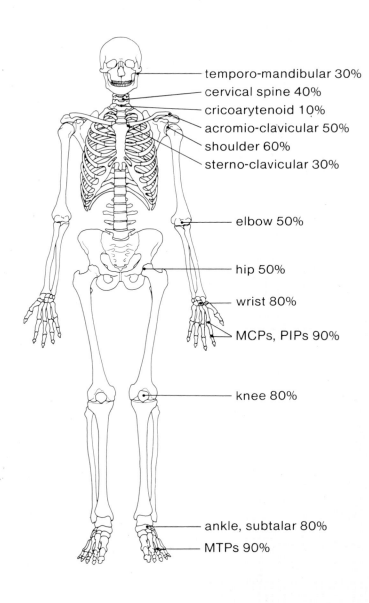

temporo-mandibular 30%
cervical spine 40%
cricoarytenoid 10%
acromio-clavicular 50%
shoulder 60%
sterno-clavicular 30%

elbow 50%

hip 50%

wrist 80%

MCPs, PIPs 90%

knee 80%

ankle, subtalar 80%
MTPs 90%

Fig. 3.6 Frequency of involvement of different joint sites in established RA.

JOINT INVOLVEMENT ON PRESENTATION OF RA

Polyarticular	75%	Monoarticular	25%
Small joints of hands and feet	60%	Knee	50%
Large joints	30%	Shoulder Wrist Hip Ankle Elbow	50%
Large and small joints	10%		

Fig. 3.5 Frequency of involvement of different joint sites at presentation in RA (approximate figures).

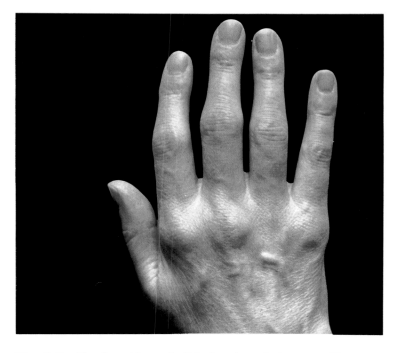

Fig. 3.7 The hand in early RA showing obvious swelling at the PIP joints together with involvement of the MCPs, which were tender on clinical examination.

Radiographs taken in the early stages of rheumatoid arthritis show swelling of soft tissues and periarticular osteoporosis, but nothing else (Fig. 3.8). Other imaging techniques, such as joint scans or thermography, will often reveal inflammation in the typical symmetrical pattern of early disease (eg. wrists, MCPs and PIPs in the hands, and MTPs in the feet) (Fig. 3.9).

The synovial fluid is usually rich in polymorphs during all stages of the disease and its volume, total cell count, and loss of normal viscosity reflect the amount of inflammation in the joint (Fig. 3.10).

Synovitis may be visualized directly, either by arthroscopy, or at arthrotomy (Figs. 3.11 & 3.12). Early disease causes a red, swollen, angry-looking joint, but as the proliferative phase develops, 'fronds' of tissue make the synovium look like seaweed, and pannus may be seen extending over the cartilage.

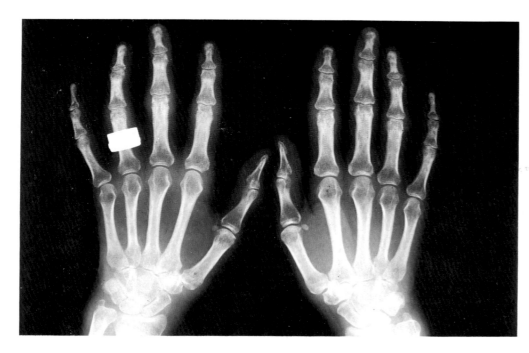

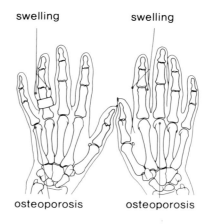

Fig. 3.8 Radiograph of the hands in early RA showing soft tissue swelling (particularly PIPs) and periarticular osteoporosis (particularly MCPs).

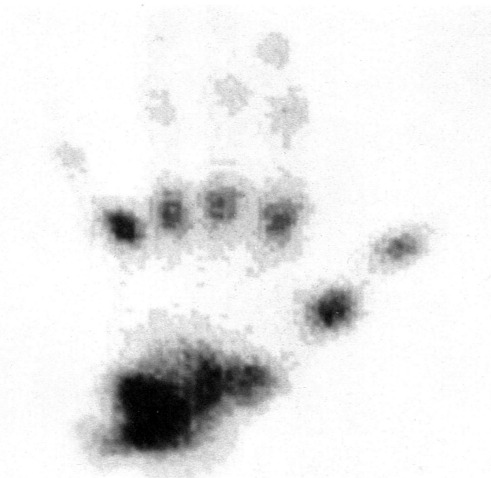

Fig. 3.9 Technetium labelled diphosphonate scan in early rheumatoid arthritis. There is increased uptake in the wrists and MCPs particularly, and less marked uptake in the PIPs.

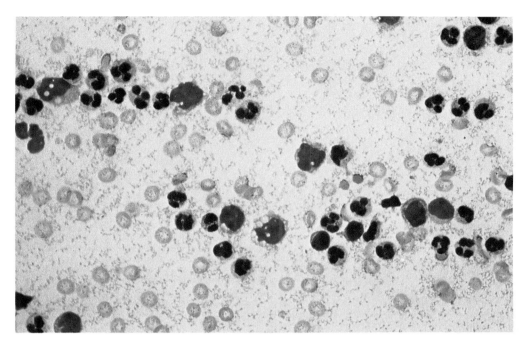

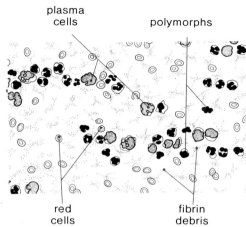

Fig. 3.10 Synovial fluid in RA showing a rich cellular exudate, hypersegmented polymorphs and mononuclear cells. Red cells and fibrin debris are also present. Grunewald-Giemsa stain, x 1500.

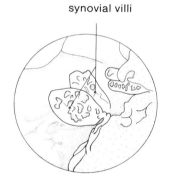

Fig. 3.11 Synovium of the knee joint at arthroscopy showing richly vascularized proliferating synovial villi. Courtesy of Dr. D. Yates.

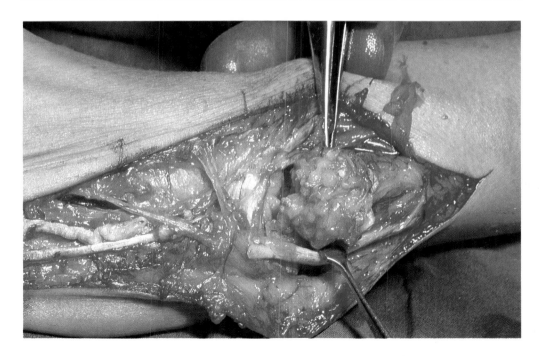

Fig. 3.12 Operative view of the elbow joint in rheumatoid arthritis showing proliferating synovium bulging out of the opened joint capsule.

There are no diagnostic features on histological examination, but the combination of synovial lining cell hyperplasia and deep infiltration with lymphocytes and plasma cells is characteristic of RA (Figs. 3.13–3.15). Immunofluorescent staining shows that many of the plasma cells in the inflamed synovium are producing

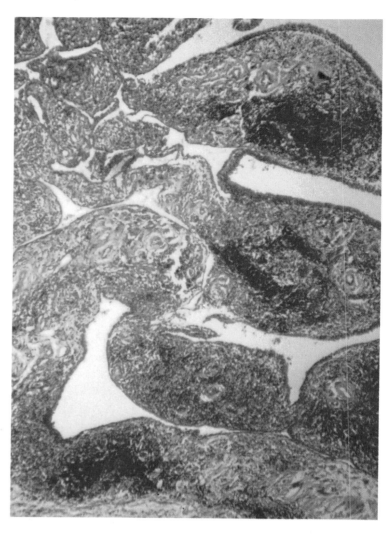

Fig. 3.13 Synovial histology in RA showing proliferating synovial lining cells on the surface of a villus. The surface fibrin contains infiltrating polymorphs and mononuclear cells. H & E stain, x 1500.

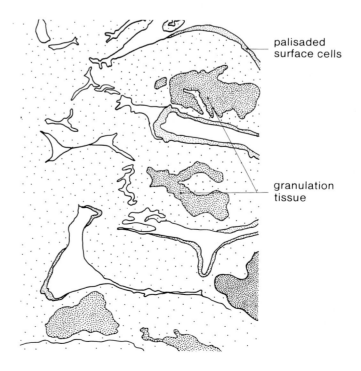

Fig. 3.14 Synovial histology in RA showing exuberant granulation tissue in proliferating villi and the deeper layers. H & E stain, x 200. Courtesy of Dr. J. Pringle.

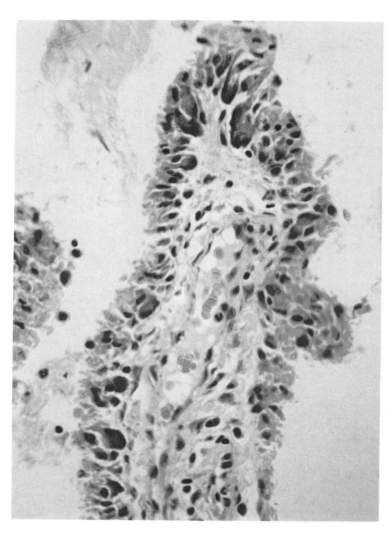

leucocytes

proliferating synovial lining cells

surface fibrin

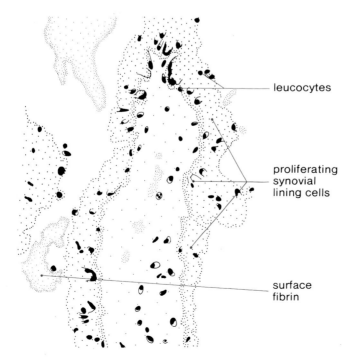

palisaded surface cells

granulation tissue

antiglobulin antibodies, and the tissue both looks and behaves rather like an active lymph node (Fig. 3.16).

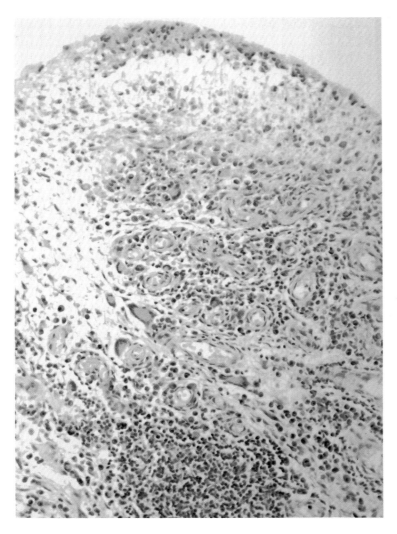

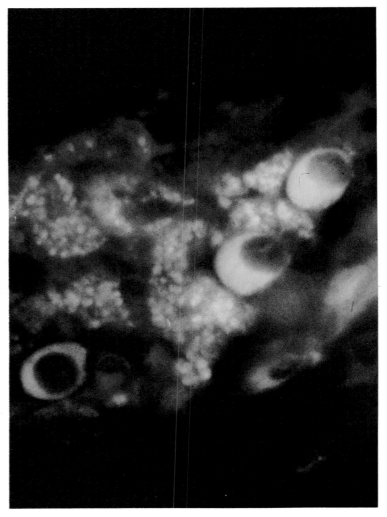

Fig. 3.15 Section across a rheumatoid synovial villus showing surface lining hyperplasia, underlying new vessel formation, and a deep infiltrate containing aggregates of leucocytes. Giemsa stain, x 640.

Fig. 3.16 Immunofluorescent staining of rheumatoid synovial tissue to show antiglobulin production in the plasma cells. Courtesy of Professor I. Roitt.

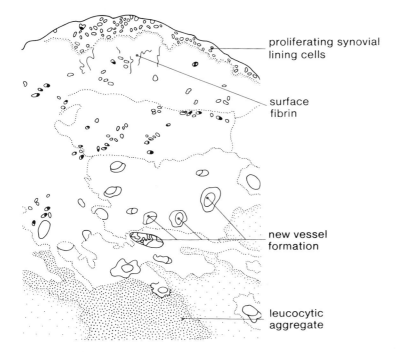

proliferating synovial lining cells

surface fibrin

new vessel formation

leucocytic aggregate

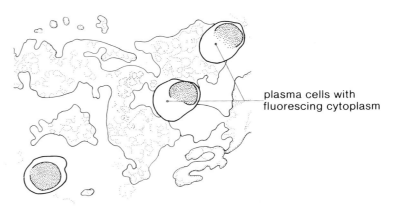

plasma cells with fluorescing cytoplasm

Joint Damage

Persistent rheumatoid synovitis usually causes destruction and deformity to the joints and periarticular tissues.

Damage occurs principally at the synovium-cartilage junction area, where the proliferating pannus of inflamed synovial tissue appears to eat into the cartilage and bone (Fig. 3.17). Radiographs show marginal erosions in bone and narrowing of the joint space due to junctional bone damage and loss of articular cartilage respectively. The radiographic features are helpful both diagnostically and in assessing the severity of the disease and its progression. Early sites of erosion include the 4th & 5th MTPs, 1st and 2nd MCPs and PIPs and the ulnar styloid (Fig. 3.18). Active erosions are characterized by periarticular

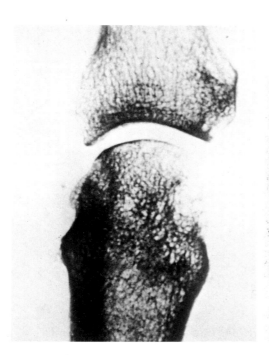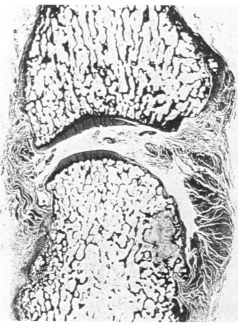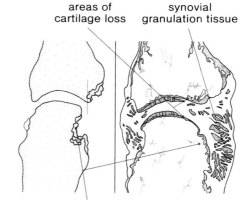

Fig. 3.17 A rheumatoid PIP joint (post mortem) showing early active erosions with loss of bone trabeculi and loss of surface cartilage both radiographically (left) and histologically (right). Courtesy of Professor E.G.L. Bywaters.

areas of cartilage loss   synovial granulation tissue

loss of bone trabeculation with infiltrating granulation tissue

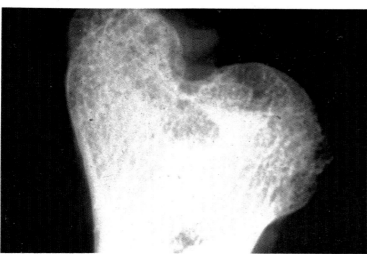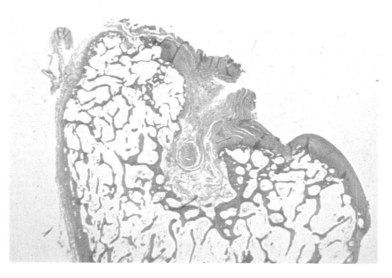

Fig. 3.18 Distal end of the ulna in rheumatoid arthritis. The radiograph shows an erosion at the base of the ulnar styloid and surface osteoporosis. The histology shows infiltrating inflammatory tissue invading the bone. H & E stain. Courtesy of Dr. D. Berens.

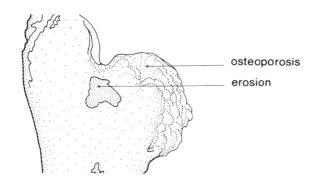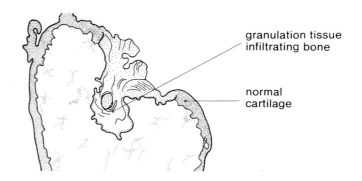

osteoporosis

erosion

granulation tissue infiltrating bone

normal cartilage

osteoporosis and a fluffy margin, whereas the old erosion looks 'punched-out', being well demarcated with a sclerotic margin (Fig. 3.19).

Tendinitis and bursitis may also cause destruction and deformity, leading to joint subluxation, laxity of periarticular tissues and tendon rupture.

These destructive changes are associated with the development of a characteristic set of clinical deformities. Ulnar drift of the fingers, Swan Neck deformities, loss of finger flexion (due to flexor tenosynovitis) and MTP and wrist subluxation are typical of some of the clinical features (Fig. 3.20).

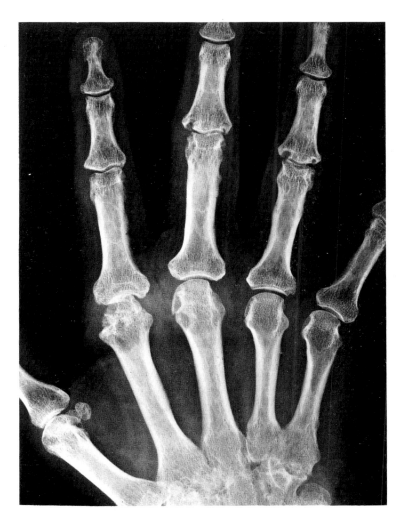

Fig. 3.19 Radiograph of the hand in RA showing both active erosions at the MCPs and old well-demarcated erosions at the PIPs.

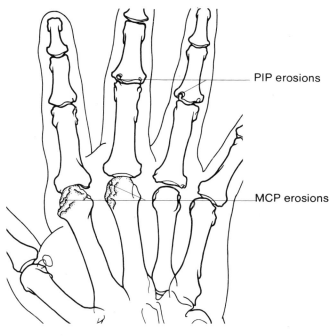

PIP erosions

MCP erosions

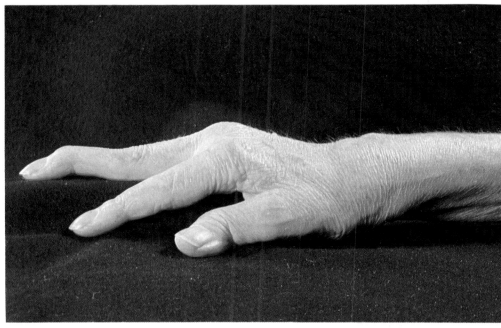

Fig. 3.20 Characteristic clinical deformities of the hand in RA including Swan Neck deformity, subluxation of the second MCP and wrist, and instability of the thumb.

Nodules

About 30% of patients with RA develop nodules. These granulomas develop in subcutaneous tissue and tendons, and may also be found in internal organs such as the heart and lung.

They have characteristic histological features: a central area of necrosis is surrounded by mononuclear cells, the macrophages aligned with their long axes pointing to the centre of the lesion, and an outer layer of fibrous tissue (Fig. 3.21).

Superficial nodules occur over pressure areas, the most common site being the ulnar border just below the elbow (Fig. 3.22). Small nodules are only found by careful examination, and are usually hard and attached to the underlying periosteum. Large ones can be hard to miss (Fig. 3.23)! High titres of serum IgM rheumatoid factor are nearly always found in nodular disease.

Vasculitis

A small proportion of patients with RA develop the third main pathological feature of the disease, vasculitis. Inflammation of the walls of small blood vessels may result in a number of different clinical and pathological features. The commonest lesions occur around the nails and may appear transiently during phases of active disease (Fig. 3.24). More persistent vasculitis may result in peripheral ulceration and even gangrene: characteristically vasculitic ulcers are very painful (Fig. 3.25). Vasculitis is a feature of severe rheumatoid disease.

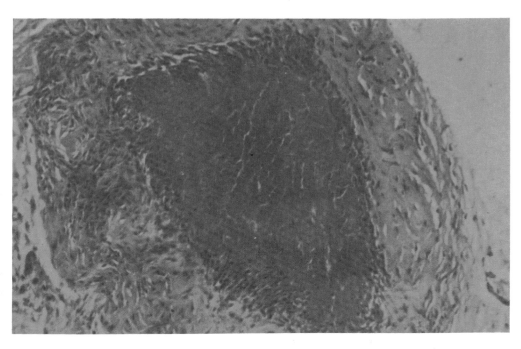

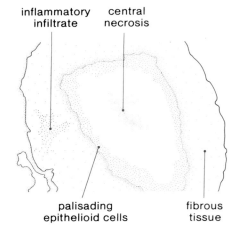

Fig. 3.21 Characteristic histological features of a rheumatoid nodule showing central necrosis, palisading epithelioid cells with some surrounding fibrous tissue and a sparse inflammatory infiltrate. H & E stain, x 20.

inflammatory infiltrate

central necrosis

palisading epithelioid cells

fibrous tissue

Fig. 3.22 A small early rheumatoid nodule at the ulnar border near the elbow.

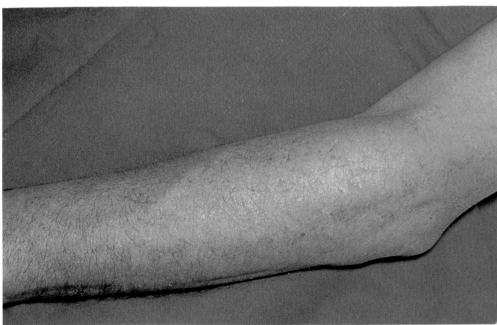

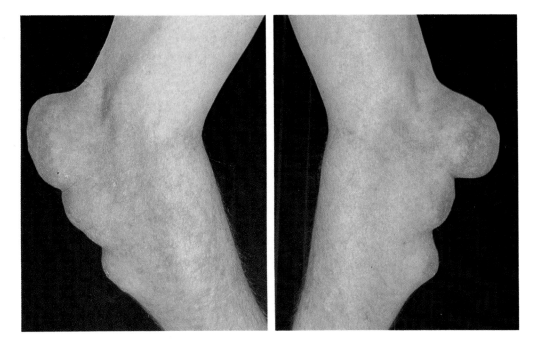

Fig. 3.23 Large nodules in RA along the subcutaneous border of the ulnae and in the wall of the olecranon bursa.

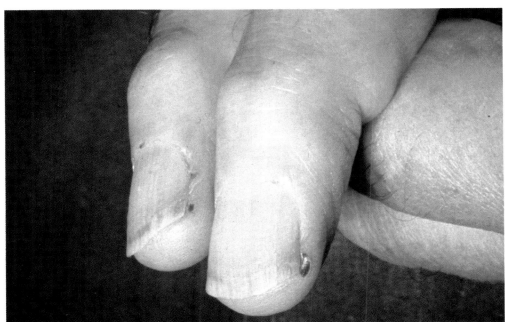

Fig. 3.24 Nail edge vasculitic lesions in RA.

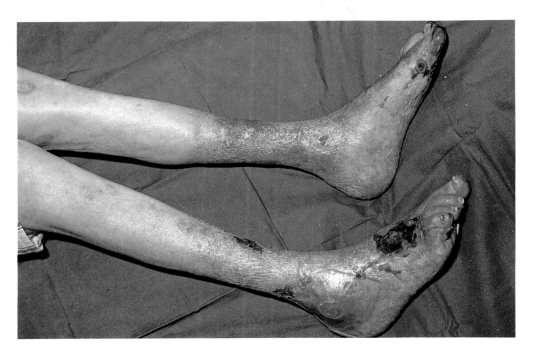

Fig. 3.25 A patient with longstanding seropositive RA with vasculitic ulceration of the legs and feet in various stages of evolution. There is some pigmentation of the skin as a result of previous ulceration.

Systemic Disease

Rheumatoid disease shows a number of systemic features including mild fever, malaise, weight loss, muscle wasting and anemia (Fig. 3.26). In addition, it also directly affects a number of different organs in the body especially in men. Serous membranes other than the synovium may be inflamed; pleural and pericardial effusions are quite common. Inflammation in the form of nodules or vasculitis can affect the eye, heart, lung, skin or peripheral nerve. Lymphadenopathy, splenomegaly, and changes in the bone marrow can contribute to hematological manifestations (Fig. 3.27). Less common secondary complications include amyloidosis and cervical cord compression.

The disease is variable in activity, with spontaneous exacerbations and remissions; it can have quite different manifestations in different patients.

Few cases of established rheumatoid disease go into complete, spontaneous remission. Some patients only have minor symptoms and signs; many develop considerable pain, stiffness and joint deformity, but remain able to lead a fairly independent life; a few become severely disabled. Life expectancy is reduced. Amyloidosis, Felty's syndrome, (the splenomegaly and leukopenia associated with RA), recurrent infections, vasculitis and cervical cord compression all carry a poor prognosis.

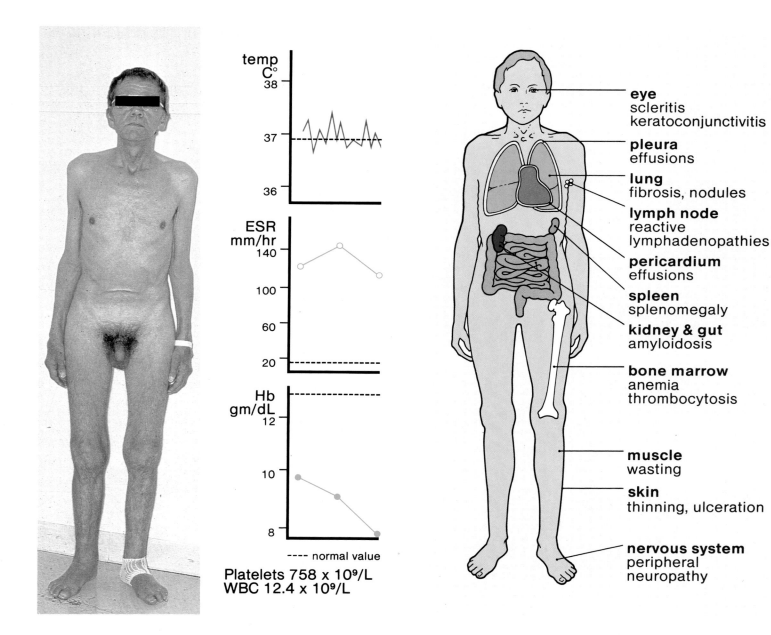

Fig. 3.26 Patient with severe active rheumatoid arthritis showing weight loss and muscle wasting as well as arthritis. The chart shows fever, high ESR, falling hemoglobin, and elevated platelet and white blood cell (WBC) count.

Fig. 3.27 Other organs commonly involved in rheumatoid disease.

4

Rheumatoid Arthritis of the Hands and Feet

The hands and feet are often the first sites to be involved in rheumatoid arthritis ('RA'). As the disease progresses a number of characteristic deformities develop and function may be impaired. Many of the extra-articular features of rheumatoid disease are also seen in the hands and feet. Radiographs of these regions are the most useful ones to aid early diagnosis and assess the progression of the disease. The clinical and radiological examination of these sites is therefore of great importance. The rheumatoid hand has been termed the patient's 'calling card', and can be the physician's guide to management.

Typical rheumatoid deformities are shown in the first two illustrations (Figs. 4.1 & 4.2). No two patients ever develop quite the same appearance, but some of the characteristic changes to look for in the hands have also been listed (Fig. 4.3). In the following pages a selection of illustrations are presented which show how these joint deformities develop. (Some of the extra-articular features are illustrated elsewhere, see 'Rheumatoid Disease'.)

Early Rheumatoid Arthritis of the Hands

The patient's first symptoms of rheumatoid arthritis often come from the hands. Early synovitis characteristically affects the proximal interphalangeal (PIP) and metacarpophalangeal (MCP) joints (Figs. 4.4 & 4.5). Swelling of these joints may lead to stiffness of the fingers and tightening of the skin; difficulty in getting rings on and off the fingers may be one of the first signs of trouble. The synovitis is often accompanied by small muscle wasting, particularly noticeable in the interossei on the dorsum of the hand (Fig. 4.6). At this stage of the disease the patient may have generalized morning stiffness (particularly severe in the hand), joint symptoms elsewhere and general malaise. Synovitis of the wrist may produce mild, diffuse swelling and some instability of the radio-ulnar joint; the physician may be able to spring the head of the ulna, causing wrist discomfort (the 'piano key' sign) (Fig. 4.6).

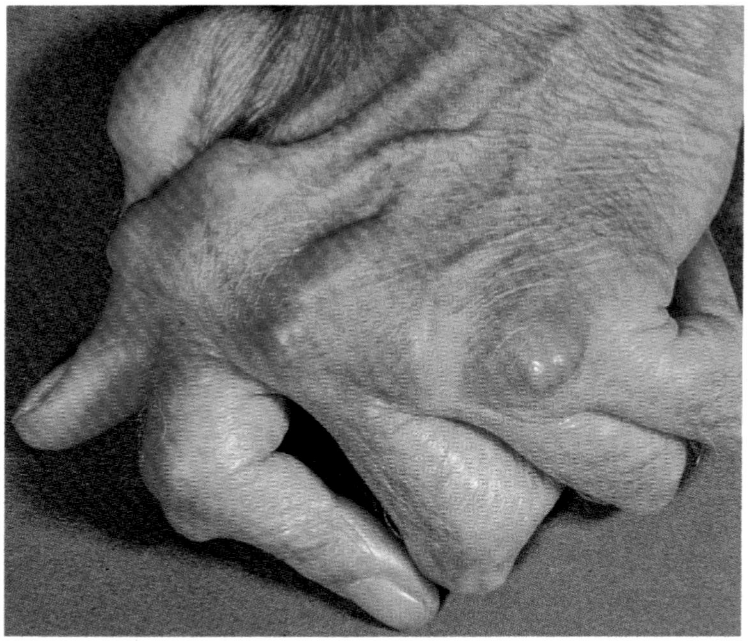

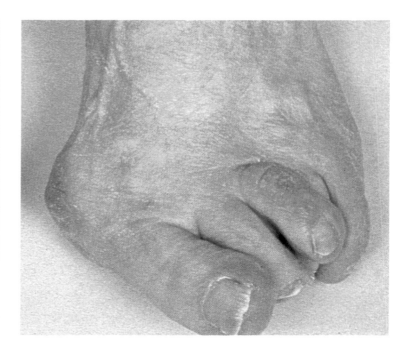

Fig. 4.1 Severe deformity in advanced RA of the hand showing muscle wasting, subluxation and ulnar deviation of the MCPs, flexion deformities of the PIPs, 'Z' deformity of the thumb and the rheumatoid nodules on tendons and in subcutaneous tissue.

Fig. 4.2 RA of the forefoot showing hallux valgus and bunion formation. There is also subluxation of the MTPs, overriding toes and 'cock-up' deformities with pressure areas over the interphalangeal joints.

Fig. 4.3 List of articular features seen in the rheumatoid hand.

SOME OF THE ARTICULAR FEATURES SEEN IN THE RHEUMATOID HAND

WRIST:	PIPs:
synovitis	synovitis and synovial cysts
prominent ulnar styloid	fixed flexion or extension deformities
subluxation and collapse of carpus	(Swan Neck or Boutonniere deformity)
radial deviation	
MCPs:	THUMBS:
synovitis	synovitis of MCP, CMC or IP joint
ulnar deviation	'Z' deformity
subluxation of joints	instability of IP joint
subluxation of extensor tendons	

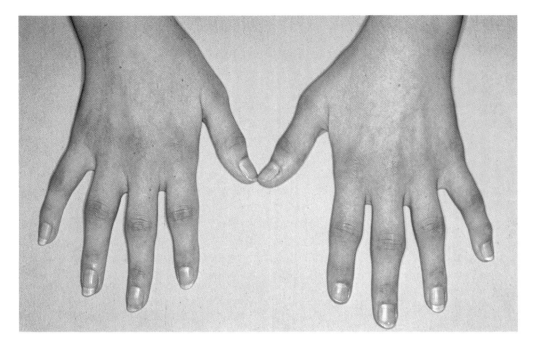

Fig. 4.4 Early RA of the hands. Synovitis is affecting the PIP joints, which results in spindling of the fingers. There is also small muscle wasting on the dorsum of the hand; the wrists are swollen, the left being more swollen than the right. Note also the erythema over the inflamed interphalangeal joints which is sometimes present. Courtesy of Dr. A. C. Boyle.

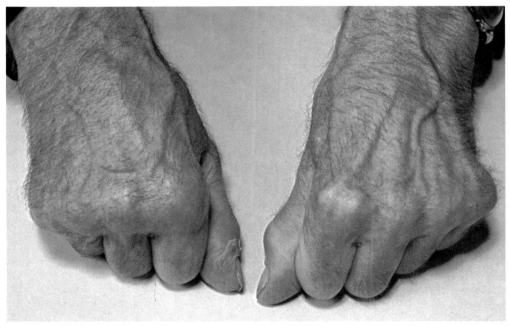

Fig. 4.5 Early synovitis of the MCP joints. This is best seen when the MCP joints are flexed. The synovitis and consequent soft tissue swelling result in a disappearance of the normal hollows between the joints. This is more apparent on the right. There is also some wasting of the dorsal interossei in the left hand.

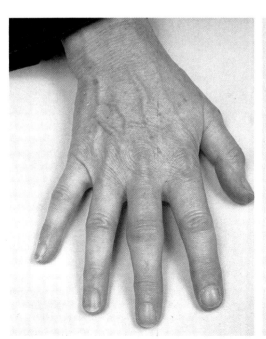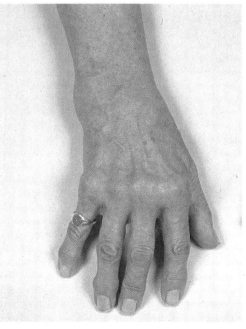

Fig. 4.6 Progression of changes in RA. The patient on the left has only had the disease for six months; swelling of the PIP joints and small muscle wasting are the only signs. The patient on the right first presented after two years of active rheumatoid disease; early subluxation of the MCP joints, the first signs of ulnar deviation, prominent small muscle wasting and synovitis of the wrist can be seen. On examination there was tenderness over the ulnar styloid which bounced up and down on pressure, due to loss of stability (the 'piano-key' sign).

In addition to joint synovitis, tenosynovitis in the hand is often an early feature of rheumatoid disease. The two most common signs are (1) dorsal sheath swellings over the wrist due to involvement of the extensor tendon sheath and (2) flexor tenosynovitis of the fingers causing restriction of movement (Fig. 4.7). 'Trigger' finger may be a presentation of rheumatoid disease; at operation the thickened synovium, which may have nodular areas trapping the tendon, can be exposed and removed (Fig. 4.8).

Another, not uncommon, presentation of rheumatoid arthritis in the hand is carpal tunnel syndrome. This is due to compression of the median nerve of the wrist. The carpal tunnel is roofed in by the flexor retinaculum of the wrist; relatively small degrees of swelling caused, for example, by the synovitis of rheumatoid disease, may produce pressure on the nerve at that site. The resulting symptoms include nocturnal parasthesia affecting the thumb and first two and a half fingers (the distribution of the sensory fibres of the median nerve) (Fig. 4.9). In more advanced cases there is wasting and weakness of the muscles on the lateral side of the thenar eminence: the abductor pollicis brevis and opponens pollicis (Fig. 4.9). Wrist splints or injection of a small quantity of local steroid may help in early cases (Fig. 4.10), but if muscle wasting and weakness occur, surgical decompression of the canal is usually necessary to relieve the pressure (Fig. 4.11). It should also be noted that the sensory symptoms of carpal tunnel syndrome do not always follow the exact anatomical distribution of the median nerve; that there are many other causes of carpal tunnel compression, and that neurological symptoms in the hand in rheumatoid arthritis can come from other causes such as ulnar nerve entrapment at the elbow (causing wasting and weakness of the interossei and hypothenar muscles, and sensory symptoms in the little finger) or disease of the cervical spine.

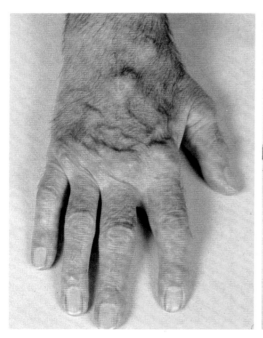
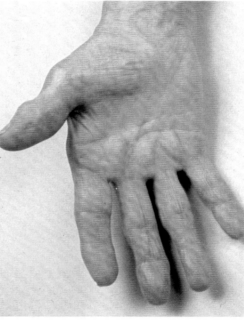

Fig. 4.7 Rheumatoid tenosynovitis. Swelling of the extensor tendon sheath (left) and of the flexor tendon sheath (right). In this patient finger flexion is painful and the middle finger tends to stick in flexion ('trigger' finger). There is muscle wasting in both hands.

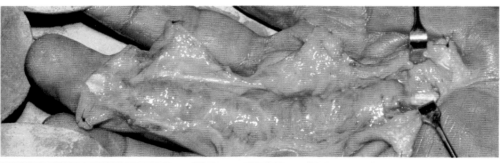
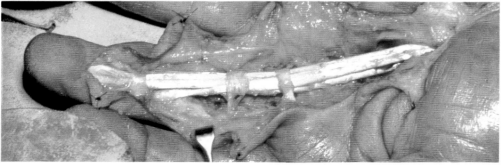

Fig. 4.8 Flexor tenosynovitis. An operation is being performed to remove synovial tissue in a case of RA causing 'trigger' finger. Exposed tendon sheath with marked synovial hypertrophy (upper); underlying tendon after removal of inflamed synovial tissue (lower). Courtesy of Mr. J. Browett.

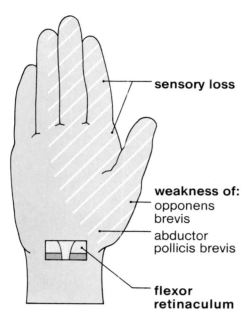

sensory loss

weakness of:
opponens
brevis

abductor
pollicis brevis

flexor
retinaculum

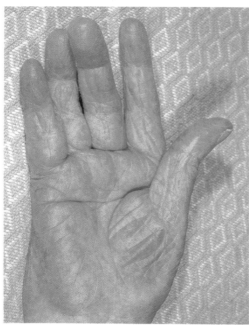

Fig. 4.9 Median nerve compression (carpal tunnel syndrome). The median nerve runs through the narrow canal below the flexor retinaculum of the wrist. It supplies the muscles of the thenar eminence and the sensory arch as shown on the diagram (left). Wasting of the abductor pollicis brevis and opponens pollicis is shown (right). Note also the palmar erythema which is often associated with RA.

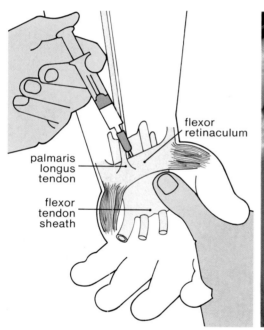

flexor
retinaculum

palmaris
longus
tendon

flexor
tendon
sheath

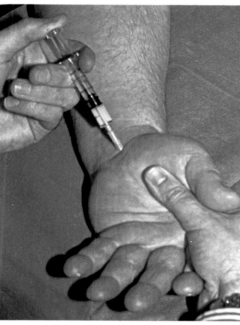

Fig. 4.10 Injection of the carpal tunnel with long-acting corticosteroids may relieve the symptoms. The needle is inserted at the level of distal palmar crease, on the radial side of palmaris longus (if present), and angled towards the fingers as shown in the diagram (left), and photograph (right).

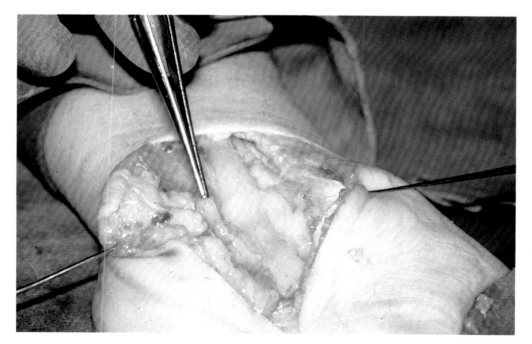

Fig. 4.11 Surgical decompression of the median nerve showing the carpal tunnel being exposed from the palmar aspect of the wrist, inflamed synovial tissue and compressed median nerve. Courtesy of Mr. J. Browett.

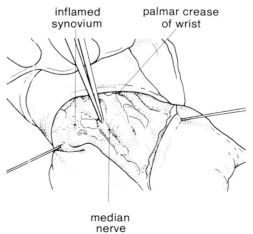

inflamed
synovium

palmar crease
of wrist

median
nerve

4.5

Rheumatoid arthritis can therefore present in the hand with synovitis, tenosynovitis or carpal tunnel syndrome. Small muscle wasting, inflammatory swelling and increased vascularity of the hand are common features. The inflamed areas feel warm to the touch, and the increased vascularity may cause palmar erythema and hyperemia of the nailfold.

Radiological features of early disease include soft tissue swelling in areas of synovitis, and marked periarticular osteoporosis (Fig. 4.12). In typical rheumatoid disease the X-ray pattern, like the clinical pattern, is usually fairly symmetrical involving the MCPs and PIPs. Intense osteoporosis may progress to a loss of definition at the margin of the joint prior to the appearance of the typical erosions at the joint margin which may be seen first on the ulnar styloid. During this early inflammatory phase the distribution of the synovitis can also be documented by other imaging techniques, such as technetium labelled diphosphonate bone scans. A diffuse increase in uptake of the isotope occurs over the inflamed areas due to their abnormal vascularity (Figs. 4.13 & 4.14).

The distribution of these early clinical and radiological changes may have some prognostic value. It has been suggested that those with early changes in the index and middle fingers have a worse prognosis than those with dominant changes in the ring and little fingers. Furthermore, the earlier the appearance of erosions after the onset of symptoms, the worse the outlook for the patient (Fig. 4.15).

Fig. 4.12 Radiograph of early RA of the hand showing soft tissue swelling and periarticular osteoporosis around the PIPs and MCPs (upper) and an early erosion at the PIP of the ring finger (lower).

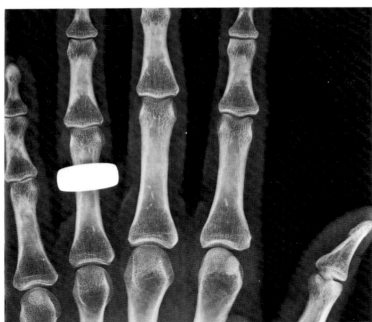

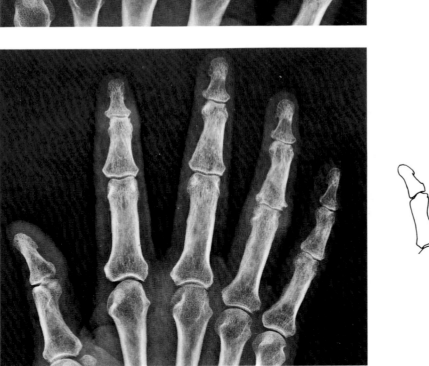

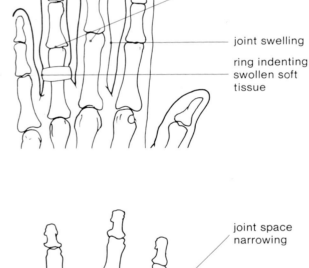

periarticular osteoporosis

joint swelling

ring indenting swollen soft tissue

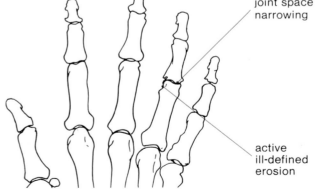

joint space narrowing

active ill-defined erosion

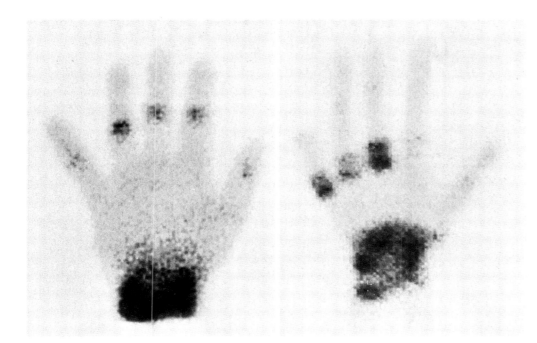

Fig. 4.13 Technetium labelled diphosphonate scans of rheumatoid hands taken in the vascular phase (within half an hour of isotope injection). There is increased isotope uptake in both wrists, and increased vascularity at the PIPs (left) and MCPs (right).

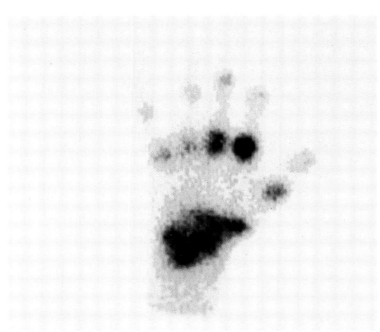

Fig. 4.14 Technetium labelled diphosphonate scan taken four hours after injection of isotope. The rheumatoid synovitis has caused isotope retention at the wrist and MCPs.

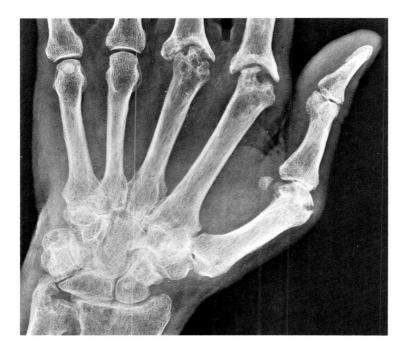

Fig. 4.15 RA two years after the onset of the disease showing florid erosive changes of the medial MCPs and carpal collapse with loss of joint space at the wrist. This distribution and severity of disease carries a poor prognosis.

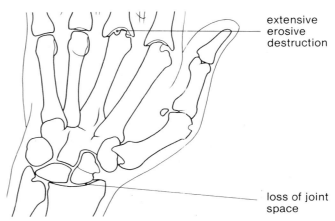

extensive erosive destruction

loss of joint space

Rheumatoid Deformities of the Wrist and Hand

The wrist and hand should be considered as a unit as they affect each other both functionally and anatomically.

Problems of the wrist arise from the synovitis (Figs. 4.16 & 4.17). The ulnar head is characteristically involved, and in addition to the early bone erosions, the ulnar collateral ligament becomes stretched and torn allowing the head of the ulna to spring up. The combination of this upward subluxation and erosive changes may lead to a prominent, ragged ulnar head which may then contribute to rupture of the extensor tendons which pass over it ('caput ulnae') (Fig. 4.18). Some subluxation of the carpal bones may also occur, and slight radial deviation of the wrist is quite common (Fig. 4.19). In advanced disease carpal collapse with extensive damage can then develop and progress, particularly in older patients, to complete fusion of the wrist (Fig. 4.20). (The wrist is one of the few sites which occasionally ankylose in rheumatoid arthritis.)

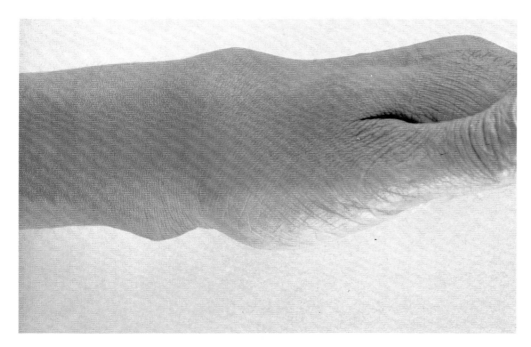

Fig. 4.16 Wrist synovitis showing extension of the synovial swelling on the dorsal and palmar aspect of the wrist.

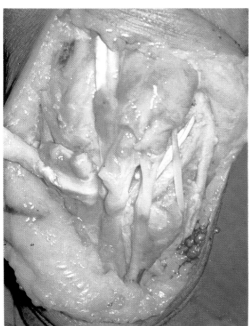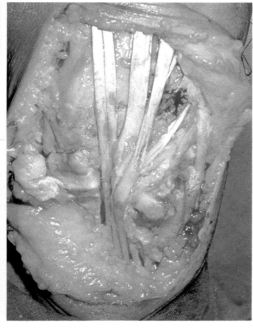

Fig. 4.17 Dorsal synovectomy of the wrist showing the bulky inflamed synovial tissue extruding from the wrist and surrounding the tendon (left) and the clean tendons after removal of the synovium (right). Courtesy of Mr. A.W. Lettin.

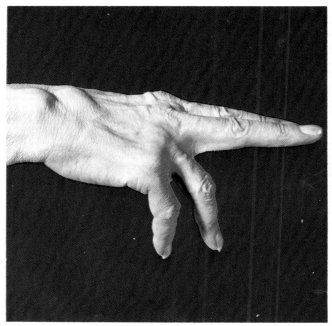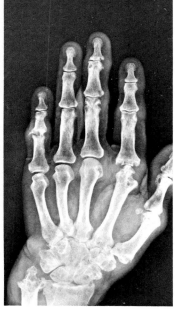

Fig. 4.18 'Caput ulnae'. The ulnar head springs up and is eroded by rheumatoid synovitis; the patient also has tenosynovitis and has ruptured two extensor tendons (left). Radiology reveals extensive rheumatoid erosions, a ragged, eroded ulnar styloid, and surrounding soft tissue swelling (right).

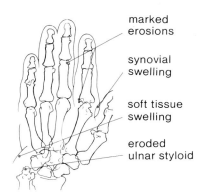

marked
erosions

synovial
swelling

soft tissue
swelling

eroded
ulnar styloid

Fig. 4.19 RA of the wrist showing volar subluxation and soft tissue swelling.

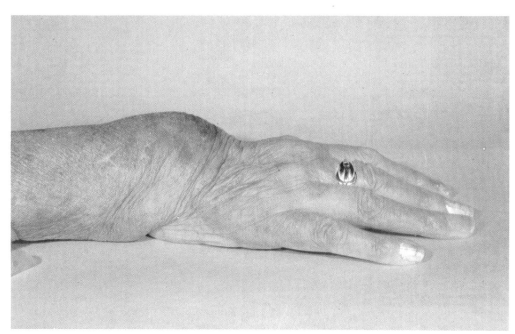

Fig. 4.20 Ankylosis of a wrist in RA. There is widespread erosive damage throughout both hands. The ulnar styloid has been surgically removed on the right. The carpal bones are fusing on both sides, but the changes are more advanced on the right.

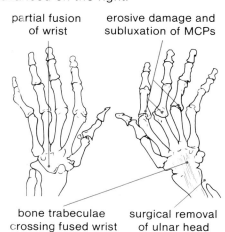

partial fusion
of wrist

erosive damage and
subluxation of MCPs

bone trabeculae
crossing fused wrist

surgical removal
of ulnar head

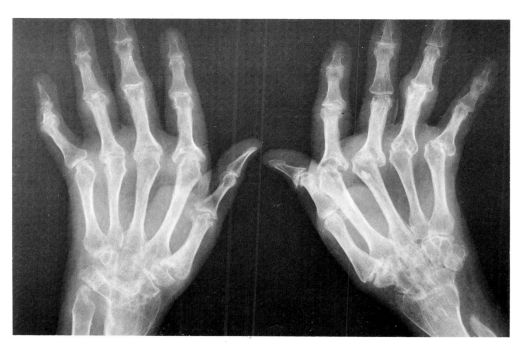

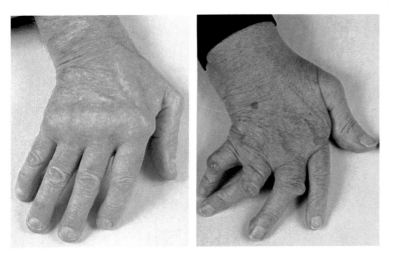

Fig. 4.21 Early ulnar deviation and MCP synovitis (left); this may progress to more marked lateral deviation with subluxation of the extensor tendons (right finger) (right).

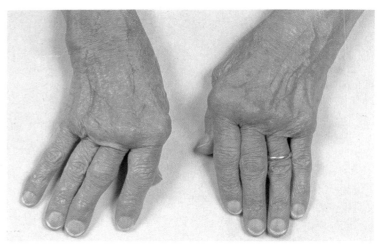

Fig. 4.22 Subluxation of the MCPs with ulnar deviation.

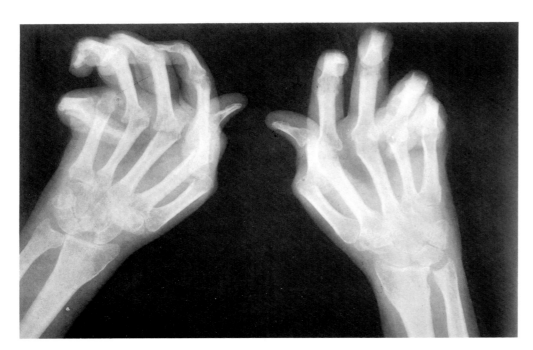

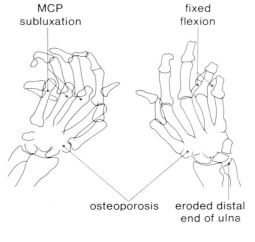

Fig. 4.23 Radiograph in 'arthritis mutilans' showing gross ulnar deviation, MCP subluxation and other changes.

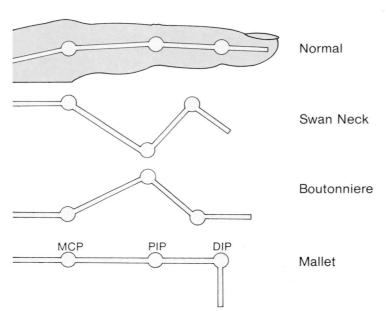

Fig. 4.24 Diagram of finger deformities in RA.

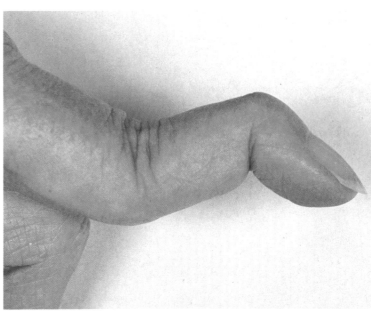

Fig. 4.25 Swan Neck deformity of the index finger showing MCP flexion, hyperextension of the PIPs and DIP flexion.

The most characteristic deformity of the fingers is ulnar deviation at the MCP (Fig. 4.21). This may be due partly to the tendency of the wrist to go into radial deviation, producing a 'zig-zag' deformity, making the tendons pull the fingers into ulnar deviation. There are many other possible explanations, including the tendency for the tendons to pull in that direction during the normal power grip, and abnormalities of the intrinsic muscle. Severe ulnar deviation may be accompanied by subluxation of the extensor tendons and by subluxation of the joints themselves (Fig. 4.22). Tendon dislocation may produce signs similar to those of tendon rupture (Figs. 4.21 & 4.23).

The three main deformities of the interphalangeal joints are (1) the Swan Neck deformity, (2) the Boutonniere deformity and rarely (3) Mallet finger (Fig. 4.24). Swan Neck deformity may develop through shortening of the interossei tending to produce flexion of the MCP accompanied by intrinsic muscle shortening tending to pull the PIP into hyperextension (Fig. 4.25). The profundus tendons then bow-string over the extended PIP contributing to the final part of the deformity, the flexion of the distal interphalangeal joint (DIP), which is probably a secondary phenomenon. Isolated flexion deformity of the DIP occurs in Mallet finger, which may be caused by avulsion of the extensor tendon.

The Boutonniere deformity is a flexion deformity of the PIP that may be accompanied by secondary hyperextension of the DIP (Fig. 4.26). Chronic inflammation and swelling allows the bone to pop out through the hood of the extensor tendon to produce the flexion deformity. The DIPs are themselves sometimes involved in rheumatoid inflammation although this rarely results in significant clinical or radiological changes (Fig. 4.27). Synovial cysts sometimes extrude from interphalangeal joints affected by rheumatoid arthritis (Fig. 4.28).

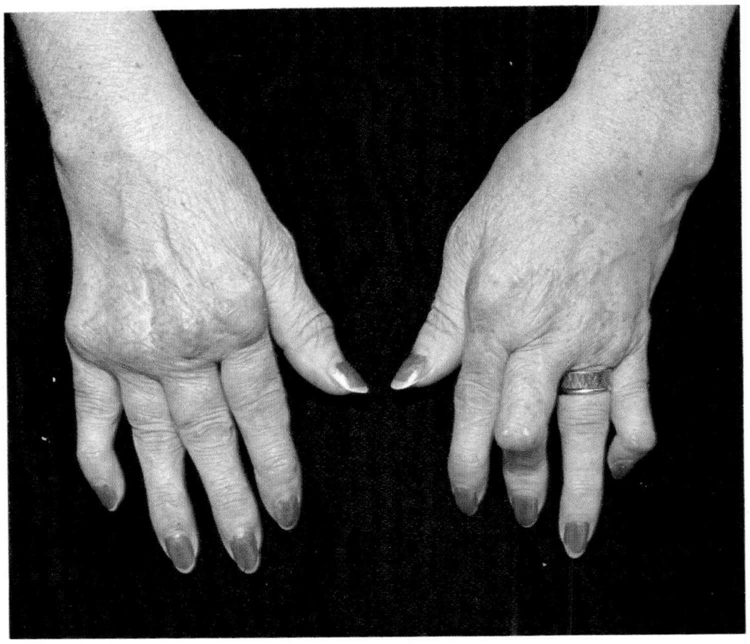

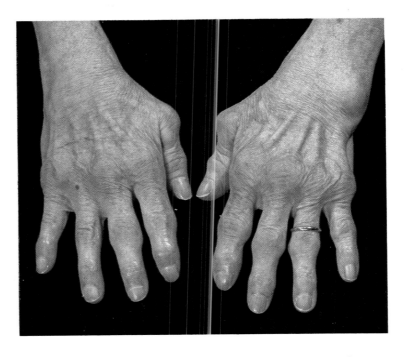

Fig. 4.27 RA involving the DIPs showing small muscle wasting, prominent ulnar styloid and swelling of the DIPs and PIPs.

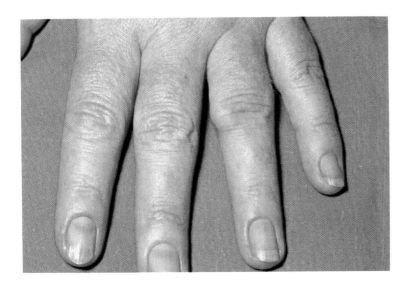

Fig. 4.26 Boutonniere deformity. The PIP of the patient's left middle finger has dislocated through the extensor tendon hood. Several other deformities are present, including radial deviation of the left wrist, early Swan Neck deformity, MCP subluxation and Mallet finger.

Fig. 4.28 A synovial cyst arising from the PIP of the ring finger. (Arthrography may be needed to confirm that the swelling communicates with the joint space.)

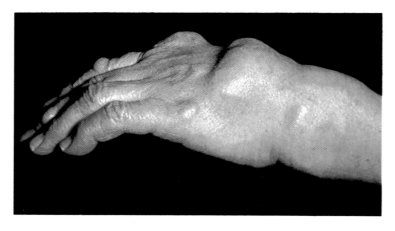

Fig. 4.29 Extensor tenosynovitis: a large extensor sheath swelling.

Progressive disease affecting tendon sheaths can lead to considerable functional loss with difficulty in moving the fingers, as well as tendon rupture (Fig. 4.29). Rupture of the extensor tendons is the most common feature and tends to occur initially in the fifth and fourth digits. A combination of tenosynovitis and the deformity of the ulnar head probably contribute to the tendon suddenly snapping. Surgical repair is often possible (Fig. 4.30).

Flexor tendons can also rupture although they do so less frequently (Fig. 4.31). Nodules may form on the tendons as well as in the subcutaneous tissue of the fingers (Fig. 4.32). These may add to the functional difficulties as well as to the unsightly appearance of the late rheumatoid hand.

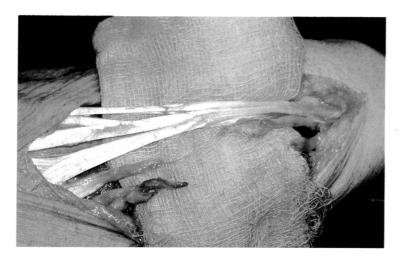

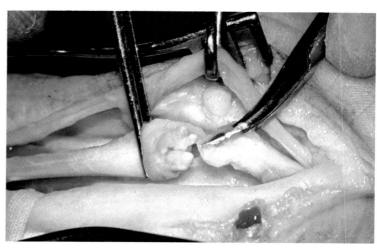

Fig. 4.30 Operative pictures of ruptured tendons showing attrition of two extensor tendons with subsequent degenerative changes (left) and repair of a ruptured flexor tendon (right). Courtesy of Mr. J. Browett.

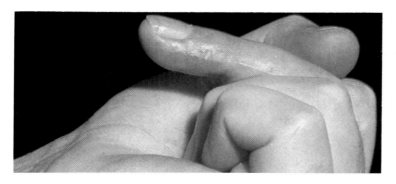

Fig. 4.31 Flexor tendon rupture. The patient cannot flex the middle finger.

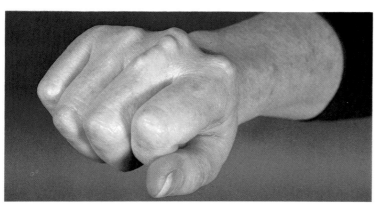

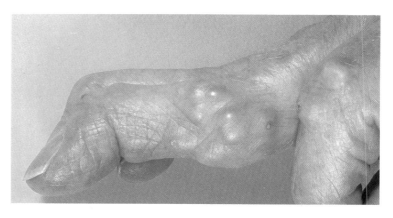

Fig. 4.32 Rheumatoid arthritis nodules on the extensor tendons of the index and middle fingers (left) and in the subcutaneous tissue of another patient (right). Note also the Swan Neck deformity and skin ulceration.

Disease of the thumb is common in rheumatoid arthritis; synovitis may affect the carpometacarpal joint (CMC) the MCP and the PIP. The characteristic deformity is the so called 'Z' thumb produced by a combination of flexion of the MCP due to inflammation, volar subluxation of the CMC and secondary hypertension of the interphalangeal joint (IPJ) (Fig. 4.33). Instability and hyperextension of the IPJ can lead to great difficulty with the pinch grip (Fig. 4.34).

Severe mutilating changes are sometimes found in late rheumatoid arthritis due to a combination of severe angulation deformity at the wrist and MCPs, accompanied by finger shortening, nodule formation, soft tissue changes, and skin abnormalities ('arthritis mutilans'). The finger shortening of late rheumatoid arthritis is usually generalized (Fig. 4.35), in contrast to the effect on individual fingers that occurs in the arthritis mutilans of psoriatic arthropathy.

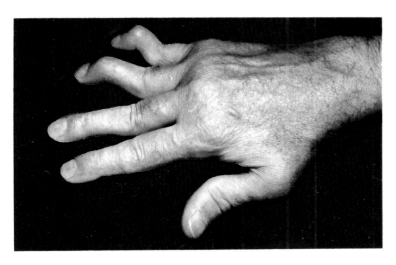

Fig. 4.33 RA of the hand showing Swan Neck deformities and swelling of the MCP joints, in addition to a typical 'Z' thumb deformity due to flexion at the MCP joint and hyperextension of the IPJ.

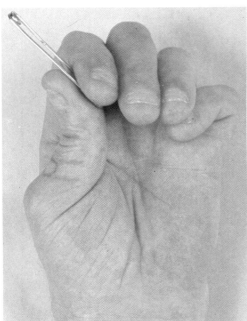

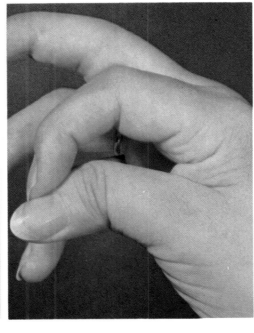

Fig. 4.34 Patients experiencing difficulty with the pinch grip due to hyperextension (left) and instability of the thumb IPJ (right).

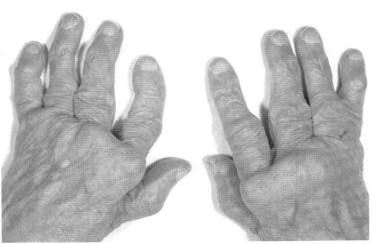

Fig. 4.35 Rheumatoid 'arthritis mutilans' showing subluxation of the MCPs and foreshortening of fingers due to bone erosion and resorption. All the fingers are involved.

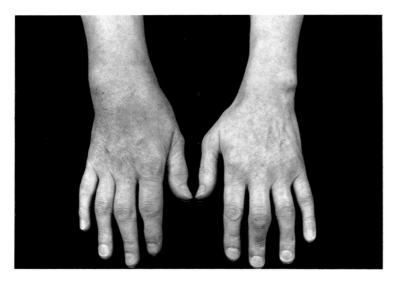

Fig. 4.36 Hand disease modified by activity. This patient had to use his right wrist at work and the disproportionate swelling of that joint is visible.

The deformity of rheumatoid hands depends on activity, often being worse in the dominant hand (Fig. 4.36). A characteristic radiological appearance can develop in men with high pain thresholds who go on working in spite of active disease (Fig. 4.37). The final outcome may also be modified by modern drug therapy, or by surgery (Fig. 4.38).

The radiological changes of established rheumatoid arthritis are characteristic (Fig. 4.39). The degree of periarticular osteoporosis, the 'fluffiness' and loss of distinction at the margins of the erosions are a guide to the activity of the erosion. The amount of joint space narrowing and degree of bone damage is a guide to severity. A sequence of radiographs taken over a period of years during the development of arthritis illustrates these points (Figs. 4.40 & 4.41).

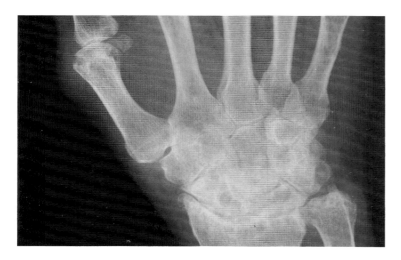

Fig. 4.37 Radiograph of 'typus robustus'. Large cysts (geodes) have formed in the bone in a patient who continued manual work in spite of active rheumatoid disease.

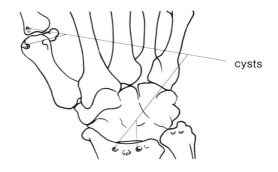

cysts

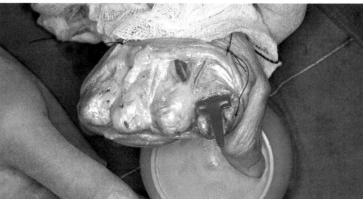

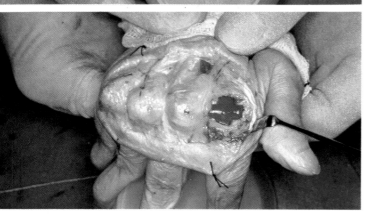

Fig. 4.38 MCP replacement. The silastic prosthesis is shown partially inserted (upper) and fully inserted (lower) across the MCP joint. The extensor tendon is retracted radially and will be pulled back and reattached over the implant. The other MCPs have subluxed and in particular it can be seen that the extensor tendon of the middle finger has slipped from its correct position and is lying between the MCPs of the third and fourth digits. Courtesy of Mr. D. Brooks.

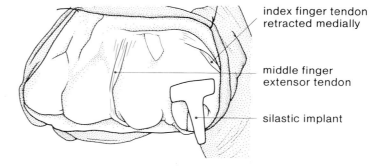

index finger tendon retracted medially

middle finger extensor tendon

silastic implant

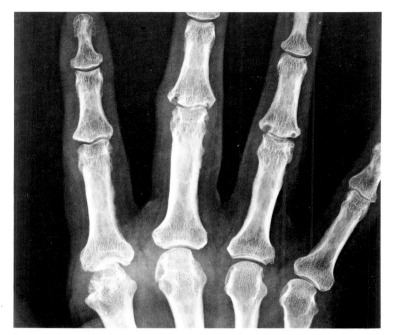

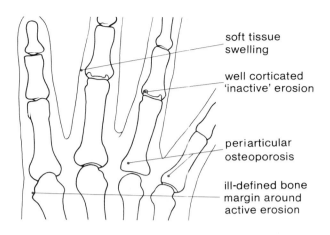

Fig. 4.39 Radiograph of the hand in advanced rheumatoid disease showing all the characteristic features.

soft tissue swelling

well corticated 'inactive' erosion

periarticular osteoporosis

ill-defined bone margin around active erosion

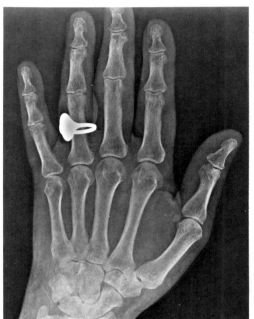

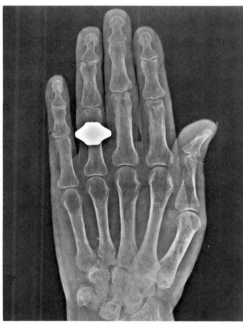

Fig. 4.40 Progressive radiological changes in rheumatoid disease: early disease showing soft tissue swelling and periarticular osteoporosis (left, 1971), followed by development of early erosions (right, 1973).

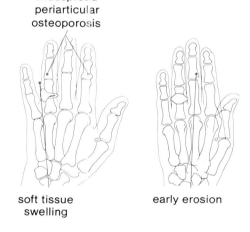

widespread periarticular osteoporosis

soft tissue swelling

early erosion

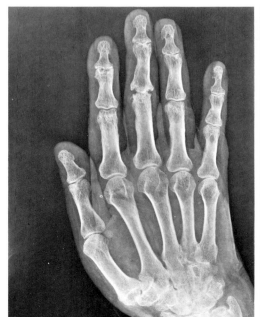

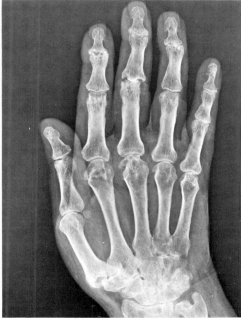

Fig. 4.41 Progressive disease showing extensive erosive damage and joint space narrowing (left, 1976; right, 1978).

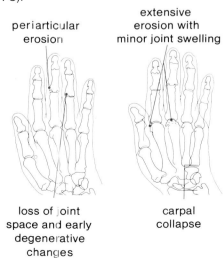

periarticular erosion

extensive erosion with minor joint swelling

loss of joint space and early degenerative changes

carpal collapse

Early Rheumatoid Changes in the Feet

The forefoot may be the first site of symptoms in rheumatoid disease. The metatarsophalangeal joints (MTPs) may also be the first areas to undergo radiological changes in this condition, even when the feet are asymptomatic.

Early symptoms include pain, stiffness and discomfort on getting up in the morning, with pain across the toes on walking and putting on shoes. This is due to synovitis of the MTPs and of the associated bursae between the bones. This explains the early signs, which include pain on lateral pressure across the joints and 'daylight' being

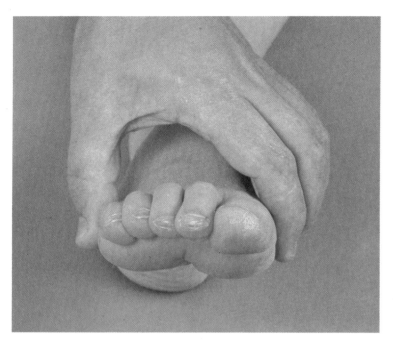
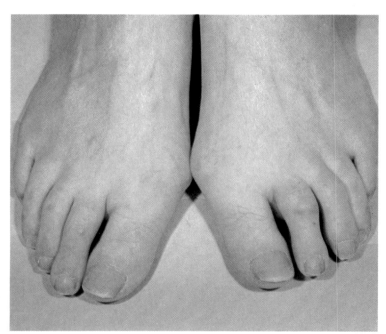

Fig. 4.42 Early RA at the MTPs. Lateral pressure may produce pain (left); the inflammatory swelling may spread the toes apart so that spaces appear between them (right) (the 'daylight sign').

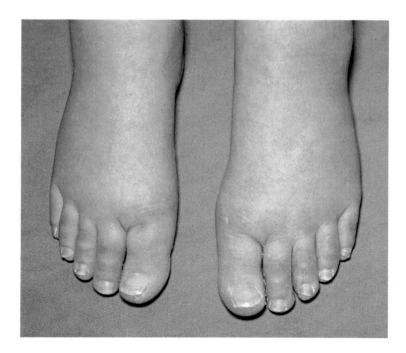
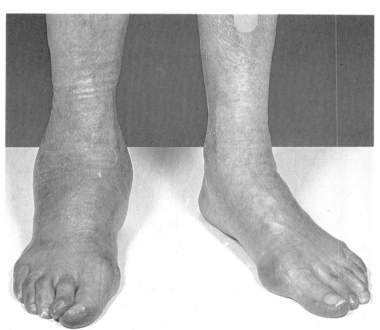

Fig. 4.43 Early RA of the feet showing the generalized edema which sometimes occurs (left) and synovitis at the ankle (right).

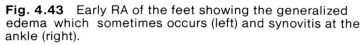

seen between the toes as they are spread out by the inflammatory swelling (Fig. 4.42).

Edema of the foot may be an early feature of rheumatoid arthritis (Fig. 4.43). Occasionally this is due to amyloidosis or other causes of hypoalbuminemia but these are rare and usually occur later on in rheumatoid disease. The reason for the early edematous phase is not clear, although an abnormality in capillary function or de-creased lymphatic drainage have been suggested. Ankle swelling due to synovitis rather than to peripheral edema can also occur (Fig. 4.43) and the disease may present as a tenosynovitis of the tibial or peroneal tendons rather than joint synovitis (Fig. 4.44). It may be possible to demonstrate the tenosynovitis by use of contrast medium (Fig. 4.45).

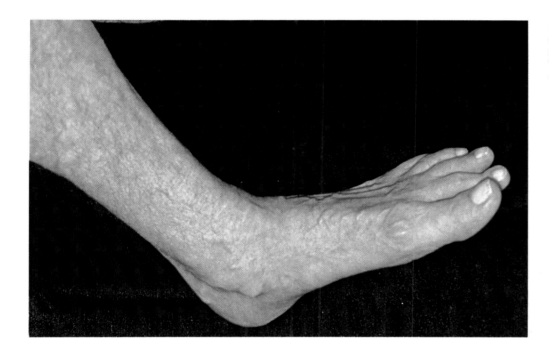

Fig. 4.44 Rheumatoid tenosynovitis at the ankle. The swelling is in the sheath of the tibialis posterior tendon. There are early rheumatoid changes in the MTP joint. Courtesy of Dr. J.D. Croft.

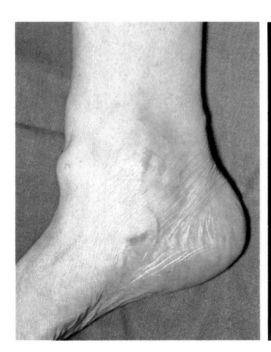 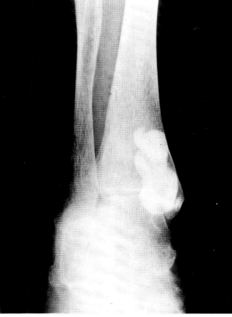 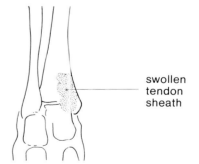

Fig. 4.45 Tenosynovitis of the tibialis anterior: the swelling seen on examination (left) and a radiograph following injection of contrast medium into the tendon sheath (right).

swollen tendon sheath

Established Rheumatoid Disease in the Feet

The hindfoot or forefoot is affected in most people with established rheumatoid disease, although it tends to predominate in one of these sites rather than damaging both in any one patient.

Forefoot disease is probably the most common, and the usual site of problems is the MTP. Following the early synovitis and inflammation, flattening and spreading of the forefoot occur followed by forward migration of the soft tissue cushion under the MTPs and dorsal subluxation of the joint itself (Fig. 4.46). This results in the head of the metatarsal becoming a weight-bearing area. This subluxation of the MTP is often palpable, and the tender areas under the forefoot are associated with callus formation (Fig. 4.47). A secondary flexion deformity of the PIPs of the toes often occurs and the 'cocked-up toe' can result in pressure over that joint from shoes (Fig. 4.48). Patients with subluxation often complain that they are walking on 'pebbles' or 'hot coals'. Examination of the shoes and the sole of the foot will give a guide to the way they are

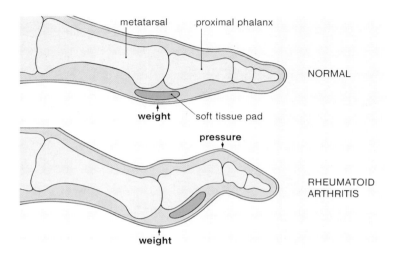

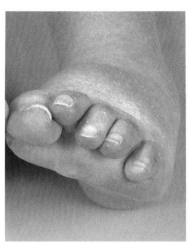 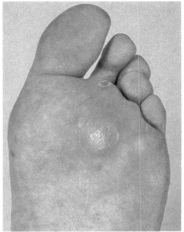

Fig. 4.46 Diagram of changes that occur at the MTP in rheumatoid disease. The weight-bearing soft tissue cushion of the foot migrates forwards and the proximal phalanx subluxes upwards. A new weight-bearing area develops over the metatarsal head and pressure from the shoes may occur over the PIP.

Fig. 4.47 MTP subluxation: the second toe often subluxes first (left) and callus forms over the weight-bearing metatarsal head (the 'center forward callosity') (right).

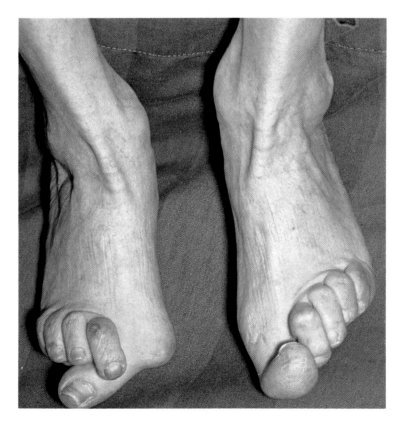

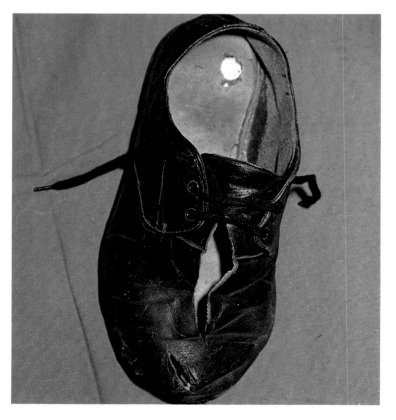

Fig. 4.48 'Cock-up' deformity: the MTPs have subluxed and there is a secondary flexion deformity at the PIP. Skin changes and ulceration due to pressure from shoes can be found.

Fig. 4.49 Examine the patient's shoes! A patient with RA has been supplied with a pair of surgical shoes, but has cut holes in the right shoe because further deformity has developed (see Fig. 4.50).

protecting the foot and to where pressure is being taken (Fig. 4.49). Hallux valgus deformities occur and this, plus the 'cock-up' toes may lead to overriding of the second or third toes on the first (Fig. 4.50).

The deformities of the toes produce new pressure areas, and 'corns', 'bunions' and ulcers are common in the rheumatoid foot. In severe disease large bursal swellings may develop underneath the forefoot and may ulcerate (Fig. 4.51). Pressure points may occur along the lateral border of the foot (Fig. 4.52).

The most important early radiological feature in the foot is periarticular osteoporosis of the MTPs (Fig. 4.53). As the condition progresses early erosions develop at the juxta-articular areas, and this may be apparent long before erosions develop elsewhere (Fig. 4.53). The feet as well as the hands should always be x-rayed when attempting to make the diagnosis and careful examination of the cortical margins of the bones may show the early lesion.

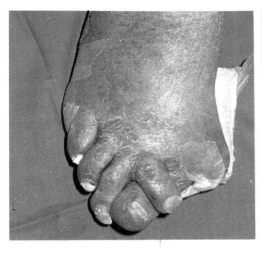
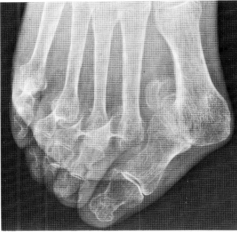

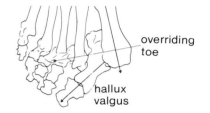

Fig. 4.50 Overriding toes. There is medial overriding of the second toe over the gross hallux vulgus (left; the same patient as in Fig. 4.49). The thin dry skin, typical of chronic rheumatoid disease, easily ulcerates. The radiograph of another patient shows lateral overriding of the second and third toes (right).

overriding toe

hallux valgus

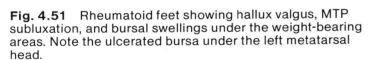
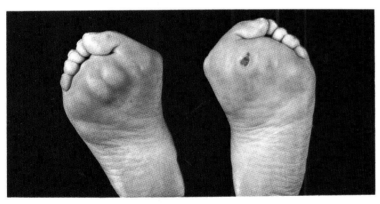
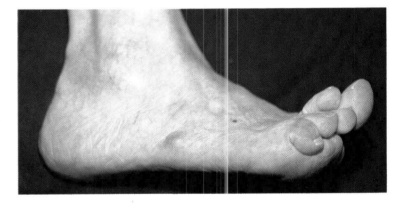

Fig. 4.51 Rheumatoid feet showing hallux valgus, MTP subluxation, and bursal swellings under the weight-bearing areas. Note the ulcerated bursa under the left metatarsal head.

Fig. 4.52 Rheumatoid arthritis of the foot. There is subluxation of the MTP joints with consequent 'cock-up' deformity and overriding of the toes. Note the pressure area on the lateral border of the foot caused by flattening of the transverse arch and widening of the forefoot. There is also a nodule on the achilles tendon.

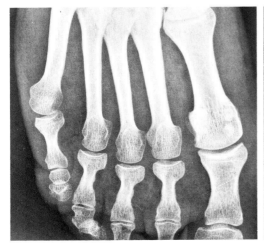
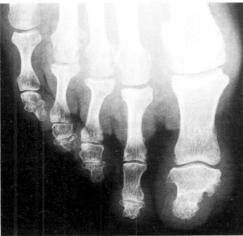

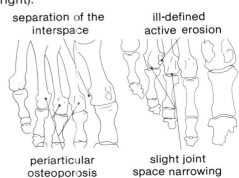

Fig. 4.53 Early RA of the MTPs: periarticular osteoporosis and widening of the foot (left) is followed by joint space narrowing and erosions (right).

separation of the interspace

ill-defined active erosion

periarticular osteoporosis

slight joint space narrowing

Disease at the hindfoot may affect the ankle, subtalar or midtarsal joints, or the tendons. The anterior tibial and peroneal tendon sheaths are often inflamed and occasionally rupture. The achilles tendon may be involved and is a not uncommon site for nodule formation which may produce pressure from the heel of the shoe (Fig. 4.54). Severe disease of the ankle itself is relatively uncommon; however the subtalar joint is often involved and disease and instability at this site leads to typical valgus deformity and loss of the arch of the foot (Figs. 4.55 – 4.57). This may lead in severe cases to the fibula abutting onto the calcaneus and to fractures of the lower end of the fibula. Midtarsal joint disease may lead to a rigid flat foot with very little flexibility, making walking on uneven surfaces extremely difficult.

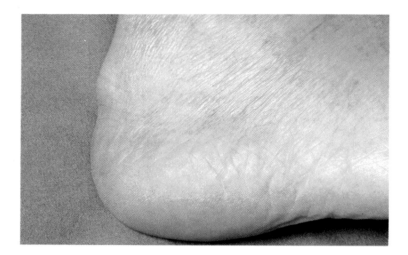

Fig. 4.54 Small rheumatoid nodule on the achilles tendon of a patient who has great difficulty wearing shoes.

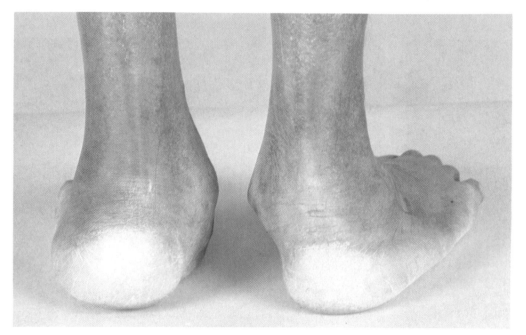

Fig. 4.55 Valgus deformity of the ankle due to subtalar disease.

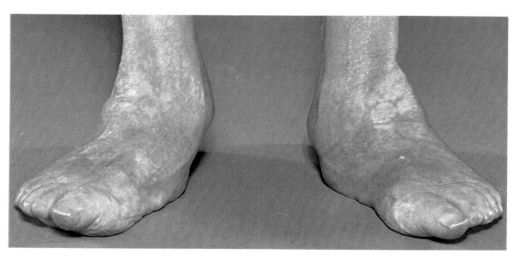

Fig. 4.56 These feet of a patient with severe RA show valgus deformities of the ankles. Midtarsal joint disease has caused collapse of transverse and longitudinal arches. The skin changes are the result of longstanding steroid therapy.

In severe advanced rheumatoid disease of the feet a combination of deformities of the hindfoot and toes with associated nodule formation and pressure from shoes produce extremely painful and unsightly deformities. Bursal swellings in the heel or forefoot may occur and fistulae occasionally develop particularly over the first MTP. Walking around on the thin bones of the rheumatoid foot may also produce march fractures.

The radiological changes in progressive rheumatoid arthritis of the forefoot are illustrated by a sequence of films taken over a period of years in one patient (Figs. 4.58 & 4.59). The abnormalities of the hindfoot are similar to those elsewhere and include loss of joint space, periarticular osteoporosis and erosions, often most apparent in the subtalar joint (Fig. 4.57).

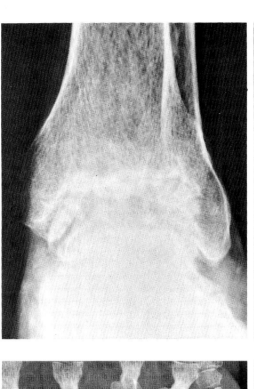
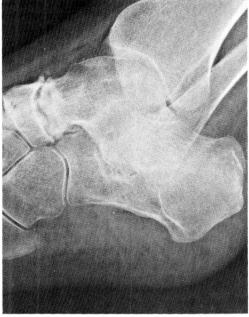

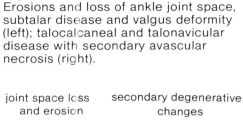

Fig. 4.57 Hindfoot disease. Erosions and loss of ankle joint space, subtalar disease and valgus deformity (left); talocalcaneal and talonavicular disease with secondary avascular necrosis (right).

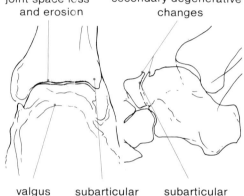

joint space loss and erosion — secondary degenerative changes

valgus hindfoot — subarticular sclerosis — subarticular collapse

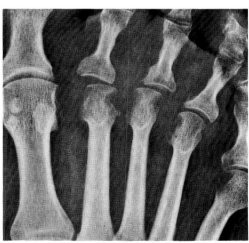

Fig. 4.58 Early rheumatoid disease of the foot showing progression from periarticular osteoporosis (left, 1972) to extensive erosive damage (right, 1973).

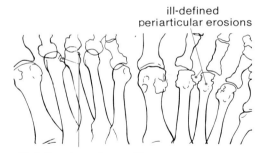

ill-defined periarticular erosions

ill-defined erosions with osteoporosis of bone

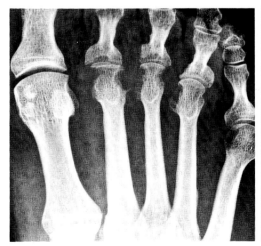
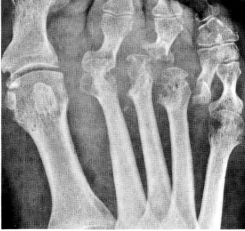

Fig. 4.59 Progressive changes in the same patient as in the previous figure showing development of extensive erosive damage and joint subluxation (left, 1975; right, 1979).

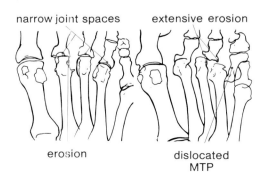

narrow joint spaces — extensive erosion

erosion — dislocated MTP

Conclusion

Some of the anatomical changes that occur in rheumatoid arthritis of the hands and feet have been illustrated. Other periarticular and soft tissue signs are shown elsewhere (see 'Rheumatoid Disease'). However, symptoms and function are more important than deformity. Function is often well maintained in the face of severe anatomical changes (Fig. 4.60), but can be severely impaired by damage at a single site. Examination of the hands and feet must include a functional appraisal as well as a description of the anatomical and inflammatory changes (see 'The Clinical Evaluation of Rheumatic Diseases').

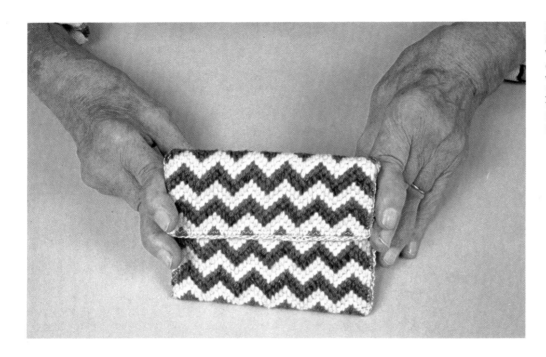

Fig. 4.60 Function may be independent of deformity. This patient who has longstanding, severe RA has developed typical hand deformities, which include subluxation of the MCP joints and Swan Neck deformity of the fingers. In spite of this she is able to do intricate work with her hands as shown here.

5

Rheumatoid Arthritis of Large Joints and Spine

With Dr. Rodney F. Waterworth

Rheumatoid arthritis is a variable and unpredictable disease which may involve any synovial joint. The common pattern is that of a peripheral onset, involving hands and feet, with a slow spread centrally to affect larger joints. However it may present as a monoarthritis of, for example, the knee. Much of the pain and disability of a patient with longstanding RA is attributable to large joint involvement with secondary mechanical damage. The spine, with the exception of the neck, is rarely involved.

In the early stages of large joint involvement, bursitis and disease of other periarticular structures may be more prominent causes of symptoms than involvement of the joints themselves. The pathology and clinical features of joint damage are similar to those seen in the hands and feet; initially there is pain, swelling and loss of range of movement and later there is destruction of cartilage and bone which result in deformity and considerable functional impairment.

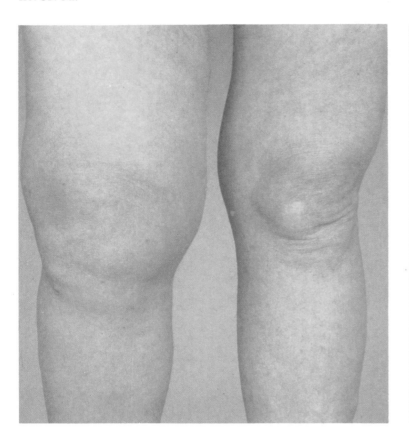

Fig. 5.1 Rheumatoid arthritis of the knee. There is swelling of the knees, much more marked on the right, due to a combination of synovial hypertrophy and fluid in the joints.

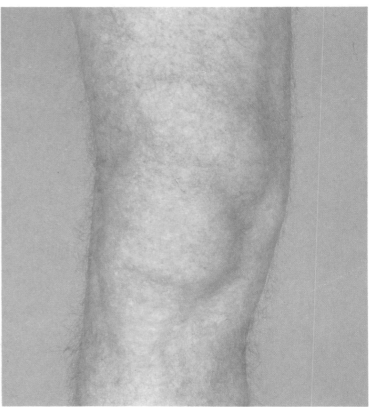

Fig. 5.2 Early rheumatoid arthritis of the knee showing extension of a small effusion into the suprapatellar pouch.

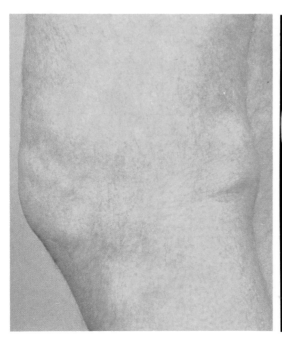
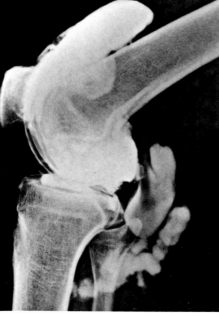

Fig. 5.3 Clinical view of a Baker's cyst (left) and an arthrogram demonstrating a ruptured cyst (right). The fluid has leaked into the soft tissue from a rupture in the wall of the cyst.

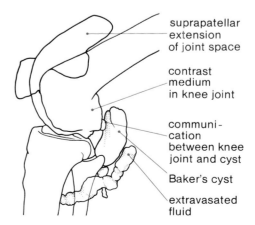

suprapatellar extension of joint space

contrast medium in knee joint

communication between knee joint and cyst

Baker's cyst

extravasated fluid

The Knee

The knee is commonly involved early in the evolution of RA and the disease may indeed present with synovitis of one or both knee joints (Fig. 5.1). Fluid may fill the suprapatellar pouch (Fig. 5.2). Intra-articular pressure in a tense swollen knee will rise considerably on flexion and thus secondary periarticular complications may appear early. These include posterior synovial protrusions (Baker's cysts) which may rupture (Fig. 5.3). Collateral and cruciate ligament laxity are common in late disease and result in joint instability (Fig. 5.4). Quadriceps wasting invariably accompanies knee disease and further predisposes to instability (Fig. 5.5). Muscle weakness may also lead to loss of full active knee extension (lag). The knee is usually less painful if rested in the flexed position, and resulting capsular fibrosis and muscle shortening result in fixed flexion deformity (Fig. 5.6).

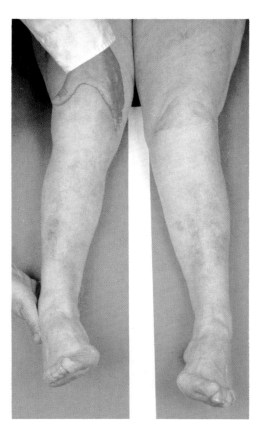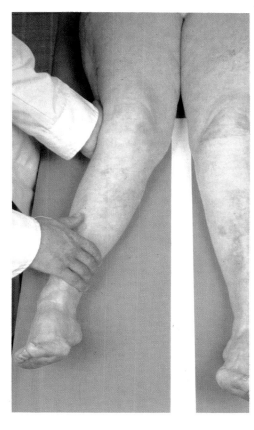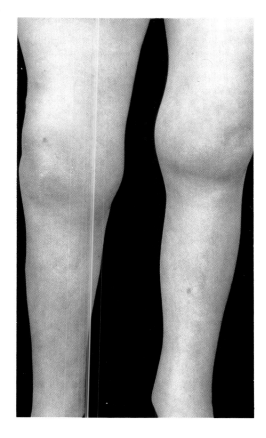

Fig. 5.4 Collateral ligament instability in established rheumatoid arthritis. Stressing the lateral collateral ligament (left) and stressing the medial collateral ligament (right). In this patient there is laxity of the medial ligament allowing the examiner to produce a valgus deformity.

Fig. 5.5 Quadriceps wasting.

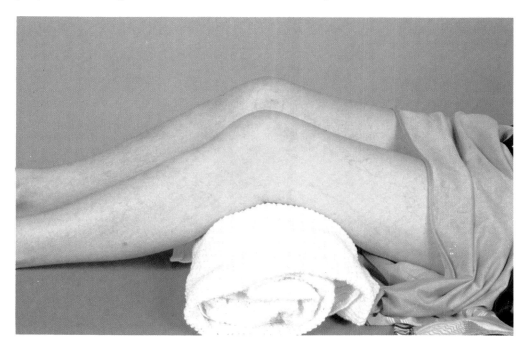

Fig. 5.6 Fixed flexion deformity of the knees. Patients with RA often find that they are more comfortable if the knees are left flexed and sleep with the knees supported on a pillow or rolled-up blankets (as here). This encourages the development of a fixed flexion deformity (here about 40°).

The radiograph or xeroradiograph in early disease shows the distension of the suprapatellar pouch, quadriceps wasting, posterior capsular distension and displacement of the fabella if present (Fig. 5.7). With established disease, weight-bearing films will show progressive loss of joint space due to cartilage loss and the development of marginal erosions. Eventually there is collapse of the tibial condyles with the development of varus

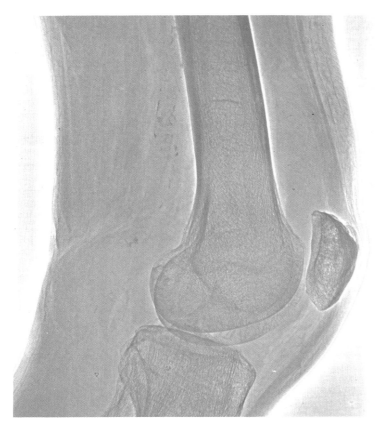

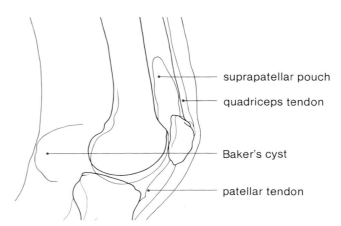

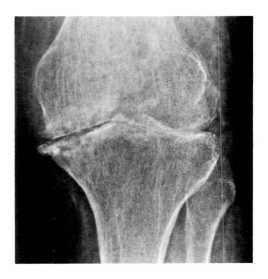

Fig. 5.7 Lateral xeroradiograph of the knee in a patient with early rheumatoid arthritis. There is a large Baker's cyst and fluid is seen distending the suprapatellar pouch. Courtesy of Dr. M. Gumpel.

suprapatellar pouch

quadriceps tendon

Baker's cyst

patellar tendon

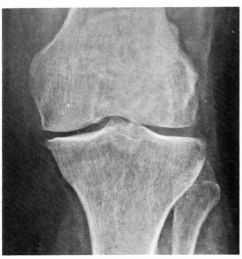

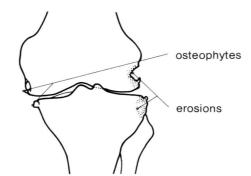

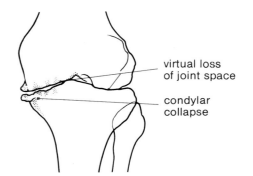

Fig. 5.8 Series of knee radiographs in RA: early disease with minimal joint space narrowing (left), further joint space narrowing, some marginal osteophytes and erosions, particularly laterally (middle), and the virtual loss of joint space and collapse of the tibial condyles with some erosive changes in the medial plateau (right).

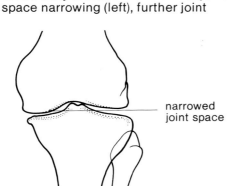

narrowed joint space

osteophytes

erosions

virtual loss of joint space

condylar collapse

or valgus deformities (Figs. 5.8 & 5.9). The occasional coexistence of varus deformity in one knee and valgus deformity in the other produces the 'windswept' knee appearance (Fig. 5.10). Angulation deformities may be exaggerated by hindfoot disease causing chronic strain on the collateral ligaments of the knee (Figs. 5.11 & 5.12).

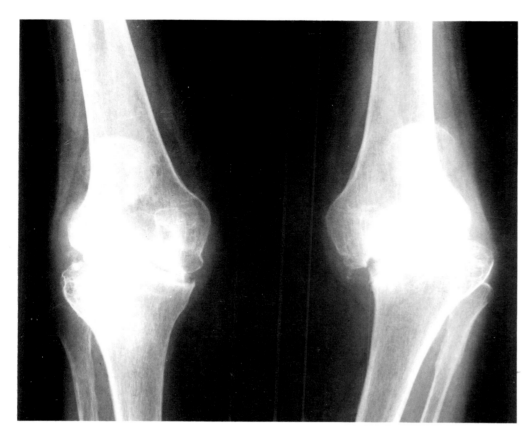

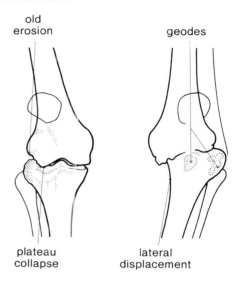

Fig. 5.9 Knee radiograph in late rheumatoid disease. There is loss of joint space, extensive erosive change, collapse particularly of the medial plateau of the left tibia resulting in varus deformity and some lateral subluxation.

old erosion   geodes

plateau collapse   lateral displacement

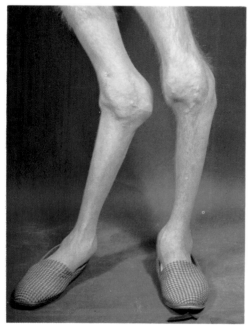

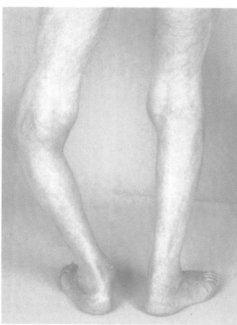

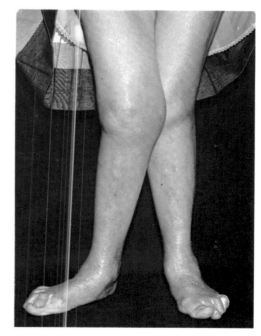

Fig. 5.10 'Windswept' knees. There is coexistent valgus deformity of the right knee and varus deformity of the left. Courtesy of Dr. M. Corbett.

Fig. 5.11 A valgus deformity of the left ankle in RA associated with severe varus deformity of the knee.

Fig. 5.12 Coincident ankle and knee deformity. There is a varus deformity of the right knee and hindfoot. Note also the overriding second toe and flattened forefoot due to rheumatoid disease.

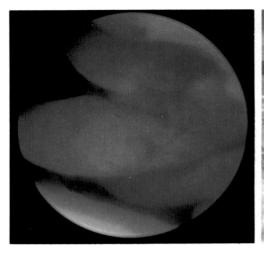 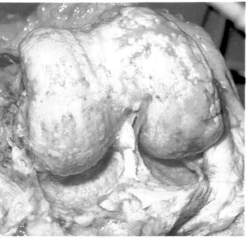

Fig. 5.13 The knee in RA: arthroscopy (left) and prior to knee replacement (right). Courtesy of Mr. A.W. Lettin.

highly vascularized proliferating synovium

articular surface of femur

cartilage   vascular synovium   cartilage loss   underlying bone erosion

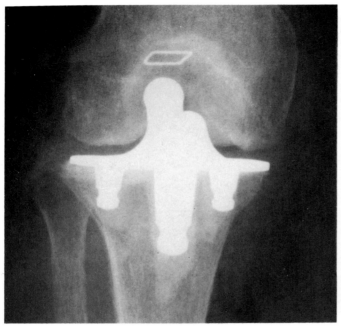 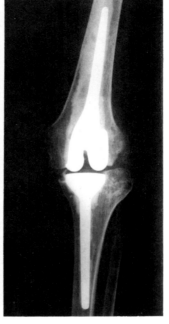

Fig. 5.14 Prosthetic surgery of the knee. A surface replacement of the Dean type suitable for patients without severe deformity and instability (left) and a long-stem Sheehan prosthesis (right). This prosthesis is unconstrained but either this or a hinge prosthesis are more suitable when there is severe joint deformity.

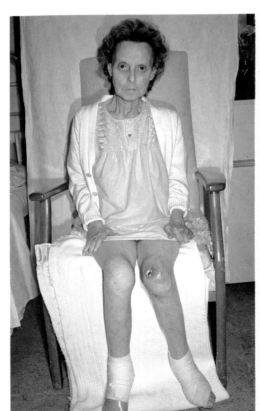 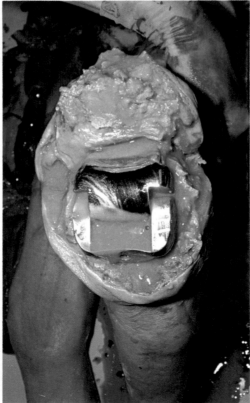

Fig. 5.15 Patient with severe rheumatoid arthritis and ulceration of the skin over the ankles which has become infected (left). Infection has spread to the knee and the metal prosthesis can be seen at the base of a deep infected ulcer. The post mortem picture from another patient who died with septicemia as a result of infection of the prosthetic joint is shown (right). Pus is invading the prosthesis.

Knee synovitis and the degree of cartilage damage may be assessed by arthroscopy or at surgery (Fig. 5.13).

Synovectomy may be useful in early disease in the absence of severe cartilage loss. Osteotomy may be appropriate in cases of predominantly unilateral compartment disease with cartilage destruction. Prosthetic surgery is required in the advanced case with extensive cartilage loss and bone damage, especially if there is significant instability or loss of extension (Fig. 5.14). Unfortunately, joint infection, which is a recognized complication of rheumatoid disease, has a predilection for the knee and if infection occurs after joint replacement it may be disastrous (Fig. 5.15).

The Hindfoot and Ankle

Forefoot involvement is very common in early RA. The hindfoot and ankle form a single functional unit which is infrequently involved in early disease. Ankle involvement may cause obvious joint swelling (Fig. 5.16). Associated periarticular disease involving the overlying tendon sheaths may contribute to the swelling. In later disease, anatomical communication between the ankle and subtalar joint and tendon sheaths often occurs. Widespread involvement of this nature causes the common valgus deformity of the hindfoot (Fig. 5.17). When associated with midtarsal joint disease severe deformity and functional impairment result (Fig. 5.18).

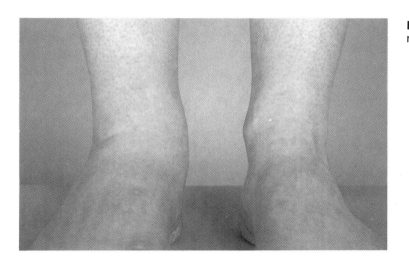

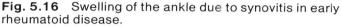
Fig. 5.16 Swelling of the ankle due to synovitis in early rheumatoid disease.

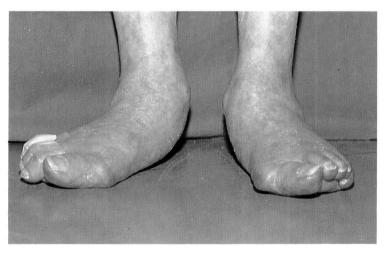

Fig. 5.17 Valgus deformity of the ankle. This patient shows such a deformity especially at the right ankle. Note also the loss of the longitudinal arch of the foot.

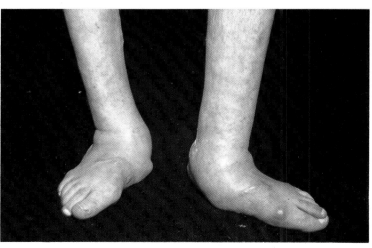

Fig. 5.18 'Hovercraft' feet in rheumatoid arthritis. There is valgus deformity of both ankles with associated midtarsal disease and collapse of the arches of the feet.

Radiographs reveal typical RA changes, and subtalar joint damage is seen to accompany ankle disease in most cases (Fig. 5.19). Valgus deformity, especially if coexistent with a valgus deformity of the knee, may provoke stress fractures in the fibula (Fig. 5.20). A valgus ankle especially if associated with loss of full dorsiflexion of the foot, may significantly impair walking.

The Hip

Pain in the hip region in early RA is often the result of bursitis, which is characterized by local tenderness (Fig. 5.21). Trochanteric bursitis is the most common; the pain over the outer aspect of the thigh in this condition is frequently and erroneously attributed by the patient to hip joint disease. Synovitis of the hip joint itself occurs

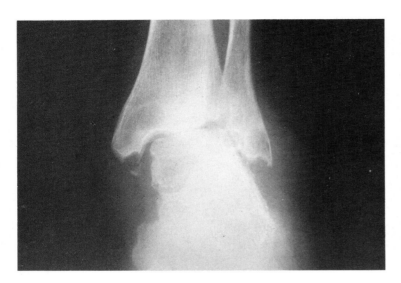

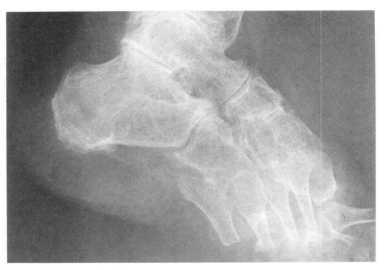

Fig. 5.19 Radiographs of the ankle in rheumatoid arthritis. There is joint space narrowing, marginal erosions, and a valgus deformity with lateral subluxation (left). The oblique lateral radiograph in another patient shows severe ankle disease with concomitant subtalar and intertarsal disease

(right). There is hyaline cartilage attrition and cortical irregularities with secondary degenerative changes including osteophytosis and subarticular sclerosis. Note also that the patient has had a forefoot arthroplasty.

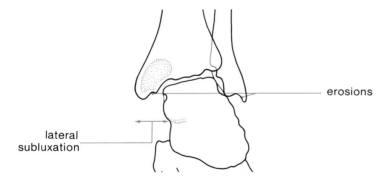

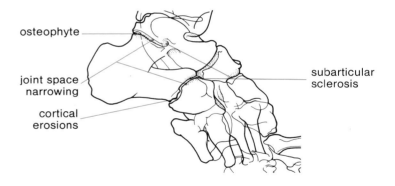

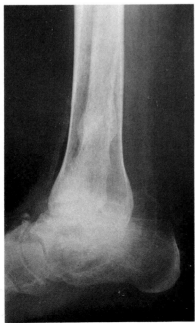

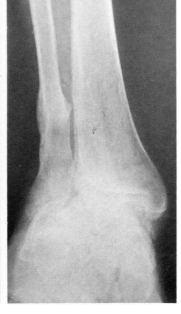

Fig. 5.20 Lateral (left) and anteroposterior (right) radiographs of the ankle in RA. There are erosions and bone necrosis in the ankle joint with an associated valgus deformity of the ankle. This has stressed the fibula and a healing angulated fracture is seen. Pes planus (flat foot) deformity is seen on the lateral view. Arterial calcification due to prolonged steroid therapy is also present.

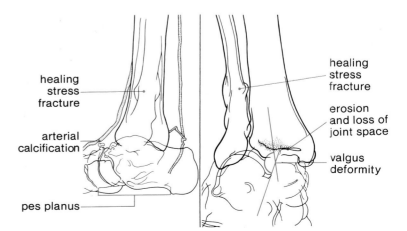

late in RA and causes anterior pain and groin pain which may radiate to the anterior thigh and knee. The earliest clinical sign of true hip involvement is loss of internal rotation (Fig. 5.22). Once hip disease is established it is usually progressive and the patient develops shortening of the limb and an antalgic gait.

The earliest radiological changes are loss of joint space – mainly central – and periarticular osteoporosis; these are followed by erosions and cystic changes, principally in the femoral head (Fig. 5.23). Collapse of the femoral head may be due to avascular necrosis which is common in RA, especially in patients on long-term steroid therapy.

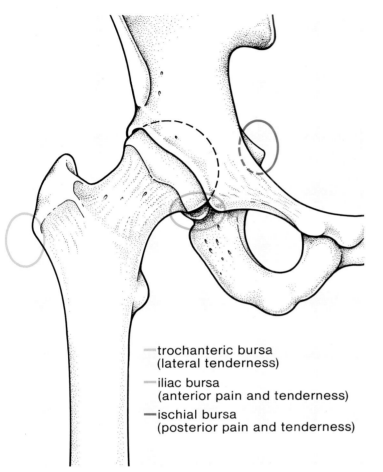

trochanteric bursa
(lateral tenderness)

iliac bursa
(anterior pain and tenderness)

ischial bursa
(posterior pain and tenderness)

Fig. 5.21 Diagram showing bursal involvement around the hip in RA.

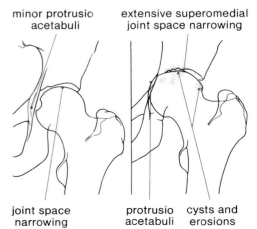

Fig. 5.22 Testing of internal rotation. With the knee flexed the examiner is abducting the ankle from the midline to test the range of internal rotation of the hip which is limited in this patient with rheumatoid arthritis.

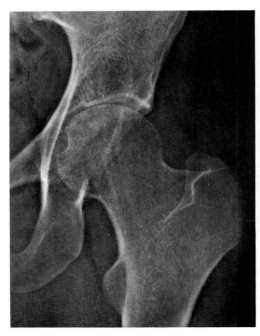

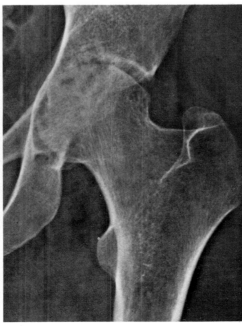

Fig. 5.23 Radiographs of the hip joint: early disease showing some central loss of joint space and early protrusio acetabuli (left). At a later stage loss of joint space is much more marked and extensive (right).

minor protrusio acetabuli

extensive superomedial joint space narrowing

joint space narrowing

protrusio acetabuli

cysts and erosions

Acetabular destruction and remodelling may result in protrusio acetabuli, which in adults is a hallmark of rheumatoid arthritis (Figs. 5.23 & 5.24). Prosthetic surgery is usually successful in restoring function and producing a pain-free joint (Fig. 5.25).

No assessment of the lower limb is complete without observing the patient's gait (Fig. 5.26). This may indicate which joint or joints are causing the greatest disturbance to function. This assessment is particularly important in the patient with severe RA in whom extensive joint surgery is contemplated, so that the most appropriate order of events can be organized.

The Shoulder

The shoulder joint and periarticular tissues are commonly involved in both early and late stages of the disease. Subacromial bursitis is common and presents with pain over the shoulder tip. The pain may radiate down the arm because of the subdeltoid extension of the bursa. Swelling of the shoulder may be apparent and movement, especially active abduction, is restricted.

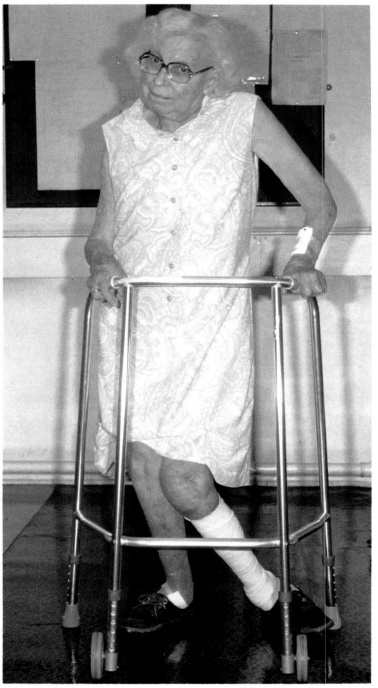

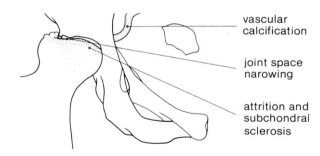

Fig. 5.24 Radiograph of the hip in advanced RA showing attrition of cartilage and bone, gross joint space narrowing and subchondral sclerosis similar to the changes seen in avascular necrosis.

vascular calcification

joint space narowing

attrition and subchondral sclerosis

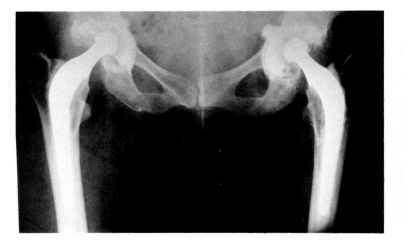

Fig. 5.25 Total hip replacement of the Charnley type.

Fig. 5.26 A patient with longstanding severe rheumatoid arthritis with multiple joint involvement. There are valgus deformities of both ankles, angulation and fixed flexion in both knees and severe wrist and elbow involvement. The combination of these deformities make it difficult for her to walk even with a wheeled Zimmer frame.

The rotator cuff tendons are frequently involved. The patient presents with a painful arc of active abduction from 50°-100° but retains full passive abduction (Fig. 5.27). These findings may be the result of inflammation or of subsequent partial or complete rupture of the supraspinatus tendon.

Plain radiographs are often normal but may show cysts or erosions in the greater tuberosity at the site of tendon attachment, and there may be upward subluxation of the humeral head. Confirmation of rotator cuff damage is obtained by arthrography; free communication may be demonstrated between subacromial bursa and the gleno-humeral joint and defects in the tendons may be outlined. Erosion of the outer end of the clavicle reflects longstanding subacromial bursitis (Fig. 5.28). Such patients usually have a long history of shoulder pain with weak active abduction.

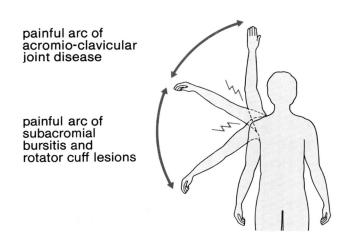

painful arc of
acromio-clavicular
joint disease

painful arc of
subacromial
bursitis and
rotator cuff lesions

Fig. 5.27 Diagram to demonstrate the typical painful arcs associated with subacromial bursitis, rotator cuff lesions and acromio-clavicular joint disease.

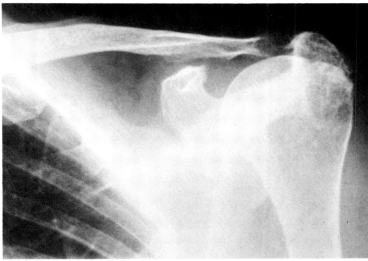

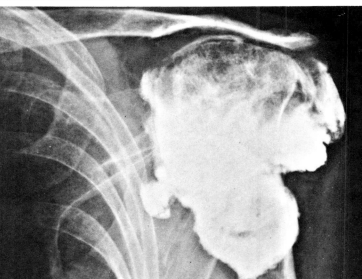

Fig. 5.28 Radiograph of the shoulder in RA showing cephalic migration of the humeral head and excavation of the acromion (upper). There is a large subarticular cyst in the humeral head, and a widened acromio-clavicular joint with erosion of the clavicle. The arthrogram in another patient shows similar bony changes with gross thinning of the acromion and clavicle secondary to pressure necrosis (lower). There is flattening of the humeral head with hyaline cartilage attrition. Contrast medium is seen in the enlarged, abnormal joint space and has extended into the subdeltoid bursa.

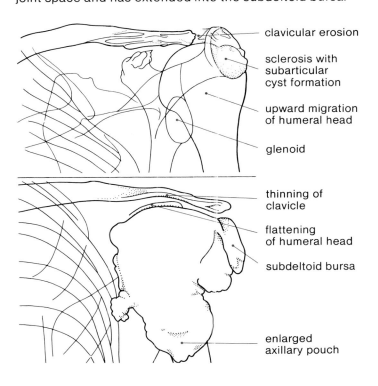

clavicular erosion

sclerosis with
subarticular
cyst formation

upward migration
of humeral head

glenoid

thinning of
clavicle

flattening
of humeral head

subdeltoid bursa

enlarged
axillary pouch

Bicipital tendinitis produces anterior shoulder pain radiating down the arm with painful restriction of shoulder abduction and internal rotation. There is tenderness over the bicipital groove, palpable with the arm externally rotated (Fig. 5.29). Stressing of the biceps by opposition of shoulder flexion is usually painful. Prolonged inflammation can end in tendon rupture (Fig. 5.30). This is uncommon but may be precipitated by local injection of steroid (Fig. 5.30).

Acromio-clavicular joint involvement may present as a painful arc of abduction which is higher than that of a rotator cuff lesion (Fig. 5.27). There is often local tenderness and swelling. Pain can be induced by forcibly raising the humerus against the fixed clavicle. A patient will often complain of night pain when lying on the affected shoulder, when similar stresses are placed on the joint. Radiographs show erosion within the joint (Fig. 5.31).

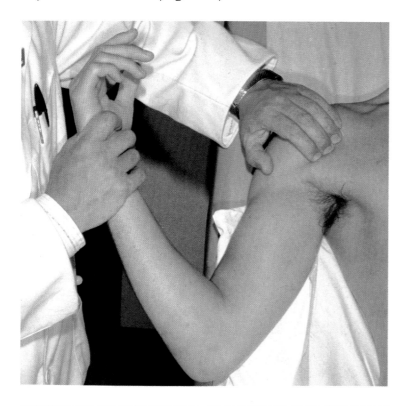

Fig. 5.29 Palpating for bicipital groove tenderness. The arm is externally rotated by the examiner to expose the biceps tendon from under the anterior part of the deltoid muscle.

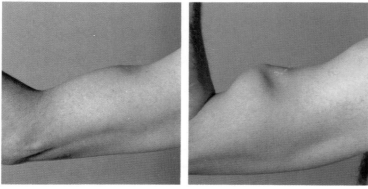

Fig. 5.30 Rupture of the long head of biceps in rheumatoid arthritis. The muscle bulk of the biceps may appear to be slightly increased (left) but on attempted flexion of the forearm the rupture becomes clearly apparent (right).

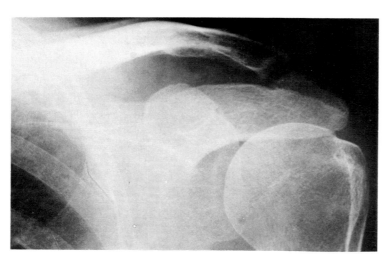

Fig. 5.31 Radiograph showing acromio-clavicular joint involvement in RA. There is widening of the joint space, surface erosion and osteoporosis of the distal end of the clavicle.

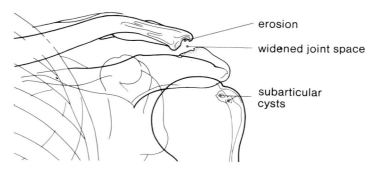

erosion

widened joint space

subarticular cysts

Patients with severe longstanding RA may develop gleno-humeral disease. The pain around the shoulder often extends into the upper arm in the distribution of the C5 nerve region which innervates the joint. There is muscle wasting and anterior effusion may be visible (Fig. 5.32). Active and passive movements in all planes are restricted. Radiographs reveal joint space narrowing due to progressive cartilage loss, and erosions may be very large and occur singly (Fig. 5.33). Bone necrosis of the humeral head is rare but is sometimes attributable to prolonged systemic steroid therapy.

Rheumatoid involvement of the sterno-clavicular joint is more common than is generally appreciated. There is local swelling and tenderness, and pain during elevation of the arm may be severe. Joint changes of narrowing, erosion and menisceal destruction are best shown by tomography (Fig. 5.34).

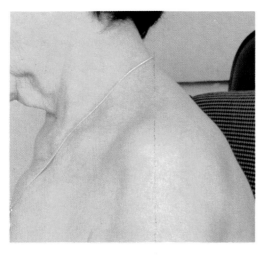
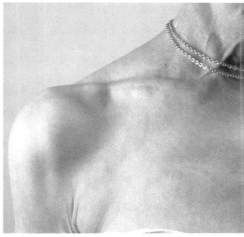

Fig. 5.32 Rheumatoid arthritis of the shoulder. This patient with gleno-humeral joint disease has visible wasting of the deltoid muscle (left). A patient with an anterior effusion is also shown (right).

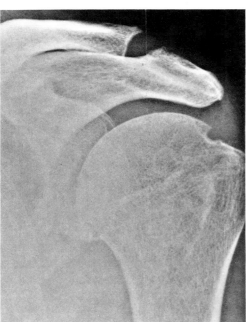
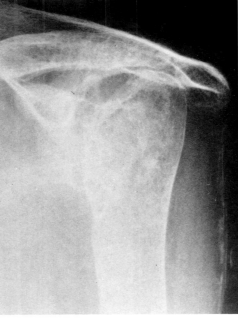

Fig. 5.33 Radiographs of the shoulder in RA showing typical marginal erosions and some loss of joint space (left). Attrition of the whole humeral head is seen in advanced end-stage rheumatoid disease (right).

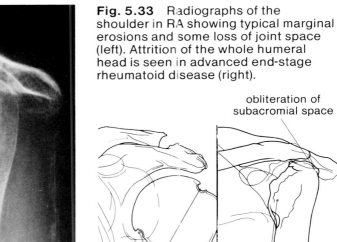

obliteration of subacromial space

periarticular erosions

irregular flattened glenoid surface

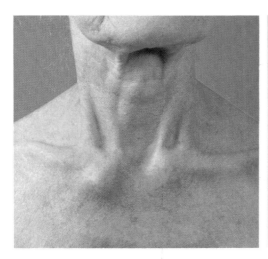
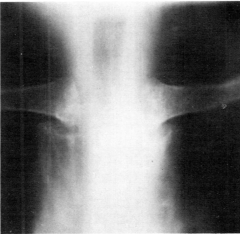

Fig. 5.34 Sterno-clavicular involvement: swelling and subluxation particularly of the right sterno-clavicular joint (left) and a tomogram (right) showing surface erosions, irregularity and sclerosis of bone, and slight excavation of the manubrium. Courtesy of Dr. E. Paice.

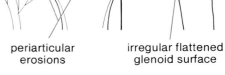
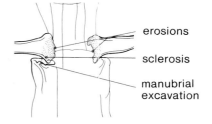

erosions

sclerosis

manubrial excavation

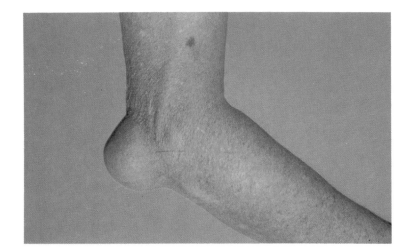

Fig. 5.35 Olecranon bursitis in early rheumatoid arthritis.

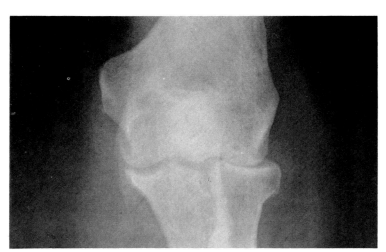

Fig. 5.36 Radiograph of the elbow in early RA. The AP view reveals joint space narrowing with some irregularity at the radio-ulnar joint.

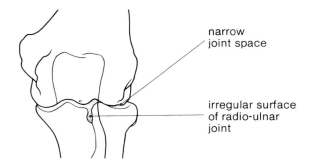

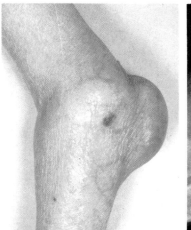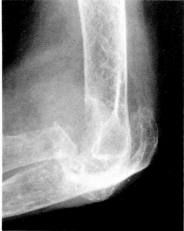

Fig. 5.37 Advanced rheumatoid disease of the elbow showing fixed flexion deformity and synovial swelling (left). The small ecchymosis is probably related to longstanding steroid therapy. The radiograph.of an elbow in advanced rheumatoid disease shows generalized osteoporosis, joint destruction and disorganization, and synovial thickening (right).

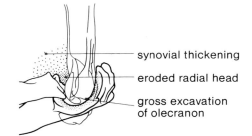

Fig. 5.38 A patient with longstanding rheumatoid arthritis with severe shoulder, elbow and wrist involvement. She is barely able to comb her hair even using a long-handled comb as provided by the occupational therapist.

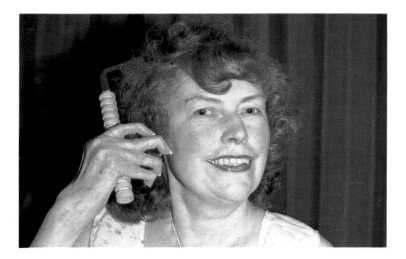

The Elbow

Periarticular involvement of the elbow is common in early RA, usually in the form of an olecranon bursitis (Fig. 5.35). Synovitis of the elbow is also frequently found and causes soft tissue swelling and limitation of movement. Loss of flexion and extension results from humero-ulnar joint involvement while loss of supination is common and results from damage to the head of the radius. The patient will complain of pain but is often unaware of a fixed flexion deformity. Further loss of pronation and supination may depend on the extent of wrist disease.

Initially radiographs show tissue plane distortion with fat pad displacement due to capsular distension (Fig. 5.36). As disease progresses there is often considerable bone destruction and deformity (Fig. 5.37). Disorganization of the elbow joint may result in an entrapment neuropathy of the ulnar nerve.

The extent of functional impairment in the upper limb depends on the involvement of wrist, elbow and shoulder. Loss of elbow extension alone has little consequence for function, but loss of flexion, especially if there is shoulder restriction, may result in the patient being unable to feed herself or comb her hair (Fig. 5.38). If internal rotation at the shoulder is impaired and supination of the forearm is lost due to elbow and wrist disease the patient may be unable to get hand to buttock and toilet hygiene becomes impossible. A simple functional assessment may therefore identify which diseased joint contributes most to disability.

The Cervical Spine

Involvement of the cervical spine is common in RA, affecting 40% of patients at some stage. In the majority of these it develops within the first two years. Synovitis occurs in the spinal joints and may damage the adjacent discovertebral junction. Apophyseal joint involvement affects vertebral alignment and predisposes to further disc damage (Fig. 5.39). The typical radiology of established disease shows narrowing of the C4/5 disc space, and often the adjacent spaces, without reactive bone formation (Figs. 5.40 & 5.41). Erosion of vertebral end plates and apophyseal joints is seen at a later stage together with sclerosis and subluxation.

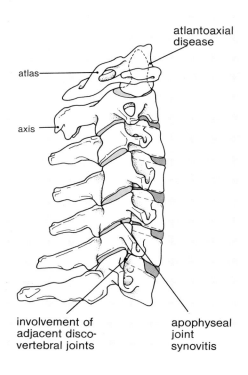

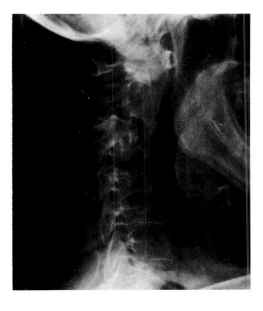

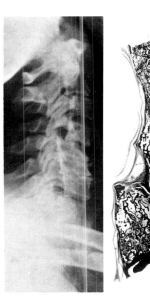

Fig. 5.39 Diagram showing sites of rheumatoid involvement in the cervical spine.

Fig. 5.40 Cervical spine involvement in rheumatoid arthritis. The two main areas of involvement are at C3/4 where there is obliteration of the disc space with some loss of bone due to a previous discitis, and the atlantoaxial region where there is gross subluxation. Note also the subluxation due to ligamentous laxity at C2/3.

Fig. 5.41 Radiograph of the cervical spine in RA showing subluxation and obliteration of the disc spaces secondary to rheumatoid disc damage (left). The sagittal section through the cervical spine shows gross disc space narrowing, some posterior fusion, and subluxation at one level (right, courtesy of Professor J. Ball).

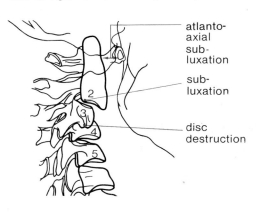

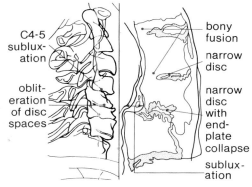

5.15

Subluxation may be subaxial, and if multiple results in a 'stepladder' appearance (Fig. 5.42). Synovitis at the atlantoaxial level causes stretching or destruction of the cruciate ligament which normally holds the odontoid peg closely to the anterior arch of the atlas. This allows atlantoaxial subluxation (Fig. 5.43). This is demonstrable radiologically on a lateral radiograph of the cervical spine in flexion, when the separation of opposed surfaces of odontoid peg and anterior arch of the atlas should be no more than 3mm (Figs. 5.44 & 5.45). Subluxation may only occur in flexion and may therefore be missed on a standard lateral radiograph. Occasionally there is fracture or destruction of the odontoid peg (Fig. 5.46). Posterior subluxation may then occur. If there is destruction of the lateral atlantoaxial bony masses or fracture of the atlas then vertical subluxation and platybasia can result (Fig. 5.47). Lateral subluxation is rare (Fig. 5.48).

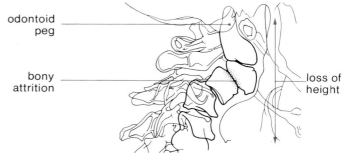

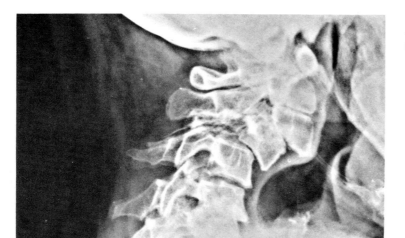

Fig. 5.42 Radiograph of the cervical spine showing cephalic migration of the (virtually intact) odontoid peg, bony attrition and a 'stepladder' deformity.

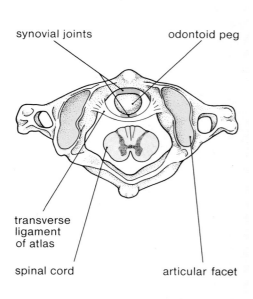

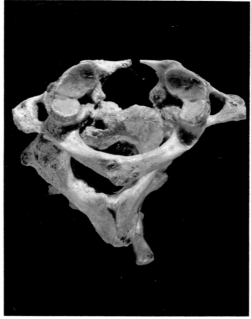

Fig. 5.43 Diagram of the anatomy of the atlantoaxial region (left), and a post-mortem specimen showing atlantoaxial subluxation (right). Note the erosion of the odontoid peg, destruction of the anterior arch of the atlas, and posterior dislocation of the axis. This resulted in gross narrowing of the spinal canal, compression of the spinal cord, and quadriplegia in this case. Courtesy of Dr. J. Bradfield.

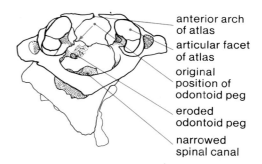

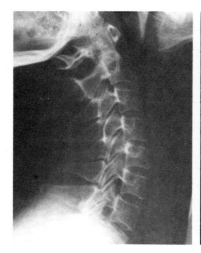

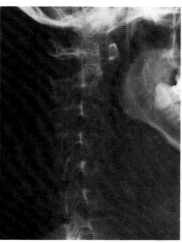

Fig. 5.44 Radiographs of the cervical spine in rheumatoid disease. The extension film shows close apposition of the odontoid to the anterior arch of the atlas (a gap of 1.5 mm) (left). The flexion film demonstrates 6mm of atlantoaxial subluxation.

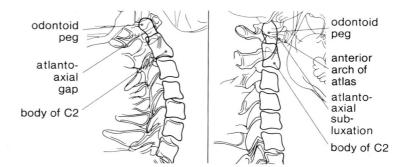

5.16

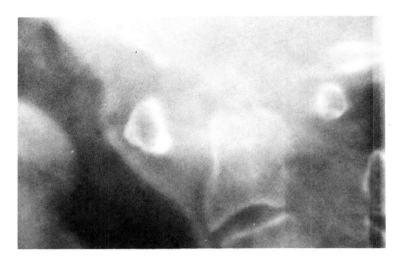

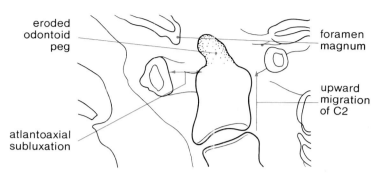

Fig. 5.45 Lateral tomogram of the atlantoaxial region clearly demonstrating atlantoaxial subluxation with erosion of the odontoid peg and upward subluxation of C2 through C1.

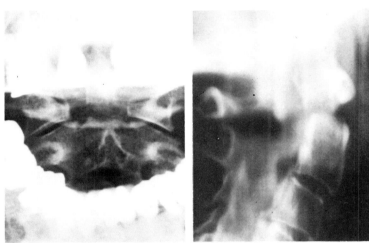

Fig. 5.46 Open mouth radiograph (left) and lateral tomogram (right) of a patient in rheumatoid arthritis. There is slight lateral displacement of the odontoid peg, and the odontoid has fractured.

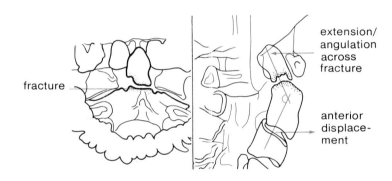

Fig. 5.47 Radiograph of the cervical spine in flexion showing atlantoaxial subluxation (left). There is disc space narrowing at C2/3. This patient's radiograph seven years later reveals severe progression with upward subluxation of C1 and C2, partial collapse of C3 and C4 and multiple subaxial subluxation (right). The patient refused admission for surgery and became paraplegic one week later.

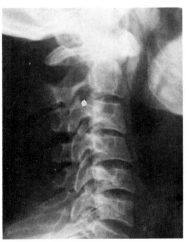

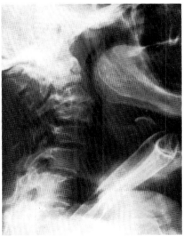

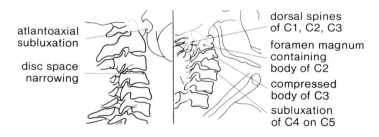

Fig. 5.48 Lateral subluxation in the cervical spine.

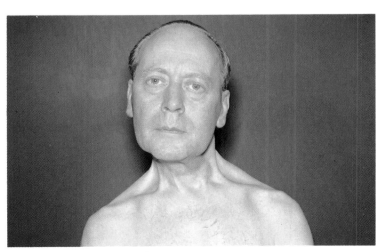

In the early stages of neck involvement there may be neck pain and stiffness. Later, neurological problems may result from atlantoaxial subluxation, subaxial subluxation (especially at C4/5 where the spinal canal is narrowest) and vertebrobasilar insufficiency (Fig. 5.49). Neurological signs may be insidious in onset and difficult to assess in the presence of peripheral joint disease. The associated vascular impairment of the circulation of the spinal cord may complicate any assessment of the level of involvement.

Patients with cervical subluxation are at risk especially when travelling; a whiplash injury can cause sudden death. Manipulation of the neck can likewise prove fatal; thus special precautions should be taken to protect the patient during induction of anesthesia for surgery. Preoperative cervical spine radiographs in flexion and extension should be taken. The patient should be sent to the operating theatre in a collar. These precautions are often overlooked (Fig. 5.50).

Major instability, or the development of progressive neurological signs, should be treated by cervical fusion with decompression, if necessary, at the appropriate level (Fig. 5.51). The aim is to avoid quadriplegia which is often irreversible and is complicated by the development of pressure sores and infection which frequently prove impossible to treat (Fig. 5.52).

Fig. 5.49 Table to show the causes of neurological problems arising from rheumatoid arthritis in the cervical spine.

NEUROLOGICAL COMPLICATIONS OF CERVICAL SPINE DISEASE

Atlantoaxial subluxation:	C2 nerve root pressure Damage to the sensory nucleus of fifth nerve (ophthalmic division) High cervical cord compression
Vertebral artery pressure:	Drop attacks Ophthalmoplegia Cerebellar signs Dizziness, nausea and vomiting
Subaxial subluxation:	Cervical root involvement (often C5) Cervical cord compression

Fig. 5.50 The radiological investigation of atlantoaxial subluxation. This patient first complained of neck pain and mild upper motor neurone symptoms following hand surgery. The flexion view of the cervical spine shows atlantoaxial subluxation of 13mm (upper left). The metrizamide myelogram shows narrowing of the spinal canal at this level due to compression by the posterior arch of C1 (upper right). The transverse CT scan at the atlantoaxial level shows posterior subluxation of the odontoid (lower).

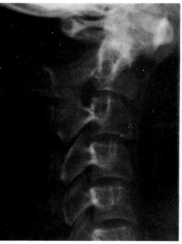
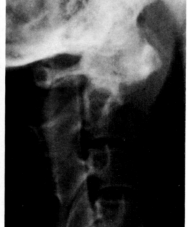
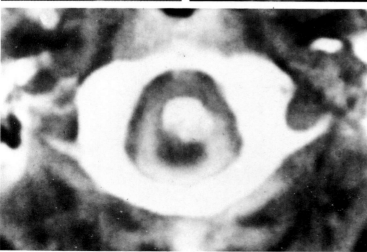

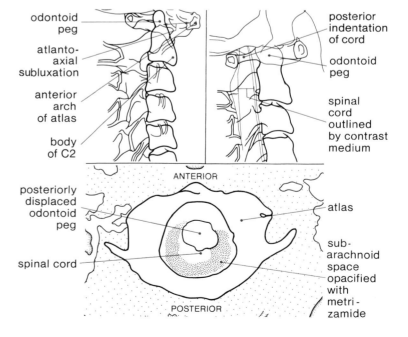

odontoid peg
atlanto-axial subluxation
anterior arch of atlas
body of C2
posterior indentation of cord
odontoid peg
spinal cord outlined by contrast medium

ANTERIOR
posteriorly displaced odontoid peg
spinal cord
atlas
sub-arachnoid space opacified with metrizamide
POSTERIOR

The Dorso-Lumbar Spine

Significant involvement of this region is very rare. Damage to intervertebral discs and apophyseal joints may occur and occasionally this is sufficient to allow vertebral subluxation. Rheumatoid nodules, cysts or granulation tissue in the epidural space can cause cauda equina compression. Costovertebreal involvement may spread and cause damage to adjacent intervertebral discs. Paravertebral bursa involvement occasionally gives rise to localized pain and tenderness.

Other Joints

Involvement of the temporomandibular joint is common.

The patient complains of ear, face or temple pain and mouth opening is painful. Crepitus is often palpable. Radiographs show joint space narrowing and condylar erosions on the mandible (Fig. 5.53). Patients with RA may have cricoarytenoid arthritis but this is usually asymptomatic. There may however be hoarseness, pain in the throat producing dysphagia, stridor or exertional dyspnea. Fixed adduction causes airway obstruction while fixed abduction may allow aspiration and result in repeated respiratory infection.

Occasionally the rheumatoid process affects the middle ear and ossicular erosion and destruction is a rare cause of deafness.

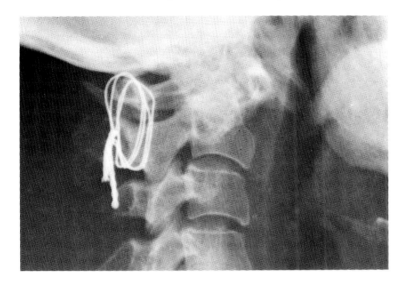

Fig. 5.51 Lateral radiograph of the cervical spine following wire fusion of the C1 and C2 posterior spinous processes.

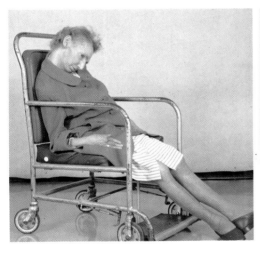

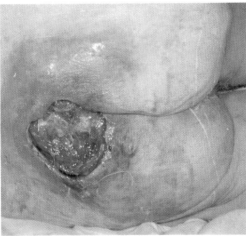

Fig. 5.52 A patient with longstanding rheumatoid arthritis at the time of admission to hospital because of developing quadriplegia (left). This pressure sore was found on clinical examination (right).

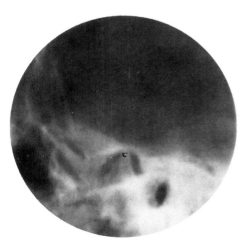

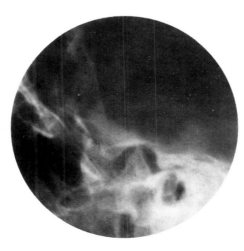

Fig. 5.53 Lateral views of the right temporomandibular joint in a patient complaining of pain on opening the mouth. There is condylar erosion and destruction and little movement between the closed (left) and open (right) views.

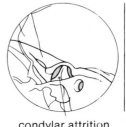

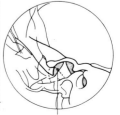

condylar attrition   usual position of condyle

Associated Bone Disease

Patients with RA may have associated changes in bone which contribute to joint damage and functional disturbance (Fig. 5.54). Periarticular bone damage contributes to local joint destruction. Generalized osteoporosis, sometimes associated with osteomalacia, may result in vertebral collapse or long bone fracture. Steroid therapy may contribute to these changes (Fig. 5.55).

Conclusion

Rheumatoid arthritis is a disease which can involve any and several joints. Many of the major functional problems of late disease and serious complications of the arthritis itself are the result of large joint or central involvement and not of the small joint polyarthritis (Fig. 5.56).

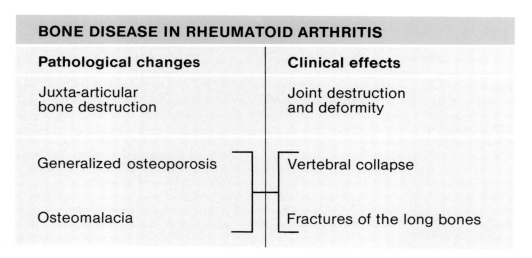

BONE DISEASE IN RHEUMATOID ARTHRITIS

Pathological changes	Clinical effects
Juxta-articular bone destruction	Joint destruction and deformity
Generalized osteoporosis	Vertebral collapse
Osteomalacia	Fractures of the long bones

Fig. 5.54 Associated bone disease in rheumatoid arthritis.

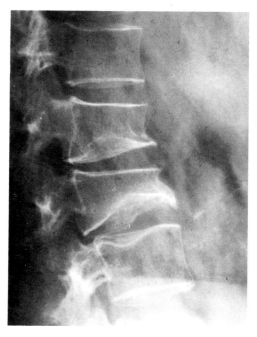

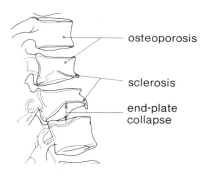

Fig. 5.55 Lateral radiograph of the thoraco-lumbar spine showing osteoporosis, vertebral collapse at several levels and sclerosis due to compression and fracture repair (left).

osteoporosis

sclerosis

end-plate collapse

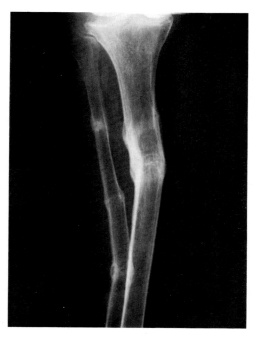

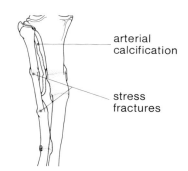

The anteroposterior radiograph of a patient with longstanding rheumatoid arthritis treated with steroid shows stress fractures of the tibia and fibula, and vascular calcification (right).

arterial calcification

stress fractures

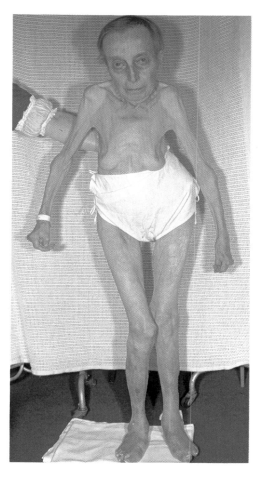

Fig. 5.56 This patient has had rheumatoid arthritis for 31 years. There is widespread joint involvement and considerable vertebral collapse which was attributed to long-term steroid therapy. Her emaciation is due to a combination of joint disease and of inability to feed herself.

6

Synovial Symptoms Outside Joints: Tendinitis, Bursitis, Serositis and Joint Rupture

Inflammation of serous membranes in rheumatoid arthritis can produce many signs and symptoms outside the joints themselves (Fig. 6.1). These may occur because of leakage of synovial fluid under pressure into the tissues around the joint – so-called joint rupture – or because of inflammation of synovial membranes lining other structures. Tendon sheath involvement produces many of the common complications of rheumatoid arthritis. The bursae may also be involved. Inflammation of the serous membranes lining the thoracic viscera constitute a less common but potentially more serious systemic manifestation of rheumatoid arthritis. It is clear that even if inflammation only involves synovial or serous membranes the term rheumatoid arthritis is a misnomer and 'systemic rheumatoid disease' is more appropriate. Other extra-articular manifestations of rheumatoid disease are dealt with in 'Extra-articular Features of Rheumatoid Arthritis'.

DISORDERS OUTSIDE JOINTS

Synovial joint extension

Acute rupture

Chronic rupture (synovial cysts)

Synovial inflammation

Tendon sheath involvement

Bursitis

Other serous membrane involvement

Fig. 6.1   Table of the disorders produced outside the joints by inflammation of serous membranes in rheumatoid arthritis.

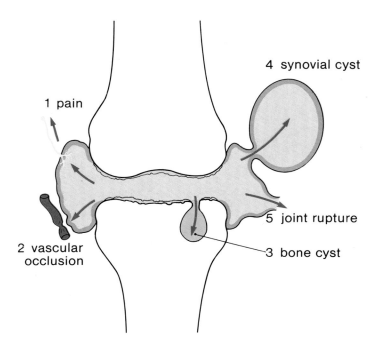

Fig. 6.2   Typical pressure/volume curves from rheumatoid and control knees injected with dextrose saline (left). Note the high pressures reached in the rheumatoid knees. This high intra-articular pressure may cause pain (1), affect the

microcirculation to the joint (2), result in the formation of synovial extensions into bone (3) or soft tissue (4), or cause joint rupture (5) (right). Adapted from data published by M.I.V. Jayson and A. St. J. Dixon.

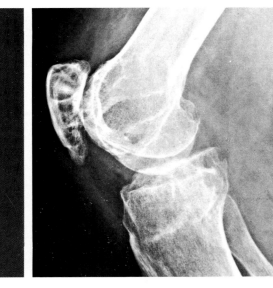

Fig. 6.3   Bone cysts and geodes around the knee joint. Geodes under the tibial plateau (left) and multiple geodes in the patella, femoral condyles and the upper part of the tibia (right).

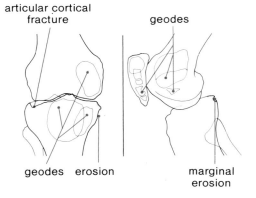

Joint Rupture

The normal joint has only trace amounts of synovial fluid. At rest the surrounding capsule is lax and the intra-articular pressure is approximately atmospheric. On exertion muscle pull distracts the joint capsule and subatmospheric pressure may be produced inside the joint. In inflammatory arthritis the volume of synovial fluid increases dramatically so that in a large joint like the knee 20 ml of fluid is very common and ten times that amount may be present. This large volume of fluid increases joint pressure directly. In addition chronic inflammation leads to fibrosis in the capsule and periarticular tissues, reducing elasticity and joint distensibility so that the volume/pressure relationship is further disturbed. The pattern of pressure changes on exercise is completely altered in the presence of an effusion (Fig. 6.2).

The rise in joint pressure in the presence of an effusion can cause rupture of the joint with extrusion of fluid into the surrounding tissues. This can occur into the bone to produce a cystic lesion known as a geode (Fig. 6.3). In the low resistance bone marrow a large subchondral cavity may occur, particularly in people with a high pain threshold who continue to use their joints vigorously in the presence of an active arthritis. Alternatively the joint fluid may extend outwards into the soft tissue surrounding the joint. This is seen most commonly at the posterior margin of the knee joint producing a popliteal or Baker's cyst. This is often palpable in the fatty tissue of the popliteal fossa and a large one may also be visible. It is most easily delineated by contrast arthrography (Fig. 6.4). The cyst does not often fill with dye unless the knee is exercised, while after injection into the cyst itself the dye does not track back into the joint, indicating that the communication is controlled by a valve mechanism (Fig. 6.5). The popliteal cyst is lined by synovial membrane so it is really a joint protrusion, probably into an existing bursa, rather than a true rupture. Ultrasound or xeroradiography may also demonstrate a popliteal cyst (Fig. 6.6).

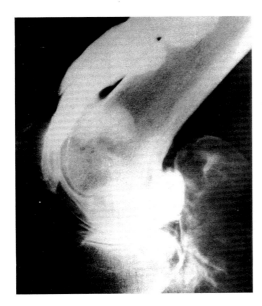

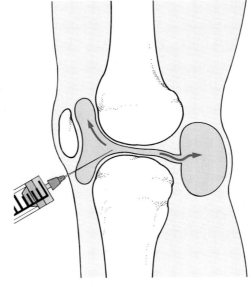

Fig. 6.4 A lateral arthrogram of the knee joint showing contrast medium in an enlarged suprapatellar pouch and extending posteriorly to outline a large popliteal cyst which contains filling defects due to fibrin.

Fig. 6.5 The valve mechanism of a popliteal cyst. Injection into the anterior synovial cavity fills both joint and

popliteal cyst (left) while injection of the cyst fails to outline the joint (right).

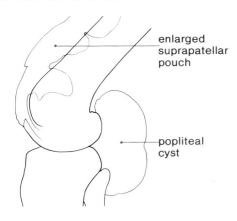

enlarged suprapatellar pouch

popliteal cyst

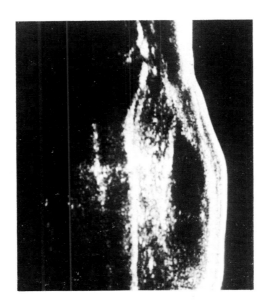

Fig. 6.6 Ultrasound scan showing a popliteal cyst (extending intramuscularly into the calf) which appears as a clear (black) area behind the tibia in this sagittal section. Courtesy of Drs. J.M. Gumpel and L.G. Darlington.

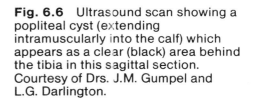

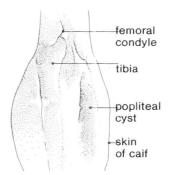

femoral condyle

tibia

popliteal cyst

skin of calf

A synovial rupture may accompany sudden rises of intra-articular pressure, as with unusual exertion in the presence of a tense effusion. Leakage of inflamed synovial fluid with a high content of proteolytic enzymes into the fascial planes of the calf produces acute inflammation in the calf with ankle edema, a picture highly suggestive of a deep venous thrombosis (DVT) (Fig. 6.7). The sudden onset of symptoms, typically during muscular exertion, and absence of edema of the foot itself make the clinical distinction from a DVT. An additional sign is discoloration around the ankle (Fig. 6.8). Contrast arthrography shows leakage into the calf (Fig. 6.9). Less commonly the rupture may occur upwards into the posterior thigh (Fig. 6.10). This is accompanied by tenderness over Hunter's canal very suggestive of an upward extension of a venous thrombosis. It is important to make the distinction. A venogram will confirm the patency of the veins (Fig. 6.11).

Chronic leakage can produce a large pseudocyst, typically in the upper calf, giving the misleading impression of a particularly well-developed calf muscle (Fig. 6.12). In longstanding cases the rupture may extend down into the lower calf even as far as the Achilles tendon (Fig. 6.13).

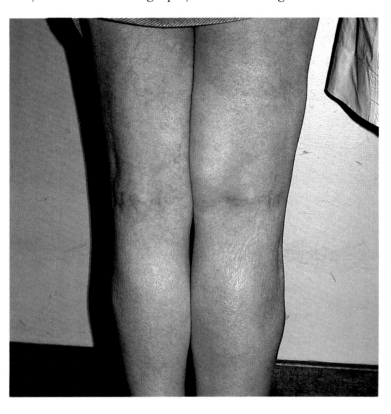

Fig. 6.7 Swollen right calf with shiny inflamed skin and local edema due to an acute synovial rupture.

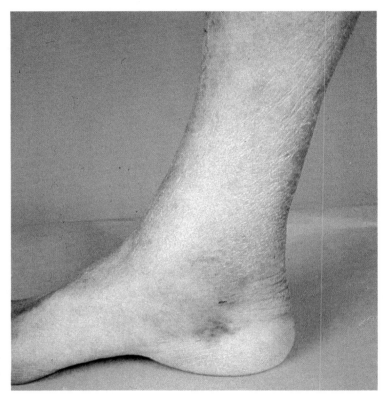

Fig. 6.8 Edema around the ankle with discoloration due to local bruising, occurring in association with an acute synovial rupture of the knee joint.

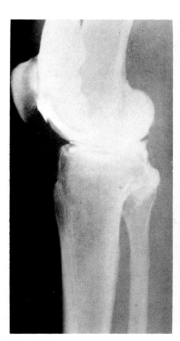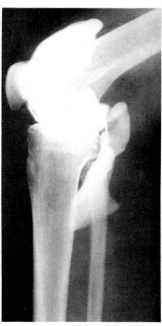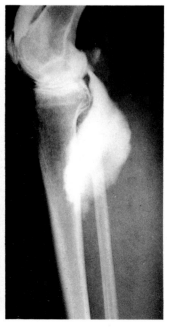

Fig. 6.9 Contrast arthogram of a knee after acute synovial rupture. Initial injection outlines the knee joint only (left). After exertion progressive leakage of fluid occurs into the muscle planes, producing a soft feathery outline (middle, right).

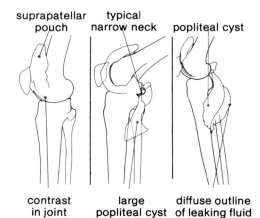

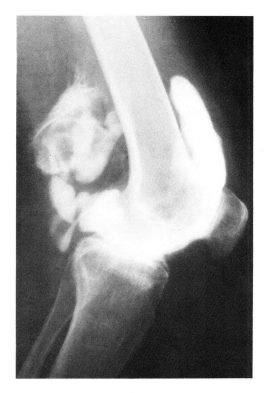

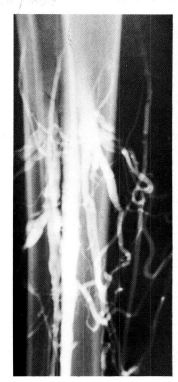

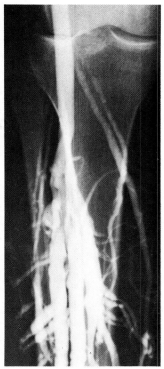

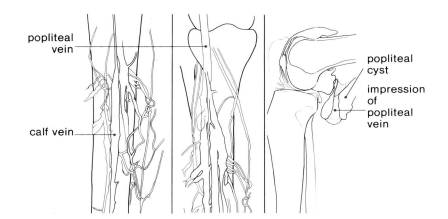

Fig. 6.10 Contrast arthrogram of the knee showing filling of the knee joint and a Baker's cyst with upward extension into the thigh.

Fig. 6.11 The differentiation from calf vein thrombosis. Venography confirms the patency of the calf veins (left, middle) and arthrography (right)

performed at the same time demonstrates a large popliteal cyst which has presumably leaked, accounting for the symptoms.

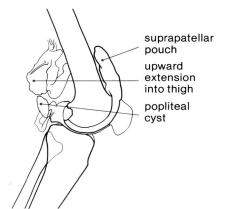

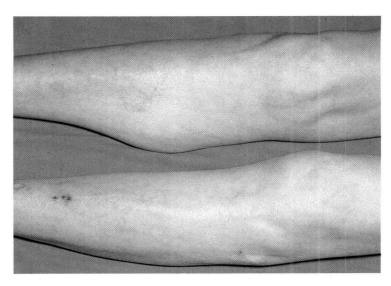

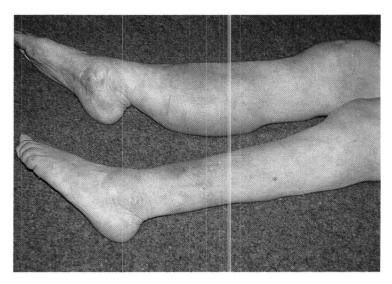

Fig. 6.12 A chronic pseudocyst producing enlargement of the calf muscle on the right in contrast to the wasting normally seen in chronic arthritis apparent in the other limb.

Fig. 6.13 Longstanding chronic synovial rupture with a large pseudocyst extending from the lower calf down to the Achilles tendon.

Contrast arthrography after exercise shows poor filling of an extensive pseudocyst (Fig. 6.14). Operation is necessary for a chronic pseudocyst and reveals thick, yellowish curd-like contents high in cholesterol and containing many rice bodies (Fig. 6.15).

The knee joint is the commonest site for joint rupture, presumably because large effusions are common in this joint and intra-articular pressures are high during weight bearing. However, joint ruptures are by no means confined to the knee joint and joint protrusions or rupture may occur in any inflammatory arthritis since they are simply a mechanical event relating to increased joint pressure. Acute joint rupture tends to occur relatively early in disease, before chronic distension of the joint produces alterations in the capsule. Chronic rupture and pseudocyst formation tend to be a later event.

Synovial leakage from the hip joint is surprisingly uncommon despite it being a weight-bearing joint. This is presumably related to the strong joint capsule and to the smaller amount of inflamed synovium usually present. Chronic synovial protrusions presenting in the upper anterior thigh can occur in uncomplicated rheumatoid arthritis and in the presence of super-added infection (Fig. 6.16).

The shoulder joint is not normally subjected to such pressures as the knee but with inflammation and capsular fibrosis intra-articular pressures may rise sufficiently to produce chronic leakage and a pseudocyst. Most commonly this presents anteriorly and is often large (Fig. 6.17). An arthrogram confirms the cystic nature and the communication with the shoulder joint (Fig. 6.17). Occasionally the joint protrusion may be upwards, presenting as a small, tense subacromial swelling in contrast to the large lax anterior cyst (Fig. 6.18).

Synovial protrusions around the elbow joint may be acute or chronic, and rupture (Fig. 6.19) may present with painful distension of the forearm muscles and edema of

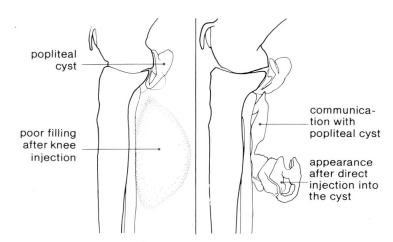

Fig. 6.14 A contrast arthrogram of a pseudocyst showing little filling after initial injection and poor filling of an extensive cyst with neither the smooth outline of a popliteal cyst nor the feathery contours of the muscle plane in acute rupture. The poor filling relates to the semi-solid contents of the pseudocyst following absorption of fluid.

Fig. 6.15 Rice bodies. The three wells in this petri dish contain different-sized particles obtained from the synovial fluid from joints of three different patients. The rice bodies consist of soft insoluble aggregates of fibrin, necrotic villi or cartilage fragments.

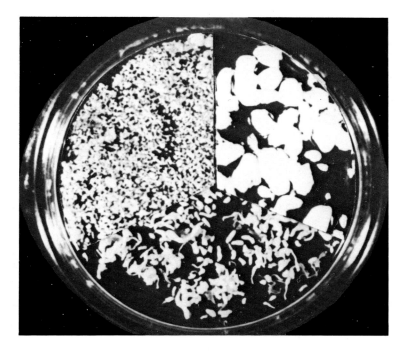

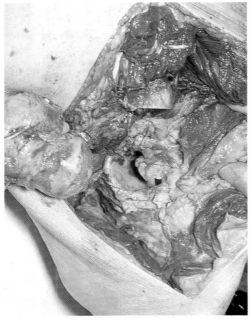

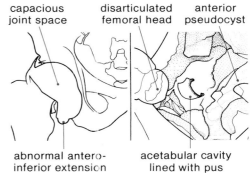

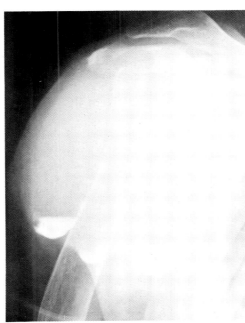

Fig. 6.16 Contrast arthrogram showing an enlarged joint space with distension of the synovium especially anteriorly (left) and an infected hip in RA which had presented with an anterior pseudocyst where purulent synovial fluid had tracked into the tissues (post mortem, right). The disarticulated femoral head shows a damaged cartilage surface.

capacious joint space   disarticulated femoral head   anterior pseudocyst

abnormal antero-inferior extension   acetabular cavity lined with pus

Fig. 6.17 A large anterior pseudocyst at the shoulder in a patient with chronic rheumatoid arthritis (left). Contrast arthrogram of the same joint showing a huge cyst (right). The apparent poor filling is simply due to the dilution of the contrast material.

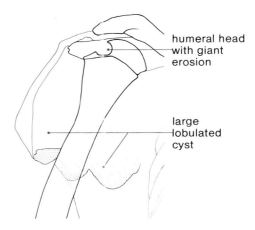

humeral head with giant erosion

large lobulated cyst

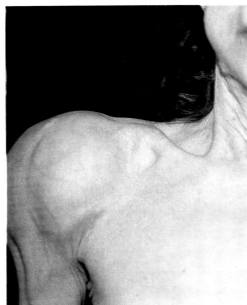

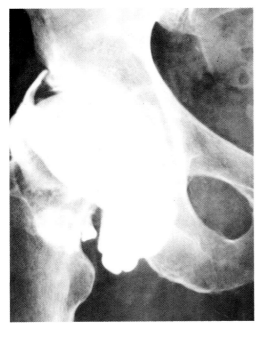

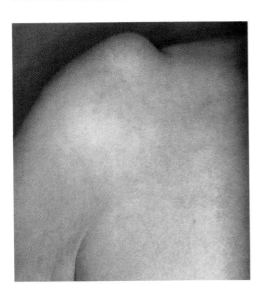

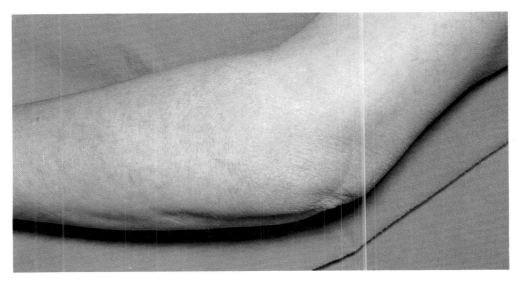

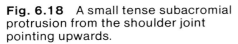

Fig. 6.18 A small tense subacromial protrusion from the shoulder joint pointing upwards.

Fig. 6.19 Painful swelling and edema of the forearm muscles due to synovial rupture from the elbow joint.

the hands. In addition the elbow is another site where a chronic leakage can either cause an anterior pseudocyst in the condylar fossa or produce large geodes in the lower end of the humerus (Figs. 6.20 & 6.21).

The wrist is an uncommon site for acute rupture. Flexor surface rupture may result in a painful red inflammatory swelling which simulates infection (Fig. 6.22). Chronic protrusion occurs more frequently and may present either laterally or more usually on the extensor (dorsal) surface of the wrist (Fig. 6.23). The wrist and metacarpal joints are also common sites for large geodes particularly in patients with vigorous occupations involving heavy manual work (Fig. 6.24). Pressures within the finger joints may also be very high on exercise and occasionally these may rupture through the dorsal capsule when a radiograph can show a surprising amount of extra-articular fluid (Fig. 6.25).

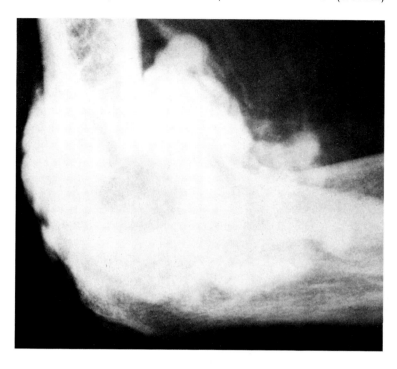

Fig. 6.20 Arthrogram showing elbow leakage in rheumatoid synovitis. Injection of contrast medium into the joint space has outlined the proliferative synovitis and demonstrated rupture of the joint capsule. Courtesy of Dr. T. Constable.

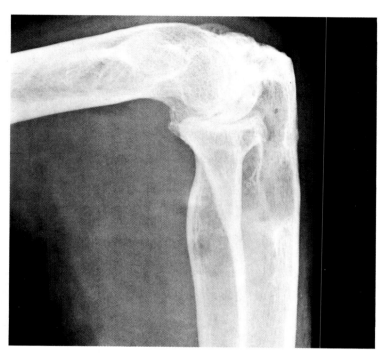

Fig. 6.21 Radiograph showing large geodes around the elbow joint, principally in the shaft of the ulna, in a patient with 'typus robustus' RA.

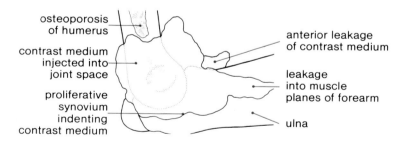

osteoporosis of humerus

contrast medium injected into joint space

proliferative synovium indenting contrast medium

anterior leakage of contrast medium

leakage into muscle planes of forearm

ulna

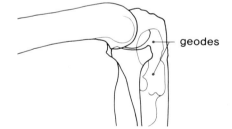

geodes

Fig. 6.22 A synovial protrusion of the wrist presenting as a tense effusion. The redness and tenderness simulates infection.

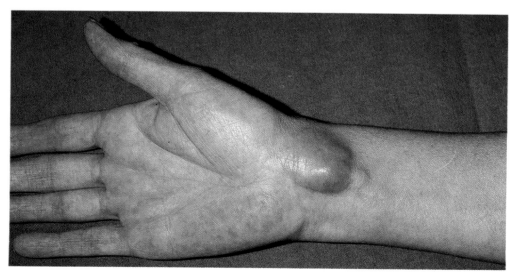

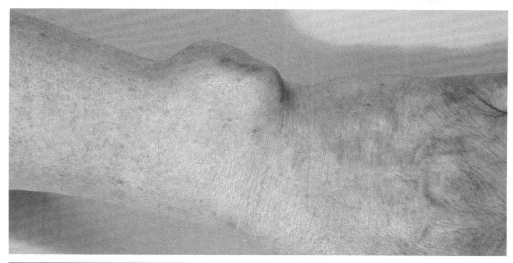

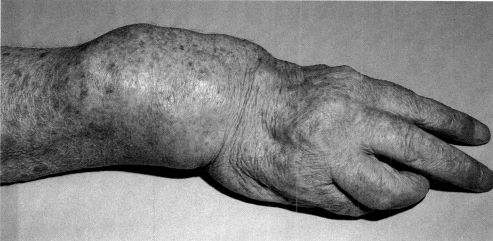

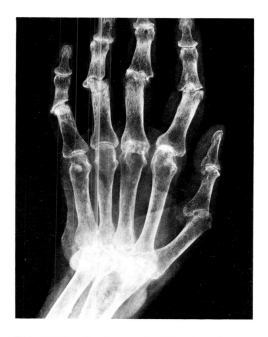

Fig. 6.24 Radiograph of the hand in a 'typus robustus' patient with chronic rheumatoid arthritis showing a large geode in the distal end of the radius and multiple geodes around the metacarpal heads. There is severe destruction of the carpus and PIP joints.

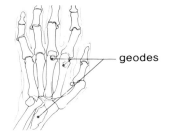

geodes

Fig. 6.23 A lateral protrusion from the wrist joint in early rheumatoid arthritis (upper) and a dorsal synovial protrusion from the wrist joint, simulating a tendon sheath effusion in chronic destructive RA (lower).

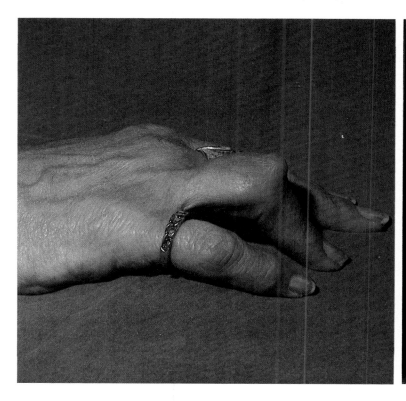

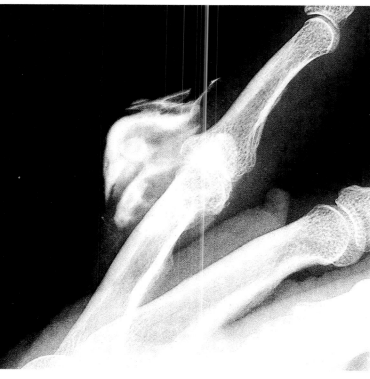

Fig. 6.25 Rupture of the PIP joint through the extensor (left) and an arthrogram of the same finger showing considerable extravasation of contrast medium from the joint through the capsule.

Joint rupture of the ankle is an uncommon complication of rheumatoid arthritis which presents as a red tender swelling with edema around and below the lateral malleolus (Fig. 6.26).

Tendinitis

Involvement of the synovium of the tendon sheaths is common in RA and may occur at any stage including at presentation. It is commonest in the flexor tendon sheaths of the wrist and the hand. In early disease rheumatoid synovitis starts directly in the tendon sheaths, just as it does in the joints. In late disease there is considerable destruction of the normal anatomy with communications between joint cavities and tendon sheath spaces as the result of longstanding inflammation (Fig. 6.27). Tendon sheath involvement in RA can produce signs and symptoms directly, with local pain or dysfunction, or indirectly. Inflamed synovium then produces involvement of local tissues either by pressure leading to nerve compression or by direct extension of the inflammation leading to tendon rupture. In the upper limb the tendon sheath of extensor carpi ulnaris is commonly involved, presenting with a large swelling which simulates a ganglion of the wrist (Fig. 6.28).

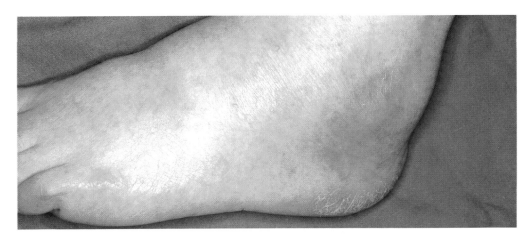

Fig. 6.26 Synovial rupture of the ankle joint producing a tender red swelling with associated edema below and posterior to the lateral malleolus.

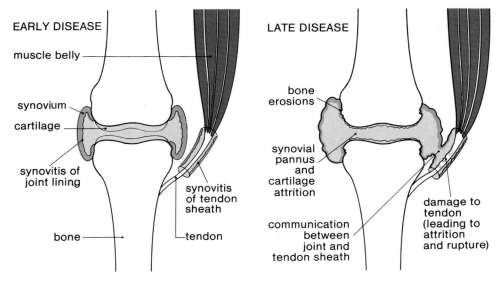

Fig. 6.27 Diagram of a joint in early and late tendinitis. In the early phase there is anatomical separation between the synovial lining of the joint and of the adjacent tendon sheath. In late disease, with synovial pannus and resultant cartilage attrition and bone erosion, there is a communication between the joint and the tendon sheath. The tendon synovitis has led to damage of the tendon itself which may progress to attrition and rupture.

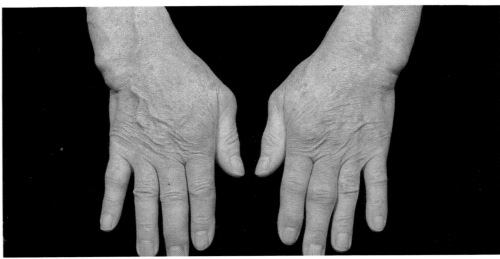

Fig. 6.28 Bilateral tendon sheath involvement of the extensor carpi ulnaris producing marked swelling adjacent to the wrist joint.

In addition the flexor tendon sheath swelling in the palm extends down into the fingers, contributing to the diffuse thickening of the proximal phalanx often seen in RA (Fig. 6.29). Injection of contrast medium into the tendon sheaths may reveal considerable anatomical distortion with abnormal communications between different flexor tendon sheaths and between tendon sheaths and adjacent joints (Fig. 6.30). Tendon sheath involvement can also occur at the ankle but is less frequent and less symptomatic than at the wrist. It can lead to local tendon swelling or to tendon rupture particularly on the medial side producing failure of active inversion of the foot.

Bursitis

There are multiple bursae in the human body, many of which are only potential spaces in a normal person. Bursae have a lining layer with many of the features of synovium and may become involved in rheumatoid arthritis (Fig. 6.31). Enlarged inflamed bursae develop abnormal communications with adjacent joints, so that the grossly distended rheumatoid joint may include what was originally bursal, as well as what was strictly articular synovial cavity (Fig. 6.32). Less commonly bursal inflammation may present symptoms directly. The commonest site for this is at the olecranon where large painful

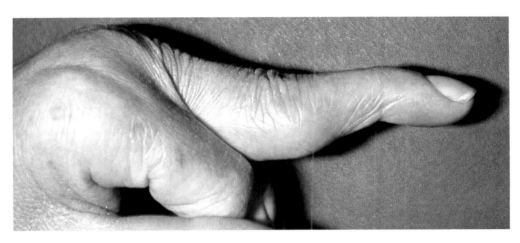

Fig. 6.29 Swelling of the proximal finger in RA due to extensive flexor tendon sheath synovitis.

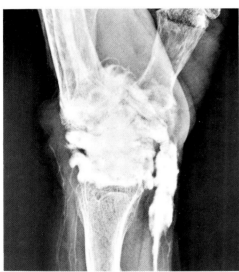

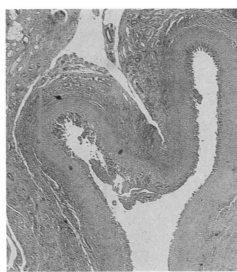

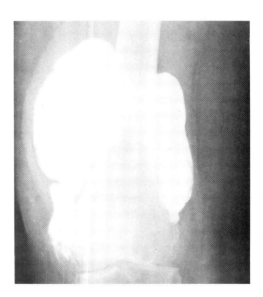

Fig. 6.30 Tenogram showing hypertrophied proliferative synovium and communication between the joint space and the tendon sheath.

Fig. 6.31 Section of chronically inflamed synovial lining of a bursa in RA showing marked hyperplasia of the lining cells, some fibrin deposition on the surface and surrounding fibrotic reaction. H & E stain, x 18.

Fig. 6.32 Arthrogram of a rheumatoid knee joint showing a huge suprapatellar bursa of the knee joint in a patient with chronic rheumatoid arthritis.

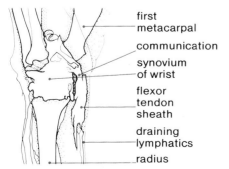

first metacarpal

communication

synovium of wrist

flexor tendon sheath

draining lymphatics

radius

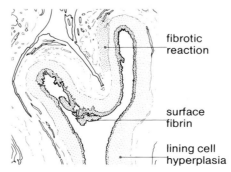

fibrotic reaction

surface fibrin

lining cell hyperplasia

effusions may develop, particularly in a rheumatoid patient who pushes up from a chair using elbows to spare his hands (Fig.6.33). An injection of contrast medium into the bursa usually fails to show fluid entering the joint itself (Fig. 6.33).

Systemic Rheumatoid Serositis

Inflammation of visceral serous membranes can occur in RA emphasizing that this is a systemic disorder. This serositis is unrelated to the musculoskeletal system but it may be relevant that inflammation of pleural and pericardial surfaces, both sites of active movement, is

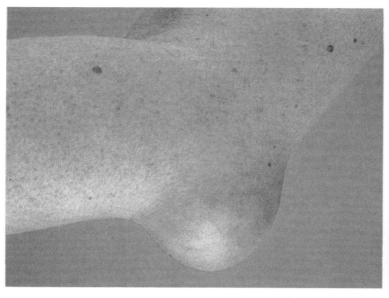
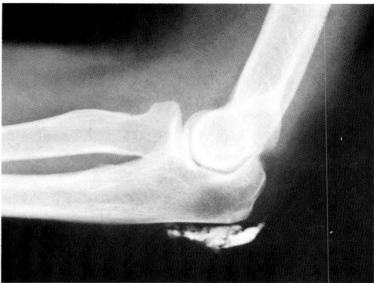

Fig. 6.33 A large olecranon bursa with nodular thickening palpable in the wall in a patient with rheumatoid arthritis (left). Contrast medium injected into an olecranon bursa shows an irregular outline due to rheumatoid synovial proliferation within the bursa. No contrast medium enters the elbow joint itself (right).

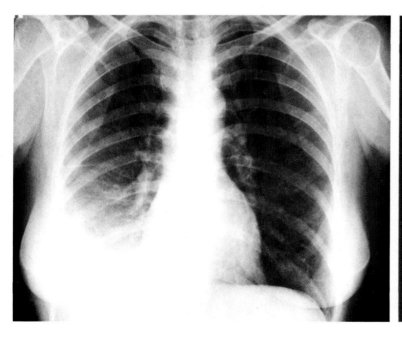
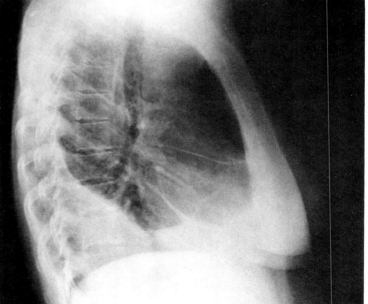

Fig. 6.34 Chest radiographs showing an asymptomatic basal pleural effusion on the right side in a patient with RA.

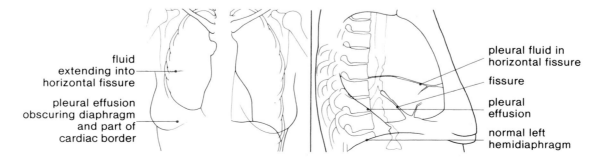

fluid extending into horizontal fissure

pleural effusion obscuring diaphragm and part of cardiac border

pleural fluid in horizontal fissure

fissure

pleural effusion

normal left hemidiaphragm

well-documented while inflammation of peritoneal membranes is virtually unknown.

Pleural effusions in rheumatoid arthritis can occur at any stage of the disease, even at presentation, but occur particularly in males with acute onset of disease. In other cases a small pleural effusion may be detected at routine radiology and may be asymptomatic (Fig. 6.34). In rare cases large chronic effusions can occur and may even cause dyspnea. They may cause diagnostic problems, particularly when a large effusion presents as a pyothorax in a patient with late and not necessarily very active arthritis, when the relationship to the RA may not be appreciated (Fig. 6.35). Aspiration of the pleural fluid reveals thick turbulent grayish fluid with a heavy deposit. In chronic cases it contains cholesterol crystals. Microscopy reveals that the debris is largely amorphous and analysis shows large quantities of immunoglobulin fragments. The cell content is high and most characteristic is the 'comet' cell (Fig. 6.36). Pleural biopsy reveals a range of histology and cell types depending upon the acuteness of the inflammation (Fig. 6.37). In chronic cases actual rheumatoid nodules may form at the surface and contain giant cells. This, together with the chronicity, may lead to a suspicion of tuberculosis. In the majority of cases pleural effusions diminish with treatment of the underlying rheumatoid arthritis, and local therapy, apart from a diagnostic tap, is unnecessary.

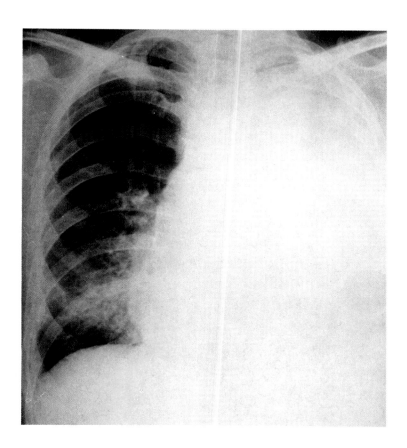

Fig. 6.35 Chest radiograph showing white-out of the pleura.

Fig. 6.36 Pleural fluid in chronic RA showing a prominent, amorphous, pinkish-staining deposit in addition to multiple phagocytic cells, both polymorphs and macrophages. The most characteristic cell is a multi-nucleate phagocytic cell, which because of its shape, with nuclei in the head and a streaming tail of cytoplasm, has been called a 'comet' cell. H & E stain, x 600.

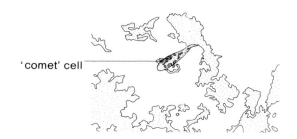

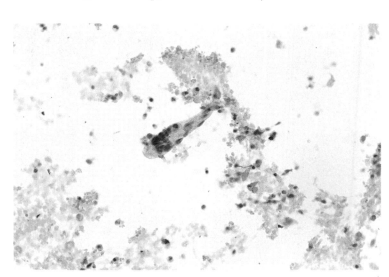

Fig. 6.37 Pleural biopsy in a case of active rheumatoid pleurisy showing fibrin deposition on the surface with enmeshed polymorphs, underlying palisading epithelioid cells and, in the deeper layers, intense chronic cellular infiltrate. H & E stain, x 60.

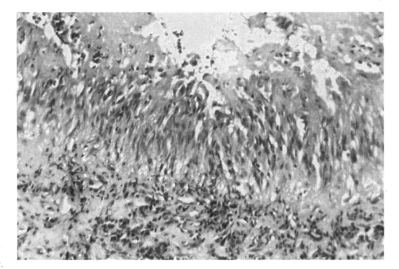

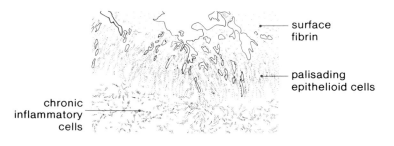

Pericardial effusions are probably quite common in rheumatoid disease even though symptoms are rare, occurring in less than one per cent of patients. Careful and repeated clinical examination, together with repeated ECGs, would demonstrate further cases. The use of diagnostic ultrasound has confirmed that small asymptomatic effusions are much commoner than is clinically suspected, being seen in as many as a third of patients (Fig. 6.38).

Rheumatoid pericarditis may rarely present symptomatically with pericardial tamponade as a late complication in a patient with multiple systemic manifestations. It shows the usual features of resistant heart failure and a markedly elevated jugular venous pressure (JVP) without the usual respiratory fall (Fig. 6.39). The grossly thickened and inflamed pericardium may embarrass cardiac action and require pericardectomy; severe pericarditis may be a fatal complication of rheumatoid disease (Fig. 6.40).

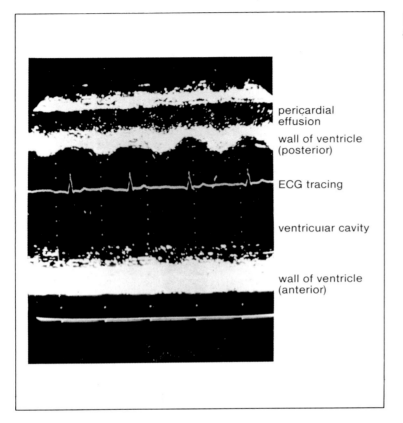

pericardial effusion

wall of ventricle (posterior)

ECG tracing

ventricular cavity

wall of ventricle (anterior)

Fig. 6.38 Echocardiogram in a patient with rheumatoid arthritis showing a large posterior pericardial effusion.

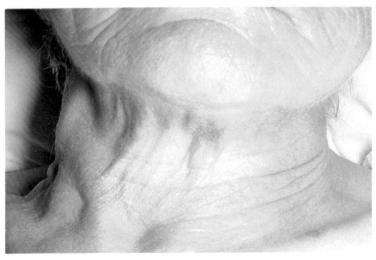

Fig. 6.39 Distended external jugular vein in a patient with markedly elevated central venous pressure due to cardiac tamponade.

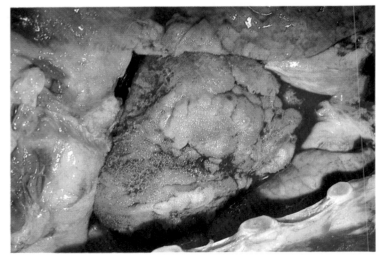

Fig. 6.40 Grossly inflamed pericardium seen at post mortem in the same patient as figure 6.39 ('Bread and Butter' pericarditis).

7

Extra-Articular Features of Rheumatoid Arthritis

In rheumatoid arthritis the patient's main complaints are directed towards the joints, as these give rise to pain. Unlike degenerative joint disease which occurs in otherwise healthy people, rheumatoid patients have in addition multiple signs of systemic disease even though these are not always overt. In rare instances the systemic manifestations are more prominent than the joint manifestations, so that some clinicians prefer the term rheumatoid disease. In virtually all cases the discerning physician will detect evidence of the disease outside the joints.

Constitutional disturbance is most marked at the onset and during a flare-up of disease. At this time low grade fever may be apparent although it is less common than with childhood arthritis. Weight loss may be a prominent feature with marked loss of muscle bulk, reducing a previously healthy active person to a state of severe functional disability even before there are fixed changes in the joints (Fig. 7.1). Feelings of helplessness and depression are common in these cases and are compounded by the lack of energy. This clinical evidence of severe constitutional disturbance is mirrored by the laboratory tests which show evidence of active inflammation, with increased levels in plasma of the acute phase proteins which of course contribute to the elevated ESR. Anemia in RA is normocytic and normochromic, may be severe and reflects bone marrow depression rather than any deficiency. Another important cause of anemia in RA is gastrointestinal bleeding. Many drugs used for pain relief, particularly the non-steroidal anti-inflammatory drugs, provoke gastric erosions (Fig. 7.2). Gastroscopy studies reveal that these occur more commonly than is clinically apparent.

Estimations of iron status in rheumatoid disease are complicated by the fact that indices such as serum ferritin may act partly as acute phase proteins and therefore also vary with disease activity. Total body iron stores may paradoxically be normal or even increased, although when bleeding has occurred bone marrow iron stores may be diminished or absent. Special stains will show large quantities of iron deposited within the rheumatoid synovium (Fig. 7.3)

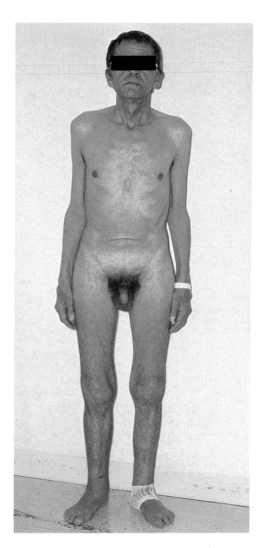

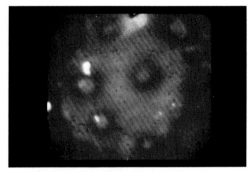

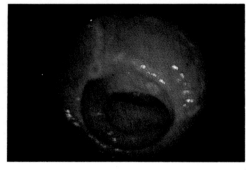

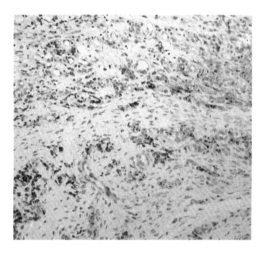

Fig. 7.3 Rheumatoid synovium showing extensive blue-staining iron deposits which are largely within the macrophages. Perl's stain, x 650.

Fig. 7.2 Acute gastric erosions on an inflamed base (upper) and acute duodenal ulcers (lower) seen at gastroscopy in rheumatoid patients on non-steroidal anti-inflammatory drugs.

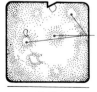

acute erosions on inflamed base

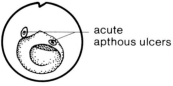

acute apthous ulcers

Fig. 7.1 A male with early rheumatoid arthritis showing severe weight loss and marked loss of muscle bulk. Three months previously he had been using a 20 lb hammer routinely.

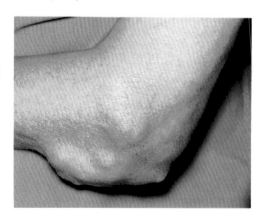

Fig. 7.4 Multiple rheumatoid granulomata occurring subcutaneously at the elbow, in association with the olecranon bursa, and on the subcutaneous border of the ulna in a patient with the 'typus robustus' form of RA.

Nodules

Nodules are chronic granulomata occurring at sites of pressure and movement, both near the body surface and internally. They are one of the most characteristic diagnostic features of rheumatoid arthritis. Rarely, similar nodules may be found in overlapping connective tissue syndromes. Nodules appear to mark the more severe end of the rheumatoid disease spectrum and are seen in approximately 30% of patients, all of whom have positive tests for rheumatoid factor. The incidence of nodular disease varies with race and geography for reasons that are not clearly established.

Rheumatoid nodules are most characteristically found subcutaneously, near the elbow joint. Tiny nodules may be a useful diagnostic feature in early disease but may come and go. Some patients develop large multiple nodules at the elbow and along the subcutaneous border of the ulna, often in association with an olecranon bursa (Fig. 7.4). This emphasizes the interrelations of synovial inflammation and rheumatoid granulomata. Large multiple nodules are sometimes seen in patients with minimal joint complaints, although radiology reveals prominent erosions and geodes. The nodules in such 'typus robustus' patients are probably determined in part by the trauma in patients who continue to use their joints despite active disease.

The histological appearance of a rheumatoid nodule is of a central avascular area of fibrinoid necrosis which is largely structureless, although it may have a sparse infiltrate of inflammatory cells, particularly in early cases (Fig. 7.5). This central area is surrounded by a palisading layer of epithelioid cells. These are tissue macrophages which have organized so as to contain and wall off the fibrinoid material. Beyond this is an area of fibrosis with a further infiltration of lymphocytes and plasma cells. Young or developing nodules may show a more fragmented appearance with multiple areas of fibrinoid necrosis.

The precise features determining nodule formation are not defined. There is little doubt that local pressure and trauma play a major part in determining the site of nodule formation which occurs at other pressure points. Thus, in severely disabled and especially bed-ridden patients, they may be found over the occiput (Fig. 7.6), or on the ear (Fig. 7.7) where the patient lies down.

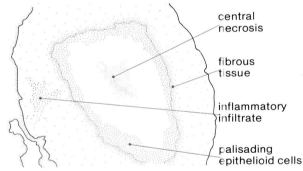

Fig. 7.5 A small rheumatoid nodule showing the gross architecture with fibrinoid material at the centre and a surrounding rim of inflammatory cells. H & E stain, x 300.

central necrosis

fibrous tissue

inflammatory infiltrate

palisading epithelioid cells

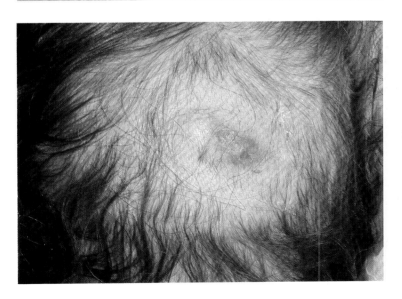

Fig. 7.6 A rheumatoid nodule, with ulceration on the surface, on the occiput of a chair-bound lady with advanced RA.

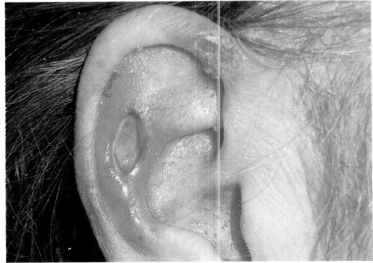

Fig. 7.7 An ulcerating rheumatoid nodule on the pinna of a patient with RA.

Multiple nodules may develop over the thoracolumbar spinous processes (Fig. 7.8), particularly in wasted patients with little subcutaneous tissue. Severe problems may be seen over the sacrum where more than one clinical pattern may occur. Multiple small nodules, close to the surface or even intracutaneous, may be seen at this site (Fig. 7.9). These are often associated with multiple finger nodules and there may be evidence of vasculitis

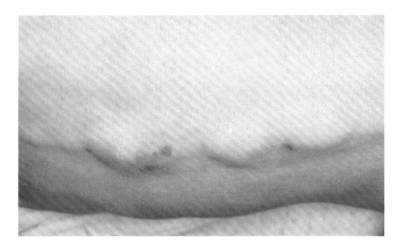

Fig. 7.8 Rheumatoid granulomata occurring at multiple subcutaneous sites in association with the posterior spinous processes in a bed-bound patient with severe weight loss.

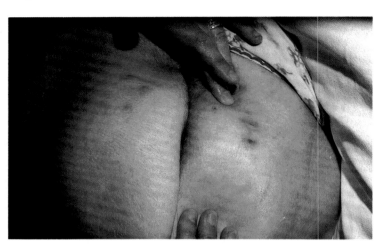

Fig. 7.9 Multiple small intracutaneous nodules, some showing surface ulceration, on the buttock of a rheumatoid patient who showed signs of vasculitis elsewhere.

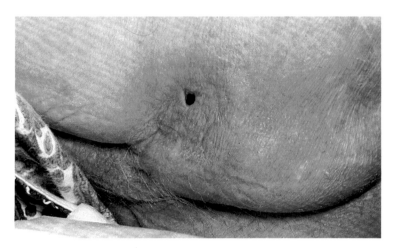

Fig. 7.10 A deep, penetrating sacral ulcer in a patient who had previously had a subcutaneous rheumatoid nodule at that site.

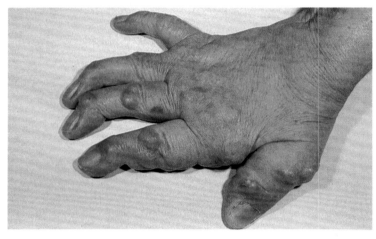

Fig. 7.11 Multiple intracutaneous nodules which had recently developed on the hands of this patient with longstanding deforming RA.

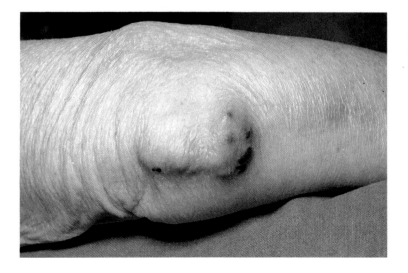

Fig. 7.12 A rheumatoid nodule at the classical site on the elbow showing apparently vasculitic lesions and surface ulceration.

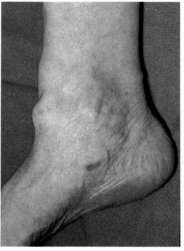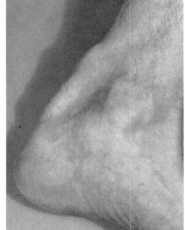

Fig. 7.13 Rheumatoid nodules in the tendon sheath at the ankle anteriorly (left) and posteriorly (right) in the achilles tendon.

elsewhere. Other patients show deeper, more characteristic, large single nodules. These may not be discovered until they present as sacral sinuses or ulcers (Fig. 7.10). Multiple nodules on the fingers (Fig. 7.11) are also small and intracutaneous but have the same histology as larger nodules. They appear and disappear more rapidly than larger nodules. The appearance of fresh crops of such small nodules is again often associated with vasculitis. Occasionally, the more characteristic large nodules, even those at the elbow, may develop multiple tiny infarcts on the surface and may even ulcerate (Fig. 7.12). Again this occurs in association with evidence of vasculitis elsewhere. Nodules may also present at sites of movement and are frequently detected in tendon sheaths. Flexor tendon sheath nodules in the palm of the hand are common. Nodules may be most easily seen around the ankle, where they may present at either anterior or posterior sites (Fig. 7.13). Another site of involvement is the eye where the characteristic discoloration of the white sclera, occurring laterally or superiorly to the iris, is known as scleromalacia (Fig. 7.14). Rarely, this can even lead to perforation of the eye (scleromalacia perforans) with leakage of contents. In the more chronic stage it may be associated with thinning of the sclera which is more apparent than real. In either case the histological appearance is that of a relatively avascular, acellular rheumatoid nodule.

Rheumatoid nodules also occur in internal organs where there is movement and thus may be seen in both the lung and the heart. In the lung they may be symptomless and present as a shadow on the chest radiograph (Fig. 7.15) which is often solitary but may be multiple. They may cause severe diagnostic problems particularly when they occur early on. Special views will often show that a solitary shadow is cavitating (Fig. 7.16) and discharge of nodule contents into the bronchus and pleural spaces has been described. Such shadows may clear completely with anti-rheumatic therapy. Invasive procedures to firmly establish the diagnosis are rarely necessary.

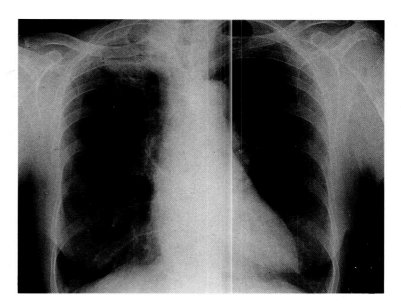

Fig. 7.15 Chest radiograph of a patient with early RA showing an obvious opacity at the right apex partly obscured by overlying bone and another rounded lesion near the left hilum partly obscured by mediastinal shadows.

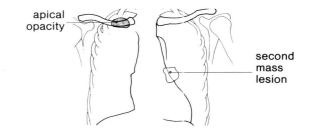

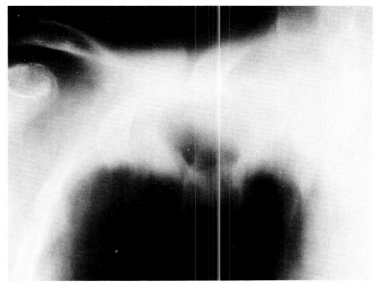

Fig. 7.16 Tomography of the right apical lesion in figure 7.15 reveals it to be cavitating. The lesion healed completely on treating the arthritis with Gold in the absence of any other therapy.

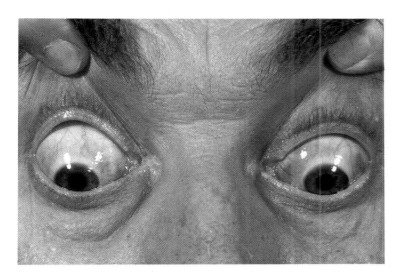

Fig. 7.14 Scleromalacia causing patches of discoloration and blueing of the normally white sclera, most marked in the lateral and superior aspects.

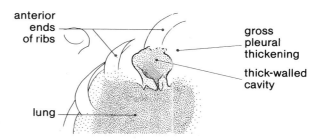

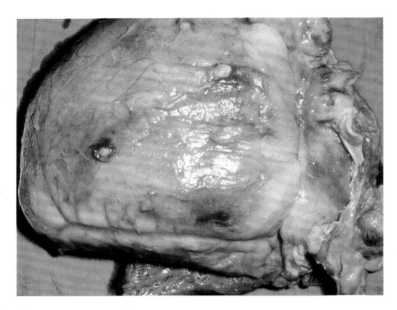

Fig. 7.17 Multiple nodules seen on the epicardial surface of the pericardium at post mortem.

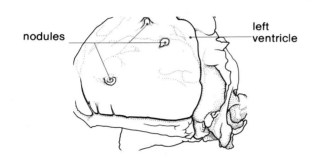

Rheumatoid nodules in the heart are detected at post mortem much more frequently than they are appreciated clinically as they rarely cause symptoms. Multiple nodules may be seen on the pericardial surface (Fig. 7.17) sometimes with other signs of pericarditis. Nodules also occur on the endocardial surface particularly at the aortic and mitral valves. Such nodules are not usually detected during life. Very occasionally aortic valve distortion, or perforation associated with the nodules (Fig. 7.18) may cause symptoms. Echocardiography may show thickening and slowing of the mitral valve leaflet (Fig. 7.19). This occurs particularly in patients with multiple subcutaneous nodules. Rheumatoid granulomata may also involve the myocardium (Fig. 7.20) where again they have essentially the same features as subcutaneous nodules (Fig. 7.21). In rare cases this involvement occurs just below the aortic root when it may involve the conducting tissue with the production of heart block.

Vasculitis

Inflammation of the blood vessels is a less common but more serious aspect of the rheumatoid disease spectrum. As with rheumatoid granulomata, the cutaneous lesions are most conspicuous but systemic manifestations are more important and are commoner than is usually clinically appreciated. Local pressure and trauma are important in determining the sites of vasculitis, particularly with cutaneous lesions. The underlying etio-

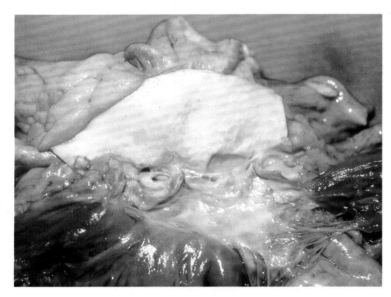

Fig. 7.18 Thickening and perforation near the free edge of two of the aortic valve cusps. Histological examination revealed rheumatoid granulomata at these sites.

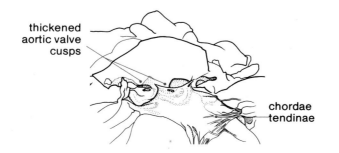

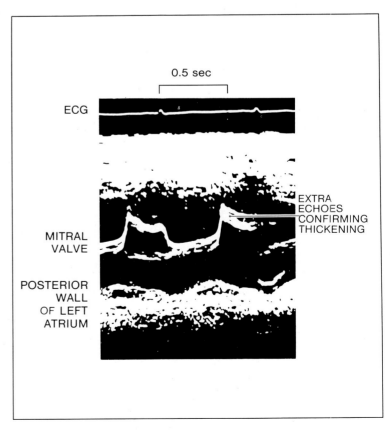

Fig. 7.19 An echocardiogram of the mitral valve anterior leaflet showing thickening with slowing of movement during diastole. Both these abnormalities were noted in patients with multiple subcutaneous nodules and are presumed to represent rheumatoid granulomata within the valve.

pathology is an inflammation involving complement-fixing immune complexes which contain rheumatoid factors. Vasculitis develops most commonly in patients with long established sero-positive and usually nodular disease, but can occur at any stage in the disease process. It is frequently seen when the synovitis is relatively inactive.

The mildest form of vasculitis is the nail edge infarct (Fig. 7.22) which may be easily missed by both clinician and patient. The site is probably trauma-determined as blanching occurs here in the normal finger on pulp pressure, as in everyday use. These lesions are in themselves relatively insignificant but may be associated in the same patient with more severe systemic vasculitis which can be fatal (Fig. 7.23). Fresh crops of such lesions should be taken seriously. Similar lesions are seen in the feet and may be associated with severe ischemia and incipient gangrene of the toes (Fig. 7.24).

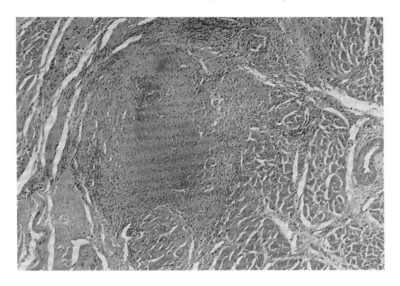

Fig. 7.20 Typical rheumatoid granuloma occurring within the myocardium at the aortic root. Post mortem specimen, H & E stain, x 80.

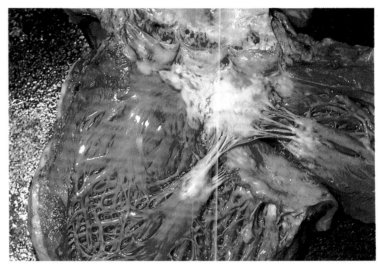

Fig. 7.21 Heart opened to show aortic valve and mitral valve chordae tendinae. Rheumatoid nodules are seen at the base of the aortic valve cusps and in the tips of the papillary muscles.

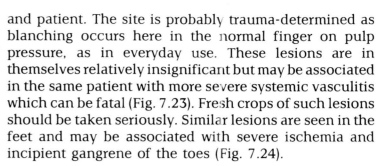

granuloma

bundles of cardiac muscle

rheumatoid nodules

thickened aortic valve cusps

papillary muscles of mitral valve

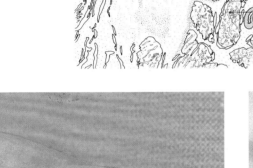

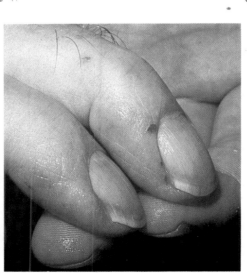

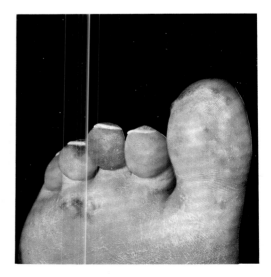

Fig. 7.22 A small nail edge infarct which may be missed. Blanching on pressure occurs in the normal finger at the same site.

Fig. 7.23 Multiple nail edge infarcts seen at post mortem in the hand of a patient who also had severe systemic vasculitis.

Fig. 7.24 Nail edge lesions on the feet occurring in association with incipient gangrene of at least two toes.

In more severe cases, with involvement of medium-sized muscular arteries, extensive gangrene may be seen which can involve large portions of one or more limb (Fig. 7.25). Unlike arteriosclerotic or thrombotic arterial occlusion the lesions may be patchy and non symmetrical. Nevertheless, if untreated they may progress sufficiently to damage the viability of the peripheral limb and necessitate amputation.

Typical vasculitic purpura (Fig. 7.26) may be seen on the lower limb or trunk, particularly at minor pressure points due to clothing. More aggressive vasculitic rashes also occur with multiple small areas of necrosis (Fig. 7.27). These may appear suddenly and progress rapidly but often clear rapidly with therapy. At the other extreme, chronic ulcers which heal poorly or enlarge slowly may also be a manifestation of vasculitis (Fig. 7.28). They also occur at atypical sites such as on the dorsum of the foot, behind the ankle, or even on the calf. When they occur at typical sites of varicose ulceration they may present diagnostic difficulties but vasculitic ulcers are usually extensive with a punched-out appearance and may contain exuberant granulation tissue. Biopsy of the lesion merely shows chronic inflammation without specific features.

Blind biopsy elsewhere may reveal a necrotizing arteritis involving muscular vessels. A good site for blind biopsy with a high diagnostic yield in such cases is the rectum (Fig. 7.29). Such a biopsy needs to be deep so as to include submucosal vessels. Serial sectioning of the tissue is important as vasculitis is frequently segmental and skip lesions may be easily missed. Rheumatoid vasculitis may involve all segments of the intestine and occasionally results in gastrointestinal bleeding or perforation. Such problems, although uncommon, carry a very high mortality.

A mononeuritis multiplex is another serious manifestation of vasculitis with a poor prognosis. This characteristically presents with a sudden wrist drop or foot drop (Fig. 7.30) in association with some degree of sensory loss. When all four limbs are involved the picture may at first appear to be a 'stocking and glove' peripheral neuropathy but an accurate history should reveal the sudden onset in one area after another. It may, of course, be associated with other manifestations such as digital gangrene and chronic ulcers. The more common but easily missed rheumatoid neuropathy is a sensory lesion involving only the sides of the fingers, often near the tips. This is associated with digital artery lesions, which can present with localized necrotic lesions in the same area (Fig. 7.31). However, in many cases all that is found is digital artery occlusion best demonstrated by brachial arteriography (Fig. 7.32). The histological appearance of this occlusion is described as 'bland intimal hyperplasia' which appears to be a non-inflammatory lesion. However, serial biopsies suggest that it is in fact the end stage of a burnt out inflammatory vasculitis. A more striking manifestation of vasculitis is an episcleritis (Fig. 7.33). In rheumatoid disease episcleritis is often asymptomatic but a persistent severe lesion is again associated with high mortality due to the related systemic vasculitis.

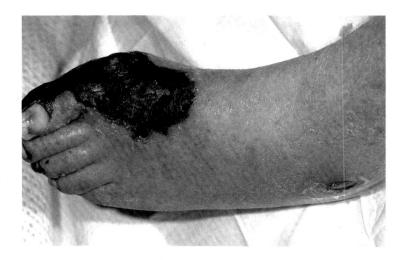

Fig. 7.25 Gangrene of the foot in rheumatoid vasculitis.

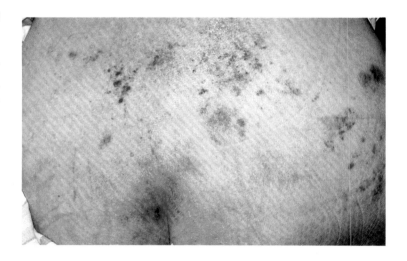

Fig. 7.26 A diffuse vasculitic purpura seen on the buttocks of a patient who showed similar lesions on both legs.

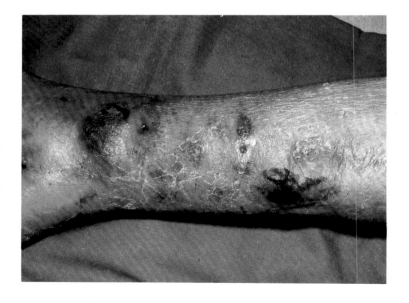

Fig. 7.27 An aggressive vasculitic rash with ulceration at some points which eventually involved all four limbs.

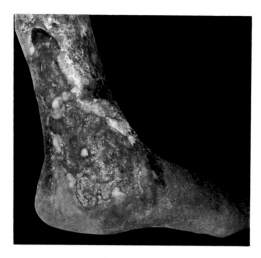

Fig. 7.28 Chronic vasculitic ulceration in a rheumatoid patient. The posterior aspect of the lower leg is affected and the more common varicose ulcer site is involved. The ulcer has deep punched-out edges. An extensive surface slough has been removed.

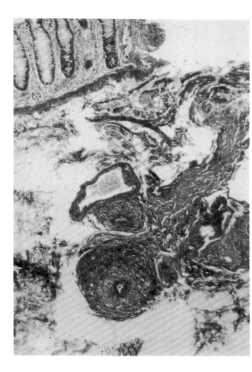

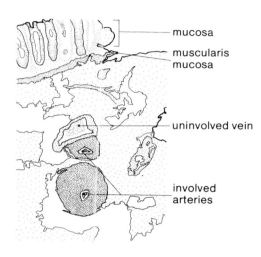

Fig. 7.29 A rectal biopsy showing vasculitis with fibrinoid necrosis and surrounding inflammatory infiltrate in the vessels deep in the submucosa. Martius Scarlet Blue stain, x 250.

- mucosa
- muscularis mucosa
- uninvolved vein
- involved arteries

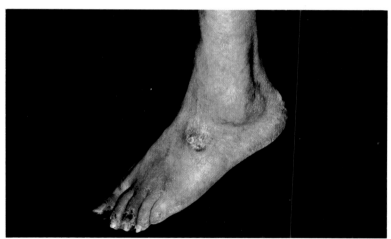

Fig. 7.30 Foot drop due to mononeuritis multiplex in a patient with rheumatoid vasculitis which also caused the gangrene of the toe and the ulcer on the dorsum of the foot.

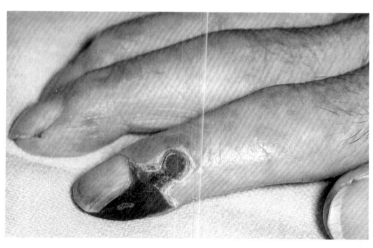

Fig. 7.31 Digital vasculitis with a necrotic lesion of one finger tip. A simple nail edge lesion is seen on the adjacent finger at the same site.

Fig. 7.32 Brachial arteriogram showing multiple areas of occlusion in the digital arteries in a patient with rheumatoid arthritis. A distal vessel has filled by collateral circulation. There was a neuropathy of the fingers.

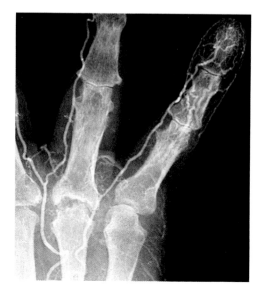

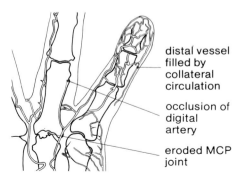

- distal vessel filled by collateral circulation
- occlusion of digital artery
- eroded MCP joint

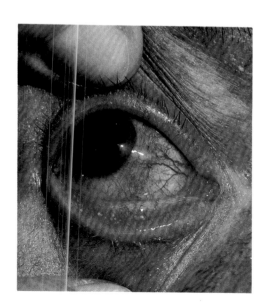

Fig. 7.33 Severe persistent episcleritis in a patient with rheumatoid disease.

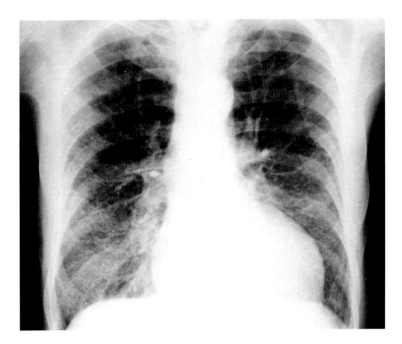

Fig. 7.34 Widespread, bilateral, basal, interstitial fibrosis involving particularly the lower and middle zones due to fibrosing alveolitis in a rheumatoid patient.

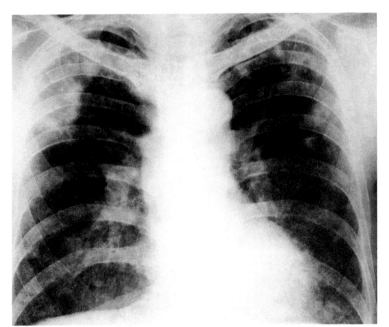

Fig. 7.35 Chest radiograph showing Caplan's syndrome in a coal miner due to complicated pneumoconiosis and rheumatoid disease. There are fibrotic mass lesions peripherally in the upper lobes (progressive massive fibrosis, PMF), multiple nodules and coarse interstitial fibrosis in the lower lobes.

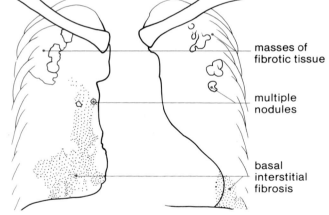

masses of fibrotic tissue

multiple nodules

basal interstitial fibrosis

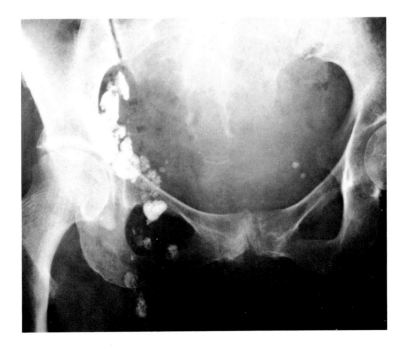

Fig. 7.36 A lymphangiogram showing enlarged iliac lymph nodes in a patient with rheumatoid arthritis with severe lower limb involvement. The granular quality is non-specific but does not suggest a lymphoma.

Other Organ Involvement and Miscellaneous Manifestations

In rheumatoid disease pulmonary involvement with serositis and granuloma have already been described and vasculitis may rarely be seen. In addition, alveolar inflammation or fibrosing alveolitis occurs more commonly in RA than would be expected and may cause widespread fibrosis seen on the chest radiograph (Fig. 7.34). Rheumatoid patients are relatively inactive due to their disabilities and may not present with dyspnea until the lesion is advanced. Screening by chest radiology of pulmonary function suggests that milder cases are commoner than clinical symptoms might indicate. A history of heavy smoking is obtained more frequently than by chance in these patients, suggesting the importance of external stimuli. In Caplan's syndrome (Fig. 7.35) the combination of pneumoconiosis and rheumatoid disease leads to prominent pulmonary changes.

Lymphadenopathy is detected clinically at accessible sites in rheumatoid patients in the vast majority of cases. The glands are small and rarely cause diagnostic confusion provided their presence is expected. Intrathoracic or intra-abdominal lymphatic hyperplasia also occurs commonly as may be documented by a lymphangiogram (Fig. 7.36). The histology of both the subcutaneous and systemic nodes show reactive hyperplasia with very prominent germinal centers (Fig. 7.37).

Splenomegaly is also observed in rheumatoid disease. Some patients with sero-positive rheumatoid disease develop Felty's syndrome in which splenomegaly is associated with neutropenia and other features (Fig. 7.38). There is a peripheral blood neutropenia although bone marrow examination usually reveals a picture of 'maturation arrest' with plentiful granulocyte precursors. The cause of the neutropenia is multifactorial. Peripheral consumption of neutrophils may be increased but neutropenia can occur in the absence of splenomegaly. Bone marrow suppression is another factor.

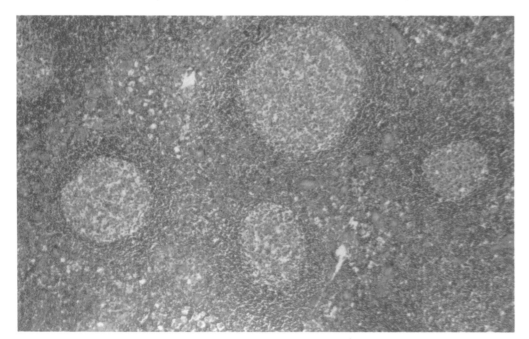

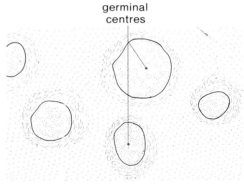

Fig. 7.37 Histological appearance of a lymph node in rheumatoid arthritis showing reactive hyperplasia with prominent germinal center formation. The size and irregularity of the germinal centres is an aid to distinguishing this from a low grade lymphoma. H & E stain, x 25.

germinal centres

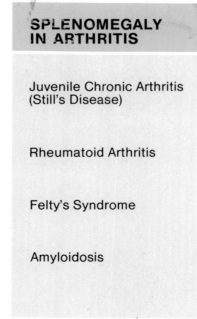

SPLENOMEGALY IN ARTHRITIS

Juvenile Chronic Arthritis (Still's Disease)

Rheumatoid Arthritis

Felty's Syndrome

Amyloidosis

Fig. 7.38 Prominent splenomegaly seen in the gross specimen at operation as can occur in juvenile and adult rheumatoid arthritis and in Felty's syndrome.

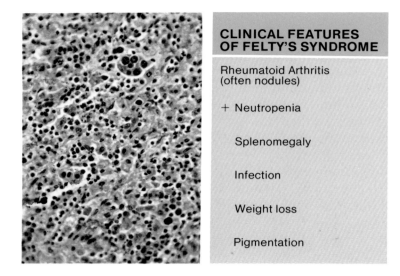

Fig. 7.39 Histological appearance of the spleen in Felty's syndrome showing plasma cell hyperplasia, extramedullary hemopoiesis and erythrophagocytosis. H & E stain, x 1300. The main clinical features of Felty's syndrome are listed.

HEPATIC CHANGES IN RHEUMATOID ARTHRITIS

CHANGES RELATED TO INFLAMMATION:-
raised synthesis of 'acute phase' proteins
   eg. C – reactive protein, serum amyloid A protein
decreased synthesis of some proteins
   eg. albumin, pre-albumin

CHANGES IN ENZYME OUTPUT:-
raised alkaline phosphatase
raised SGOT or γGT

HISTOLOGY:-
usually normal, occasional minimal changes
in Kupffer cells

Fig. 7.40 The main laboratory abnormalities suggesting liver involvement in rheumatoid arthritis. Histological abnormalities are scanty or absent.

The histology of the spleen shows prominent non-specific immunological reactivity, akin to the germinal center hyperplasia of lymph nodes. Erythrophagocytosis may also be a feature (Fig. 7.39). The original description of the syndrome included the observations of weight loss (which is common) and leg ulcers and pigmentation (which are not). Splenomegaly also occurs in juveniles as part of the disease. Amyloidosis may cause splenic enlargement in both juvenile and adults.

Hepatomegaly is not common in rheumatoid arthritis but abnormalities of so-called liver function tests are frequently seen (Fig. 7.40). Marked elevations of acute phase proteins (which are produced in the liver), particularly CRP, occur together with an inverse fall in serum albumen levels. Alkaline phosphatase is frequently increased in active rheumatoid disease, but elevation of cellular enzymes such as SGOT and gamma glutamyl transpeptidase (γGT) may also occur. In such cases liver biopsy shows minimal histological change with occasional infiltrating lymphocytes or no gross abnormality.

Bone involvement in rheumatoid arthritis produces the radiological appearance of osteopenia. When severe, this may produce vertebral collapse (Fig. 7.41). The causes are several; steroid-induced osteoporosis, inactivity osteoporosis, a contribution from active rheumatoid inflammation, and in some cases osteomalacia. Elderly, house-bound rheumatoid patients, particularly in Northern climates, may have both a dietary deficiency of Vitamin D and an absence of exposure to sunlight. Biochemical changes may be minimal but osteopenia is seen in hand radiographs together with the more characteristic pseudofractures, or even undisplaced total fractures produced by minimal trauma, in the long bones (Fig. 7.42).

Renal involvement in rheumatoid disease itself is notable for its rarity, although very occasionally both vasculitis and glomerulitis have been observed. The more usual changes are attributable either to therapy or to amyloidosis. The nephropathy induced by gold or penicillamine is usually reversible. Renal failure with small shrunken kidneys may be due to analgesic nephropathy with necrosis and even sloughing of renal papillae

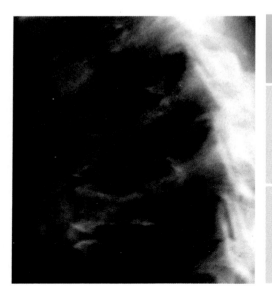

POSSIBLE CAUSES OF
VERTEBRAL WEDGING
RELATED TO RA

OSTEOPOROSIS

Active Rheumatoid Disease
Steroid Therapy
Inactivity

OSTEOMALACIA

Dietary Deficiency
Immobility causing
lack of sun exposure

Fig. 7.41 Radiograph showing vertebral wedging occurring at multiple sites in the dorsal spine. Causative mechanisms are listed.

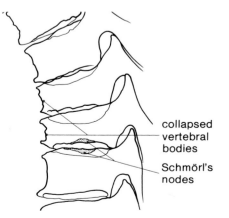

collapsed
vertebral
bodies

Schmörl's
nodes

producing a characteristic picture in the gross specimen (Fig. 7.43). Amyloidosis presents with chronic renal failure or with a nephrotic syndrome. A renal biopsy may show involvement of glomeruli (Fig. 7.44) and other areas of the kidney. Renal involvement is the most serious aspect of amyloidosis in the majority of cases; nevertheless amyloid is deposited widely throughout the tissues. Rectal biopsy is a safer way to establish the diagnosis and gives a high diagnostic yield (Fig. 7.44). In a few cases the clinical presentation may relate to amyloid deposition in the gastrointestinal tract resulting in diarrhoea and malabsorption.

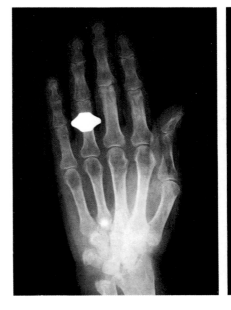

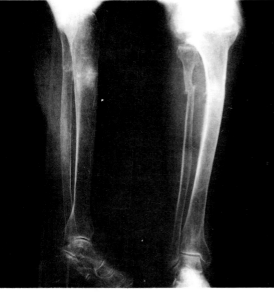

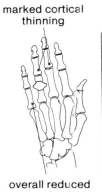

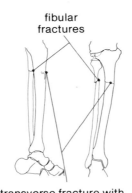

Fig. 7.42 Radiographs showing severe osteopenia in the hand with marked thinning of the cortical bone (left) and a non-displaced fracture of the tibia and fibula (right) due to osteomalacia in a rheumatoid patient.

marked cortical thinning   fibular fractures

overall reduced bone density   transverse fracture with slight valgus angulation

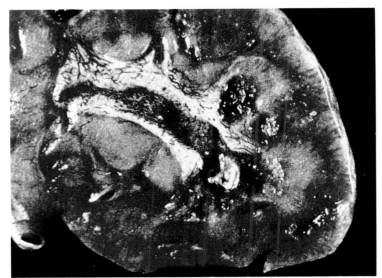

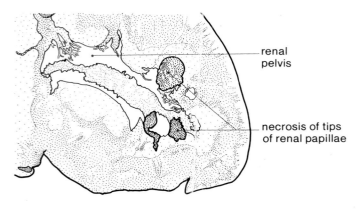

Fig. 7.43 Gross anatomy of the cut surface of the kidney at post mortem in a patient with analgesic nephropathy showing necrosis of several of the renal papilli.

renal pelvis

necrosis of tips of renal papillae

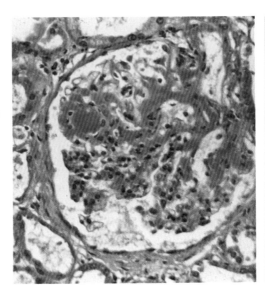

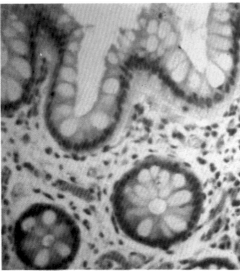

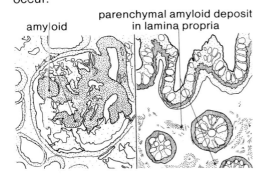

Fig. 7.44 Reactive amyloidosis. Glomeruli deposition (left, Methyl Violet, x 900) and a rectal biopsy showing the amorphous pink-staining amyloid deposits in the lamina propria (right, Sirius Red stain, x 1000). Both mucosal and vascular deposition may occur.

amyloid   parenchymal amyloid deposit in lamina propria

7.13

Secondary Sjögren's or the sicca syndrome is another associated manifestation of rheumatoid disease. This may present with enlargement of the salivary glands, most obviously of the parotid gland; clinically this gives rise to a dry mouth although the patients may not complain of this (Fig. 7.45). Biopsy of one of the minor salivary glands of the lip can establish the diagnosis by showing the characteristic lymphocytic infiltration of the glands (Fig. 7.46). Sialography shows a characteristic pattern of duct abnormality with strictures and dilated central ducts. More important manifestations of the sicca syndrome occur in the eye, although again dry eyes may not give rise to clinical complaints even when severe. The degree of lacrimal gland involvement may be crudely assessed by insertion of standardized filter paper as in the Schirmer test. The extent of the resultant keratitis may be easily demonstrated by the insertion of Rose Bengal or fluorescein into the conjunctival sac (Fig. 7.47).

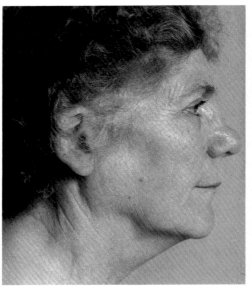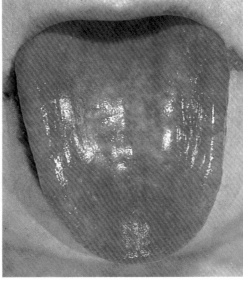

Fig. 7.45 A rheumatoid patient showing parotid enlargement with secondary Sjögren's syndrome (left) and the dry tongue with mucosal atrophy (right).

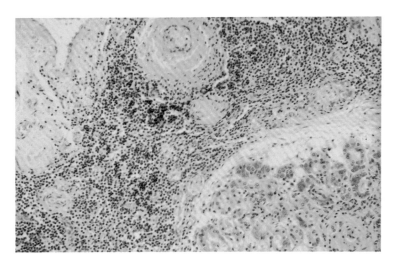

Fig. 7.46 Histological appearance of one of the minor salivary glands in the sicca syndrome showing lymphocytic infiltration and glandular destruction. H & E stain, x 680.

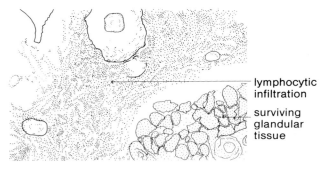

lymphocytic infiltration

surviving glandular tissue

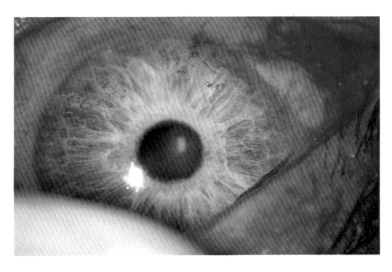

Fig. 7.47 Keratitis in a patient with sicca syndrome demonstrated by Rose Bengal staining. Courtesy of Mr. Paul A. Hunter.

8

Systemic Lupus Erythematosus

with Drs. John H. Klippel
and Joseph D. Croft Jr.

Systemic lupus erythematosus is an uncommon, serious idiopathic disease characterized by acute and chronic inflammation which can involve many organs. It is often relapsing and can lead to chronic pathology. There is a significant morbidity and a diminishing but still important mortality. The disease occurs predominantly in females in the reproductive years with a predilection for black and certain other races. Patients of any age or either sex may be affected. Genetic factors may be important in the disease and studies of monozygotic twins have demonstrated a very high frequency of disease concordance (Fig. 8.1). Family studies have found clinical or more often serological abnormalities suggestive of lupus in about 10% of the relatives of lupus patients. In many families these would appear to be associated with the histocompatibility markers HLA-DR2 and DR3 (Fig. 8.2).

Environmental factors such as sunlight, infection and stress can trigger flares in established disease. Whether such factors may initiate lupus *de novo* in genetically predisposed people awaits further research.

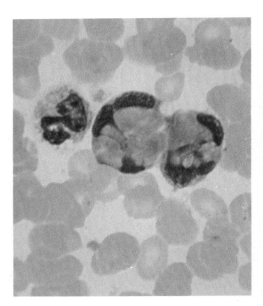

Fig. 8.1 Facial lesions in twins highlighting the importance of genetic factors in disease pathogenesis. Courtesy of Dr. R. Klofkorn.

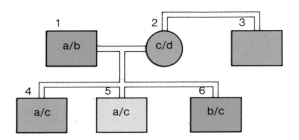

HLA haplotype			
	A	B	DR
a =	30	51	2
b =	11	35	4
c =	1	37	3
d =	3	7	2

Fig. 8.2 Family chart in SLE. Studies of families with multiple cases of SLE (patients 2, 3, 4) often identify patients with subclinical serologic abnormalities suggestive of lupus (patient 5). These studies reveal evidence of inheritence of disease susceptibility with HLA-D region genetic markers, in this case DR 2/3.

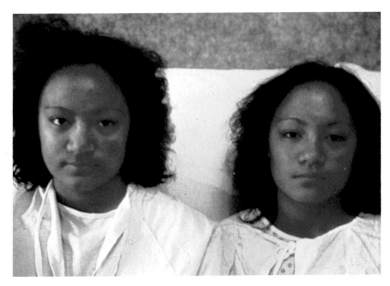

Fig. 8.3 The LE cell. The LE cell is produced *in vitro* by the phagocytosis by neutrophils of nuclear fragments reactive with anti-nuclear antibodies. *In vivo* LE cells may form in bone marrow, synovial, pleurocardial or cerebro-spinal fluid. Courtesy of Professor I.M. Roitt.

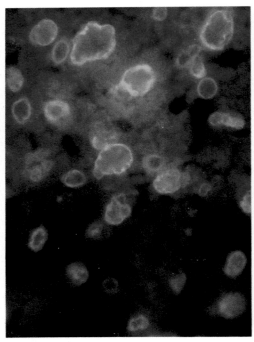
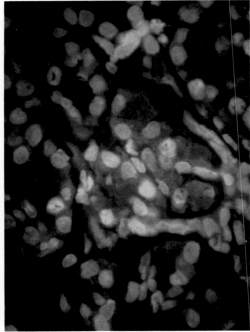

Fig. 8.4 Patterns of anti-nuclear antibody immunofluorescence produced by antibodies of different specificities. Rim or peripheral pattern (left) and diffuse or homogenous pattern (right). Courtesy of Dr. N. Rothfield.

Immunology

The ready detection of numerous antibodies to cellular components of the nucleus, cytoplasm and cell membrane has led to the concept that lupus is an autoimmune disease. The major immune response appears to be directed against nuclear antigens. These anti-nuclear antibodies are responsible for the LE cells and immuno-fluorescence on tissue sections (Figs. 8.3 & 8.4). Tests for anti-nuclear factors are extremely valuable in establishing the diagnosis as they are positive in over 90% of patients but they are not specific. Serum antibodies to one nuclear antigen, deoxyribonucleic acid (DNA), are more disease specific. They can be measured directly by several techniques. Antibodies to native (double-stranded) DNA can be quantitated using indirect immunofluorescent assay using the protozoa *Crithidia luciliae* (Fig. 8.5). This test is often used in conjunction with other immunological studies such as levels of serum complement in the serial assessment of disease activity (Fig. 8.6). When DNA antibodies complex with nuclear antigens and are deposited within tissues, an immune-mediated inflammatory reaction may result. There is evidence of serum as well as tissue-fixed complexes containing nuclear antigen and anti-nuclear antibodies (Fig. 8.7).

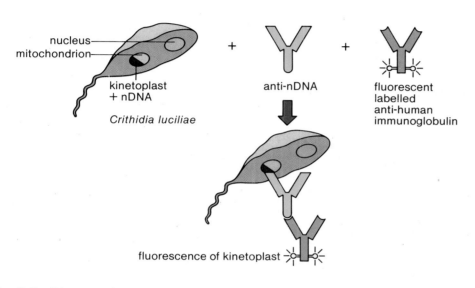

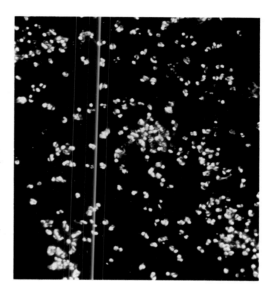

Fig. 8.5 Diagram showing the method of quantifying anti-nDNA antibodies (left). A positive test for anti-nDNA using the *Crithidia luciliae* technique (right). Courtesy of Dr. P. Maddison.

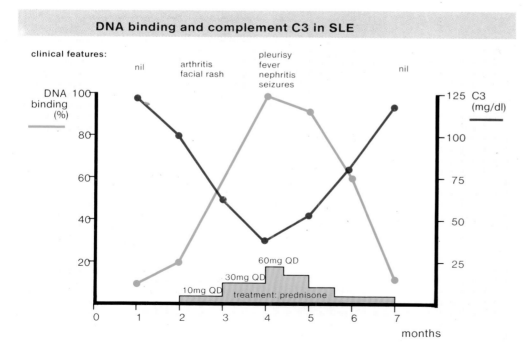

Fig. 8.6 A graph showing the levels of DNA binding and complement C3 in SLE. Rising serum titers of antibodies to DNA and falling levels of complement proteins often precede a flare in clinical lupus activity.

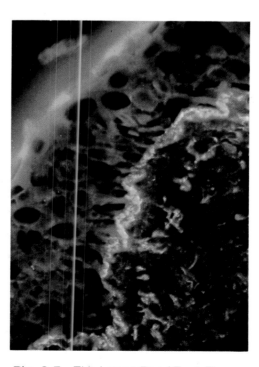

Fig. 8.7 The Lupus Band Test. The green band of IgG at the dermal-epidermal junction is the characteristic finding.

Symptomatology

The symptomatology of SLE is highly varied. Non-specific constitutional sysmptoms such as fatigue, anorexia, weight loss and fever are common and typically accompany periods of active disease and flares. Although the severity of involvement of a single organ system may dominate the clinical presentation at any one time, variable involvement of multiple organs becomes apparent as the disease progresses. Over 90% of patients experience rashes or joint complaints during the course of the disease. Inflammation of serosal surfaces and renal or CNS disease all show a lower frequency but carry a more serious prognosis. Typical figures for the percentage involvement of different organs at the presentation and during the course of the disease are tabulated in figures 8.8 and 8.9.

Skin and Mucous Membranes

The spectrum of skin manifestations of lupus is immense as virtually any layer of the skin from epidermis to subcutaneous fat can be affected. The two types of rash regarded as characteristic are the erythematous maculopapular eruption and the discoid lesion. The erythematous variety frequently develops on the bridge of the nose and malar eminences leading to the well-known 'butterfly rash' (Fig. 8.10). The rash frequently follows sun exposure and resolves without scarring or pigmentary changes. More diffuse erythematous rashes develop on the face and in other sun exposed areas such as the arms, neck and upper trunk (Fig. 8.11). Discoid lesions begin as erythematous maculopapular eruptions which progress through stages of induration, hyperkeratosis, follicular dilatation and then atrophy with scarring. The central portions of the lesions become

CLINICAL FEATURES ON PRESENTATION IN SLE	
Arthritis or arthralgia	55%
Skin involvement	20%
Nephritis	5%
Fever	5%
Other	15%

Fig. 8.8 Incidence of clinical features on presentation in SLE.

ORGAN INVOLVEMENT IN SLE	
Joints	90%
Skin	
– rashes	70%
– discoid lesions	30%
– alopecia	40%
Pleuropericardium	60%
Kidney	50%
Raynaud's	20%
Mucous membranes	15%
CNS (psychosis/convulsions)	15%

Fig. 8.9 Organ involvement during the course of disease.

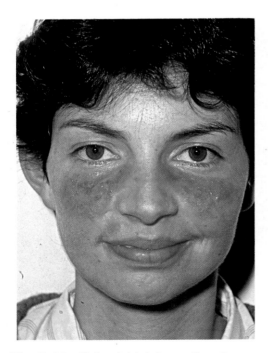

Fig. 8.10 Raised, blotchy erythematous eruption over the bridge of the nose extending over malar regions ('butterfly rash').

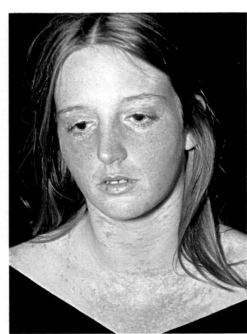

Fig. 8.11 Diffuse erythematous rash.

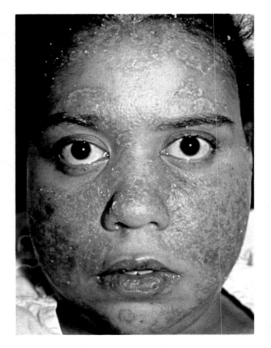

Fig. 8.12 Discoid lesions on the face with a central, atrophic hypopigmented area, with telangiectasia and adherent scale. The expanding margins reveal active inflammation with erythema, induration and increased pigmentation.

depressed with loss of pigment but the expanding peripheral portions become more active; these areas are often raised and hyperpigmented. Typical locations for discoid lesions include the face, scalp, ears, upper arms and sun exposed areas of the trunk (Fig. 8.12).

A vascular pathology underlies several of the cutaneous manifestations. This is particularly evident in the hands with inflammation of the nailfold capillaries, periungual infarcts (Fig. 8.13) and tender erythematous nodules in the pulp of the digits and palms (Fig. 8.14). The latter appear identical to the vasculitis described in bacterial endocarditis (Osler's nodes and Janeway lesions). Palpable purpura with normal platelet levels may develop on the upper or lower extremities. Livedo reticularis, especially in the legs, may reflect disease activity (Fig. 8.15). Vasomotor instability produces Raynaud's phenomenon (Fig. 8.16).

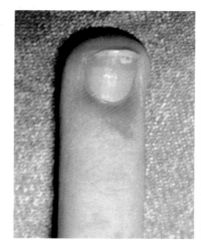
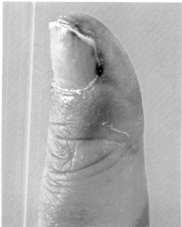

Fig. 8.13 Periungual erythema with dilatation of nailfold capillaries and cutaneous vessels (left) and infarction (right) resulting from vasculitis of small blood vessels.

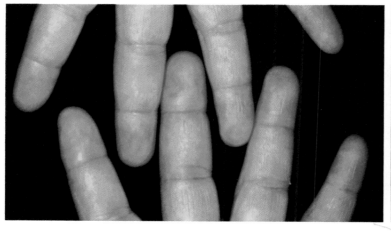

Fig. 8.14 Vasculitis of the pulp of the digits ('Osler's nodes') (left) and palm ('Janeway lesions') (right) which are painful and lead to tissue atrophy.

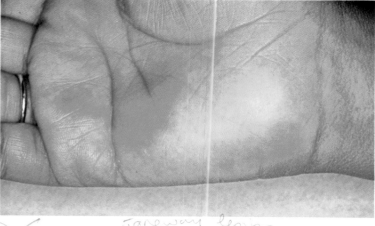

Fig. 8.15 Livedo reticularis. Courtesy of Dr. D.G.I. Scott.

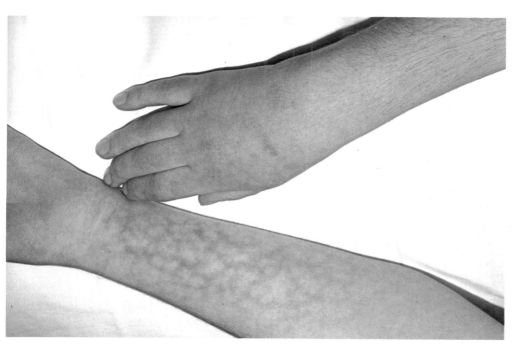

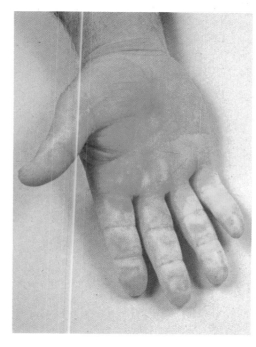

Fig. 8.16 Raynaud's phenomenon. This is often limited to a few digits and frequently occurs in SLE overlap syndromes.

In severe cases progression to digital atrophy and infarction may occur, particularly in patients with lupus overlap syndromes.

Hair loss in the absence of overt scalp inflammation may lead to diffuse or patchy alopecia (Fig. 8.17). The hair usually grows back as the activity of the disease subsides. The new hair growth may be of a different color than the original and have a brittle ragged appearance. In contrast, discoid lesions of the scalp may produce severe irreversible alopecia as a result of atrophy and loss of hair follicles (Fig. 8.18).

Mouth ulcers may also be more common in active disease. In SLE ulceration of the mucous membranes of the mouth, nose and genital mucosa is typically painless and is often detected only by careful physical examination (Fig. 8.19). Mucous membranes may also be affected by discoid types of lesion (Fig. 8.20). The denuded mucosa is particularly susceptible to secondary infection, often with *Candida spp*.

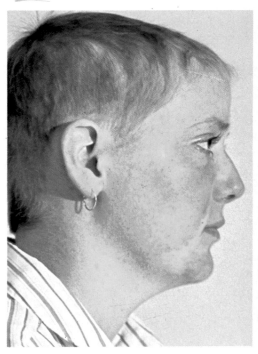 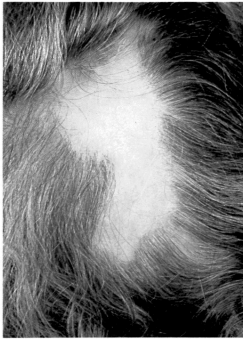 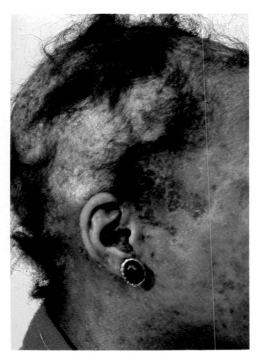

Fig. 8.17 Hair loss which may accompany disease flares leading to diffuse (left) or localized (right) alopecia.

Fig. 8.18 Scarring produced by discoid involvement of scalp leading to permanent alopecia.

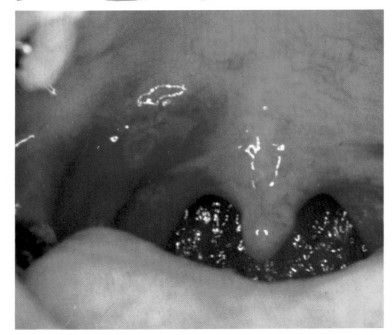 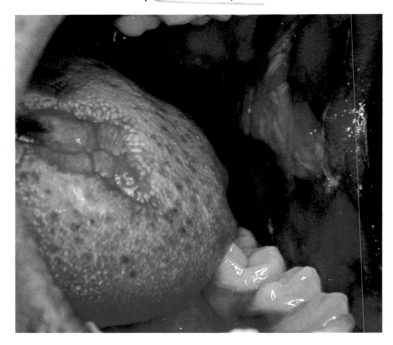

Fig. 8.19 Shallow ulceration of the palate.

Fig. 8.20 Discoid involvement of the buccal mucosa.

Joint and Bone Involvement

Arthropathies in systemic lupus erythematosus are of several types. Arthralgia, with severe pain in large joints, often occurs. The most characteristic arthritis is an acute intermittent swelling involving the entire hand or foot; it is often unilateral (Fig. 8.21). Polyarthritis commonly involves the small as well as the large joints and may be confused with rheumatoid arthritis (Fig. 8.22). There is a symmetrical distribution, morning stiffness and even occasionally small nodules (Fig. 8.23). However, on follow-up the fixed joint deformities characteristic of

rheumatoid do not usually develop. Tendon sheaths also show recurrent episodes of synovitis which in the hands results in laxity of the joint capsules and surrounding ligaments. This can lead to deformity and ulnar deviation of the metacarpophalangeal joints (Fig. 8.24) and flexion/extension abnormalities of the digits. These deformities are usually easily reducible and not associated with radiological evidence of erosion. This clinical and radiographic picture is similar to the joint disease described with chronic rheumatic fever (Jaccoud's

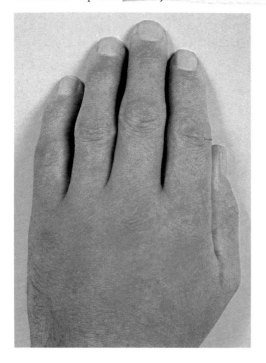

Fig. 8.21 A swollen hand in SLE.

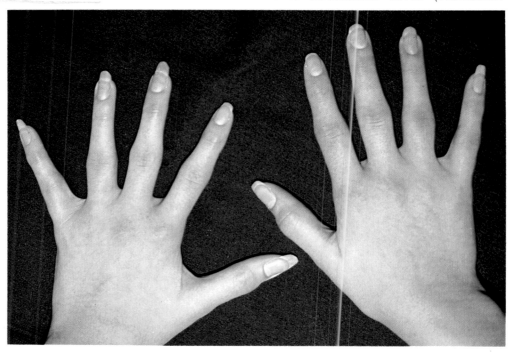

Fig. 8.22 Arthritis of the hands in SLE.

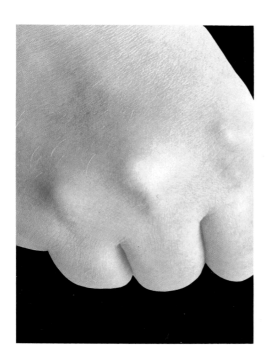

Fig. 8.23 Nodules present in a patient with SLE.

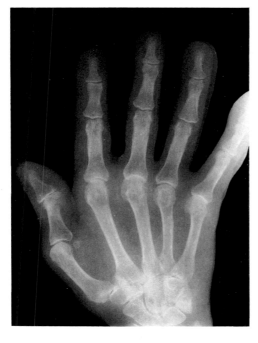

Fig. 8.24 Hand radiograph showing ulnar deviation of the metacarpophalangeal joints. There is cartilage thinning but no evidence of an erosive arthritis.

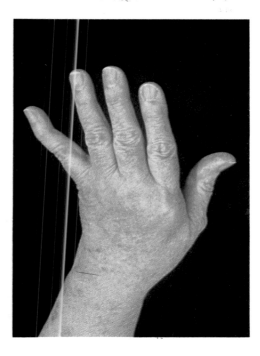

Fig. 8.25 Jaccoud's arthritis.

arthritis (Fig. 8.25). Chronic monoarthritis suggests either infection, or more likely osteonecrosis. Osteonecrosis may occur in as many as one third of lupus patients especially those on high dose steroids. It most commonly involves the head of the femur, the head of the humerus (Fig. 8.26), medial or lateral epicondyles of the distal femur (Fig. 8.27), and the superior margin of the talus. Any other bone may also be involved. Early on, in the absence of radiographic changes, suspected osteonecrosis should be evaluated by a bone scan which reveals an area of absent uptake at the site of the infarcted bone surrounded by a region of increased uptake (Fig. 8.28). If repair of the necrotic area is inadequate to support the cartilage surface, collapse and disruption of the joint surface occurs. The established lesion shows bone collapse and destruction of the joint surface which can lead to significant pain and functional impairment.

Heart and Lung Involvement

Acute inflammation of serosal surfaces leads to pleuritis, pericarditis and, rarely, peritonitis. Pleural and pericardial effusions may be quite large (Fig. 8.29). Echocardiography may demonstrate pericardial effusion in the absence of a grossly abnormal cardiac shadow on the radiograph (Fig. 8.30). Analysis of the fluid may be required to exclude infection or another etiology. The serosal effusions in lupus are sterile exudates with pH greater than 7.3 with normal levels of LDH and glucose. The cell content is variable, but can be high and occasionally LE cells are seen in the pleural fluid.

Pulmonary infiltrates with profound dyspnea may develop due to lupus involving the lung itself. A number of secondary processes, especially infection, but also congestive cardiac failure, drug toxicity or uremia may also cause dyspnea and pulmonary shadows. A careful history and physical examination and laboratory studies will usually define the cause. In difficult cases cardiac studies, pulmonary lavage or biopsy may be required. In lupus lung, intra-alveolar hemorrhage is a frequent finding. Immunofluorescent stains may reveal deposits of immunoglobulin and complement along the alveolar lining (Fig. 8.31). Similar evidence of immune-mediated damage can be found in the pulmonary arterioles and bronchioles. Elevation of both diaphragms, often with linear basal atelectasis ('shrinking lung') is another cause of dyspnea very typical of SLE (Fig. 8.32).

Cardiac involvement is of four basic types – pericarditis, endocarditis, myocarditis and coronary artery disease.

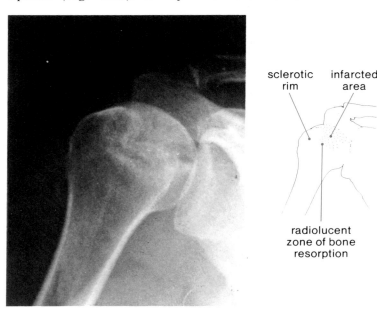

Fig. 8.26 Shoulder radiograph in avascular necrosis showing an established infarct in the humeral head. The infarcted area is bounded by a zone of radiolucency indicating bone resorption and a rim of sclerosis representing repair. There is a loose fragment of avascular bone.

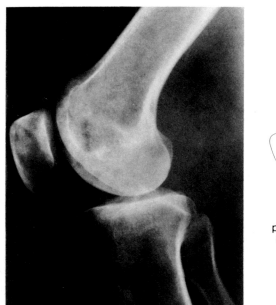
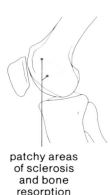

Fig. 8.27 Knee radiograph in avascular necrosis showing subtle changes in the distal femur: there is a diffuse increase in medullary sclerosis with patchy areas of bone resorption.

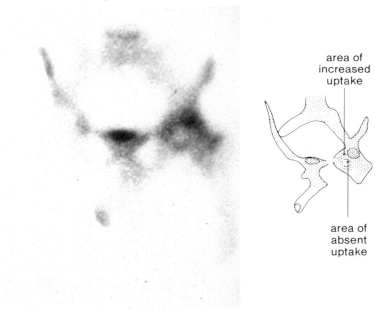

Fig. 8.28 Isotope bone scan of the pelvis showing the typical appearance of avascular necrosis. There is an area of absent uptake surrounded by an area of increased uptake.

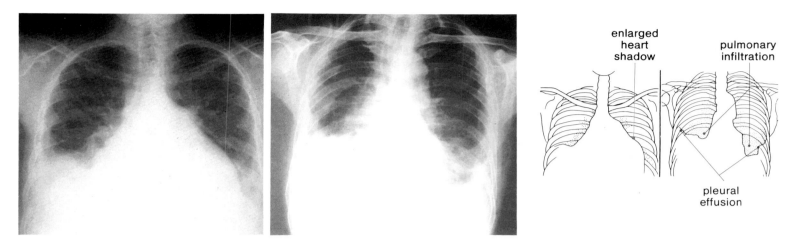

Fig. 8.29 Chest radiographs showing pericardial effusion (producing a hugely enlarged heart shadow) and pleural effusion (left) and more marked pleural effusion and pulmonary infiltration (right).

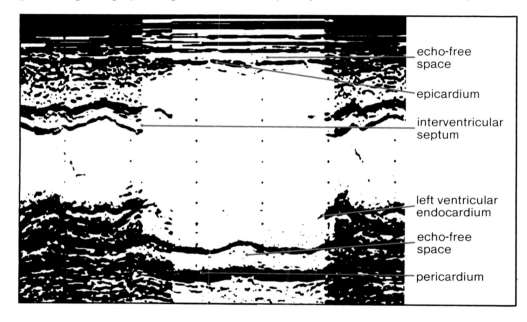

Fig. 8.30 Echocardiogram showing a pericardial effusion. There is an echo-free space both anterior to the right ventricle and posterior to the left ventricle.

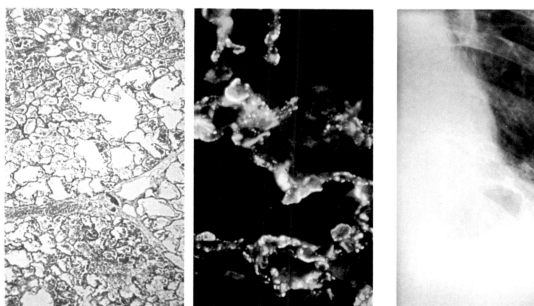

Fig. 8.31 Intra-alveolar hemorrhage (left). This process can produce hemoptysis and severe dyspnea. Immunofluorescent stains of lung tissue demonstrate immunoglobulins and complement along the alveoli (right) suggesting immune mediated damage. Courtesy of Dr. E Lewis.

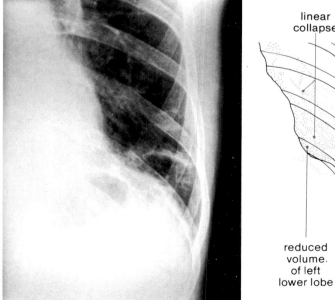

Fig. 8.32 Chest radiograph showing multiple areas of linear collapse with shrinkage of the left lower lobe.

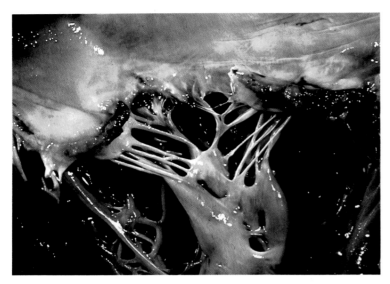

Fig. 8.33 Vegetations (Libman-Sacks endocarditis) on the cusps of the mital valve.

Vegetations on the undersurface of the mitral or aortic valve leaflets (Libman-Sacks endocarditis) can cause murmurs but rarely lead to hemodynamically significant dysfunction (Fig. 8.33). Inflammation of the myocardium may be suspected clinically by finding a resting tachycardia and evidence of congestive cardiac failure. Cardiac enzymes may be elevated and the ECG shows conduction defects and ST-T wave changes. Coronary arteritis is occasionally seen during acute flares. In late SLE occlusive disease of major coronary arteries is increasingly recognized (Fig. 8.34). The relationship between corticosteroids, vasculitis, hypertension and these arteriosclerotic changes has not been clearly defined. Complications arising from these changes are important causes of morbidity.

Lupus Nephritis

Clinically apparent nephritis develops in 40-75% of

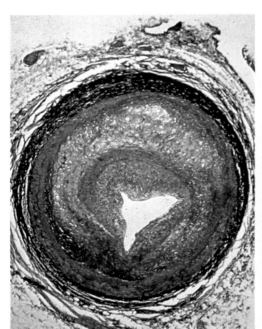

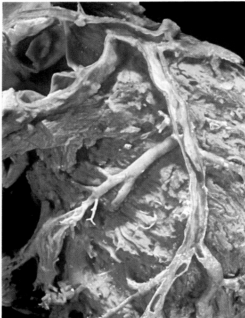

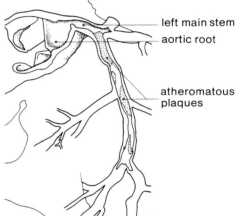

Fig. 8.34 Histology showing occlusion of the major coronary artery by atheroma (left, H&E stain). The anterior descending coronary artery showing multiple sites of obstructive arteriosclerotic disease (right, courtesy of Professor A.E. Becker).

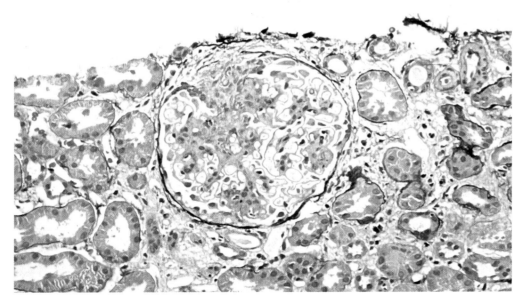

Fig. 8.35 Renal histology showing focal and mesangial proliferative glomerulonephritis with small crescents. H&E stain, x 500. Courtesy of Professor D. Brewer.

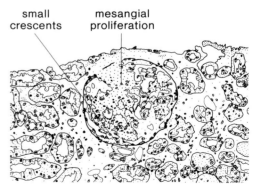

patients with SLE mostly within five years of onset and is a major cause of morbidity and mortality. Almost all patients with SLE have some glomerular abnormality on renal biopsy. Why some develop florid and progressive renal disease and others do not remains unclear. Despite abundant evidence that many of the lesions of lupus nephritis are a result of the glomerular localization of immune complexes, attempts to correlate the development of the different types of lupus nephritis with the levels or biological properties of circulating immune complexes have been inconclusive.

The female:male sex ratio of 10:1 and the peak age of onset of lupus nephritis of 20-30 years is no different from SLE as a whole. The majority of patients present with proteinuria as the main feature, accompanied by a full nephrotic syndrome in over half. Most patients have microscopic hematuria and urinary microscopy often shows a 'telescoped' sediment containing all types of casts; hyaline, granular and red blood cell. The glomerular filtration rate is frequently depressed by the time renal disease is noticed and occasionally patients present with a rapidly progressive glomerulonephritis (Fig. 8.35).

Histologically, lupus nephritis is characterized by variation in glomerular morphology seen on light microscopy and the frequent simultaneous occurrence of extensive subendothelial, subepithelial and mesangial deposits on electron microscopy (Fig. 8.36). On immunofluorescent microscopy granular deposits of IgG (Fig. 8.37), IgA and IgM (Fig. 8.38) are regularly present and in the majority C3 and the classical component pathway proteins C1q and C4 are also found.

Although the classification of renal biopsies is difficult, this provides the best guide to the severity of nephritis. A mild mesangial proliferative glomerulonephritis is found in approximately 20% of patients. Light microscopy shows mesangial expansion and hypercellularity, and

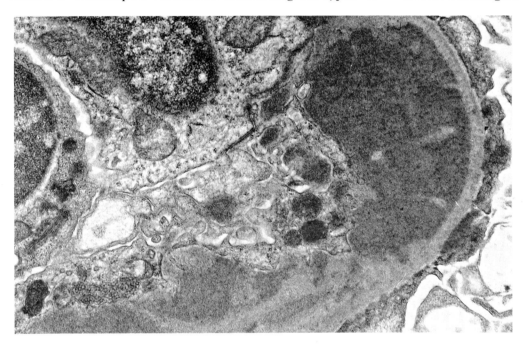

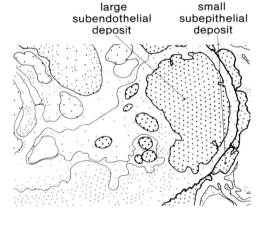

Fig. 8.36 Electron micrograph in lupus membranous glomerulonephritis showing the large subendothelial as well as small subepithelial deposits. x 20,000. Courtesy of Professor D. Brewer.

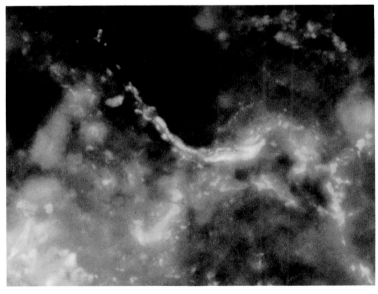

Fig. 8.37 Immunofluorescent photomicrograph showing granular deposits of IgG on the tubular basement membrane in a patient with a lupus tubulo-interstitial nephritis. Courtesy of Professor D. Brewer.

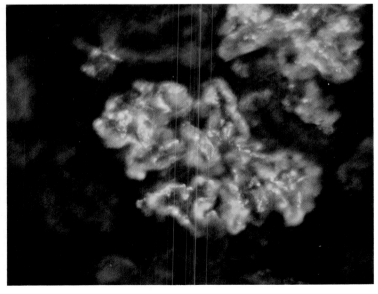

Fig. 8.38 Immunofluorescent photomicrograph showing granular deposits of IgM on capillary loops and also in the mesangium. Courtesy of Professor D. Brewer.

immune deposits can often be identified in the mesangial areas by immunofluorescent or electron microscopy. Lupus membranous nephropathy is found in some 10-15% of patients (Fig. 8.39). In addition to diffuse regular subepithelial deposits there are usually immune deposits in the mesangium and in subendothelial sites, and often mesangial or focal segmental proliferation (Fig. 8.40). These latter features are uncommon in idiopathic membranous nephropathy.

The commonest histological lesion in lupus nephritis is a proliferative glomerulonephritis found in 60-70% of cases (Figs. 8.41 & 8.42). This may be focal or segmental, affecting a minority of glomeruli and often less than half the glomerular area, or severe and diffuse. Ultrastructural studies of the diffuse proliferative lesion reveal extensive subepithelial, subendothelial and mesangial deposits. The combination of large subepithelial and subendothelial deposits in the same capillary loop produces the 'wire-loop' lesion. Extensive extracapillary proliferation (crescent formation) is common in diffuse proliferative glomerulonephritis and may be followed by a rapid deterioration of renal function. In some glomeruli an appearance indistinguishable from mesangiocapillary glomerulonephritis may be seen (Fig. 8.43). A tubulo-interstitial nephritis with immune deposits in the basement membranes of the renal tubules may be the dominant feature of the nephritis and present as tubular acidosis or aminoaciduria.

The renal histology of lupus nephritis is not static. Transformation of initially mild disease into severe progressive glomerulonephritis has been observed and the severe forms of nephritis may regress to less severe varieties following treatment with corticosteroids and immunosuppressants. The effects of treatment and the potential for histological transformation reduces the predictive accuracy of renal biopsy for prognosis.

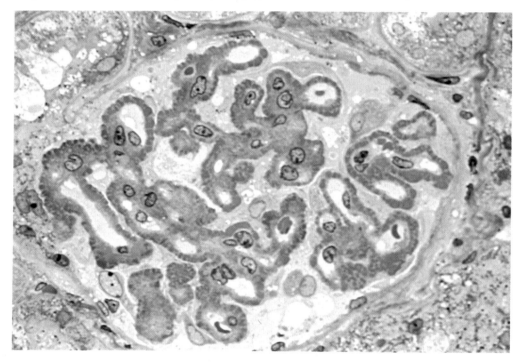

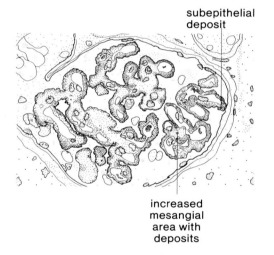

Fig. 8.39 Section stained with toluidine blue showing regular sub-epithelial and some mesangial deposits in a patient with lupus membranous glomerulonephritis. x 2,400. Courtesy of Professor D.R. Turner.

subepithelial deposit

increased mesangial area with deposits

Fig. 8.40 Histology showing focal segmental proliferative glomerulo-nephritis. H&E stain, x 500. Courtesy of Professor D. Brewer.

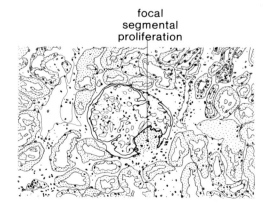

focal segmental proliferation

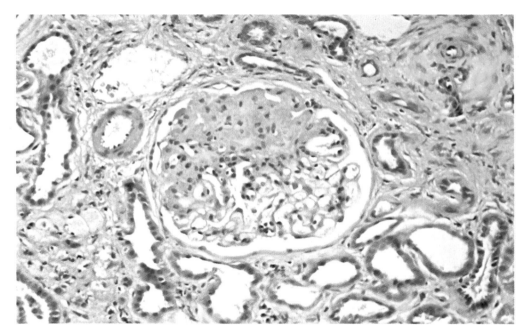

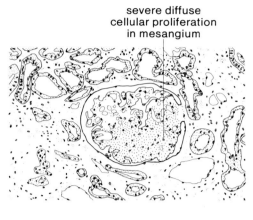

Fig. 8.41 Histology showing diffuse mesangial proliferative glomerulo-nephritis. H&E stain, x 1,250. Courtesy of Professor D. Brewer.

severe diffuse
cellular proliferation
in mesangium

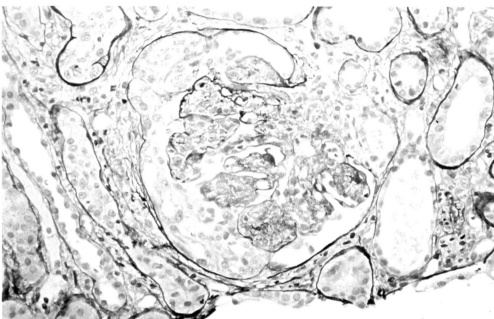

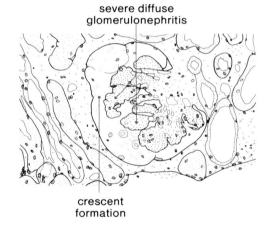

Fig. 8.42 Histology showing diffuse proliferative glomerulonephritis with extracapillary proliferation and crescent formation. PA Silver stain, x 1,250. Courtesy of Professor D. Brewer.

severe diffuse
glomerulonephritis

crescent
formation

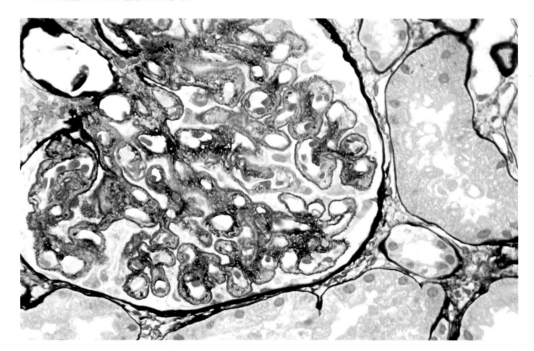

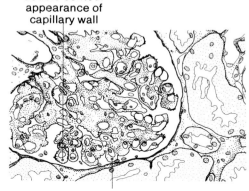

Fig. 8.43 Histology showing the mesangiocapillary pattern of lupus glomerulonephritis. Note the sub-epithelial spikes, chunky subendothelial deposits in some capillary loops and tramline appearance of some capillaries. PA Silver stain, x 2,000. Courtesy of Professor D. Brewer.

double contour
appearance of
capillary wall

subendothelial deposit

Neurological Disease

Central and peripheral nervous system involvement is another common feature of SLE which makes an important contribution to the morbidity of this disease. There is a broad spectrum of neurological manifestations (Fig. 8.44). Secondary events contributing to a neurological disorder (uremia, hypertension, infection and drug therapy) may further complicate diagnosis and treatment. Routine investigations (CSF examination, EEG, brain scan, etc) may reveal non-specific abnormalities, or be entirely normal. No single characteristic pathological lesion has been identified, although micro-infarcts are common. The diversity of manifestations are probably related to immune-mediated injury at different specific anatomical locations but the pathogenesis is not clear. Organ and non-organ psychiatric syndromes are common and are important clinical features of SLE.

Prognosis

The apparent prognosis of SLE has improved steadily over the last half century (Fig. 8.45). This is partly accounted for by the increasing recognition of milder cases of the disease. The development of renal lesions in particular affect the prognosis adversely and are an indication for more aggressive therapy (Fig. 8.46).

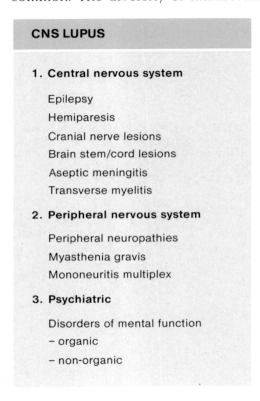

CNS LUPUS

1. **Central nervous system**

   Epilepsy
   Hemiparesis
   Cranial nerve lesions
   Brain stem/cord lesions
   Aseptic meningitis
   Transverse myelitis

2. **Peripheral nervous system**

   Peripheral neuropathies
   Myasthenia gravis
   Mononeuritis multiplex

3. **Psychiatric**

   Disorders of mental function
   – organic
   – non-organic

Fig. 8.44 Neuropsychiatric manifestations of SLE.

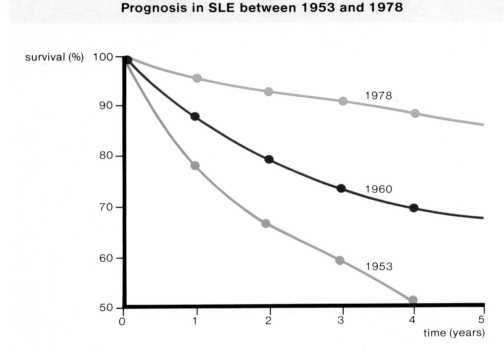

Prognosis in SLE between 1953 and 1978

Fig. 8.45 Graph showing the apparent improved prognosis in SLE between 1953 and 1978.

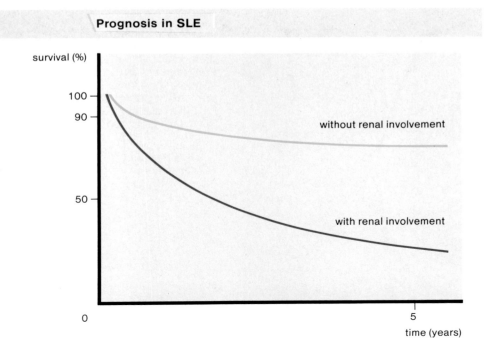

Prognosis in SLE

Fig. 8.46 Graph showing the differential prognosis in patients with and without renal involvement.

8.14

9

Systemic Lupus Erythematosus Variants

with Dr. Peter J. Maddison

A number of variants of systemic lupus erythematosus (SLE) have been described which may differ in clinical manifestations, serology and prognosis. These important subsets may not be recognized by rheumatologists. They often present to dermatologists, and the usual serological screening tests may be negative.

VARIANTS CHARACTERIZED BY CUTANEOUS MANIFESTATIONS
Discoid Lupus
Chronic discoid cutaneous lupus has for a long time been distinguished from SLE. In fact, the distinction between discoid lupus erythematosus (DLE) and SLE is arbitrary and controversial, and many physicians view DLE as a part of the spectrum of lupus erythematosus in which the lupus process is confined to the skin with few or no systemic lupus signs and symptoms.

The discoid lupus lesion starts as a circumscribed indurated erythematous plaque which develops a central area of hyperkeratosis, follicular plugging and atrophy. Plaques generally occur on the face, behind the ears and on the scalp but may be widespread (Figs. 9.1–9.5).

The histological picture is characterized by epidermal atrophy, liquefaction degeneration of the basal layer of the epidermis and a mononuclear cell infiltrate (Fig. 9.6). Direct immunofluorescence of the lesion demonstrates granular deposition of immunoglobulin and complement at the dermo-epidermal junction (Fig. 9.7) but in contrast to SLE, immunofluorescence of uninvolved skin is negative (ie. the lupus band test is negative).

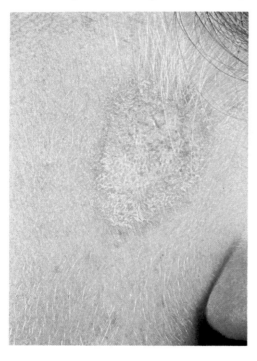
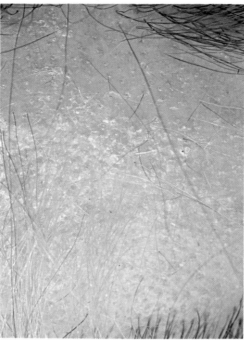

Fig. 9.1 Early discoid lupus lesion on the side of the face.

Fig. 9.2 Chronic discoid scalp lesion showing atrophy with hair loss and follicular plugging (left) and a lesion in a negro showing depigmentation (right).

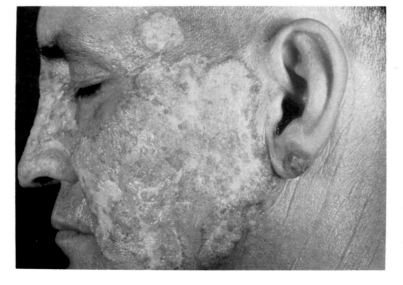
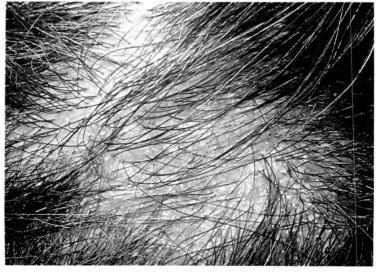

Fig. 9.3 Widespread chronic discoid lupus lesions on the face and neck demonstrating hyperkeratosis.

Fig. 9.4 Early discoid lesion on the scalp.

9.2

The lesions of DLE may be photosensitive, and mucous membrane lesions may occur (Figs. 9.8 & 9.9). A small percentage of patients with DLE subsequently develop features of SLE, but most have a low incidence of systemic complications, and autoantibodies characteristic of SLE (especially antibodies to native DNA) are absent.

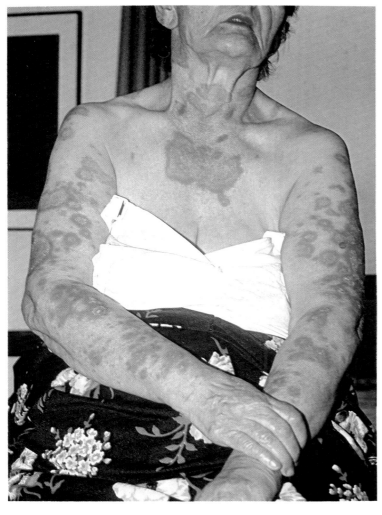

Fig. 9.5 Multiple discoid lupus lesions on the arms.

Fig. 9.6 The histological appearance of discoid lupus showing epidermal atrophy, liquefaction degeneration of the basal layer of the epidermis and a mononuclear cell infiltrate. H&E stain, x 300.

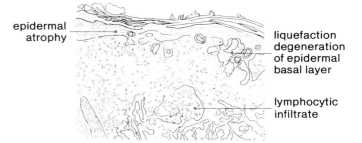

epidermal atrophy

liquefaction degeneration of epidermal basal layer

lymphocytic infiltrate

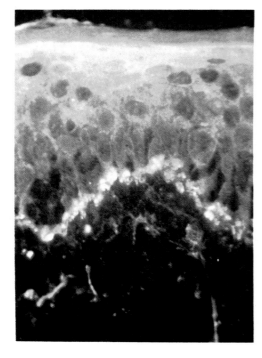

Fig. 9.7 Direct immunofluorescence of a discoid lesion showing granular deposition of IgG at the dermo-epidermal junction.

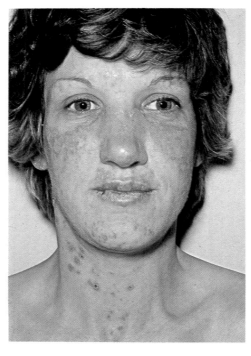

Fig. 9.8 Photosensitive discoid lupus lesion in sun-exposed areas.

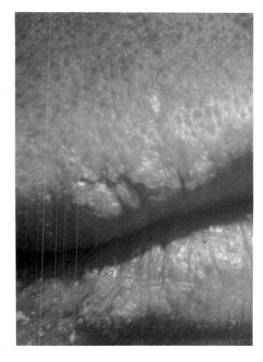

Fig. 9.9 Discoid lupus lesions involving the mucous membranes of the lips.

Perniotic Lupus

Perniotic lupus describes infiltrated lesions on the ends of the fingers or nose (Fig. 9.10). Early on these lesions resemble chilblains and are aggravated by cold but later they become obvious discoid lupus lesions. This entity is quite distinct from lupus pernio of Besnier which is due to the tubercle bacillus.

Subacute Cutaneous Lupus Erythematosus

Subacute cutaneous lupus erythematosus (SCLE) identifies a subset of lupus patients with a characteristic recurring non-scarring dermatitis. These patients exhibit a wide distribution of lesions, with the face, arms and trunk being frequently affected. The lesions are often photosensitive and two morphological forms are described, annular and papulosquamous (Figs. 9.11 & 9.12). These patients often present first to a dermatologist but most have a mild systemic illness, and the majority have positive tests for anti-nuclear antibody (ANA). Serious organ involvement, however, is less frequent than in 'classical' SLE, and patients with SCLE have a low incidence of renal disease. This may be related to the low prevalence of antibodies to DNA. These patients are characterized by the presence of antibody to the cytoplasmic ribonucleoprotein Ro(SSA), and the homogeneity of the group is further demonstrated by the majority having the B cell alloantigen HLA-DR3 (Fig. 9.13).

Lupus Profundus

The term lupus profundus applies to patients who develop soft, non-tender subcutaneous nodules, one to several centimetres in diameter, usually on the forehead, cheek or chin (Fig. 9.14). The overlying skin is often involved, either as a lesion of chronic DLE or with erythema. Histological examination reveals inflammation of the deeper parts of the corium and subcutaneous tissues. The lesions are chronic and heal with subcutaneous atrophy leaving a depressed area in the skin. These lesions may be the sole manifestation of the disease or occur in association with other features of SLE. They respond well to antimalarial drugs such as hydroxychloroquine.

Relapsing, nodular non-suppurative panniculitis is occasionally a feature of SLE and may be the presenting manifestation. Indurated tender or non-tender nodules similar to those seen in Weber-Christian disease occur, especially on the trunk and extremities. At times the overlying skin ulcerates; this heals leaving depressed scars (Fig. 9.15).

VARIANTS CHARACTERIZED BY ATYPICAL SEROLOGY

SLE is characterized by the presence of serum antibodies to a wide variety of cellular constituents. During the past two decades a great deal of progress has been made in developing tests for autoantibodies commonly associated with these diseases to aid clinical diagnosis. These tests include the detection of ANA by indirect immunofluorescence (IMF), of antibodies to native DNA (nDNA) and of antibodies to soluble cellular ribonucleoproteins including nRNP, Sm, Ro(SSA) and La(SSB) by immunodiffusion (Fig. 9.16).

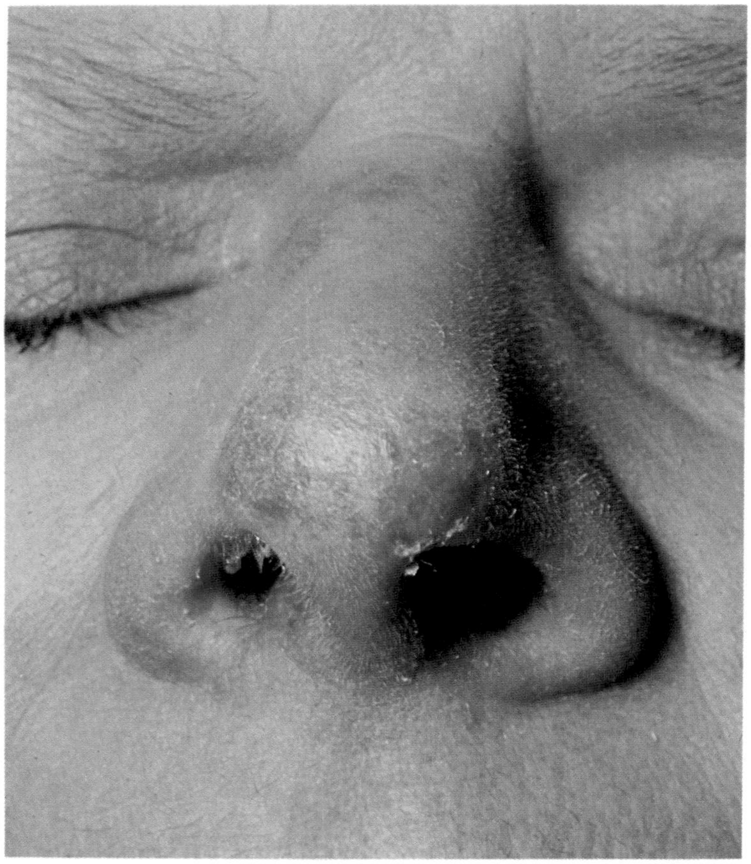

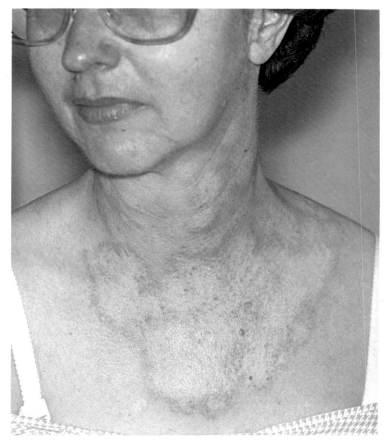

Fig. 9.10 A typical example of lupus pernio.

Fig. 9.11 Subacute cutaneous lupus erythematosus: annular variety.

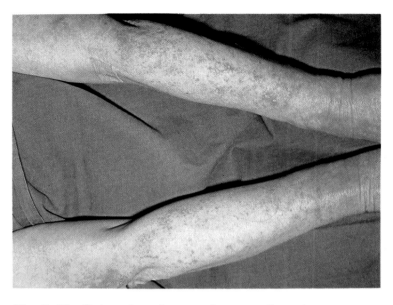

Fig. 9.12 Subacute cutaneous lupus erythematosus: papulosquamous variety.

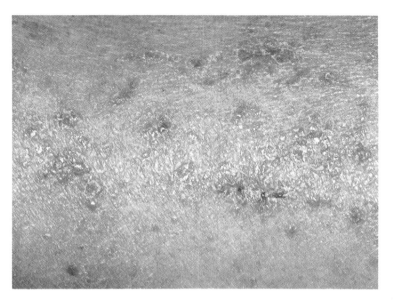

SUBACUTE CUTANEOUS LUPUS ERYTHEMATOSUS

Widespread, non-scarring
but often photosensitive rash

Annular or papulosquamous morphology

Mild systemic disease common
but renal involvement rare

Positive ANA in most patients, but anti-DNA uncommon

Antibody to Ro (SSA) in two thirds of patients

HLA-DR3 present in the majority of patients

Fig. 9.13 Clinical and laboratory features of subacute cutaneous lupus erythematosus.

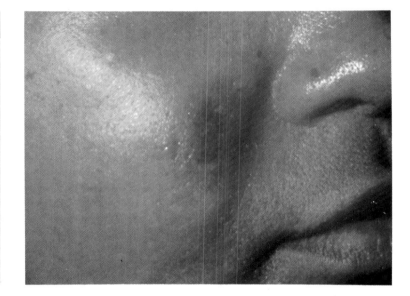

Fig. 9.14 Lupus profundus: subcutaneous nodule on the cheek with erythema of overlying skin.

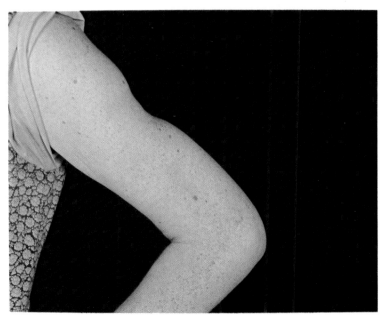

Fig. 9.15 Depressed scars left by nodular non-suppurative panniculitis.

SEROLOGICAL TESTS TO AID DIAGNOSIS OF SLE

Test	% positive in SLE
ANA by indirect immunofluorescence	95
Antibody to nDNA	60
Antibodies to soluble ribonucleoproteins by immunodiffusion	80
anti nRNP	30
anti Sm	20
anti Ro (SSA)	30
anti La (SSB)	10

Fig. 9.16 Serological tests to aid diagnosis of SLE.

ANA by Indirect Immunofluorescence

Detection of ANA by IMF is the most sensitive screening test for SLE. Approximately 95% of patients with SLE have a positive test. Four patterns of anti-nuclear staining are commonly recognized. These are homogenous, peripheral (rim), speckled and nucleolar patterns and reflect the predominant antibody species in the serum (Fig. 9.17). The peripheral pattern is related to the presence of antibody to DNA, but in fact these patterns have limited ability to predict the specificities of antibodies present in the serum.

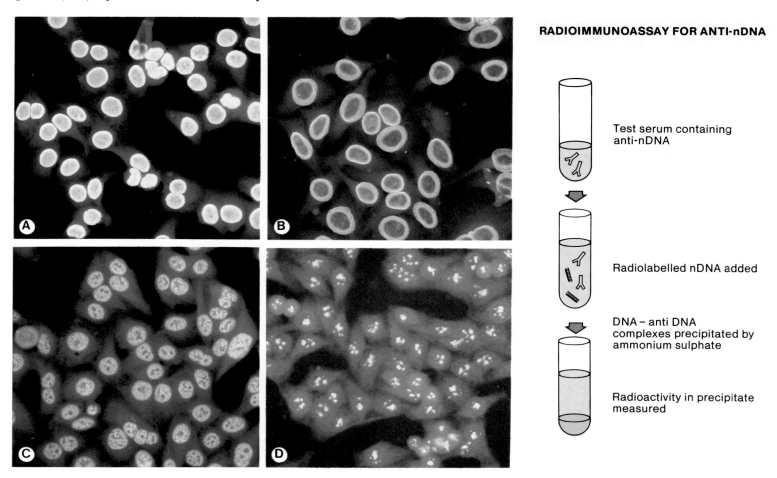

Fig. 9.17 The four common patterns of anti–nuclear staining: homogenous (A), peripheral (B), speckled (C) and nucleolar (D).

RADIOIMMUNOASSAY FOR ANTI-nDNA

Test serum containing anti-nDNA

Radiolabelled nDNA added

DNA – anti DNA complexes precipitated by ammonium sulphate

Radioactivity in precipitate measured

Fig. 9.18 Summary of the radio-immunoassay technique for demonstrating anti– nDNA.

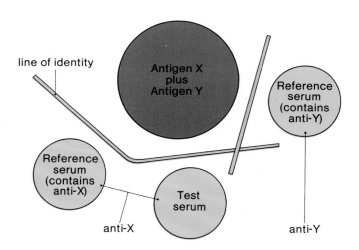

line of identity

Antigen X plus Antigen Y

Reference serum (contains anti-Y)

Reference serum (contains anti-X)

Test serum

anti-X

anti-Y

Fig. 9.19 The Ouchterlony technique of passive immunodiffusion. A test serum thought to contain anti-X or anti-Y is allowed to diffuse with reference sera against X and Y. In this case, the test serum contains anti-X and the precipitin line fuses with anti-X reference serum line, forming a line of identity. If the test and reference sera are not identical then the lines will cross.

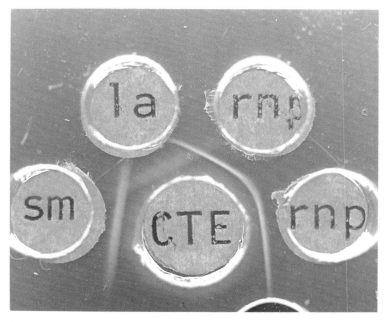

Fig. 9.20 Immunodiffusion detecting antibodies to nRNP, Sm and La(SSB). CTE is calf thymus extract.

Fig. 9.21 Some reasons for a negative IMF test for ANA in SLE.

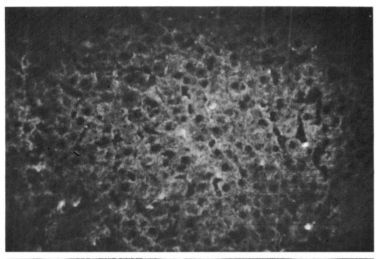

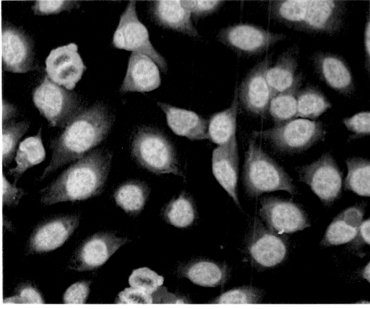

Fig. 9.22 Serum containing antibody to the nuclear ribonucleoprotein La(SSB) given a negative IMF test on mouse liver sections (upper) but a positive test on HEp-2 cells (lower).

Antibody to DNA

Antibody to nDNA is present in two-thirds of SLE patients and is rarely found in other conditions. It is generally detected by a sensitive radioimmunoassay employing ^{125}I-labelled DNA (Fig. 9.18). The test serum is incubated with radiolabelled DNA, and if anti-DNA is present complexes containing ^{125}I-labelled DNA are formed and can be separated from free DNA by techniques such as precipitation with 50% ammonium sulphate or the addition of an anti-human globulin antiserum. The radioactivity in the precipitate formed by either of these techniques is then measured in a gamma counter.

Antibody to nDNA can also be detected using the immunofluorescence technique with *Crithidia luciliae*, a hemoflagellate with a kinetoplast-containing circular (native) DNA (see 'Systemic Lupus Erythematosus'). This technique, which is simple though not so sensitive as radioimmunoassay, has the advantage of permitting the detection of complement-fixing antibodies. The presence of complement-fixing anti-DNA antibodies shows a good correlation with lupus nephritis.

Antibody to Soluble Ribonucleoproteins

Individuals with SLE make antibody to a variety of soluble nuclear and cytoplasmic constituents that can be detected by the Ouchterlony method of passive immunodiffusion (Fig. 9.19). In this technique double diffusion is performed in 0.6% agarose. Test and reference sera are allowed to diffuse against a source of antigen, usually a concentrated saline extract of mammalian tissue such as calf thymus or human spleen. The presence of antibody is indicated by a precipitin line. If the antibody systems in the test and reference serum are identical they will fuse (reaction of identity) whereas if they are not identical they will cross. This simple test system can be used to detect antibodies to nRNP, Sm, Ro(SSA) and La(SSB) (Fig. 9.20).

ANA-Negative SLE

There are occasions when the ANA test is negative in SLE (Fig. 9.21). Technical reasons include a prozone effect (when sera containing very high titres of ANA fail to produce immunofluorescence staining until sufficiently diluted), and the fact that a substrate used for the immunofluorescence test may lack the nuclear constituent in question. The La(SSB) nuclear antigen for example, is not expressed in mouse liver sections, but is expressed in human tumour cell lines such as HEp-2 cells (Fig. 9.22). Negative tests may occur in patients after prolonged treatment with corticosteroids or immunosuppressive agents, or in patients with end stage renal disease. The ANA test may be transiently negative when anti-nuclear antibodies are present but bound in the serum in the form of immune complexes, or rarely when anti-nuclear antibodies are lost through the kidney in patients with profuse proteinuria. However, it is the persistent finding of a negative test for ANA in active, untreated disease that has given rise to the concept of 'ANA-negative' SLE.

CLINICAL AND SEROLOGICAL FEATURES OF ANA-NEGATIVE SLE

Prominent photosensitive dermatitis

Rare renal and neuropsychiatric manifestations

Antibodies to Ro (SSA) in 60% of patients

Antibodies to ss DNA alone in 30% of patients

Fig. 9.23 Clinical and serological features of 'ANA-negative' SLE.

Such patients constitute approximately 5% of the lupus population. 'ANA-negative' SLE patients are characterized by a high incidence of severe photosensitive dermatitis and a lower frequency of severe lupus complications such as nephritis and neuropsychiatric disease (Figs. 9.23 & 9.24). The majority of these patients do have serological abnormalities characteristic of SLE. Antibodies to the cytoplasmic ribonucleoprotein, Ro(SSA), can be detected in the sera of two-thirds and the majority of the remainder have antibodies to single-stranded DNA (ssDNA) (Fig. 9.25). The failure of anti-ssDNA to stain the interphase nuclei of epithelial tissue in the IMF test is well known.

SLE Associated with C2 Deficiency

A lupus-like disease occurs in patients with the rare

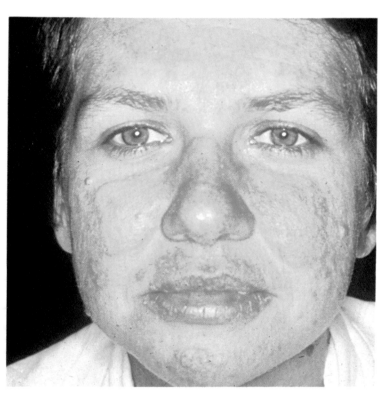

Fig. 9.24 Photosensitive facial rash in an 'ANA-negative' SLE patient.

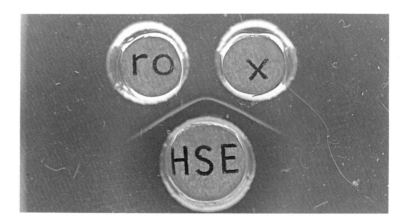

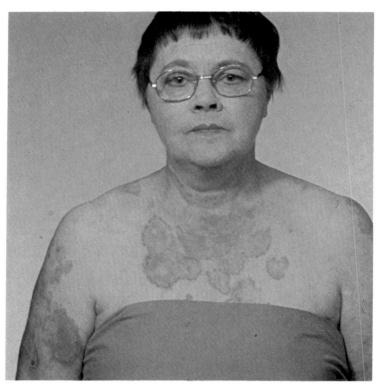

Fig. 9.26 Lupus rash in a patient with homozygous C2 deficiency.

Fig. 9.25 The serum (X) of a patient with 'ANA-negative' SLE on an immunodiffusion plate. HSE is human spleen cell extract and Ro a reference serum containing anti-Ro(SSA) antibodies. The formation of a line of identity indicates their presence in serum X.

CLINICAL AND SEROLOGICAL FEATURES OF SLE IN PATIENTS WITH C2 DEFICIENCY

Prominent cutaneous manifestations

Low frequency of lupus nephritis

ANA test often negative

Low prevalence of antibodies to nDNA

Antibodies to Ro (SSA) in the majority of patients

Fig. 9.27 Clinical and serological features of SLE in patients with C2 deficiency.

genetically-determined deficiency of the complement component C2. These patients predominantly have cutaneous manifestations with marked photosensitivity and there is a low incidence of lupus nephritis (Figs. 9.26 & 9.27). The majority of these patients have some antibodies to Ro(SSA) but there is a low titre of antibodies to nDNA and ANA is often absent. However this condition represents only a tiny proportion of 'ANA-negative' disease.

CLINICAL FEATURES OF NEONATAL SLE

The human placenta is hemochorial, that is, the syncytiotrophoblast is in direct contact with maternal blood in the intervillous spaces. IgG is transported across the placenta by specific receptors which differ from Fc receptors on other cell surfaces because they bind monomeric, uncomplexed IgG (Fig. 9.28). The placenta therefore permits transfer of IgG autoantibodies including ANA to the fetal circulation. These then disappear from the child's circulation over the next six months as the maternal IgG is degraded. The transfer of maternal ANA is usually not associated with observable effects on the baby, but occasionally newborn babies of SLE mothers develop transient features of lupus. These include photosensitive skin rashes with histological features typical of SLE (Figs. 9.29 & 9.30). The most important manifestation in the newborn is complete heart block which, unlike the rashes, generally persists and may need insertion of a pacemaker. This may be the commonest cause of congenital heart block. Babies born to mothers with subclinical disease but with antibody to Ro(SSA) in their serum appear to be more at risk of developing these manifestations.

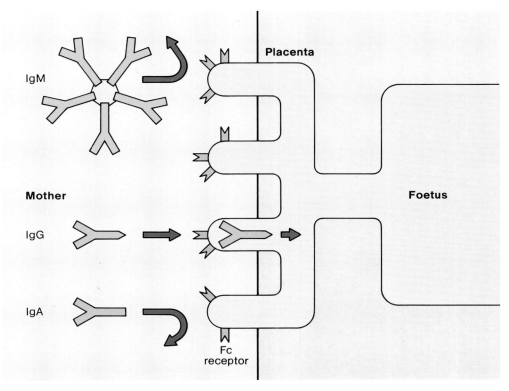

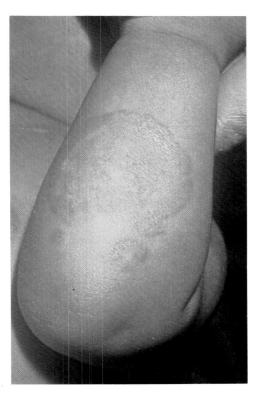

Fig. 9.28 Transport of maternal IgG across the placenta via specific Fc receptors. Antibody of the IgG class is transported in preference to other classes.

Fig. 9.29 Photosensitive rash in a neonate of an SLE mother.

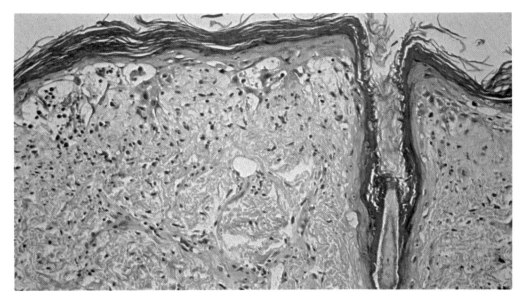

Fig. 9.30 Typical SLE histology in neonatal rash showing liquefaction degeneration of the epidermal basal layer and lymphocytic infiltration. H&E stain, x 400.

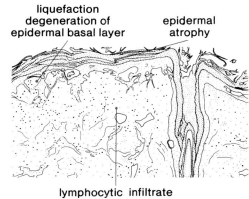

SLE IN THE ELDERLY

Approximately 15% of SLE patients develop the disease after the age of 60 years (Figs. 9.31 & 9.32). Age appears to modify the disease: with increasing age the mode of onset is more insidious and the pattern of organ involvement is different, with a greater incidence of interstitial lung disease but with much less neuropsychiatric or renal involvement.

OVERLAP SYNDROMES

The classification of connective tissue diseases depends upon identifying certain patterns of clinical and laboratory abnormalities. There is, however, considerable overlapping of these disorders and many patients do not fit into traditional diagnostic categories. In the majority there is difficulty only in the early stages of the disease when the presenting features are those common to a number of connective tissue diseases, such as fever, malaise, arthralgia, Raynaud's phenomenon and positive tests for ANA and rheumatoid factor. Usually one pattern gradually emerges. Less commonly, features of two or more diseases coexist and the mixed syndrome persists indefinitely. Commonest amongst these are disorders with features of scleroderma combined with those of SLE

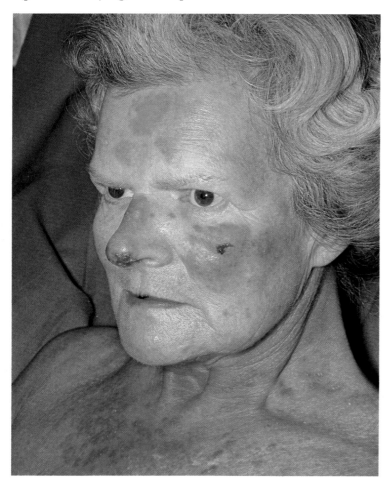

Fig. 9.31 SLE developing in an elderly woman.

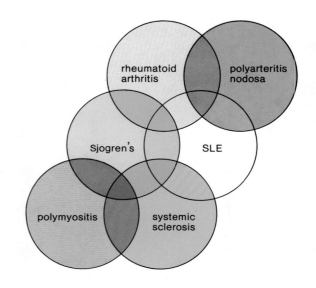

Fig. 9.33 Connective tissue disease overlaps.

SLE IN THE ELDERLY

In 15% of cases, disease begins after 60 years of age

Onset is often insidious

Age modifies pattern of organ involvement:
   interstitial lung disease is common
   neuropsychiatric and renal disease is uncommon

CLINICAL AND LABORATORY FEATURES OF MCTD

Polyarthritis

Raynaud's phenomenon

Swollen hands or sclerodactyly

Abnormal esophageal motility

Myositis

Low incidence of lupus nephritis

Hyperglobulinemia

Positive ANA (often speckled pattern)

Antibody to nRNP

Fig. 9.32 Characteristics of SLE developing in the elderly.

Fig. 9.34 Clinical and laboratory features of MCTD.

and of polymyositis, or of rheumatoid arthritis associated with those of SLE (Fig. 9.33). A proportion of patients with overlap syndromes are characterized by the presence of high titres of serum antibodies to nRNP. These patients have been designated as having mixed connective tissue disease (MCTD).

Mixed Connective Tissue Disease

Clinical and laboratory features commonly described in MCTD are shown in figure 9.34. Most reported cases are women with a mean age of onset in the fourth decade. It occurs in children, and childhood disease appears to be more severe with more renal, cardiac and hematological complications.

The clinical picture is variable, especially at the start. Usually patients present with an 'SLE-like' picture in which non-deforming arthritis, erythematous rashes, serositis and fever are present (Fig. 9.35).

Raynaud's phenomenon is prominent, often precedes other manifestations by months or years and is sometimes severe (Figs. 9.36 & 9.37). Skin manifestations of SLE are frequently seen but many patients also develop 'scleroderma-like' features such as swollen fingers or sclerodactyly (Figs. 9.38 & 9.39).

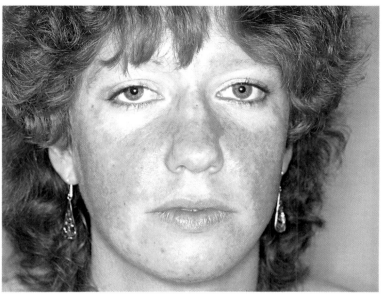
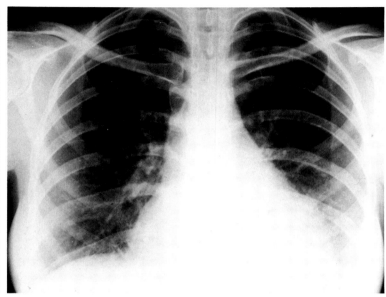

Fig. 9.35 An 'SLE' presentation of MCTD with facial rash (left) and pleuropericarditis (right).

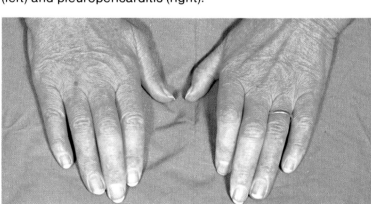
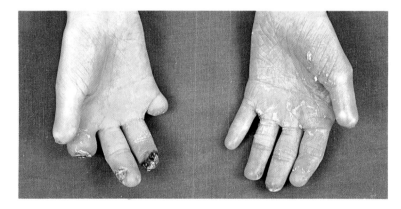

Fig. 9.36 Raynaud's phenomenon in MCTD.

Fig. 9.37 Loss of digits in a patient with MCTD.

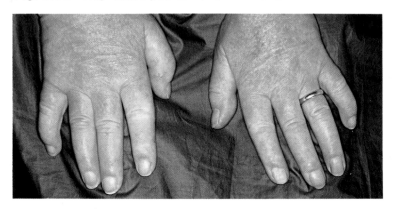
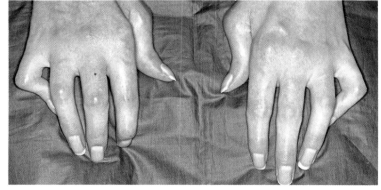

Fig. 9.38 Sausage fingers in MCTD.

Fig. 9.39 Sclerodactyly in MCTD.

Abnormal esophageal motility is common (Fig. 9.40) and interstitial pulmonary fibrosis may occur (Fig. 9.41), but diffuse scleroderma and serious systemic complications of systemic sclerosis affecting the intestine, heart, lung and kidney are rare. Myalgia is common, often accompanied by a moderate increase in serum levels of muscle enzymes such as creatine phosphokinase. Occasionally a severe proximal myopathy occurs and the muscle biopsy shows a typical myositic picture (Fig. 9.42).

Non-deforming polyarthritis is common but in some cases the joint disease suggests rheumatoid arthritis with subcutaneous nodules (Fig. 9.43), radiological erosions (Fig. 9.44) and positive tests for rheumatoid factor.

Laboratory characteristics include an ANA test positive in high titre, often with a speckled pattern of fluorescence, and the presence of high titres of antibodies to nRNP (Fig. 9.45), with relative absence of the typical SLE antibodies to other nuclear antigens such as native DNA.

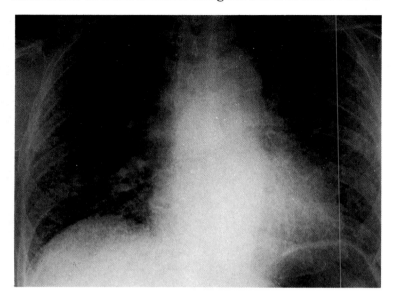

Fig. 9.41 Chest radiograph showing interstitial pulmonary fibrosis in MCTD.

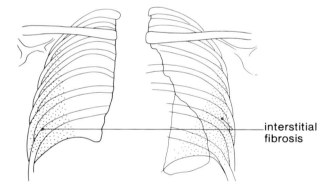

interstitial fibrosis

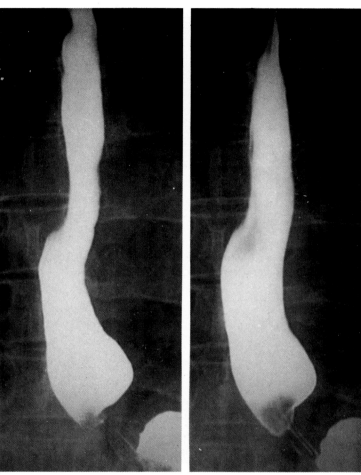

Fig. 9.40 Barium swallow showing complete lack of peristalsis in the esophagus in a patient with MCTD.

Fig. 9.42 Muscle histology in MCTD showing necrotic muscle fibers and interstitial and perivascular infiltation by lymphocytes and plasma cells in MCTD. H&E stain, x 1200.

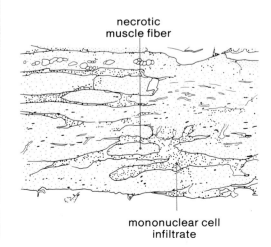

necrotic muscle fiber

mononuclear cell infiltrate

Fig. 9.43   Subcutaneous nodule in MCTD.

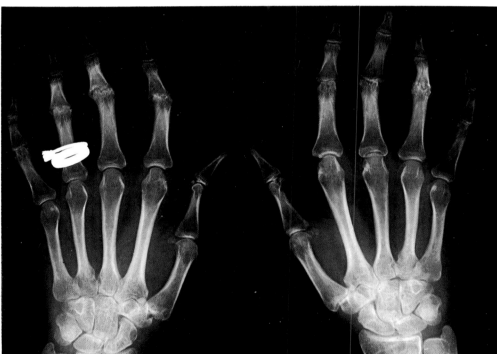

Fig. 9.44   Hand radiograph showing erosions in MCTD.

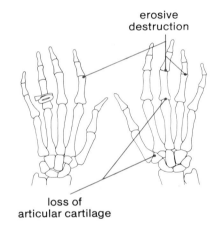

erosive
destruction

loss of
articular cartilage

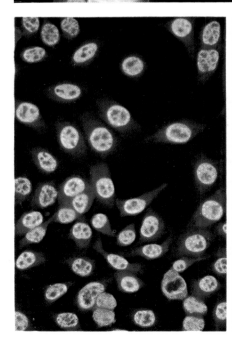

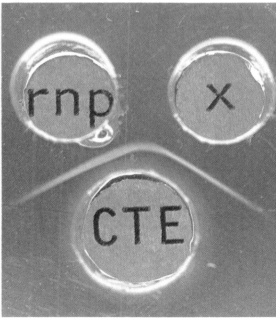

rnp

x

CTE

Fig. 9.45   A positive ANA test showing the speckled pattern of fluorescence (left) and antibody to nRNP demonstrated by immunodiffusion (right).

DRUG-INDUCED SLE

A variety of drugs may precipitate features of SLE (Fig. 9.46). Associations are best documented with procainamide and hydralazine and to a lesser extent with isoniazid and certain anticonvulsants. Anti-nuclear antibodies develop in 50 to 75% of patients taking procainamide or hydralazine in sufficient doses for 9 to 12 months. Of these, half develop clinical features. Drug-induced lupus occurs more readily in slow-acetylators and hydralazine-induced lupus shows a close association with HLA – DR4 (Fig. 9.47).

Drug-induced lupus occurs more often in the elderly and the clinical picture is similar to idiopathic lupus in this age group with prominent cutaneous, joint, pericardial, pleural and pulmonary manifestations: renal involvement is rare (Fig. 9.48).

ANA are present in high titre. These can be shown to react predominately with histones, especially the H_2 fraction. Antibodies characteristic of idiopathic lupus such as anti-native DNA and antibodies to soluble cellular antigens such as nRNP, Sm, Ro(SSA) and La(SSB) are only rarely present, and serum complement levels usually remain normal.

Discontinuation of the offending drug usually results in rapid resolution of the symptoms, although ANA may persist for several months.

CONCLUSION

These variants of lupus enlarge the concept of the disease by suggesting a wide disease spectrum often with a more benign prognosis than classical SLE. The association of more benign clinical variants with different autoantibodies in the absence of antibodies to native DNA, with complement deficiencies, or with HLA markers, may help unravel the complex etiopathology of multisystem SLE.

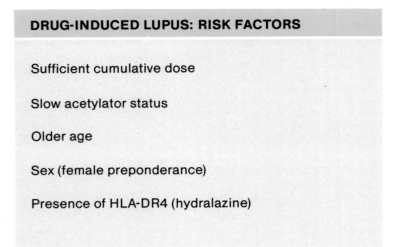

DRUG-INDUCED LUPUS: RISK FACTORS

Sufficient cumulative dose

Slow acetylator status

Older age

Sex (female preponderance)

Presence of HLA-DR4 (hydralazine)

Fig. 9.47 Risk factors in drug-induced lupus.

DRUG-INDUCED LUPUS

Frequent Association

Procainamide	Anticonvulsants
Hydralazine	Chlorpromazine
Isoniazid	

Rare Association

Oral contraceptive	Prazosin
Chlorthalidone	Propylthiouracil
Griseofulvin	Quinidine
Levodopa	Reserpine
Methyldopa	Streptomycin
Methysergide	Sulphonamides
Penicillin	Tetraclyline
Pencillamine	

DRUG-INDUCED LUPUS: CLINICAL FEATURES

COMMON

Polyarthritis

Rash

Pleurisy/pericarditis

Pulmonary infiltrates

High titre ANA (mainly to histones)

Resolution when drug stopped

RARE

Renal and neuropsychiatric disease

Anti-nDNA

Low serum complement levels

Fig. 9.46 Some drugs which may induce a lupus syndrome.

Fig. 9.48 Clinical features of drug-induced lupus.

10

Scleroderma, Dermatomyositis and Polymyositis

with Dr. Carol M. Black

SCLERODERMA

Scleroderma is an uncommon generalized connective tissue disease of unknown etiology and pathogenesis. Its clinical variants range from the self-limiting and localized to the progressive and intractable forms. It is characterized by hardening of the skin: there is excessive deposition of collagen in both the skin and internal organs. Vascular changes occur and involve the microvessels and small arteries. The relationship between the fibrosis and the vascular abnormalities remains to be determined. Raynaud's phenomenon also occurs in 80 to 90% of patients.

Scleroderma is distributed widely both geographically and racially. The peak onset is in the third to fifth decades. Females predominate over males three to one and in the child-bearing years ten to one. Five year survival varies from one-third to two-thirds of patients. The poor prognosis is related to age, race and cardiopulmonary and kidney diseases.

The increasing number of familial cases reported suggests that genetic and environmental factors may be important in the etiology. Chromosomal abnormalities have been reported together with a weak association with certain HLA antigens.

Environmental toxins such as polyvinyl chloride and 'Spanish oil' may induce fibrosis or a scleroderma-like syndrome in people with a similar genetic background (Fig. 10.1).

Classification of Scleroderma

Classification is difficult because of clinical diversity and the similarity of changes seen in many other disorders. The main distinction is between disease without systemic involvement (localized) and that with such involvement (systemic sclerosis) (Fig. 10.2).

Scleroderma occurring in childhood shows a variable cutaneous picture but systemic involvement is rare. Tendon contractures and subcutaneous nodules are frequent (Fig. 10.3). Linear scleroderma is common and may involve subcutaneous tissue, muscle and even bone (Fig. 10.4).

Pathology of Scleroderma

The pathological changes in scleroderma occur in skin, internal organs and blood vessels. The sequential changes of inflammation, fibrosis and atrophy are most common in the skin (Figs. 10.5 & 10.6), but occur to a lesser extent in the gut, heart, lungs and kidneys.

Characteristic features of the vascular lesion are concentric proliferation and thickening of the intima with little change in the media and fibrosis of the adventitia (Fig. 10.7). Basement membrane thickening is also common.

SCLERODERMA

An uncommon idiopathic disease

Peak onset 20–50

Female : male 3:1

Predisposing factors include:

Genetic
HLA – A₁, B₈, DR₃, DR₅

Environmental:
chemical agents
eg. vinyl chloride, rape seed oil
drugs eg. pentazocine, bleomycin

Fig. 10.1 Some features and predisposing factors in scleroderma.

CLASSIFICATION OF SCLERODERMA

1. Localized:
    morphea: plaque like, guttate, generalized
    linear scleroderma
    scleroderma 'en coup de sabre'
    (± facial hemiatrophy)
2. Generalized:
    with diffuse visceral involvement
    CREST syndrome
    overlap with other connective tissue disease
3. Chemical-induced scleroderma–like conditions
    eg. vinyl chloride disease
4. Diseases with skin changes mimicking scleroderma
    eg. scleredema
5. Eosinophilic fasciitis

Fig. 10.2 Classification of scleroderma.

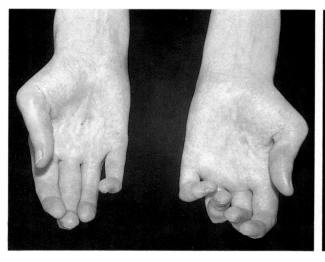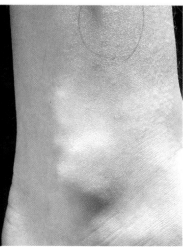

Fig. 10.3 The hands and ankle of a patient with scleroderma. Note the tight appearance of the skin and also the flexed fingers which are the result of tendon contractures (left). The ankle has several subcutaneous nodules just posterior to the malleolus (right).

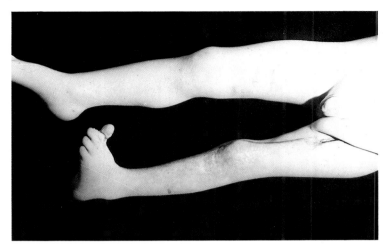

Fig. 10.4 Linear scleroderma. There is involvement of the skin and subcutaneous tissues in the left leg producing considerable contracture and deformity.

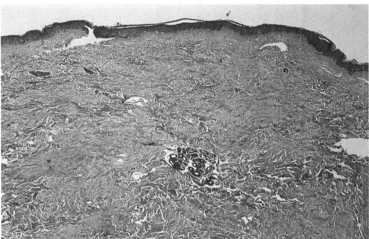

Fig. 10.5 Skin histology in scleroderma. The normal dermal-epidermal junction is replaced by collagen which surrounds the sweat glands. H&E stain, x 25. Courtesy of Dr. A.B. Price.

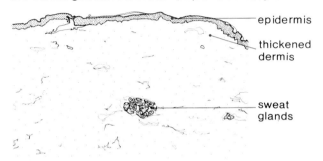

epidermis

thickened dermis

sweat glands

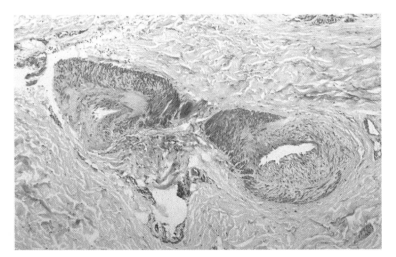

Fig. 10.6 Histology of the skin showing intimal thickening of the small arterioles. H & E stain, x 80.

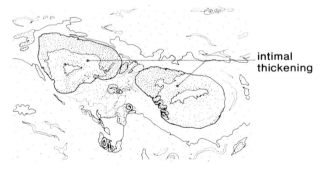

intimal thickening

Fig. 10.7 Histology of the lung in scleroderma showing arteriolar intimal thickening, alveolar destruction and degeneration of elastic tissue. Elastic stain, x 80.

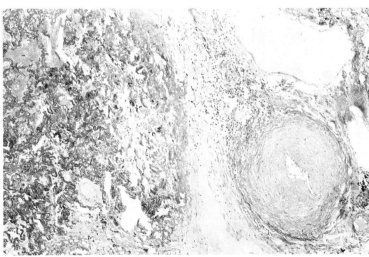

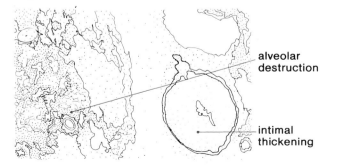

alveolar destruction

intimal thickening

These changes occur in medium-sized arteries, small arteries and arterioles throughout the body. Capillaries are also involved, most prominently at the nail fold. With a wide angle microscope they are seen to be disrupted and distorted with enlargement and dilatation of the sparse capillary loops (Fig. 10.8).

Localized Scleroderma (Morphea)

This is a disorder limited to the cutis, subcutis and muscles, occurring more frequently in females than males. The linear form, more common in childhood, includes frontoparietal lesions which can cause severe deformity (Fig. 10.9). A plaque form typically occurs in

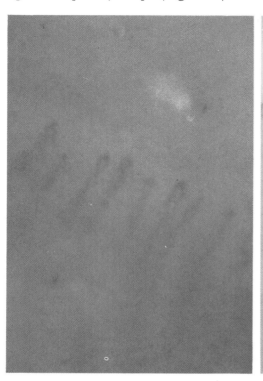 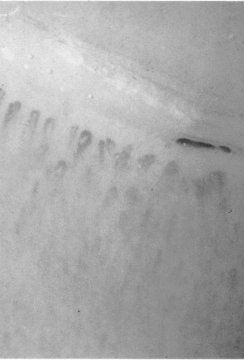 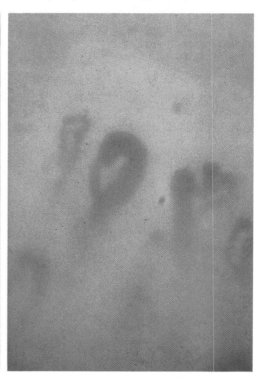

Fig. 10.8 Nail fold capillary photography. Normal regularly-formed capillary loops resembling hairpins (left). Capillary loops in scleroderma: the outlines are fainter and less regular and there is subcuticular capillary hemorrhage (middle). Another patient (right) has one large dilated loop and one of a bizarre shape. Courtesy of Dr. M.F.R. Martin.

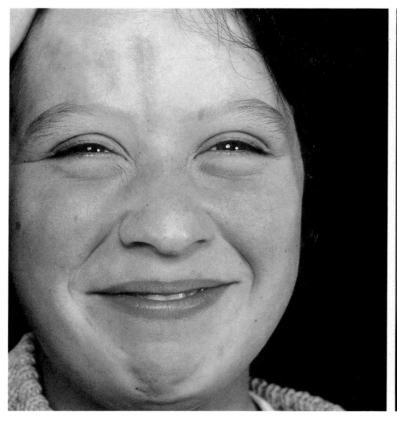 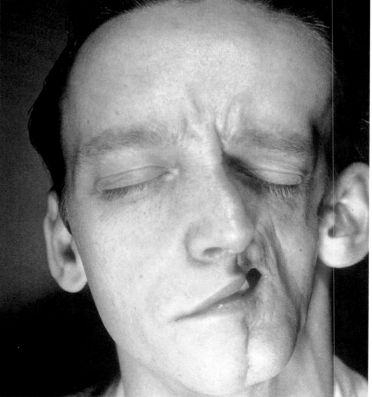

Fig. 10.9 Morphea. A patient with a linear frontal lesion at the early stage (left). Severe involvement of the left side of the face producing considerable distortion (right).

adult life (Fig. 10.10). It is usually self-limiting. The hardening of the skin in the localized forms is similar to that of systemic sclerosis but the relationship is controversial (Fig. 10.11). Raynaud's and visceral involvement are absent but transition to the systemic form may occur and antinuclear antibodies are occasionally found.

Systemic Sclerosis

Systemic sclerosis has a variable prognosis and severity with a spectrum ranging from restricted skin changes, often limited to the face and hands, to widespread cutaneous thickening with rapidly advancing visceral involvement. Attempts have been made to divide systemic sclerosis into several clinical patterns; these provide useful guides to prognosis but are not absolutely predictive. A limited scleroderma together with calcinosis, Raynaud's, esophageal involvement and telangiectasia is known as the CREST syndrome.

Cutaneous Involvement

There are three stages in the evolution of skin disease. (1) The edematous phase causes bilateral painless pitting edema of the hands and may also involve the feet, legs, arms and face.

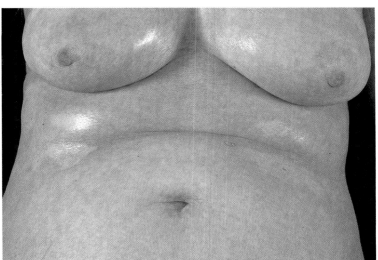

Fig. 10.10 Morphea en plaque. Confluent lesions with linear streaking (left) and well-localized pale, shiny lesions on the breasts and trunk (right).

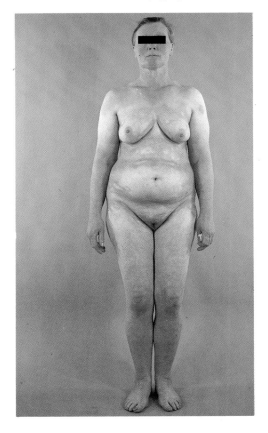

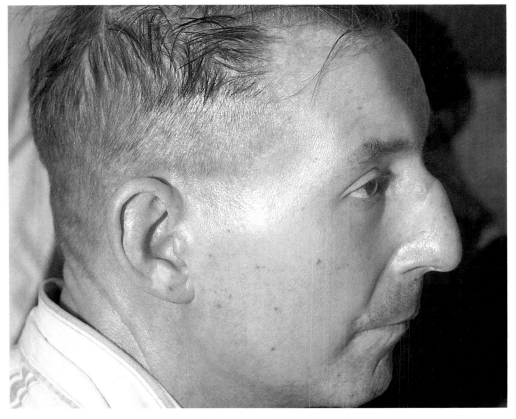

Fig. 10.11 A patient with generalized morphea involving the upper arms, trunk and face.

Fig. 10.12 Systemic sclerosis. This patient illustrates a typical tight appearance to the facial skin together with alopecia.

10.5

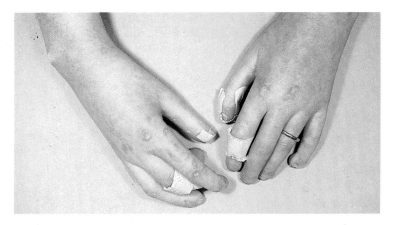

Fig. 10.13 The hands in scleroderma. There is edema, particularly of the left hand, the skin appears tight and there is superficial ulceration on many digits.

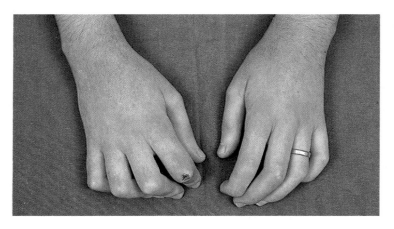

Fig. 10.14 Contractures and ulceration in scleroderma. This patient with late disease has tight skin over the fingers with developing contractures and some ulceration. Note also the loss of hair from the dorsum of the fingers.

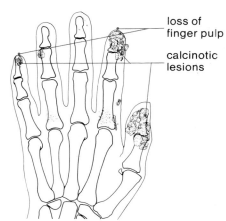

Fig. 10.15 Scleroderma involving the trunk and face.

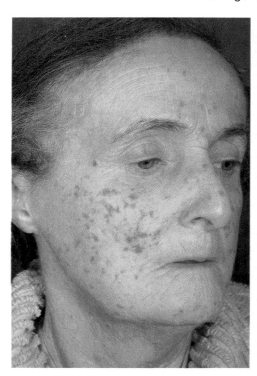

Fig. 10.16 The face in scleroderma showing the typical microstomia with angular creases and tightness of the facial skin with telangiectasia on the cheek and the forehead. This patient also has some temporal alopecia.

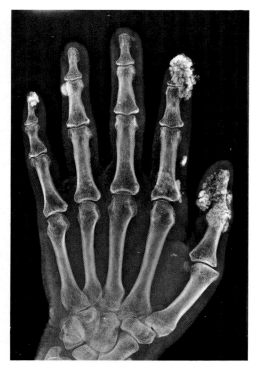

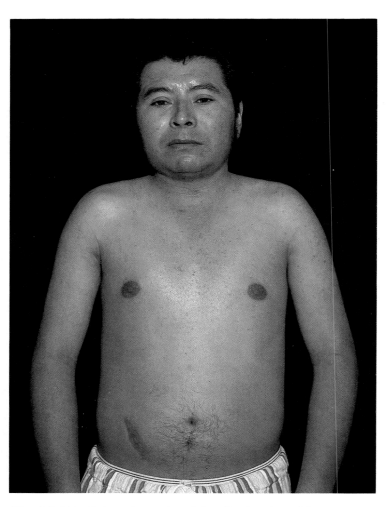

loss of finger pulp

calcinotic lesions

Fig. 10.17 Hand radiograph in scleroderma showing loss of tissue at the fingertips (in particular in the index and little fingers) with numerous calcinotic lesions in the soft tissues.

Acro = extremity

(2) The edema is gradually replaced by thickening and tightening of the skin. This is most frequently found to involve the fingers, face (Fig. 10.12) and hands (Figs. 10.13 & 10.14), spreading in varying degrees to the limbs and trunk (Fig. 10.15).

(3) Atrophy occurs later and hardening of the tissues can lead to limb contractures. The face becomes immobile and pinched, microstomia develops (Fig. 10.16) and alopecia may occur. Radiographs taken at this stage may show finger pulp atrophy, often associated with calcinosis, and acro-osteolysis (Figs. 10.17 & 10.18).

Intracutaneous and subcutaneous calcification occurs most commonly in patients with the CREST syndrome, and affects the fingertips, the extensor surface of the forearms, the prepatellar bursa (Fig. 10.19) and the olecranon bursa. The calcinotic lesions vary in size from tiny deposits to large masses and ulceration of the overlying skin may occur (Figs. 10.20 & 10.21).

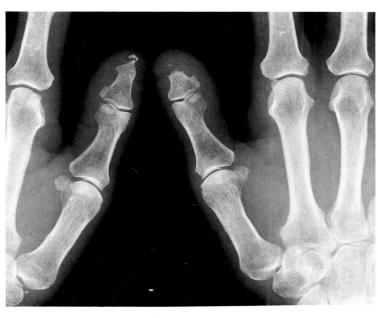

Fig. 10.18 Hand radiograph in scleroderma showing severe acro-osteolysis involving the terminal phalanges of both thumbs.

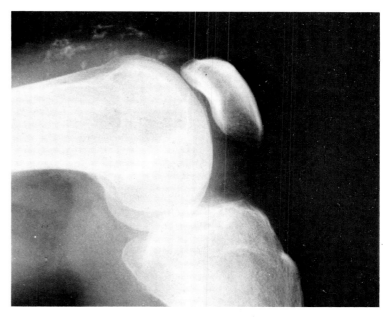

Fig. 10.19 Knee radiograph in a patient with the CREST syndrome showing calcinotic deposits in the prepatellar bursa of the knee.

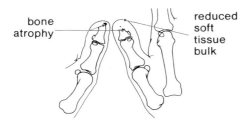

bone atrophy — reduced soft tissue bulk

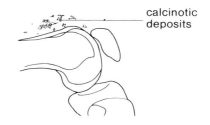

calcinotic deposits

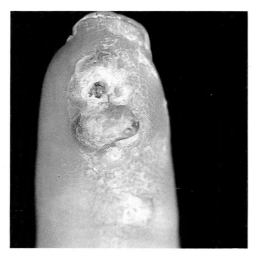

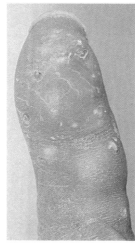

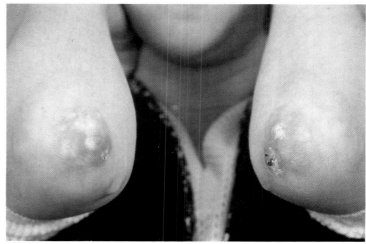

Fig. 10.20 The finger of a patient with the CREST syndrome showing large ulcerating calcinotic masses in the finger pulp.

Fig. 10.21 Calcinotic lesions in a patient with the CREST syndrome involving the thumb (left) and elbows (right).

Vascular Changes

These are both structural and vasospastic (Raynaud's phenomenon). Over 95% of patients with scleroderma have Raynaud's phenomenon affecting the fingers and often the toes. This usually precedes other cutaneous changes and by as much as 30 years. Raynaud's phenomenon occurs in several connective tissue diseases, of which scleroderma and the mixed connective tissue disease (MCTD) are by far the commonest (Fig. 10.22). The risk of patients with Raynaud's developing systemic sclerosis is less than 2% in females and about 6% in males. Despite the poor perfusion seen clinically and on thermography (Fig. 10.23), arteriography may show patent vessels. However, Raynaud's in systemic sclerosis may be complicated by small areas of ischemic necrosis and ulceration of the fingertips, which subsequently leads to pitting scars (Fig. 10.24). These lesions may be difficult to treat; gangrene may follow (Fig. 10.25), and they may become secondarily infected.

Cold-induced vasospasm can also contribute to the ischemic process in kidney, heart and lung tissue. Dilated capillary loops and venules (telengiectasia) are

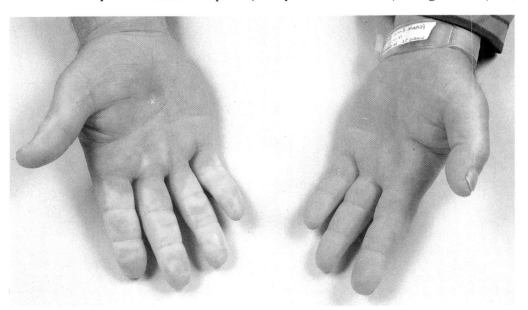

RAYNAUD'S PHENOMENON IN MUSCULOSKELETAL DISORDERS

Scleroderma	90%
Overlap or mixed	85%
SLE	25%
DM or PM	20%
RA	10%

Fig. 10.22 The prevalence of Raynaud's phenomenon in different musculoskeletal disorders (left). The hands of a patient with severe Raynaud's showing the typical white appearance of the fingers (right). The left index finger has been amputated due to previous gangrene.

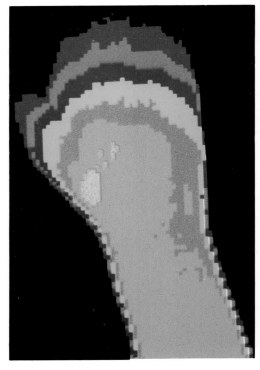
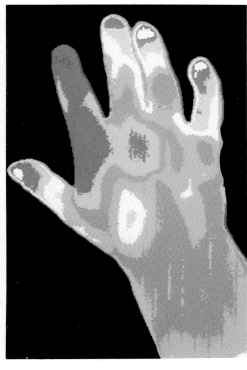
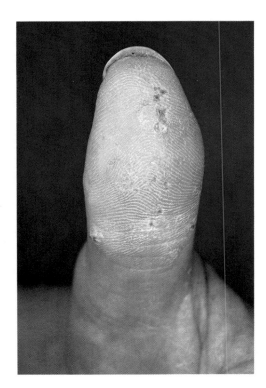

Fig. 10.23 Thermograms of the hands in Raynaud's phenomenon before and after cold stress. Cold stress (1 minute at 20°C) results in loss of perfusion of the fingers ('thermal amputation', left). During this phase the fingers appear white. Increased perfusion develops during the recovery phase (reactive hyperemia, right), although in this case the index finger has remained cool. Courtesy of Mr. E.F.J. Ring.

Fig. 10.24 Severe Raynaud's phenomenon in a patient with scleroderma, which has led to the development of ischemic necrosis with resulting pitted scars.

10.8

common on the hands, lips, tongue and mucous membranes. They are often found in patients with the CREST syndrome (Fig. 10.26).

Locomotor Involvement

Primary myositis is frequent and often insidious, presenting clinically with easy fatigability rather than specific muscle weakness. Clinical examination may reveal muscle atrophy with proximal weakness (Fig. 10.27). Laboratory abnormalities include significant elevation of muscle enzymes while EMG shows polyphasic potentials. Muscle biopsy may show predominantly interstitial changes with increased deposition of collagen and degenerate myofibrillar changes, but florid inflammation is uncommon.

Tendon involvement causes friction rubs and flexion contractures. Polyarthralgia and arthritis are often early manifestations of systemic sclerosis and are seen at some time in the majority of the patients. The arthritis is occasionally progressive and erosive (Fig. 10.28).

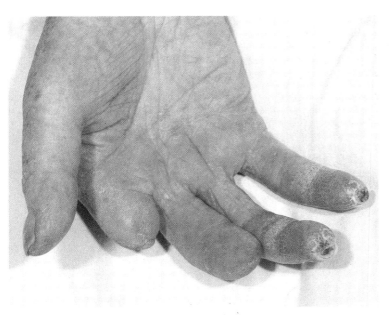

Fig. 10.25 Severe Raynaud's phenomenon. This patient has ulcerating lesions and gangrene in the ring and little fingers. Previous gangrene has necessitated amputation of the index and middle fingers.

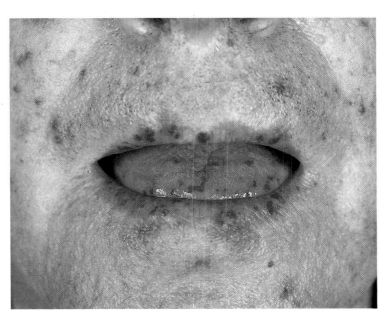

Fig. 10.26 A patient with the CREST syndrome showing the typical telangiectasia in the perioral region and the tongue.

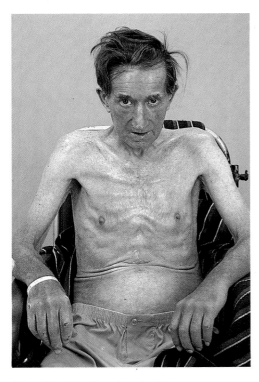

Fig. 10.27 A patient with severe proximal muscle wasting due to myositis. Note the waxy tight appearance of the skin over the fingers with several small ulcers.

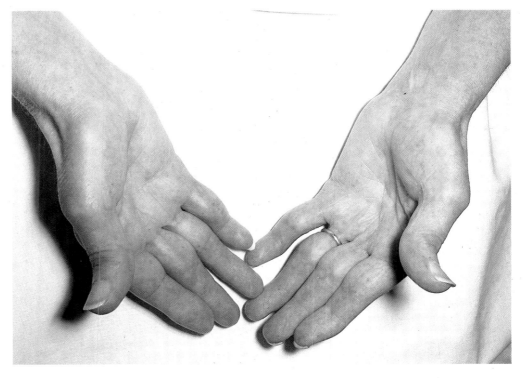

Fig. 10.28 A patient with scleroderma who has developed a destructive arthritis of the small joints of the hands with resultant Swan Neck deformities of the fingers.

Gastrointestinal Tract Involvement

The gut is the second most common organ system after the skin to be involved in systemic sclerosis. Involvement can cause serious morbidity and death. Esophageal involvement occurs in the majority of patients although it may be asymptomatic. Dysphagia for solid foods and heartburn are the commonest complaints. Barium swallow characteristically shows decreased or absent peristalsis in the lower portion of the esophagus and distal esophageal dilation (Fig. 10.29). A hiatus hernia or stricture may also be found. The histology of the esophagus may be normal early in the disease but later on there is smooth muscle atrophy and widespread fibrosis (Fig. 10.30).

The stomach is rarely involved but small bowel disease is seen in up to half the patients. Symptoms of intestinal stasis and/or malabsorption (relating to bacterial overgrowth) include abdominal pain, distension, nausea, vomiting, pseudo-obstruction, diarrhoea and weight loss. The pathological findings are similar to those described in the esophagus with atrophy and fibrosis (Fig. 10.31). Characteristic radiological changes of dilatation and barium flocculation are most frequent in the duodenum and proximal jejunum (Fig. 10.32).

Large bowel involvement is more common radiologically than is clinically appreciated. The radiological appearance of a wide-mouthed colonic diverticulum is almost pathognomic of scleroderma (Fig. 10.33).

Other Visceral Involvement

Renal, cardiac, and pulmonary involvement are separately associated with a decreased survival, renal scleroderma having the worst prognosis. The patterns of injury in the kidney, heart and lung are similar, consisting of excessive deposition of collagen, vascular change and possibly cold-induced vasospasm.

Pulmonary Involvement

The commonest symptom of lung involvement is dyspnea on exertion. It is often insidious and therefore underestimated but occurs in up to half the patients. Coughing and chest pain occur less frequently. Basal fine inspiratory rales are the most frequent findings. Clubbing rarely occurs. Other findings may include cysts in the middle or lower lobes, pleural thickening (Fig. 10.34) and adhesions, vascular lesions and occasionally alveolar cell carcinoma.

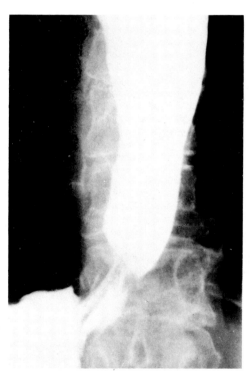

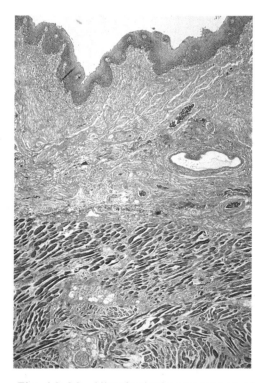

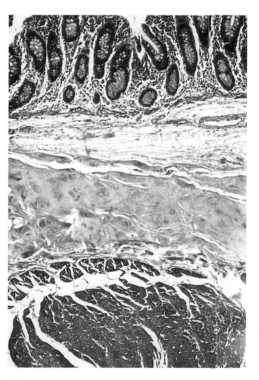

Fig. 10.29 Barium swallow in a patient with scleroderma.

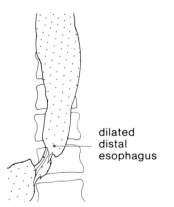

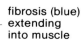

dilated distal esophagus

Fig. 10.30 Histological appearance of the esophagus in scleroderma. There is extensive and excessive collagen deposition in the submucosa and early involvement of the muscle coat. Martius scarlet blue stain, x25. Courtesy of Dr. A.B. Price.

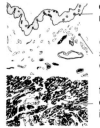

esophageal mucosa

dense submucosal collagen

fibrosis (blue) extending into muscle

Fig. 10.31 Histological appearance of the colon in scleroderma showing dense hyalinized collagen in the submucosa. Trichrome stain, x75.

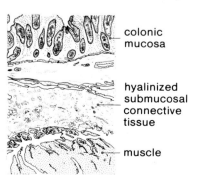

colonic mucosa

hyalinized submucosal connective tissue

muscle

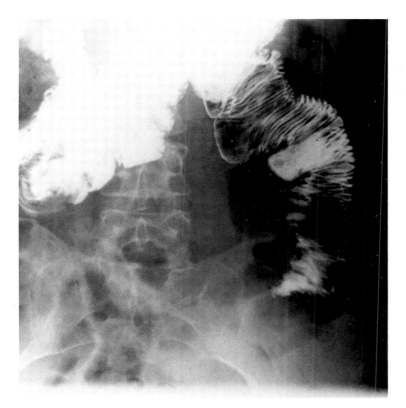

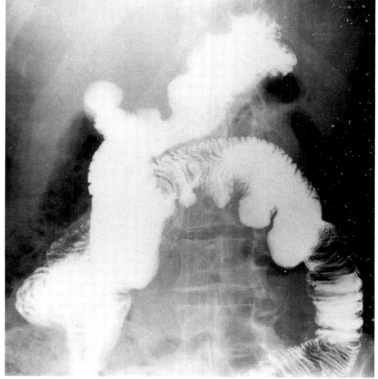

Fig. 10.32 Barium follow-through examination showing dilatation of the duodenum and jejunum with a 'wire spring' appearance. Flocculation of the barium is due to impaired intestinal mobility.

Fig. 10.33 Barium study showing wide-mouthed colonic diverticula.

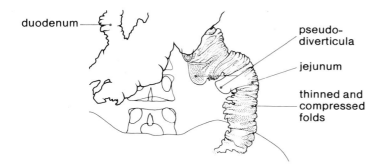

duodenum

pseudo-diverticula

jejunum

thinned and compressed folds

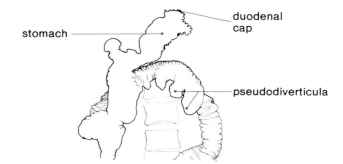

stomach

duodenal cap

pseudodiverticula

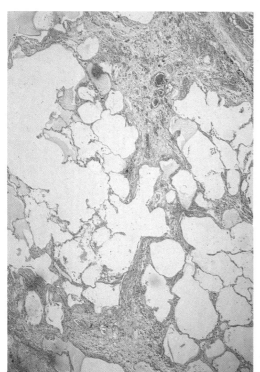

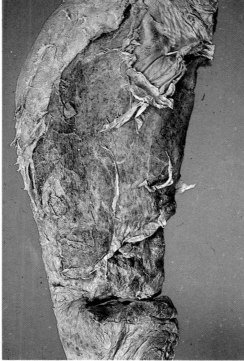

Fig. 10.34 Histology of the lung showing developing fibrosis with destruction of the normal alveolar architecture (left, H & E stain, x30). Post mortem specimen of the lung showing pleural fibrosis and adhesions (right).

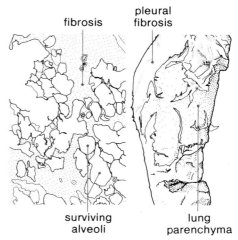

fibrosis

pleural fibrosis

surviving alveoli

lung parenchyma

10.11

The earliest radiological changes are an increase in fine interstitial markings confined to the lung base, later progressing to the lower two-thirds but sparing the apices (Fig. 10.35). There may be associated cystic changes. Pulmonary function tests show an almost equal incidence of obstructive and restrictive disease patterns. Patients with dyspnea commonly have impairment of diffusing capacity for carbon monoxide. Up to half of scleroderma patients have elevated pulmonary artery pressure, particularly those with CREST syndrome, and pulmonary hypertension may cause disproportionate dyspnea.

Cardiac Involvement

This occurs in up to 80% of patients. It is often asymptomatic but may present with arrhythmia, conduction defects, pericarditis, pericardial effusion, chronic congestive cardiac failure, angina or sudden death. The echocardiogram (Fig. 10.36) or chest radiograph may show an enlarged heart. A restrictive pericarditis or restrictive cardiomyopathy may be present. The characteristic pathological lesions are myocardial fibrosis and focal necrosis (Fig. 10.37).

Renal Involvement

This is the major cause of death in systemic sclerosis. Autopsy studies show a higher incidence than clinical surveys. About 40% of patients have clinical manifestations, the onset being acute or chronic. Chronic renal disease usually causes proteinuria and mild hypertension, and the pathology shows an adventitial cuff of collagen around small interlobular arteries. Acute renal disease has a dramatic onset with malignant hypertension, rapid renal failure and microangiopathic hemolytic anemia. The small interlobular arteries show characteristic concentric internal proliferation, and fibrinoid necrosis of small arteries and afferent arterioles may be seen (Fig. 10.38). Other changes include deposition of intramural fibrin and smooth muscle degeneration. The glomerulus may show mesangial proliferation, obliteration of the tufts, thickening of basement membranes or arteriolar proliferative changes.

DERMATOMYOSITIS AND POLYMYOSITIS

Dermatomyositis (DM) is an inflammatory disease of muscle characterized by symmetrical proximal muscle weakness and typical cutaneous lesions. Polymyositis (PM) is an identical myopathy occurring in the absence of rash. Both may occur in childhood and both have been linked to malignant disease. The etiology is unknown, but a virus-triggered mechanism in a genetically predisposed host leading to a self-perpetuating lymphocyte-mediated autodestructive process has been suggested. Several viruses, including rubella, influenza and Coxsackie A or B, which can cause acute myositis, have also been implicated in chronic polymyositis. Cytotoxic lymphocytes from patients with DM have been shown to kill muscle cells. PM and DM have been classified into 5 subgroups (Fig. 10.39) and analysis suggests a series of diagnostic criteria (Fig. 10.40).

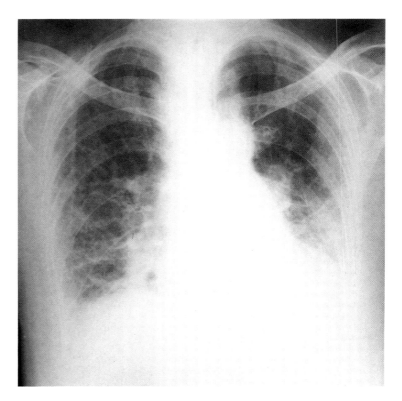

Fig. 10.35 Chest radiograph in scleroderma showing increased interstitial markings in the lower two-thirds and associated cystic changes.

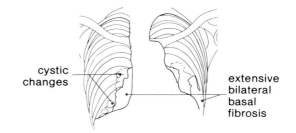

cystic changes

extensive bilateral basal fibrosis

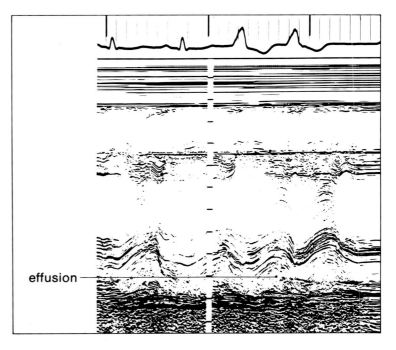

effusion

Fig. 10.36 Echocardiogram of a patient with scleroderma and cardiac involvement showing two extra systoles and a pericardial effusion. The extrasystoles seen here reflect the myocardial damage.

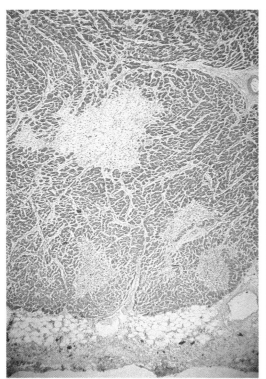

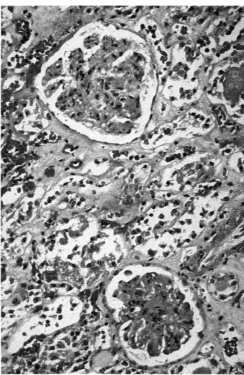

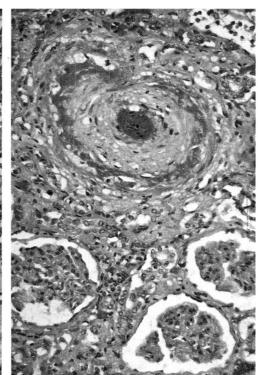

Fig. 10.37 Histology of cardiac muscle in systemic sclerosis showing focal areas of necrosis. H & E stain, x 20.

Fig. 10.38 Histology of renal cortex showing focal thickening and polymorphs in the glomerular tuft (left) and an arteriole with fibrinoid necrosis

and intimal thickening (right). There is obliteration of the glomeruli by diffuse thickening of the capillary basement membrane. H & E stain, x 25.

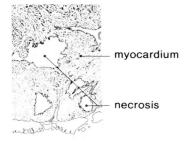

myocardium

necrosis

extensive
tubular damage

obliteration
of glomerulus

fibrinoid
necrosis

mucoid intimal
fibrosis of
arterioie

obliteration of
glomerulus

CLASSIFICATION OF DERMATOMYOSITIS (DM) AND POLYMYOSITIS (PM)

1. Primary idiopathic DM

2. Primary idiopathic PM

3. DM (or PM) associated with neoplasia

4. Childhood DM (or PM) with vasculitis

5. DM (PM) in collagen–vascular disease

Fig. 10.39 A classification of dermatomyositis and polymyositis.

DIAGNOSTIC CRITERIA OF DERMATOMYOSITIS AND POLYMYOSITIS

Symmetrical progressive proximal weakness

Muscle biopsy showing inflammatory changes

Elevated muscle enzymes (eg.CPK)

Electromyographic abnormalities (eg.polyphasic potentials)

Characteristic dermatological changes

Fig. 10.40 Criteria for the diagnosis of dermatomyositis and polymyositis.

Muscle Involvement

The characteristic clinical feature is progressive proximal weakness, often insidious in onset, usually painless, and in acute disease sometimes associated with initial cutaneous edema and erythema. Typical presenting complaints are difficulty in climbing stairs and weakness of the neck muscles. With progressive disease, muscle wasting and atrophy occur and muscle contractures are a major problem (Fig. 10.41).

Arthralgia and myalgia occur in 25% of patients and Raynaud's phenomenon in 12%. An EMG may be useful in establishing the diagnosis and in distinguishing myositis from steroid myopathy. Abnormalities on EMG may aid diagnosis but do not correlate with disease activity. Muscle enzymes are useful diagnostically in following the course of the disease and predicting relapses. They should be measured serially. Muscle weakness may be documented objectively by strain gauge myometry. Changes often lag behind the changes in enzyme levels. Muscle biopsy can be helpful in making the diagnosis and serial needle biopsies can be used to follow the progression of DM (Fig. 10.42).

Cutaneous Lesions

The characteristic dermatological features of dermatomyositis include:
(1) an erythematous rash causing lilac (heliotrope) discoloration of the eyelids and periorbital edema (Fig. 10.43). This rash often spreads onto the shoulders and chest and may include the arms and hands (Fig. 10.44).
(2) a scaly erythematous dermatitis involving the dorsum of the hands, knuckles and extensor surfaces of other joints (Goddron's patches') (Fig. 10.45). Nail fold changes, periungual erythema, cuticular hypertrophy and infarcts may occur as in other connective tissue disorders (Fig. 10.46). In a small group of patients with underlying malignancy the cutaneous signs become a major manifestation of disease and there is 'malignant erythema' – a fiery red suffusion overlying the more chronic lesion of DM (Fig. 10.47).

The relationship of polymyositis and dermatomyositis to malignancy is controversial. When strict diagnostic criteria are applied, about 90% of patients have associated malignancy – most commonly of breast or stomach.

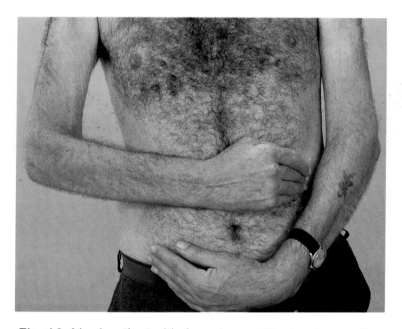

Fig. 10.41 A patient with dermatomyositis showing wasting of the proximal arm muscles with a fixed flexion deformity of 90° in the right elbow due to muscle contracture.

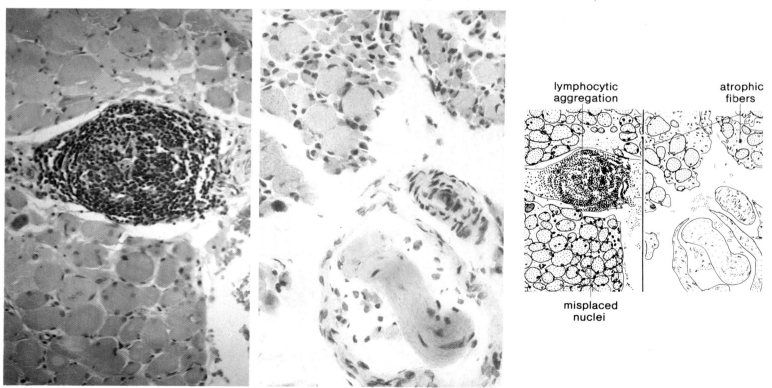

Fig. 10.42 Muscle histology in dermatomyositis. Individual muscle fibers have taken up varying amounts of stain and their nuclei are misplaced (left). A large aggregation of lymphocytes is seen. The section on the right shows perifascicular fiber atrophy. H & E stain, x 300.

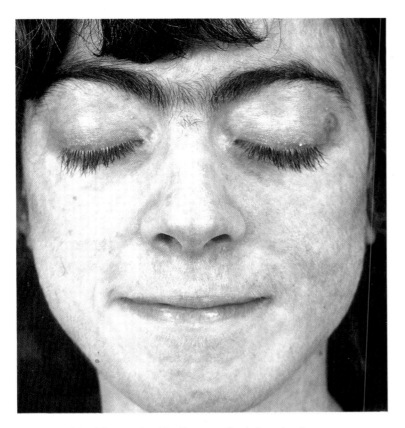

Fig. 10.43 The typical heliotrope facial rash of dermatomyositis.

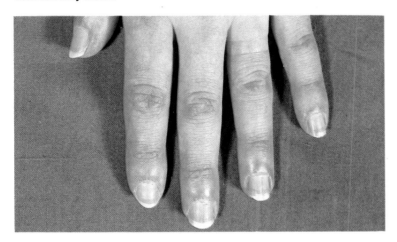

Fig. 10.44 An erythematous rash on the hand in dermatomyositis.

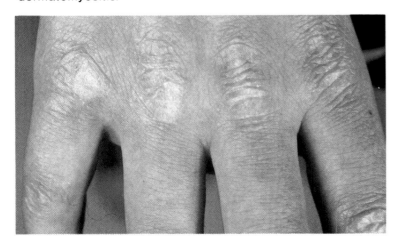

Fig. 10.45 Erythematous dermatitis (Goddron's patches) on the knuckles in dermatomyositis.

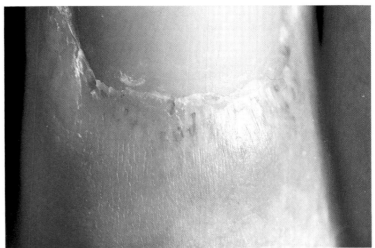

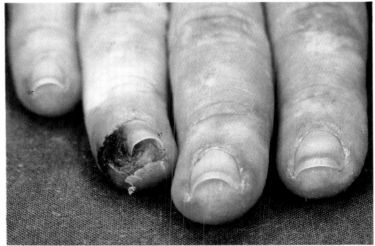

Fig. 10.46 Periungual edema and capillary hemorrhage in the nailbed (upper) and severe changes with terminal ulceration of the finger (lower) in dermatomyositis.

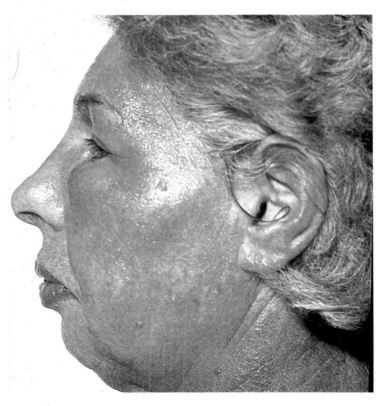

Fig. 10.47 The fiery red appearance of malignant erythema.

10.15

Calcinosis of subcutaneous tissue and the fascial planes between muscles can be dramatic and troublesome especially in chronic disease. It is more common in children (Figs. 10.48 & 10.49).

Vasculitis may involve the skin, resulting in Raynaud's phenomenon, livedo reticularis, gangrene or ulceration (Figs. 10.50 & 10.51). It can also occur in the internal organs, notably the gastrointestinal tract, leading to hematemesis, ulceration and perforation, especially in childhood disease.

Systemic Involvement

Involvement of cardiac muscle occurs in up to 20% of patients and can cause dysrhythmias and congestive cardiac failure.

Pulmonary involvement is the worst prognostic sign in polymyositis. It takes two forms. Weakness of the respiratory muscles, often associated with a dysphagia, may result in ventilatory failure or aspiration pneumonia. Fibrosing alveolitis may also occur. Pulmonary function tests should be performed routinely.

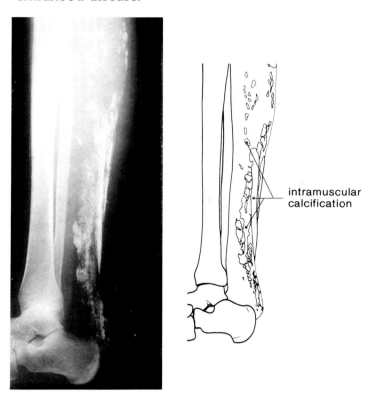

Fig. 10.48 Radiograph of the leg showing extensive calcification in the calf muscles.

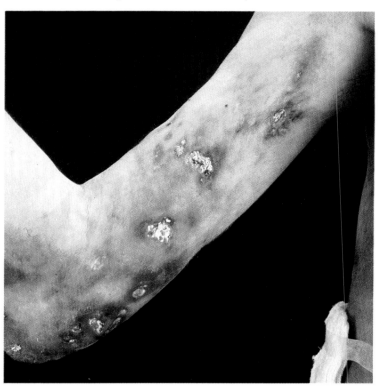

Fig. 10.49 An adolescent with dermatomyositis. There is considerable muscle wasting and numerous calcinotic lesions, some of which have ulcerated.

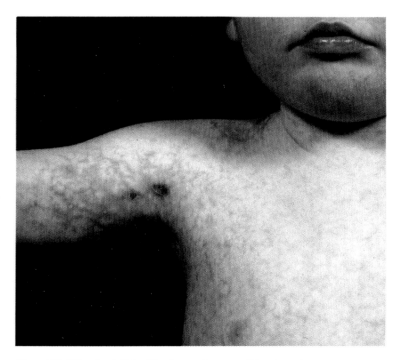

Fig. 10.50 A child with dermatomyositis showing livedo reticularis and subcutaneous calcinosis together with two small ulcers just anterior to the axilla.

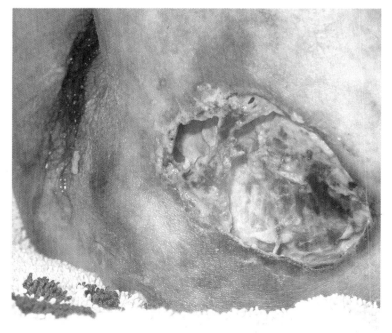

Fig. 10.51 Cutaneous vasculitis in a child with dermatomyositis: a huge ulcerating lesion on the buttock has developed.

11

Vasculitis

with Dr. David G. I. Scott

The vasculitides are a mixed group of diseases characterized by inflammatory infiltration of blood vessels. Many classifications have been unsatisfactory due to the variety of clinical syndromes of vasculitis. The most useful classification is simple and based on pathology and vessel size (Fig. 11.1). The inclusion of group 1a recognizes the difficulty in distinguishing classical idiopathic polyarteritis nodosa (PAN) from necrotizing arteritis: the appearances of PAN may occur in association with hepatitis B infection, with malignancy, or even with connective tissue diseases. The inclusion of group 1b emphasizes the important role of systemic necrotizing arteritis in conditions such as Churg-Strauss syndrome and Wegener's diseases, although these are characterized by the occurrence of granulomata; the coexistence of these two lesions within the same syndrome needs to be emphasized.

Various clinical syndromes are included in the different groups (Fig. 11.2) though there is some overlap both clinically and pathologically (Fig. 11.3).

The relationship between vasculitis and granulomatosis is a spectrum ranging from pure arteritis without granulomatosis to pure granulomatosis without vasculitis (Fig. 11.4). Thus classical polyarteritis nodosa and the arteritis of rheumatoid arthritis are at one end of the spectrum while rheumatoid nodules and midline granulomata lie at the other end.

CLASSIFICATION OF VASCULITIS

1   Systemic necrotising arteritis
       a) of the polyarteritis nodosa type
       b) with granulomatosis

2   Hypersensitivity or small vessel vasculitis

3   Giant cell or large vessel arteritis

Fig. 11.1   A simple classification of vasculitis based on vessel size and histology.

EXAMPLES OF VASCULITIC SYNDROMES

1a)   PAN ± hepatitis B_s antigen, malignancy, etc.,
      Arteritis of RA, SLE, MCTD, etc.,
      Kawasaki's disease

1b)   Churg-Strauss syndrome
      Wegener's granulomatosis

2   Henoch-Schönlein purpura
      Vasculitis of RA, SLE, MCTD, etc.,
      Cryoglobulinemic vasculitis

3   Giant cell arteritis
      Takayasu's arteritis

Fig. 11.2   Clinical examples of systemic necrotizing arteritis of the polyarteritis nodosa type (group 1a), or with granulomatosis (group 1b), small vessel vasculitis (group 2) and large vessel arteritis (group 3). Overlap features of vasculitis associated with rheumatoid arthritis (RA), systemic lupus erythematosus (SLE) and mixed connective tissue disease (MCTD) lead to inclusion in group 1a and group 2.

Fig. 11.3   Diagram showing the size of vessel involved in the different classification groups. There is considerable overlap between groups 1a and 1b, slight overlap between groups 1 and 2, but very little overlap between group 3 and the other groups.

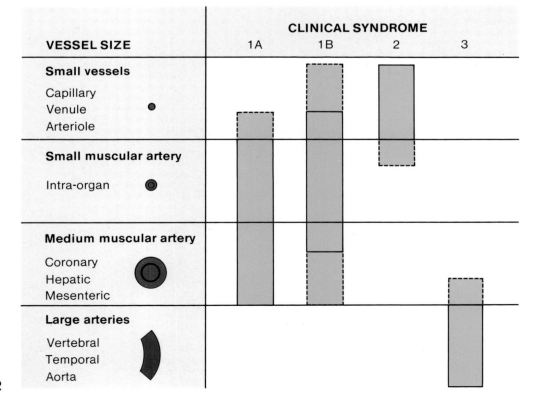

Pathology

Biopsy is central to the diagnosis of vasculitis. The value of some commonly used biopsy sites varies for both classification and diagnosis (Fig. 11.5). Nasopharyngeal biopsy is particularly useful for the diagnosis of Wegener's granulomatosis but of little value in Churg-Strauss syndrome. Angiography may demonstrate particular vascular abnormalities and the size of vessel involved, which are important for diagnosis (Fig. 11.6). Typical changes include aneurysm formation, stenosis or attenuation of arteries; these may occur in renal or coeliac axis vessels. These changes have been demonstrated most commonly in polyarteritis nodosa but micro-aneurysms have also been described in the other diseases associated with systemic necrotizing arteritis (ie. groups 1a and 1b). Arch aortography is necessary for the diagnosis of the large vessel vasculitis of Takayasu's arteritis but angiography is of little value in giant cell arteritis.

Biopsy may reveal aneurysms as well as acute necrotizing arteritis. The histological expression of vasculitis may be similar at different biopsy sites and examples

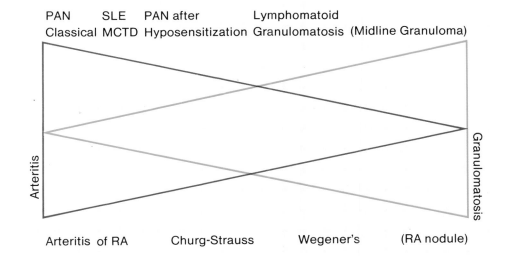

RELATIONSHIP BETWEEN ARTERITIS AND GRANULOMATOSIS
(ie. groups 1A and 1B)

PAN   SLE   PAN after   Lymphomatoid
Classical MCTD Hyposensitization Granulomatosis (Midline Granuloma)

Arteritis   Granulomatosis

Arteritis of RA   Churg-Strauss   Wegener's   (RA nodule)

Fig. 11.4 The relationship between arteritis and granulomatosis. Diseases associated with pure arteritis include classical PAN and the arteritis of RA, whereas RA nodules are examples of pure granulomatous disease. Many vasculitic syndromes show some features of both. (After Alarcon-Segovia, 1980.)

VALUE OF BIOPSY SITES FOR DIAGNOSIS AND CLASSIFICATION

	1A	1B	2	3
Skin	±	+	+++	−
Kidney	++	++	+	−
Muscle	+	+	−	−
Sural nerve	++	+	−	−
Testis	+	+	−	−
Rectum	++	+	−	−
Temporal artery	±	−	−	+++
Naso-pharynx	−	++	−	−
Angiography	+++	++	−	+++

Fig. 11.5 The value of different biopsy sites for the diagnosis and classification of vasculitis. They range from − (no value) to +++ (most value). Angiography is a useful method of diagnosis for groups 1a, 1b and 3.

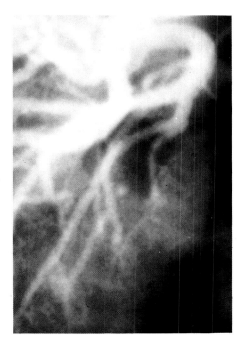

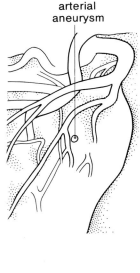

arterial aneurysm

Fig. 11.6 Right renal angiogram showing typical small micro-aneurysms in a patient with PAN. It is important when performing angiography to include both renal arteries and the coeliac axis for the demonstration of such aneurysms.

include the rectum (Fig. 11.7) and testis (Fig. 11.8). A similar picture of aneurysm formation with fibrinoid necrosis of an artery may also be seen at renal biopsy (Fig. 11.9). Arteritis can be detected in approximately 50% of renal biopsies in patients with PAN. However, even if affected vessels are not found in tissue obtained at renal biopsy, this site may still be helpful for diagnosis, as there are characteristic changes associated with renal vasculitis, including focal segmental glomerulonephritis, which is seen in about two-thirds of patients (Fig. 11.10) and ischemic changes. These occur in any disease associated with vasculitis which affects the kidney and represents small artery or arteriolar involvement. Immunofluorescence may help differentiate between different vasculitic syndromes. Negative immunofluorescence (for the presence of immunoglobulin or complement) is characteristic of PAN, Wegener's granulomatosis and Churg-Strauss vasculitis (group 1). By contrast, deposits of immunoglobulin and complement are characteristically seen in the glomerulus in diseases such as systemic lupus erythematosus and Henoch-Schönlein purpura.

The sural nerve is another useful site for biopsy and vasculitis is commonly detected at this site in patients with mononeuritis multiplex or peripheral neuropathy (Fig. 11.11).

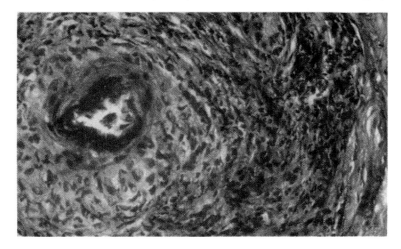

Fig. 11.7 Rectal biopsy from a patient with systemic necrotizing arteritis. There is inflammation of a small artery with fibrinoid necrosis of the intima and extensive inflammatory cell infiltration through all layers of the vessel walls. Martius Scarlet Blue, x 570.

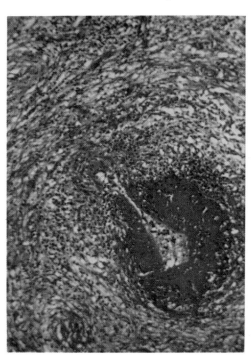

Fig. 11.8 Testicular biopsy showing polyarteritis nodosa. The small artery in the centre has developed a large aneurysm with fibrinoid necrosis in the aneurysm wall. There is extensive inflammatory infiltration surrounding and infiltrating the artery and aneurysm. H&E stain, x 420.

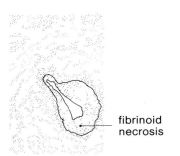

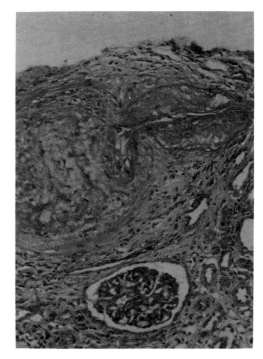

Fig. 11.9 Renal biopsy showing polyarteritis nodosa. The artery has developed an aneurysm filled with a blood clot. Note the normal glomerulus despite the prominent arterial involvement. PAS stain, x 280.

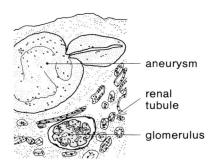

aneurysm

renal tubule

glomerulus

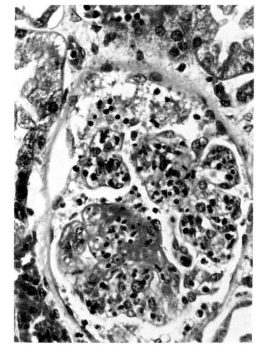

Fig. 11.10 Renal biopsy from a patient with systemic necrotizing arteritis. There is a segmental area of fibrinoid necrosis in the glomerulus but the rest of the glomerulus is normal (focal segmental glomerulonephritis). H&E stain, x 700.

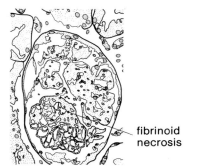

fibrinoid necrosis

Skin biopsies often only contain small arterioles, venules or capillaries. This site is therefore most useful for the diagnosis of small vessel or hypersensitivity vasculitis, though such a diagnosis should also depend on the absence of larger vessel involvement in other affected organs. One characteristic feature of *acute* small vessel vasculitis in skin is the presence of nuclear debris from polymorphonuclear leucocytes (leucocytoclasis) and thus a common histological term for such small vessel involvement especially in the skin is acute leucocytoclastic vasculitis (Fig. 11.12).

With healing of vasculitic lesions, the inflammatory infiltrate in the blood vessels subsides. In the late stage of vasculitis the most prominent histological change is disruption or rupture of the internal elastic lamina (Fig. 11.13).

Fig. 11.11 Sural nerve biopsy from a patient with necrotizing arteritis and neuropathy. A small artery shows fibrinoid necrosis with inflammatory infiltrate throughout the vessel wall and in surrounding tissue. Three nerve bundles are also clearly shown. H&E stain, x 220.

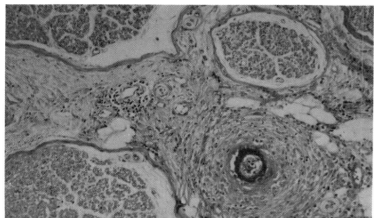

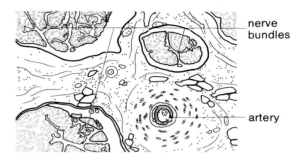

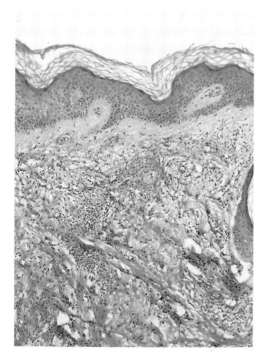

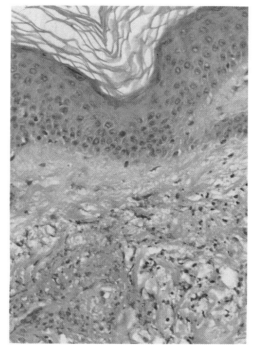

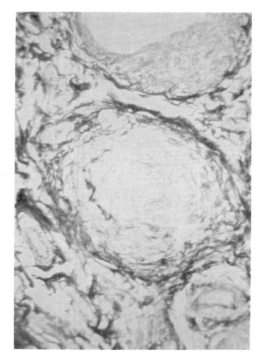

Fig. 11.12 Skin biopsy showing acute leucocytoclastic vasculitis. The low power view shows widespread inflammatory cell infiltrate in the subdermis (left, x 280) and the high power view reveals small capillaries surrounded by inflammatory cells and fragmented nuclei (right, x830). H&E stain.

Fig. 11.13 Biopsy stained to show the internal elastic lamina. The small artery in the middle of this picture shows obliteration of the lumen together with complete disruption of the internal elastic lamina. There are few inflammatory cells. This represents old or 'burnt out' chronic arteritis. Van Gieson Elastic stain, x 560.

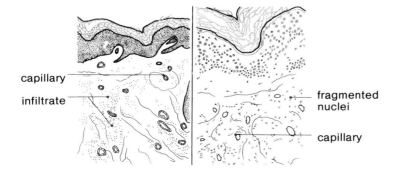

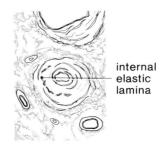

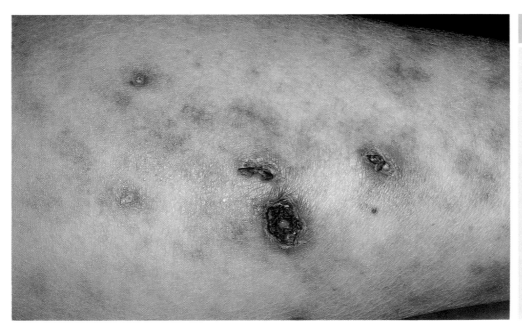

FEATURES OF CLASSICAL PAN	
Systemic	80%
Renal	75%
Arthritis/myalgia	60%
Cutaneous	55%
Neurological	50%
Abdominal	45%

Fig. 11.14 Systemic necrotizing arteritis of the PAN type: example of cutaneous involvement showing small necrotic patches due to small arterial involvement (left) and the common clinical manifestations (right).

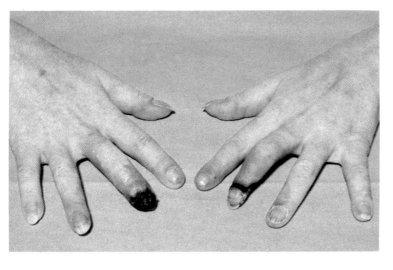

Fig. 11.15 Severe peripheral gangrene affecting the fingers in a patient with PAN.

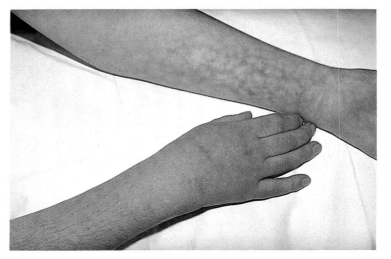

Fig. 11.16 Typical livedo reticularis on the arm of a patient with PAN. The reticular pattern of discoloration is typical of this condition.

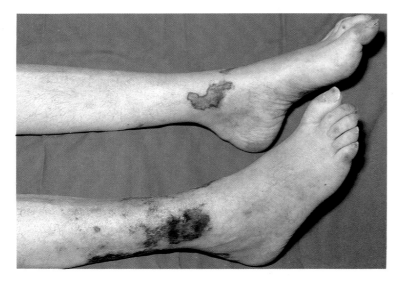

Fig. 11.17 Extensive muscle wasting and bilateral foot drop due to mononeuritis multiplex in a patient with PAN. In addition note the skin ulceration due to co-existent cutaneous vasculitis. Courtesy of Dr. M. Walport.

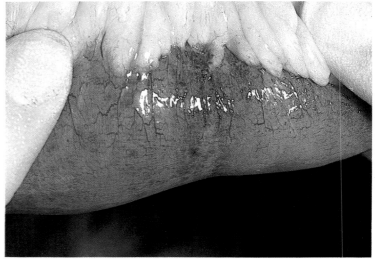

Fig. 11.18 Typical circumferential infarction of the intestine due to arteritis affecting the mesenteric arcuate artery in a patient with PAN. This frequently results in perforation of the bowel wall. Courtesy of Professor G. Slaney.

Clinical Syndromes – Systemic Necrotizing Arteritis (Group 1)

The PAN group of systemic necrotizing arteritis may be associated with a variety of cutaneous as well as systemic features (Fig. 11.14). Systemic symptoms include fever, myalgia and weight loss. Renal involvement is also common and renal failure is an important cause of morbidity and mortality. The clinical features include hematuria, loin pain, acute and chronic renal failure and hypertension. Typical renal histology has been described above. It is important to rheumatologists to note the high incidence of musculoskeletal involvement (60%) and that arthritis is seen in at least 40% of patients.

Other cutaneous manifestations of systemic necrotizing arteritis include peripheral gangrene (Fig. 11.15), cutaneous rashes and livedo reticularis (Fig. 11.16).

A variety of neurological manifestations occur. The commonest is mononeuritis multiplex which may affect all four limbs (Fig. 11.17), followed by a symmetrical sensori-motor neuropathy.

Abdominal pain is a common presenting symptom and may reflect severe life-threatening arteritic involvement due to gastrointestinal, renal or other intra-abdominal organ infarction. Smaller arteries may also be involved, particularly mesenteric arteries, resulting in characteristic circumferential infarcts (Fig. 11.18).

Arteritis is occasionally a complication of connective tissue diseases including rheumatoid arthritis and systemic lupus erythematosus. The clinical features of arteritis may be identical to those described above. Connective tissue diseases are also associated with small vessel vasculitis and further descriptions of vasculitis in connective tissue disease are included in group 2.

Kawasaki's disease (also known as the mucocutaneous lymph node syndrome) is an acute systemic illness of infants and children. The characteristic features include conjunctival congestion (Fig. 11.19), fever, exanthematous rash and cervical lymphadenopathy. The disease is usually self-limiting although a small number (up to 2%) of cases are fatal due to rupture of a coronary artery aneurysm (Fig. 11.20). Histology shows typical necrotizing

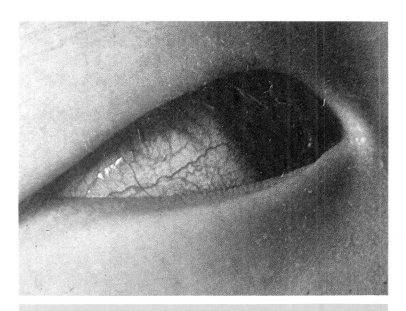

FEATURES OF KAWASAKI'S DISEASE

Fever	95%
Conjunctival congestion	90%
Exanthema	90%
Oral mucosa involvement	90%
Desquamation	90%
Cervical lymphadenopathy	75%

Fig. 11.19 Typical conjunctival congestion of Kawasaki's disease and the characteristic clinical manifestations.

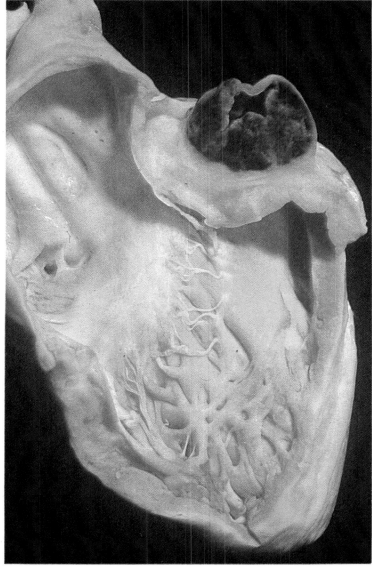

Fig. 11.20 Necropsy specimen from a patient with Kawasaki's disease showing a ruptured aneurysm of the right coronary artery. Courtesy of Professor A.E. Becker.

arteritis. Coronary arteritis may also be detected angiographically in up to 60% of children with Kawasaki's disease. This arteritis is identical to that seen in infantile PAN but the mucocutaneous involvement and lymphadenopathy confirm Kawasaki's disease as a distinct clinical syndrome. Because of the systemic nature of Kawasaki's disease and the mucous membrane involvement, children usually look ill and extremely miserable (Fig. 11.21). Desquamation especially affecting the extremities is another common feature (Fig. 11.22).

Churg and Strauss described a vasculitic syndrome that differed from classical PAN — pulmonary vessels were frequently affected and there was a wider range of vessel involvement (see Fig. 11.4). Histological findings include intra- and extra-vascular granulomata often with eosinophilic infiltrates (Fig. 11.23) as well as necrotizing arteritis. Common clinical associations are the development of asthma in adult life and marked eosinophilia in the peripheral blood (Fig. 11.24). It is important to note that the only significant clinical difference from classical PAN is the high incidence of pulmonary involvement; cutaneous, neurological, renal and joint involvement may thus be identical to that seen in PAN.

The most common cutaneous manifestation in Churg-Strauss vasculitis is a non-thrombocytopenic purpura due to small vessel or capillary vasculitis (Fig. 11.25). In addition to the histological and clinical features of pulmonary involvement radiological changes are often seen. The most frequent finding is a transient pulmonary infiltration (Fig. 11.26).

Wegener's granulomatosis is often classified separately from the other systemic necrotizing arteritides. This is because of the severity of pulmonary, sinus and nasopharyngeal symptoms. However, vasculitis is a common feature and the range of vessels involved is similar to that seen in Churg-Strauss syndrome. Both granulomatous and necrotizing arteritis may be detected in biopsies, particularly of the nasopharynx and lung (Fig. 11.27).

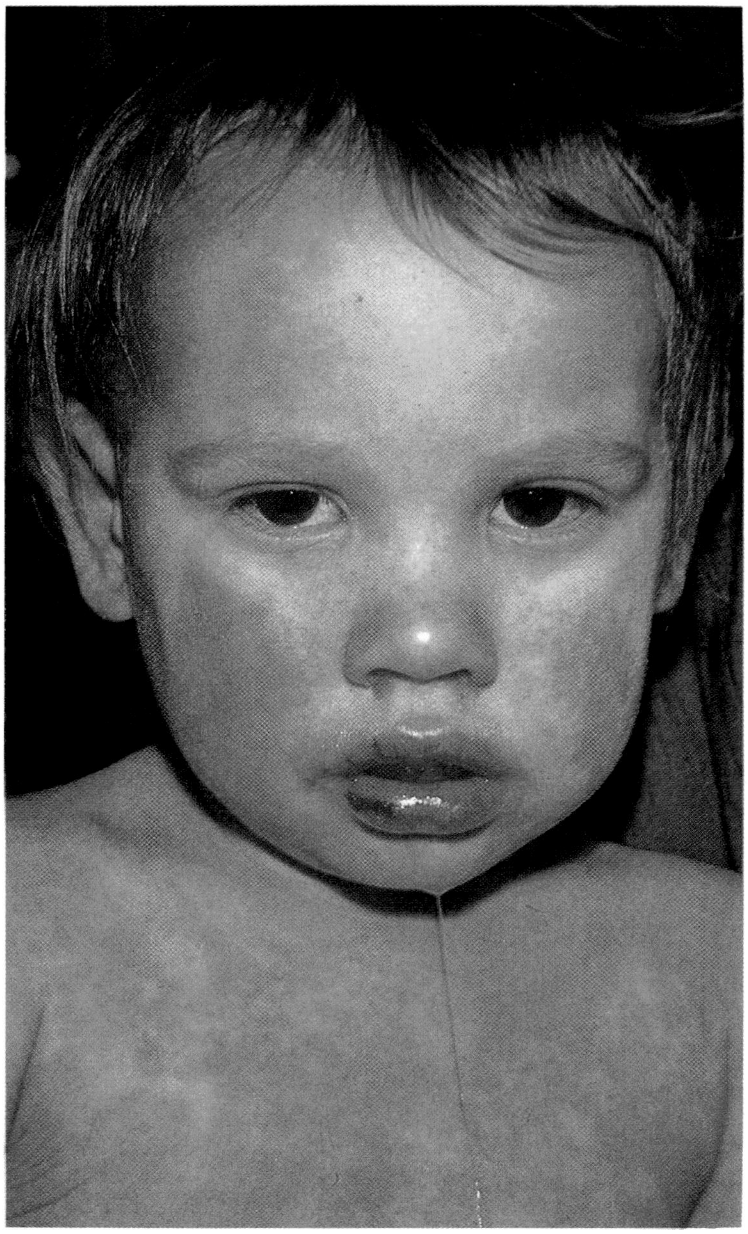

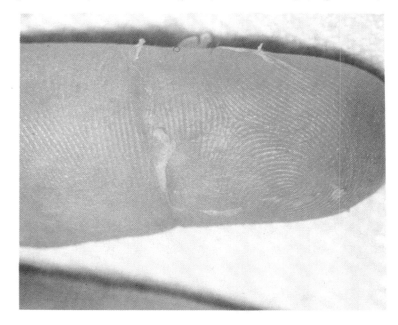

Fig. 11.22 Typical desquamation of the finger tips in a patient with Kawasaki's disease.

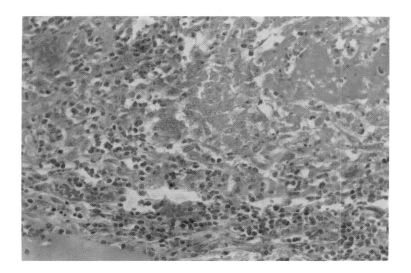

Fig. 11.23 Churg-Strauss syndrome: the edge of a granuloma which is surrounded by an intense infiltration with eosinophils. H&E stain, x 740.

Fig. 11.21 A child with Kawasaki's disease. Note the erythematous rash and the severe mucous membrane involvement.

FEATURES OF CHURG-STRAUSS SYNDROME

Vasculitis:	
Pulmonary	100%
Cutaneous	70%
Renal	60%
Neuropathy	60%
Arthritis	40%

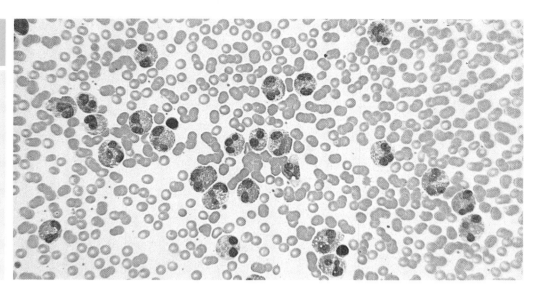

Fig. 11.24 Churg-Strauss syndrome: the major clinical manifestations (left). Note the frequency of pulmonary involvement compared with classical PAN. The peripheral blood smear (right) from a patient with Churg-Strauss syndrome shows numerous eosinophils. Giemsa stain, x 2000.

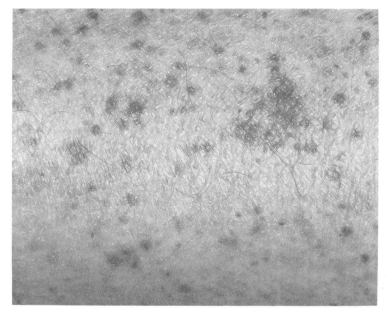

Fig. 11.25 Churg-Strauss syndrome: non-thrombocytopenic purpura due to leucocytoclastic capillaritis.

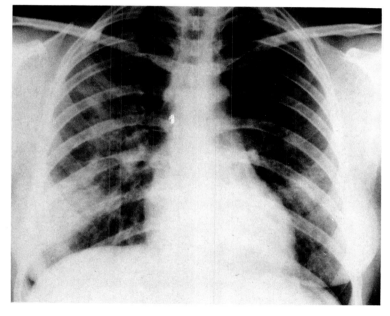

Fig. 11.26 Chest radiograph showing fluffy pulmonary infiltrates in a patient with Churg-Strauss syndrome. Courtesy of Professor M. Turner-Warwick.

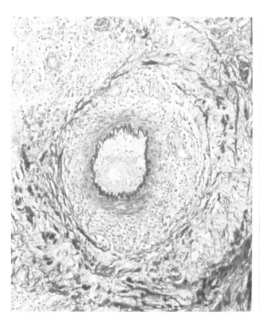

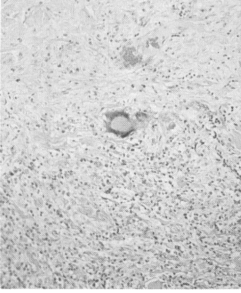

Fig. 11.27 Wegener's granulomatosis: arteritis of a medium-sized artery with intense inflammatory infiltration (left, Van Gieson Elastic stain, x 280) and the edge of a granuloma, showing a large giant cell from the same specimen (right, H&E stain, x 420).

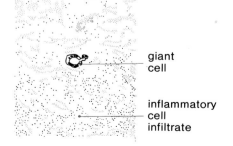

giant cell

inflammatory cell infiltrate

The major difference between Wegener's granulomatosis and Churg-Strauss syndrome is the lack of blood or tissue eosinophilia, or allergic history, in patients with Wegener's granulomatosis.

Saddle-nose deformity is common and is due to destruction of nasal cartilage by granulomata (Fig. 11.28). The other characteristic lesions in Wegener's granulomatosis are very similar to those seen in the PAN type of systemic necrotizing arteritis. Ophthalmic involvement, especially anterior uveitis, is slightly commoner and neuropathy slightly rarer than in classical PAN. It is worth noting again the frequency of arthritis in patients with Wegener's granulomatosis.

Vascular lesions or granulomata may affect any part of the upper respiratory tract and oral mucosa. Gingivitis and stomatitis are common and destructive ulceration in the oropharynx can occur (Fig. 11.29).

The commonest cutaneous lesion is a vasculitic purpura (Fig. 11.30). Histological examination usually reveals a leucocytoclastic capillaritis with or without granulomata. When larger vessels are involved cutaneous infarction may ensue (Fig. 11.31).

Ophthalmic involvement may be severe. Lesions include proptosis due to granulomatous infiltration as well as episcleritis and scleritis (Fig. 11.32).

Radiological abnormalities are commonly seen in the lung and facial bones. Pulmonary nodules or infiltrates, which are frequently bilateral, may progress to cavitation (Fig. 11.33). When facial bones are involved there is often marked destruction detected radiologically (Fig. 11.34).

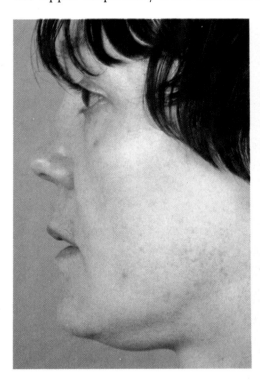

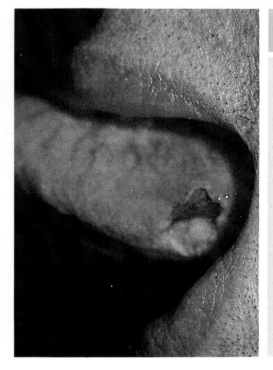

WEGENER'S GRANULOMATOSIS – SITES OF INVOLVEMENT	
Pulmonary	100%
Sinus/nasopharynx	90%
Renal	80%
Arthralgia/arthritis	60%
Cutaneous	50%
Ophthalmic	40%
Neurological	30%

Fig. 11.28 Typical saddle nose deformity in Wegener's granulomatosis due to destruction of nasal cartilage.

Fig. 11.29 Wegener's granulomatosis: a large vasculitic ulcer on the tongue and a table showing the common clinical manifestations.

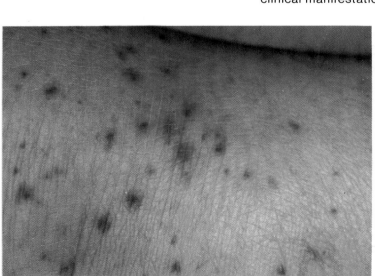

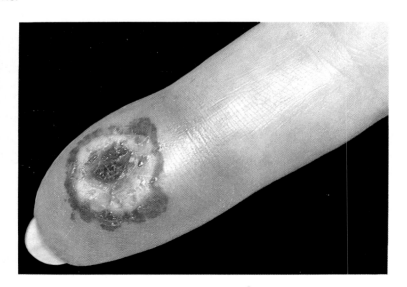

Fig. 11.30 Vasculitic purpura in a patient with Wegener's granulomatosis.

Fig. 11.31 Larger vessel involvement in Wegener's granulomatosis resulting in a destructive vasculitic ulcer.

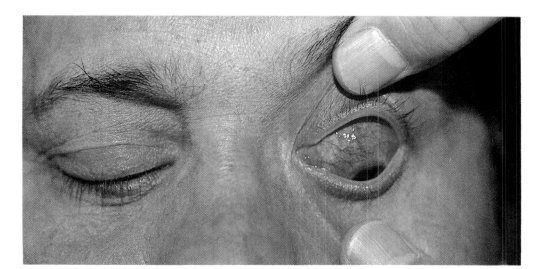

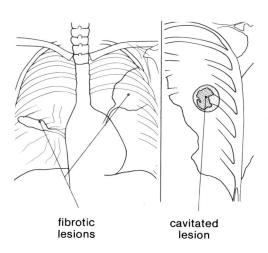

Fig. 11.32 Scleritis in a patient with Wegener's granulomatosis.

fibrotic
lesions

cavitated
lesion

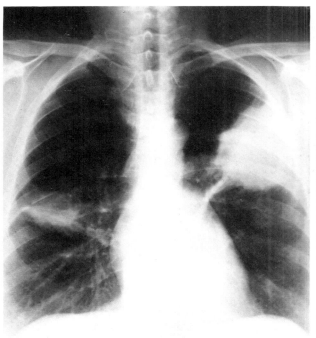

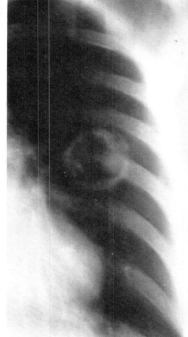

Fig. 11.33 Chest radiograph (left) and tomogram (right) in Wegener's granulomatosis. The radiograph shows two large peripheral lesions with irregular outlines. The larger lesion on the patient's left abuts the pleura. Fibrotic strands are radiating to each lesion from the hilar shadows. The tomogram from another patient shows a solitary lesion which has cavitated. Note the irregular thick wall.

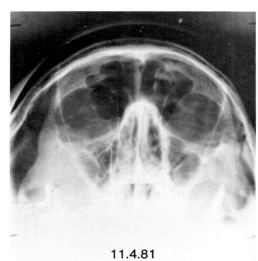

11.4.81

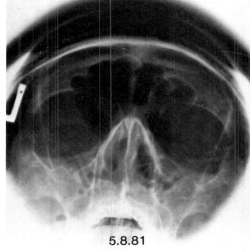

5.8.81

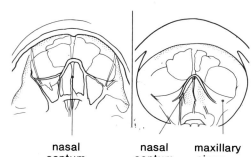

nasal
septum

nasal
septum

maxillary
sinus

Fig. 11.34 Skull radiographs in Wegener's granulomatosis, taken four months apart, showing destruction of the nasal septum and gross mucosal thickening. The maxillary sinuses have become radio-opaque.

Clinical Syndromes – Small Vessel Vasculitis (Group 2)

Hypersensitivity or small vessel vasculitis is a feature of a number of different clinical diseases including the connective tissue disorders such as rheumatoid arthritis (RA), systemic lupus erythematosus (SLE) and mixed connective tissue disease (MCTD). There are also a number of distinct clinical syndromes characterized by small vessel vasculitis including Henoch-Schönlein purpura (HSP) and cryoglobulinemic vasculitis.

Small digital arteries and arterioles are commonly affected in connective tissue diseases. Histology shows a bland intimal proliferation which is thought to represent old vasculitis. These lesions are still clinically important as they are often associated with vascular lesions elsewhere. The clinical manifestations include digital infarcts (Fig. 11.35), nailfold infarcts (Fig. 11.36) and nail edge infarcts (Fig. 11.37). When larger peripheral arteries are involved in patients with connective tissue disease ischemia of the whole finger (Fig. 11.38) or frank gangrene (Fig. 11.39) may result.

In SLE, small vessel vasculitis is commoner than necrotizing arteritis and occurs in a large number of patients with active disease. However, it is the necrotizing arteritis which is associated with the most serious problems such as peripheral gangrene or gangrenous patches on the skin (Fig. 11.40), peripheral neuropathy, mononeuritis multiplex or severe CNS disease. In addition, spinal cord infarction is a rare but serious problem especially when the cervical cord is involved (Fig. 11.41).

Raynaud's syndrome is common to all connective tissue diseases particularly SLE, scleroderma and dermatomyositis. It is thought to be due to vasospasm potentiated by temperature change (particularly cold) and results in a characteristic pallor of the fingers (Fig. 11.42).

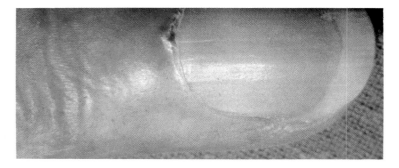

Fig. 11.36 Small nailfold infarct in a patient with SLE.

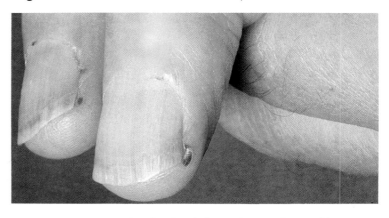

Fig. 11.37 Typical nail edge infarcts in a patient with rheumatoid arthritis, complicated by vasculitis. In the index finger there is also a small nailfold infarct.

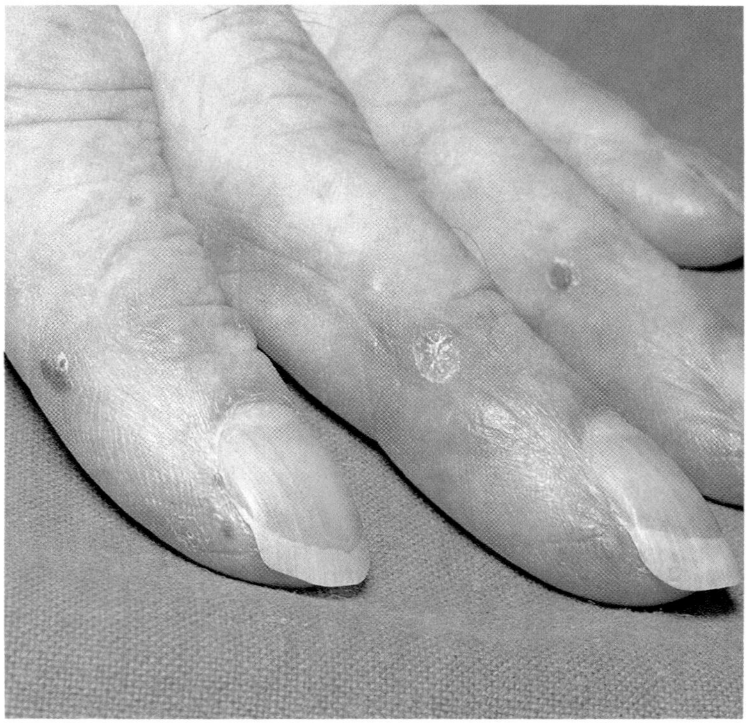

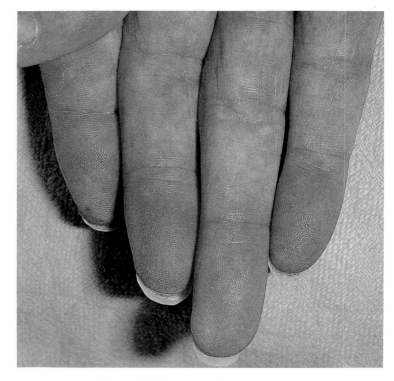

Fig. 11.35 Typical digital infarcts in a patient with connective tissue disease. The small infarcts are in the territory of the digital arteries.

Fig. 11.38 Severe ischemia and incipient gangrene affecting the index, middle and ring fingers in a patient with rheumatoid arthritis. The dorsum of his hand also showed typical nail fold and nail edge infarcts. This patient, therefore, showed vasculitis in different sizes of vessel.

Although angiography may show occlusion in some of these cases there is no evidence that inflammatory changes of blood vessels play a part in Raynaud's syndrome.

The most characteristic feature of small vessel vasculitis is a non-thrombocytopenic purpura. This is caused by inflammation of small cutaneous capillaries and is more common in dependent parts of the body.

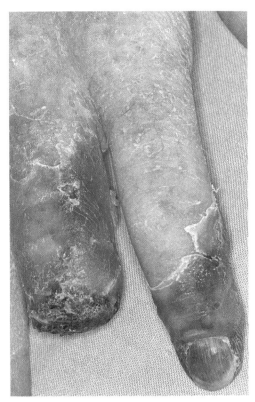

Fig. 11.39 Frank gangrene requiring amputation in a patient with MCTD.

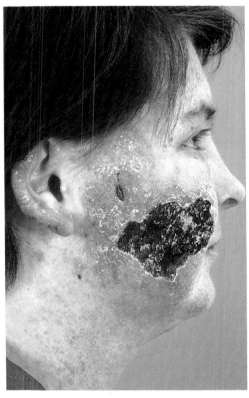 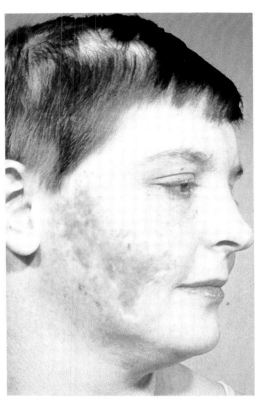

Fig. 11.40 Severe scarring of the face due to arteritis in a patient with SLE (left). The appearance three months later is also shown (right). Note also the marked alopecia.

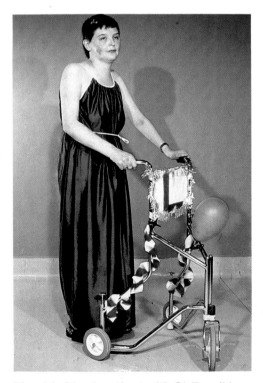

Fig. 11.41 A patient with SLE walking with a frame (the same patient as shown in figure 11.40). She had developed an arteritic lesion of her cervical cord at the level of C3 which presented clinically as a Brown-Sequard syndrome.

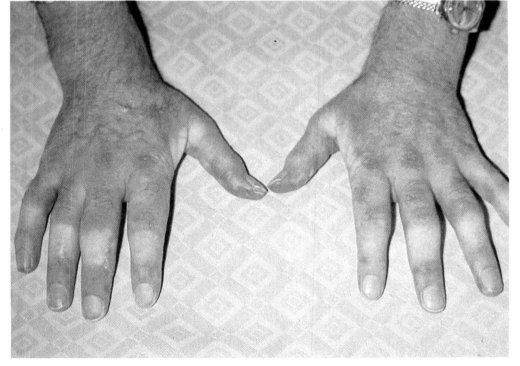

Fig. 11.42 Severe Raynaud's phenomenon in a patient with dermatomyositis/scleroderma overlap syndrome. There is extreme pallor of some fingertips. In addition, this patient has dry erythematous patches over his metacarpophalangeal joints characteristic of skin involvement in dermatomyositis.

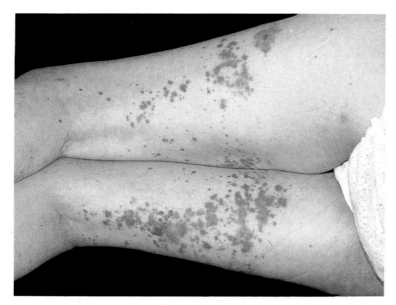

Fig. 11.43 Extensive non-thrombocytopenic purpura in a patient with rheumatoid arthritis. This is due to capillaritis but, when these are extensive, lesions can coalesce and even result in cutaneous infarction.

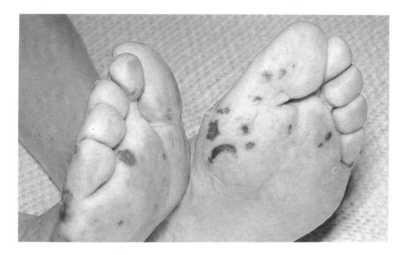

Fig. 11.44 Vasculitic lesions on the soles of the feet in a patient with essential mixed cryoglobulinemia.

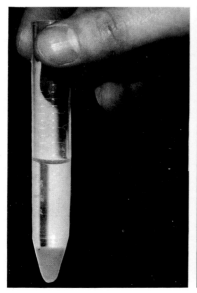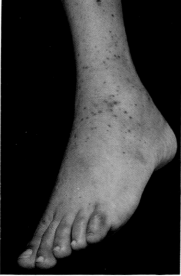

Fig. 11.45 Essential mixed cryoglobulinemia: the typical precipitation of cryoglobulins in a test tube kept at 4° C (left) and the characteristic purpuric vasculitic rash affecting the lower extremities (right).

This may in part be caused by increased hydrostatic pressure. If enough purpuric lesions develop these may coalesce and also result in cutaneous infarction (Figs. 11.43 & 11.44).

Cryoglobulinemic vasculitis may result in any of the lesions described above. However, the most characteristic is a non-thrombocytopenic purpura (Fig. 11.45). Cryoglobulins are proteins which precipitate in the sera in the cold. They are thought to represent circulating immune complexes and may be associated with many different vasculitic diseases including PAN, rheumatoid vasculitis and vasculitis associated with SLE. They may also occur in the absence of a recognized clinical syndrome when the term essential mixed cryoglobulinemia is often used. Clinical features also include systemic involvement such as neuropathy, renal vasculitis and arthritis.

Behçet's syndrome is characterized by recurrent episodes of oral and genital ulcers. A number of other organs may be involved including the eye, joints and the brain stem. The underlying pathology is a vasculitis usually involving only venules. However, larger vessels may be involved. Oral ulcers are the most common feature and are severe. They are deep, punched-out and usually heal with scarring (Fig. 11.46). Uveitis is the commonest ocular manifestation of Behçet's syndrome and may result in a hypopyon (Fig. 11.47). Vasculitis may also be detected in the retina. It is characterized by areas of non-perfusion and may be confirmed by fluorescein angiography (Fig. 11.48).

Henoch-Schönlein purpura is a distinctive clinical syndrome characterized by a non-thrombocytopenic purpura, arthritis usually affecting large joints, abdominal pain sometimes associated with gastrointestinal haemorrhage and renal disease. It commonly affects young children but has been reported in adults. The purpura is caused by a vasculitis affecting small capillaries and thought to be due to deposition of IgA-containing immune complexes. Immunofluorescence shows IgA

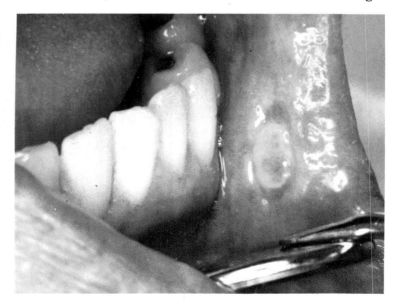

Fig. 11.46 Behçet's syndrome: a large deep ulcer of the oral mucosa which in time will heal with scarring.

deposition in the walls of cutaneous blood vessels and also in the glomerulus when the kidney is affected. Henoch-Schönlein purpura represents the most common systemic vasculitis in which only small vessels are involved (Fig. 11.49). There are a wide number of other, rarer vasculitic diseases. Pyoderma gangrenosum (Fig. 11.50) is associated with a number of different conditions especially Crohn's disease and ulcerative colitis but it has also been described in association with rheumatoid arthritis.

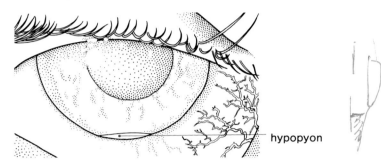

Fig. 11.47 Small sterile hypopyon in the eye of a patient with Behçet's syndrome. Courtesy of Dr. S. Lightman.

hypopyon

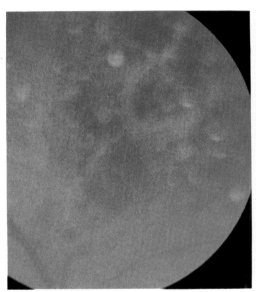 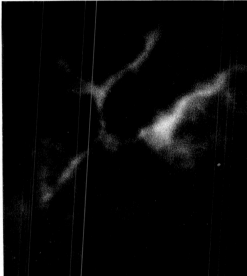

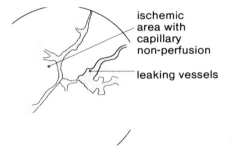

Fig. 11.48 Retinal vasculitis in a patient with Behçet's syndrome. These pictures show an area of ischemia detected at ophthalmoscopy (left) and confirmed by fluorescein angiography (right). Courtesy of Dr. S. Lightman.

ischemic area with capillary non-perfusion

leaking vessels

Fig. 11.48 Retinal vasculitis in a patient with Behçet's syndrome. These pictures show an area of ischemia detected at ophthalmoscopy (left) and confirmed by fluorescein angiography (right). Courtesy of Dr. S. Lightman.

FEATURES OF HENOCH-SCHÖNLEIN PURPURA	
Purpura	100%
Arthritis	71%
Gastrointestinal involvement	68%
Renal involvement	45%
Fever	75%
Hypertension	13%

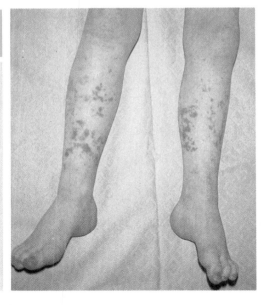

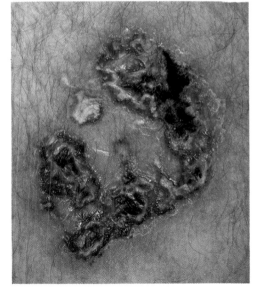

Fig. 11.49 Henoch-Schönlein purpura (HSP): the major clinical manifestations (left) and the typical rash on the legs of a child who also had a mild arthritis affecting his left knee (right).

Fig. 11.50 Typical ulcer of pyoderma gangrenosum showing slightly raised purplish edges and areas of severe necrosis but with some central sparing.

Clinical Syndromes – Large Vessel Arteritis (Group 3)

Large vessel or giant cell arteritis is really restricted to two major clinical syndromes.

Giant cell arteritis is a panarteritis predominantly affecting elderly patients. Although almost any large artery may be involved, the majority of clinical signs result from involvement of the carotid artery or its branches. The characteristic presenting feature is severe headache due to temporal artery involvement (hence the term, temporal arteritis). Examination may reveal a thickened, tender, non-pulsatile temporal artery (Fig. 11.51). The histological appearance is characterized by giant cells and other inflammatory cells, which affect all layers of the artery (Fig. 11.52). It is important to remember the segmental nature of arteritis especially in giant cell arteritis. Biopsies should therefore include as long a piece of artery as possible.

In Takayasu's arteritis giant cells are rarely detected and this disease affects young women who present with a systemic disease with features of malaise, weight loss, fever and arthralgia. The arteritis usually involves the aortic arch and its branches and clinical examination may reveal bruits over the affected vessel. The most important sequel of such inflammation is the development of stenosis which may be detected at angiography (Fig. 11.53). Aortic arch angiography is essential for diagnosis as laboratory features are relatively non-specific. The most commonly involved vessels are the subclavian, carotid and renal arteries.

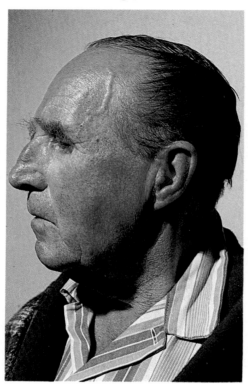

Fig. 11.51 Prominent left temporal artery in a patient with giant cell arteritis. The artery was tender and non-pulsatile.

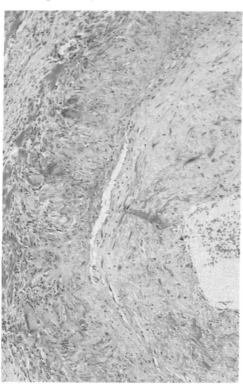

Fig. 11.52 Temporal artery biopsy showing inflammatory infiltration throughout all layers of the arterial wall with destruction of the elastic lamina. Small numbers of giant cells can also be seen in the outer part of the muscle coat. H&E stain, x 400.

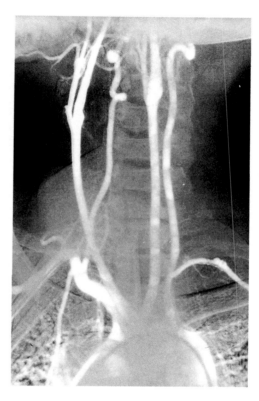

Fig. 11.53 Aortic arch angiogram in a patient with Takayasu's disease showing severe narrowing of the left subclavian artery with narrowing at its origin from the left vertebral artery. In addition, the right subclavian artery is tapered and narrower than normal. Examination of the abdominal aorta also revealed some narrowing of the left renal artery at its origin.

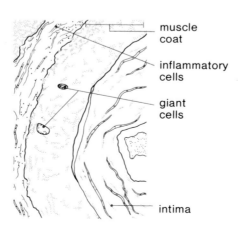

muscle coat
inflammatory cells
giant cells
intima

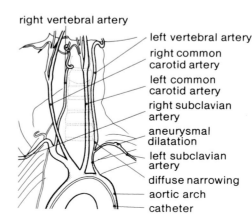

right vertebral artery
left vertebral artery
right common carotid artery
left common carotid artery
right subclavian artery
aneurysmal dilatation
left subclavian artery
diffuse narrowing
aortic arch
catheter

| 12 |

Ankylosing Spondylitis

with Dr. Ian Haslock

Ankylosing spondylitis is a common inflammatory arthropathy most frequently occurring in young men. The inflammation affects chiefly the sacroiliac joints and the spine and usually starts at the bottom of the back and works its way to the top. Peripheral inflammatory synovitis and enthesopathy can also occur. It is one of the group of inflammatory polyarthropathies, with a predilection for the spine and absence of serum rheumatoid factor, known as the seronegative spondarthritides.

There are few diseases so easily recognizable as advanced spondylitis (Figs. 12.1 & 12.2). The diagnosis can be made at a glance if a patient with a bamboo spine is passed in the street. Such extreme deformity should become increasingly rare as ankylosing spondylitis is one of the most successfully treatable of the rheumatic diseases.

Pathology

The pathological findings in synovial joints are those of an inflammatory synovitis similar to that seen in rheumatoid arthritis. A more characteristic feature is the development of enthesopathy; inflammation occurs at the bone/ligament junction (the enthesis) producing erosion of bone and destruction in the ligament (Figs. 12.3 & 12.4). Inflammatory infiltration occurs in the vessels of the ligament and subsequent healing is by bone deposition (Fig. 12.5). A similar process takes place at the junction of the annulus fibrosus with the vertebral body (Fig. 12.6).

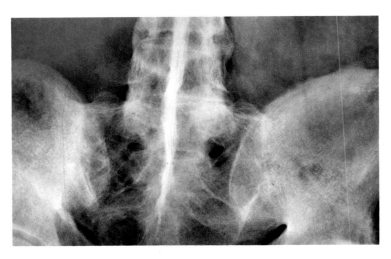

Fig. 12.2 Pelvic radiograph in severe ankylosing spondylitis showing fusion of the sacroiliac joints, syndesmophytes and spinous processes.

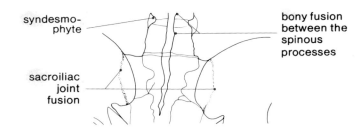

syndesmophyte

sacroiliac joint fusion

bony fusion between the spinous processes

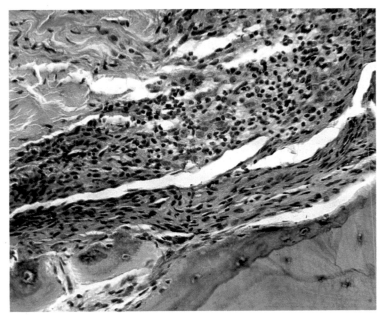

Fig. 12.3 Histological appearance in active iliac enthesopathy. An inflammatory lesion has destroyed the attachment of the ligament to the ilium. H&E stain, x 150. Courtesy of Professor J. Ball.

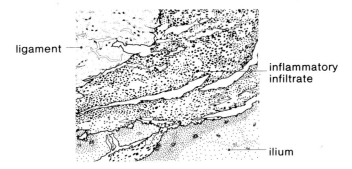

ligament

inflammatory infiltrate

ilium

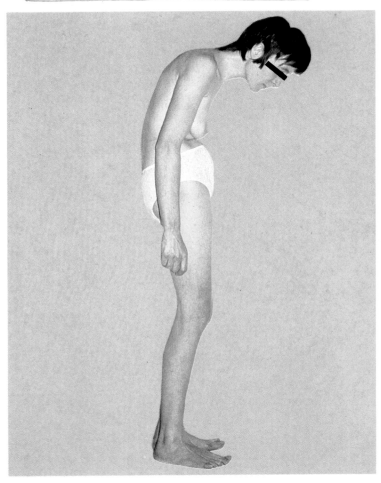

Fig. 12.1 A patient with severe ankylosing spondylitis (AS). Characteristic features of her posture include flattened lumbar lordosis, severe dorsal kyphosis, prominent abdominal folds and flexed knees.

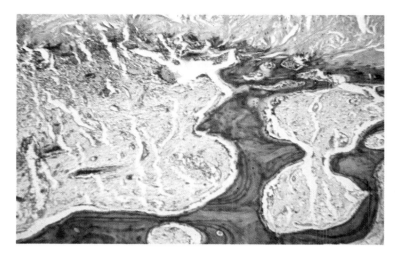

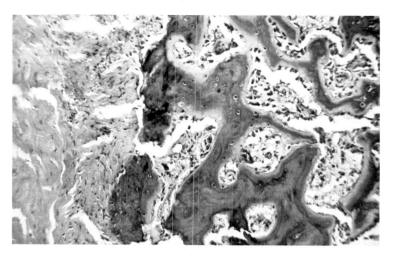

Fig. 12.4 Appearance of severe enthesopathy at the greater trochanter. The attachment of the ligament to the bone is destroyed and replaced by inflammatory tissue containing reactive (woven) bone spicules. Repair of the attachment by new bone can be seen. H&E stain, x 150. Courtesy of Professor J. Ball.

Fig. 12.5 Deposition of reactive (woven) bone in another part of the biopsy shown in the previous figure. The reactive new bone has joined up with the ligament to form a new enthesis and a bony spur. H&E stain, x 180. Courtesy of Professor J. Ball.

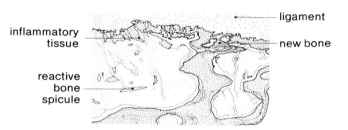

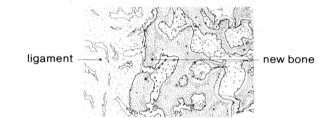

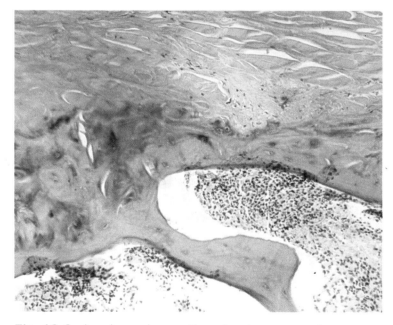

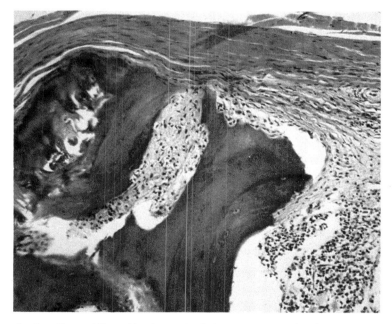

Fig. 12.6 Lumbar spine section showing a normal attachment of the outer annulus to the vertebral body near the vertebral rim (left). The same area in a patient with AS shows destruction of the attachment of the outer annulus by inflammatory tissue (right). H&E stain, x 220. Courtesy of Professor J. Ball.

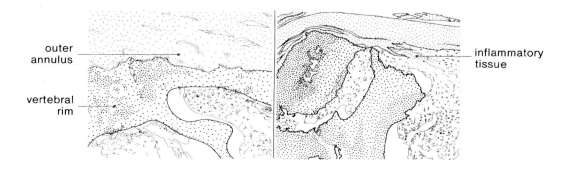

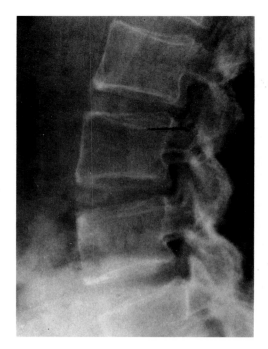

Fig. 12.7 Lumbar spine radiograph showing vertebral squaring. Note the erosion and sclerosis at the vertebral corners.

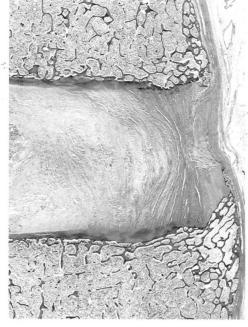

Fig. 12.8 Lumbar spine section showing early healing of anterior spondylitis with formation of a syndesmophyte. H&E Stain, x 5. Courtesy of Professor J. Ball.

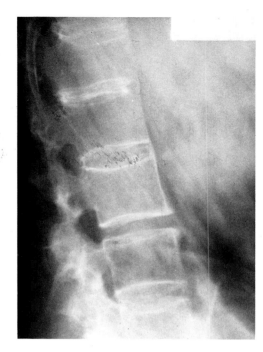

Fig. 12.9 Lumbar spine radiograph showing intervertebral bony ankylosis along the anterior margins and vertebral squaring.

sclerosis

squared outline

vertebral rim

syndesmophyte

bony fusion

'squared' vertebral outline

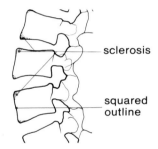

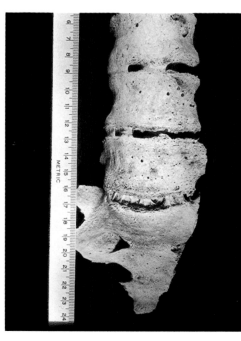

Fig. 12.10 Post-mortem specimen of lumbosacral spine in longstanding ankylosing spondylitis showing bony bridging between adjacent vertebrae and fusion across the articular surfaces of the sacroiliac joint. Courtesy of Professor B. Vernon-Roberts.

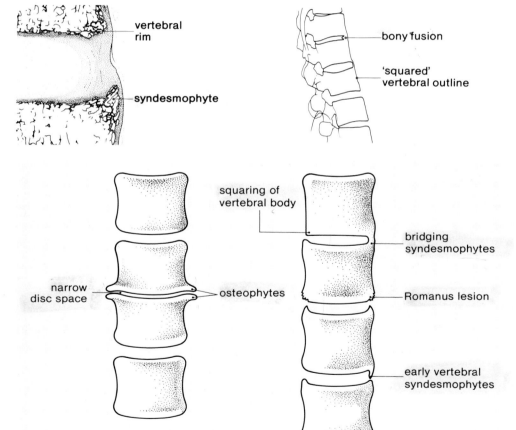

squaring of vertebral body

narrow disc space

osteophytes

bridging syndesmophytes

Romanus lesion

early vertebral syndesmophytes

degenerative disease   ankylosing spondylitis

Fig. 12.11 Diagram showing some of the essential differences between vertebral changes due to degenerative joint disease and ankylosing spondylitis.

These early changes may be detected on radiographs or isotope bone scans. Progression of these erosions leads to loss of the normal bony contour at the junction between the vertebrae and the discs, producing the characteristic vertebral squaring (Fig. 12.7).

As inflammation progresses, healing takes place behind the leading edge with bony deposition (syndesmophyte formation) (Fig. 12.8). The process takes place at the disc margin resulting in intervertebral bony ankylosis (Figs. 12.9 & 12.10). The characteristic vertical alignment of syndesmophytes contrasts with the horizontal disposition of osteophytes found in spinal spondylosis (Fig. 12.11). In advanced ankylosing spondylitis there is bony deposition around the synovial joints of the spine producing fusion of the sacroiliac joints and capsular ossification of the facet joints (Figs. 12.12 & 12.13). Continuing ossification produces the 'bamboo spine' of severe disease. A similar pathological process may occur in entheses elsewhere especially around the pelvis and the heel, leading to erosion and ossification (Fig. 12.14). An inflammatory synovitis of the peripheral joints, especially of the shoulders and hips, can occur and is pathologically indistinguishable from other inflammatory arthropathies (see Fig. 12.3).

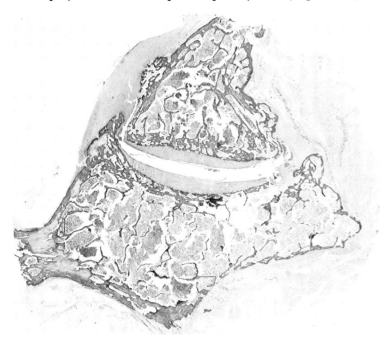

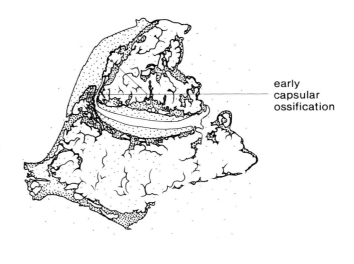

Fig. 12.12 Lumbar facet joint section showing early capsular ossification. H&E stain, x 3. Courtesy of Professor J. Ball.

early capsular ossification

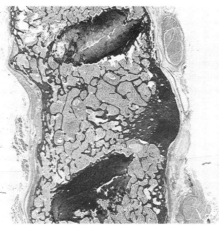

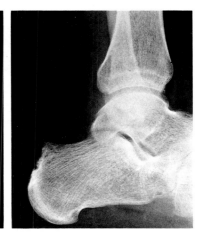

Fig. 12.13 Longitudinal section of two facet joints showing capsular ossification with enchondral ossification of residual articular cartilage. H&E stain, x 5. Courtesy of Professor J. Ball.

Fig. 12.14 Hip radiograph showing enthesopathy in AS (left). There is extensive new bone formation at muscle and ligament insertions. Note the fused sacroiliac joints and intervertebral fusion. The lateral heel radiograph shows erosion and new bone formation at the insertion of the Achilles tendon.

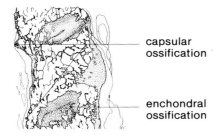

capsular ossification

enchondral ossification

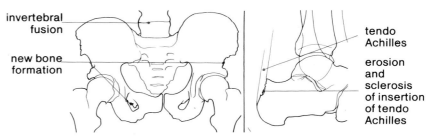

invertebral fusion

new bone formation

tendo Achilles

erosion and sclerosis of insertion of tendo Achilles

Clinical Features

If treatment is to be maximally effective and deformities prevented then early diagnosis is vital. This will only be made when a careful clinical and radiological examination is undertaken whenever suspicion of the disease arises.

Early Ankylosing Spondylitis

HISTORY Many spondylitics present with low back pain. If this arises from the sacroiliac joints it is often felt in the buttocks especially while seated; patients may, for example, report inability to sit through a cinema film. Sacroiliac pain may also radiate down the back of the thigh as far as the popliteal fossa and is often misdiagnosed as 'sciatica' despite the absence of signs of nerve root irritation (Fig. 12.15). Back pain in ankylosing spondylitis is of the inflammatory type, that is, with morning stiffness which slowly abates with activity, the stiffness and pain recurring after periods of inactivity during the day. Pain around the chest wall may occur early in the course of the disease and a history of iritis may be obtained. Heel pain may be present and a family history of ankylosing spondylitis or another seronegative spondarthritis may be found (Fig. 12.16).

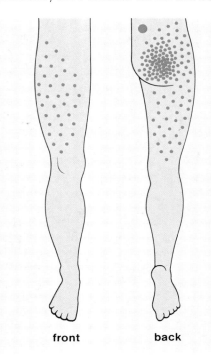

front   **back**

Fig. 12.15 The distribution of sacroiliac joint pain. The density of stippling indicates the frequency of pain perception in different areas.

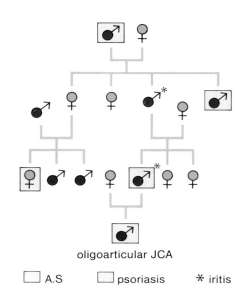

oligoarticular JCA

☐ A.S   ☐ psoriasis   ✳ iritis

Fig. 12.16 Family tree showing the hereditary component to ankylosing spondylitis. One uncle and the grandfather of the index case had AS and the patient's son, aged 10, has oligoarticular JCA. Note also the association with iritis and psoriasis in the extended family.

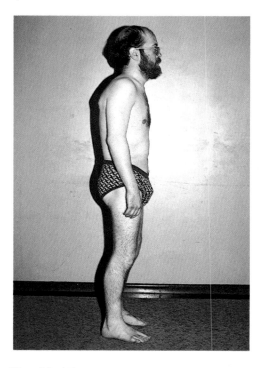

Fig. 12.17 A young man with early ankylosing spondylitis showing loss of lumbar lordosis and accentuation of the dorsal curve.

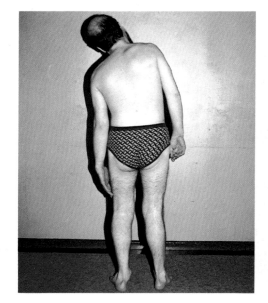

Fig. 12.18 The same patient as in the previous figure attempting to bend to one side. There is almost no lateral flexion in the lumbar spine.

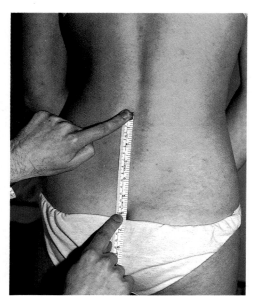

Fig. 12.19 Measurement of forward flexion. With the patient erect the lumbosacral junction is identified between the dimples of Venus. A mark is made 10cm above the lumbo-sacral junction and one

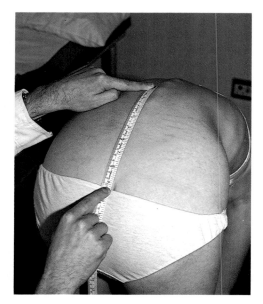

5cm below it. The tape measure is held along this 15cm line (left). When the patient bends forward the distance between the marks increases, in this case to 22cm (right).

Although the disease is most common in young men it has recently become appreciated that the incidence in women is higher than was previously thought. In female patients the disease is often mild and restricted to the sacroiliac joints and lower lumbar spine. A high index of suspicion and a careful history and clinical examination are especially important in this group.

EXAMINATION In many patients spinal posture alters before radiological signs of the disease are present. The normal lumbar lordosis is lost and the dorsal curve is accentuated (Fig. 12.17). Lumbar spine movement is restricted in all directions and examination must include observation of back movement. Lateral flexion is characteristically reduced first, a useful sign in differential diagnosis (Fig. 12.18). Measurement is usually made only of forward flexion using Macrae's modification of Shober's method (Fig. 12.19). Measurement of the finger-floor distance is inadequate as a patient with a fused spine may be able to touch the toes if the hips are mobile (Fig. 12.20). Several methods of clinical assessment for sacroiliitis exist, some of which are illustrated here (Figs. 12.21 & 12.22). There is considerable doubt about their diagnostic accuracy and the overall contribution they make to diagnosis is small. Discomfort felt around the chest wall,

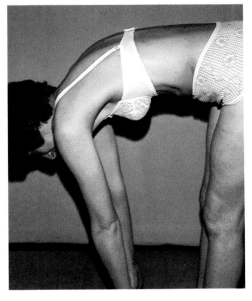

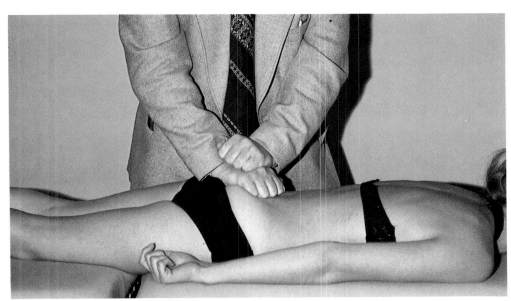

Fig. 12.20 A woman with ankylosing spondylitis who can touch her toes despite rigidity of her lumbar spine. Because her hips are mobile, this test appears normal.

Fig. 12.21 Clinical assessment of sacroiliitis. Direct pressure is applied over the sacrum with the patient lying prone.

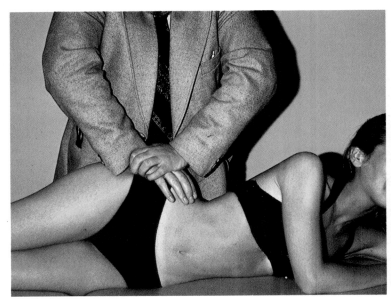

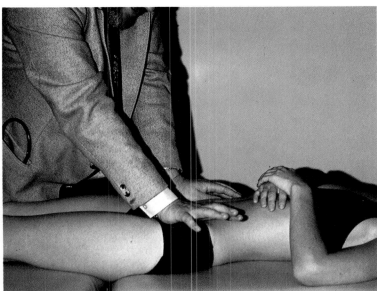

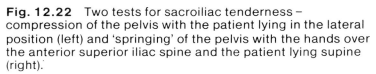

Fig. 12.22 Two tests for sacroiliac tenderness – compression of the pelvis with the patient lying in the lateral position (left) and 'springing' of the pelvis with the hands over the anterior superior iliac spine and the patient lying supine (right).

particularly when exertion necessitates deep breathing, is often perceived early in the course of ankylosing spondylitis. Examination of chest expansion may reveal restriction of rib movement (Fig. 12.23). This should be related to the subject's age and sex rather than taking the arbitrary 2.5cm expansion suggested by some diagnostic criteria. Thoracic spine rotation may also be reduced (Fig. 12.24). Examination of the eyes may reveal signs of past or present iritis (Fig. 12.25). Peripheral joints are sometimes involved early in the disease and presentation of ankylosing spondylitis with a swollen knee is not uncommon (Fig. 12.26).

INVESTIGATIONS The key investigation is the radiograph. Usually the sacroiliac joints are involved first. Symmetrical involvement of the whole joint is typical. The changes include widening of the joint space and erosions, sclerosis and eventually joint space narrowing and fusion (Figs. 12.27 & 12.28). It is preferable to use pelvic radiographs to assess the sacroiliac joints, rather than a view coned down

to the joints, if only because of the extra information given by the pelvic film. It is especially important to observe whether the epiphyses on the iliac crest have fused as the adolescent sacroiliac joint is particularly difficult to interpret and may appear wide and irregular in normal subjects. Erosive changes in the pubic symphysis and calcification at tendinous insertions into the pelvis may also be seen on the full pelvic radiograph and the condition of the hips can also be examined (Fig. 12.29).

Sacroiliitis may take many years to become radiologically apparent. In an attempt to make an earlier diagnosis, quantitative sacroiliac scintigraphy, usually using 99m technetium methylene diphosphonate, has been introduced and thermography has also been used. The use of these techniques remains controversial and although they may aid the diagnosis in some adults they are of little value in the adolescent group as high uptake may be seen in normal joints. Clinical suspicion and careful examination therefore remain the cornerstones of diagnosis.

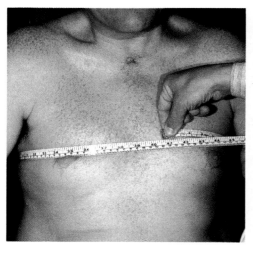

Fig. 12.23 Examination of the chest. The tape measure is usually applied just above the nipple line.

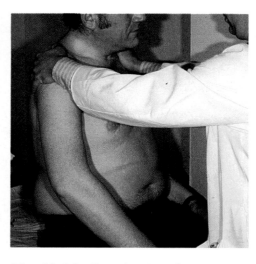

Fig. 12.24 Examination of rotation in the thoracic spine. The patient is seated on a couch to immobilize the pelvis and

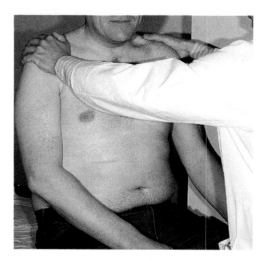

his shoulders are then rotated by the examiner.

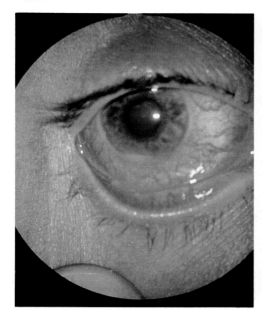

Fig. 12.25 Iritis in a patient with ankylosing spondylitis. In this severe case there is considerable conjunctival injection and a hypopyon is also present.

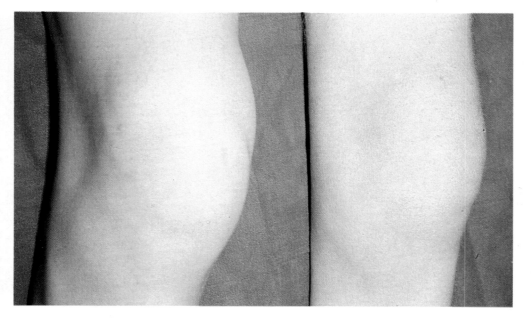

Fig. 12.26 The knees of a teenage boy showing large effusions, particularly on the right. He

subsequently developed inflammatory type back pain and was found to have changes in the lumbar spine.

Marginal erosions and early syndesmophytes may be seen on spinal radiographs (see Fig. 12.7). A common site for the first syndesmophyte is at the dorsolumbar junction which is often poorly seen on conventional radiographs (Fig. 12.30). A film centred on this region may be of diagnostic value.

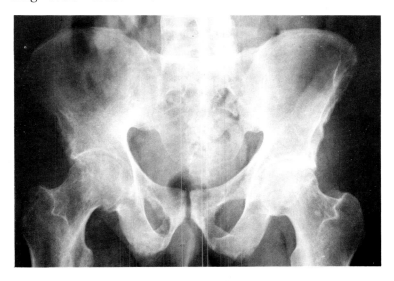

Fig. 12.27 Pelvic radiograph showing widening of the joint spaces; erosions and marginal sclerosis on both sides of the sacroiliac joints. Note also similar changes in the pubic symphysis.

Fig. 12.28 Pelvic radiograph in advanced ankylosing spondylitis. The sacroiliac joints are barely distinguishable as they have now fused. Typical changes are seen in the lumbrosacral spine. Note also the bony proliferation around the pelvis, fluffy erosions at the origins of the adductor muscles and hip involvement.

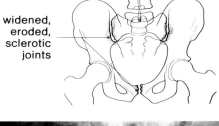

widened, eroded, sclerotic joints

fused sacroiliac joints — intervertebral fusion — secondary bone proliferation

erosion and new bone at tendon insertions

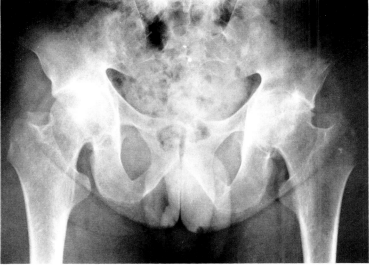

Fig. 12.29 Pelvic radiograph showing sacroiliac joint fusion at the top and erosions at the lower margins. Note also joint space narrowing in both hips with erosive damage on the left in particular.

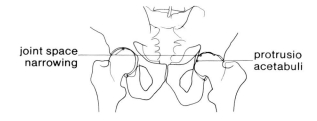

joint space narrowing — protrusio acetabuli

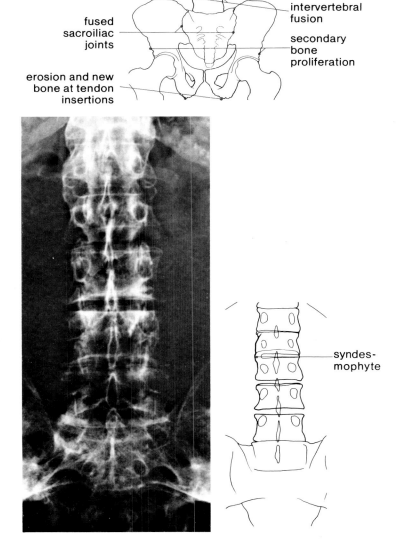

syndes-mophyte

Fig. 12.30 Lumbar spine radiograph showing a syndesmophyte at L 1/2.

The ESR or plasma viscosity are often raised in ankylosing spondylitis but are inconsistent and do not always provide a good measure of inflammatory activity. No diagnostic biochemical abnormalities exist. The majority of patients have the tissue type HLA-B27 but as the most extreme estimates suggest that only 20% of people with B27 will develop a seronegative spondarthritis this is not of value as a diagnostic test.

Progressive Ankylosing Spondylitis

Clinically advancing disease is characterized by increasing stiffness of the spine. The dorsal stoop becomes more prominent with consequent restriction of the chest, and neck pain and stiffness occur. Some patients have an apparently asymptomatic progression to this stage of severe spinal stiffness (Fig. 12.31). Such patients usually seek attention when stiffness in the neck makes activities such as driving difficult. Examination reveals the extent of rigidity elsewhere.

The radiology of progressive disease reveals advancing sacroiliitis and extending new bone formation which forms bridges between adjacent vertebrae (Fig. 12.32).

Severe Ankylosing Spondylitis

The spinal disease may spread to involve the entire spine with bony fusion from neck to sacrum (Figs. 12.33 & 12.34). The thoracic kyphosis increases at this stage and the patient may be able to see in front of him only by using

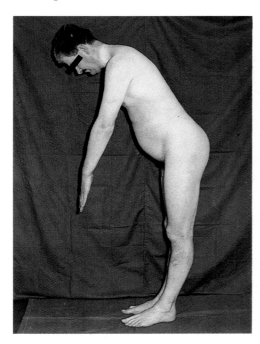

Fig. 12.31 Progressive ankylosing spondylitis. This patient with severe limitation of lumbar flexion was asymptomatic for many years.

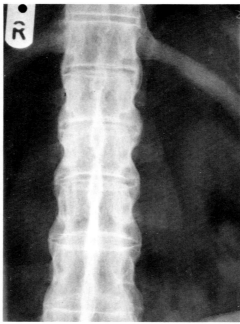

Fig. 12.32 Lumbar spine radiograph showing extensive bony ankylosis in a typical 'bamboo spine' pattern. Note also the ossification of the dorsal interspinous ligament and fusion at the costovertebral joints at T12. The changes are symmetrical at all levels.

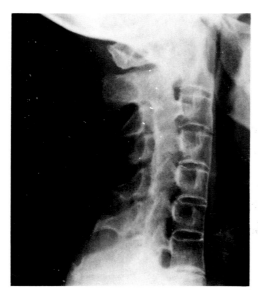

Fig. 12.33 Cervical spine radiograph showing severe changes with vertebral squaring and anterior fusion and obliteration due to fusion of the facet joints.

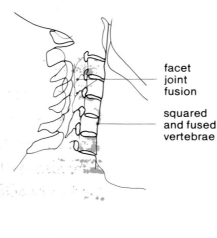

Fig. 12.34 A patient with severe ankylosing spondylitis showing fused spinal processes in the dorsal spine (which is kyphotic).

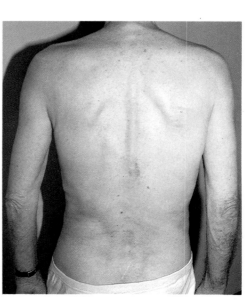

12.10

prismatic spectacles. Two-thirds of patients have hip disease and one-third have shoulder involvement (Figs. 12.35 & 12.36). Trauma is a considerable problem to the advanced spondylitic. His lack of trunk mobility makes him prone to falls and his rigid spine is vulnerable, fractures often taking place through bony bridges. Occasionally inflammatory changes involving the intervertebral disc give rise to 'discitis' which causes local pain accompanied by radiological evidence of considerable disc space narrowing and irregularity. This occurs particularly when an isolated disc level is unaffected by bony ankylosis with a consequent excess of movement at that point (Fig. 12.37).

Extra-articular Manifestations

The main extra-articular manifestations of ankylosing spondylitis are listed in figure 12.38. They increase with disease duration but do not correlate with the activity or severity of the spondylitis.

Iritis is the commonest extra-articular manifestation and eventually occurs in about 20% of spondylitic patients (see Fig. 12.25). It may be recurrent and if not promptly treated can lead to extensive ocular damage. Pulmonary problems also occur. A restrictive pattern of respiratory function tests is produced by chest wall rigidity and the lung apices are particularly poorly aerated in spondylitic patients. This probably contributes to the development of fibrosis in the upper zones which occurs in about 1.5%

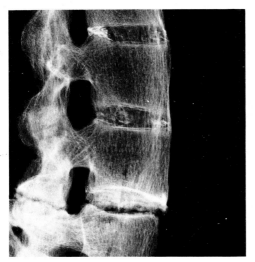

Fig. 12.35 Pelvic radiograph in severe ankylosing spondylitis showing obliteration of the sacroiliac joints and erosion of the adductor tendon insertions. There is also severe hip involvement with loss of joint space, new bone formation and marginal sclerosis, secondary to old inflammation.

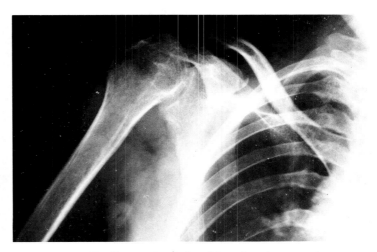

Fig. 12.36 Radiograph of shoulder showing erosive changes over the lateral aspect of the humeral head, narrowing of the joint space and upward migration of the humeral head due to rotator cuff damage.

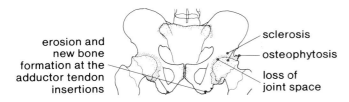

erosion and new bone formation at the adductor tendon insertions

sclerosis

osteophytosis

loss of joint space

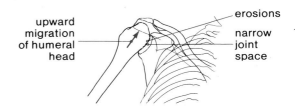

upward migration of humeral head

erosions

narrow joint space

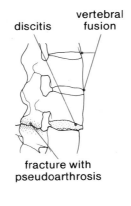

discitis

vertebral fusion

fracture with pseudoarthrosis

Fig. 12.37 Radiograph (post mortem) showing discitis, intervertebral fusion and pseudoarthrosis at a fracture site.

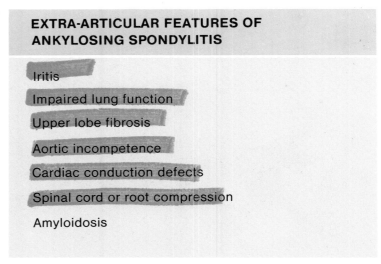

EXTRA-ARTICULAR FEATURES OF ANKYLOSING SPONDYLITIS

- Iritis
- Impaired lung function
- Upper lobe fibrosis
- Aortic incompetence
- Cardiac conduction defects
- Spinal cord or root compression
- Amyloidosis

Fig. 12.38 Table listing the major extra-articular manifestations of ankylosing spondylitis.

of cases (Fig. 12.39). Spondylitic patients may also be prone to chest infections. Aortic incompetence is an uncommon but well recognized complication, and cardiac conduction defects may also occur.

Neurological damage may arise from spinal trauma or atlanto-axial subluxation. The cauda equina syndrome can develop and is associated with arachnoid cysts in some patients.

The widespread use of spinal irradiation in the 1940s and 1950s has produced an increased incidence of leukaemia and of basal cell carcinoma in irradiated areas together with typical skin changes of pigmentation and telangiectasis (Figs. 12.40).

Management

Physiotherapy with a regular daily regime of home exercises is the key to management of spondylitis (Fig. 12.41). Hydrotherapy is also beneficial (Fig. 12.42). Non-steroidal anti-inflammatory drugs may be a useful adjunct to this therapy as they decrease symptoms. The major extra-spinal manifestations such as iritis also require prompt diagnosis and early treatment. If the diagnosis is made early and the patient is made aware of the condition and its treatment, deformity and disability can be prevented. A full understanding of the clinical features, diagnosis and management of this condition is therefore vital for physicians.

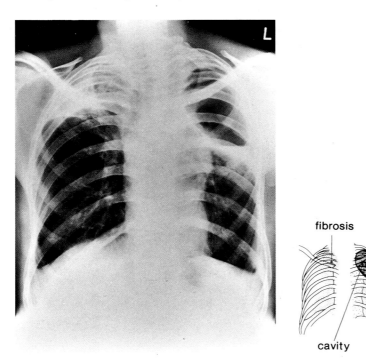

Fig. 12.39 Chest radiograph showing cavitation in a previous area of fibrosis with some fluid in the cavity. Although no aspergilloma is visible, the patient had strongly positive skin tests for aspergillosis. There is also fibrosis in the right upper zone.

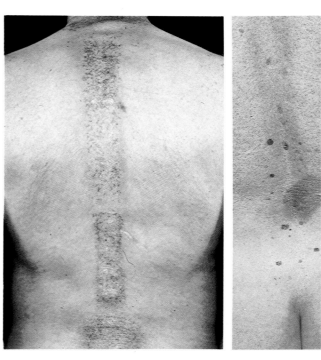

Fig. 12.40 A patient with severe ankylosing spondylitis who had been treated with radiotherapy 30 years previously. Widespread telangiectases are obvious in the original radiation field (left). A patient who had radiotherapy for AS has developed multiple carcinomata (right). Courtesy of Professor R.J. Berry.

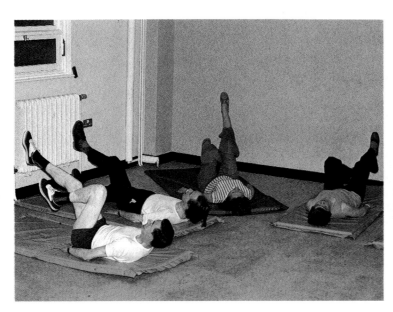

Fig. 12.41 A physiotherapy class at the famous Royal National Hospital for Rheumatic Diseases, Bath, UK.

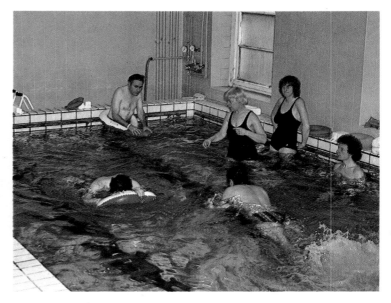

Fig. 12.42 Hydrotherapy pool for the treatment of the ankylosing spondylitis.

13

Seronegative Spondarthritis

with Dr. Ian Haslock

The term seronegative spondarthritis refers to a group of distinct diseases which have a number of characteristics in common (Fig. 13.1). These include the absence of rheumatoid factor or other autoantibodies, involvement of the spine and a peripheral inflammatory arthritis. There is a high incidence of the HLA antigen B27 in many diseases in this group and family studies have revealed a network of interconnections amongst them. Finally, many members of the group share similar extra-articular features. This colligative concept of a disease group has important diagnostic, therapeutic and etiologic implications (Fig. 13.2). The group includes ankylosing spondylitis, psoriatic arthritis, Reiter's disease and the arthritis associated with inflammatory bowel disease. Many cases of 'reactive arthritis' and some forms of juvenile chronic arthritis should also be included. It is not clear whether Behçet's or Whipple's disease belong in this group. Despite the strong links and overlaps between the members of this group, they will be considered separately.

PSORIATIC ARTHRITIS

About 7% of patients with psoriasis develop an arthropathy. A peripheral arthritis shows three main patterns, each of which may be complicated by sacroiliac and/or spinal involvement (Fig. 13.3).

Distal Psoriatic Arthritis

Distal interphalangeal joint (DIP) involvement is usually accompanied by disease of the associated nail giving rise to the term 'topographical psoriatic arthritis' (Fig. 13.4). Clinically, the involved joints show signs of inflammatory synovitis which may progress to produce a characteristic deformity (Fig. 13.5). The nails may show pitting, or severe onycholysis mimicking fungal infection (Fig. 13.6). Radiologically, there are erosive changes which may be severe and share characteristics with the other forms of psoriatic arthritis (Fig. 13.7).

CHARACTERISTICS OF SERONEGATIVE SPONDARTHRITIDES

Absence of rheumatoid factor	Familial clustering
Involvement of sacroiliac and spinal joints	Increased incidence of HLA-B27
Peripheral arthritis (predominantly lower limb)	Common spectrum of extra-articular features (predominantly muco-cutaneous)
Enthesopathy	

Fig. 13.1 Table of common characteristics of diseases included in the group of seronegative spondarthritides.

SERONEGATIVE SPONDARTHRITIS

Ankylosing spondylitis

Psoriasis

(Whipple's disease)

Ulcerative colitis

Crohn's disease

Reiters disease

(Behçets syndrome)

Reactive arthritis

Fig. 13.2 Table of diseases included in the group of seronegative spondarthritides.

PATTERNS OF PSORIATIC ARTHROPATHY

Distal interphalangal joint disease with associated nail lesions

Seronegative polyarthritis often variable and asymmetrical, may develop transient 'sausage digits'

Deforming arthritis ('arthritis mutilans')

Spondylitis

Fig. 13.3 Table showing the patterns of involvement in psoriatic arthritis.

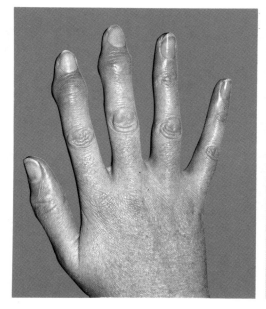

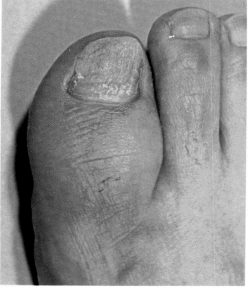

Fig. 13.4 DIP arthritis in psoriasis: involvement of the index and middle fingers (left) and a great toe showing nail involvement (right) with arthritis of the interphalangeal joint.

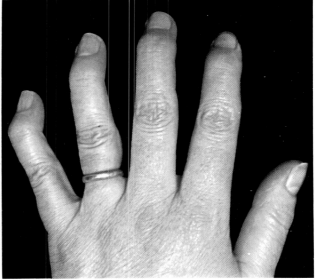

Fig. 13.5 Deformity of the hands arising from longstanding psoriatic arthritis. The other small joints of the hands are uninvolved despite the advanced deformity of the DIPs.

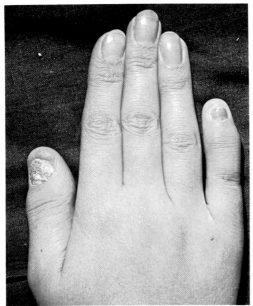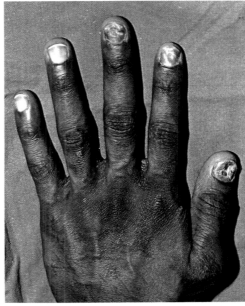

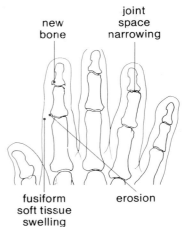

Fig. 13.6 Psoriatic nail dystrophy (left) and fungal nail dystrophy (right).

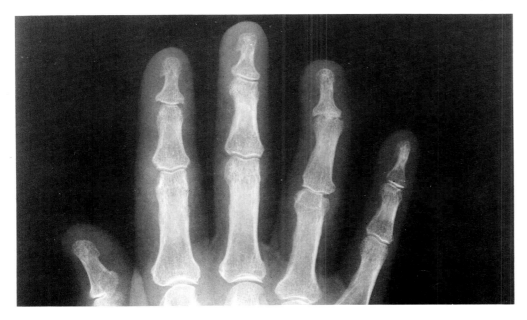

Fig. 13.7 Hand radiograph in psoriatic arthritis showing DIP erosions and associated bone proliferation. Joint space narrowing is present together with fusiform soft tissue swelling of the fingers.

new bone

joint space narrowing

fusiform soft tissue swelling

erosion

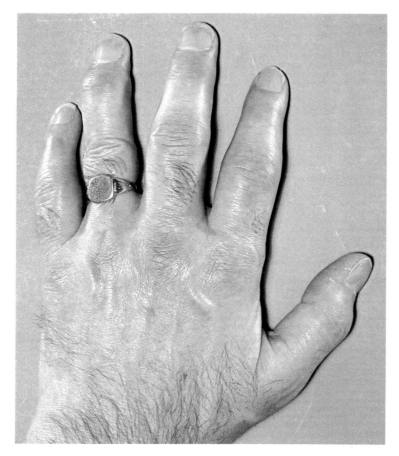

Fig. 13.8 Polyarticular arthritis, in particular at the left ring DIP.

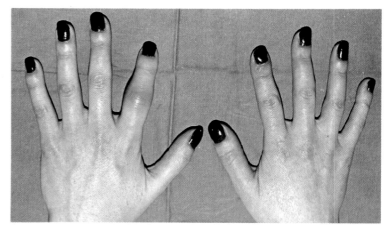

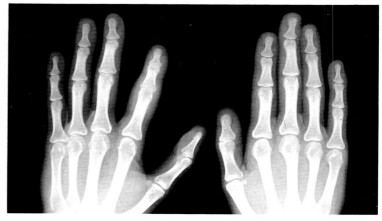

Fig. 13.9 'Indistinguishable' psoriatic arthritis involving the left index PIP joint. Note the lack of periarticular osteoporosis despite joint space narrowing.

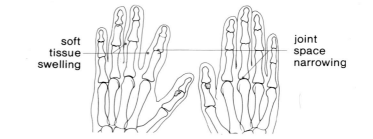

soft tissue swelling

joint space narrowing

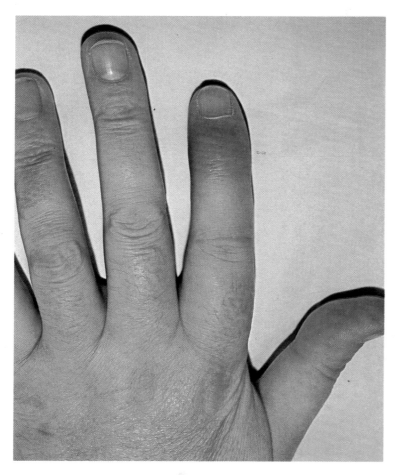

Fig. 13.10 Sausage finger.

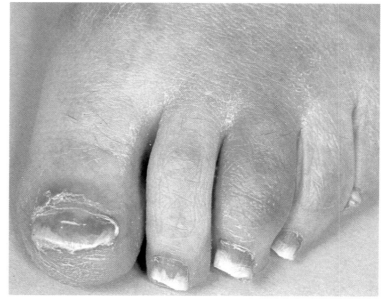

Fig. 13.11 Sausage toes with associated nail dystrophy.

'Indistinguishable' Psoriatic Arthritis

This is the most common form of psoriatic arthritis and is so named because of its resemblance to rheumatoid arthritis. However, it is more asymmetrical and particular joint activity may fluctuate considerably (Figs. 13.8 & 13.9). A characteristic feature is the 'sausage digit' which is diffusely swollen in comparison with the spindle-shaped swelling of rheumatoid arthritis (Fig. 13.10). It occurs because inflammation involves both the proximal and distal interphalangeal joints and the flexor tendon sheaths. Involvement of fingers and toes is equally common (Fig. 13.11).

Other joints may suffer severe temporary exacerbations with large effusions (Fig. 13.12). In common with other seronegative spondarthritides psoriatic synovitis may involve tendons.

Deforming Psoriatic Arthritis

The first description of arthritis mutilans was in psoriatic arthritis. Although this is rare, occurring in only 5% of patients, it is extremely disabling with active synovitis of many joints in the hands and feet being accompanied by severe erosive changes and osteolysis (Figs. 13.13 & 13.14). The end result is an asymmetrical, grossly deforming arthritis with gross destructive changes seen radiologically (Fig. 13.15).

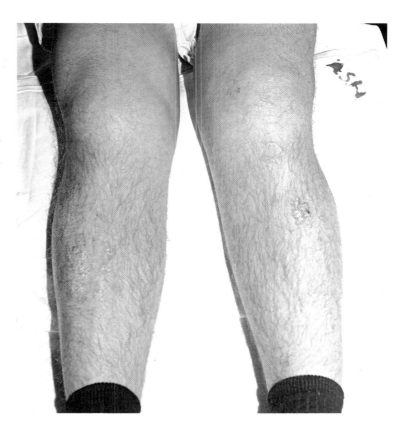

Fig. 13.12 Effusion of the right knee. Note the psoriatic lesions on both shins.

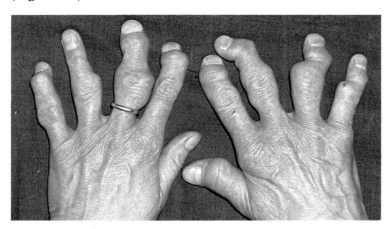

Fig. 13.13 Psoriatic arthritis mutilans. This patient has gross joint destruction which has led to telescoping of the fingers. Note the nail pits, particularly in the index and little fingers.

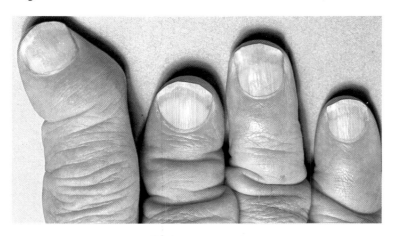

Fig. 13.14 Psoriatic arthritis mutilans. This patient has severe joint damage with distortion due to old (asymmetrical) synovitis. Courtesy of Dr. M. Corbett.

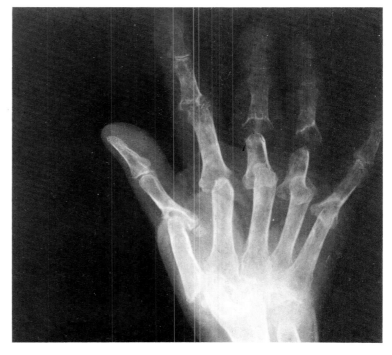

Fig. 13.15 Hand radiograph is psoriatic arthritis mutilans showing pencil-in-cup deformities and shortening of the digits.

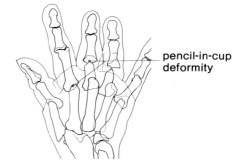

pencil-in-cup deformity

Psoriatic Spondylitis

Each pattern of psoriatic arthritis may be complicated by sacroiliitis and spondylitis (Fig. 13.16), although this is most frequently associated with the deforming type and least so with the distal type. Isolated spinal disease in the absence of peripheral joint manifestations may also occur in

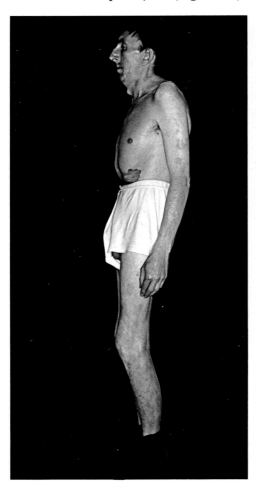

Fig. 13.16 A patient with spondylitis and psoriasis.

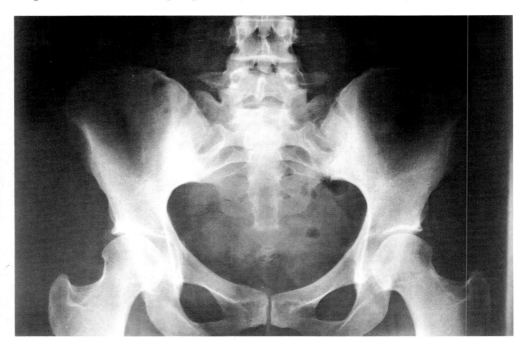

Fig. 13.17 Pelvic radiograph showing asymmetrical sacroiliitis predominantly involving the lower two-thirds of the joints, particularly on the right.

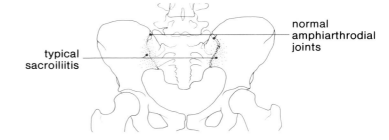

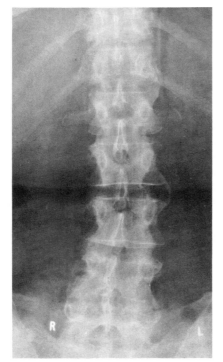 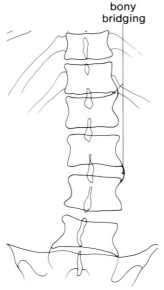

Fig. 13.18 Lumbar spine radiograph showing asymmetrical syndesmophyte formation with bony bridging.

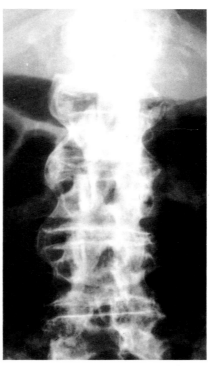 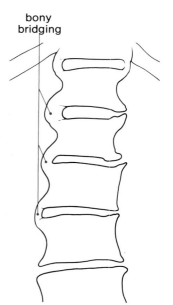

Fig. 13.19 Lumbar spine radiograph in severe psoriatic spondylitis showing asymmetrical involvement and, in particular, coarse new bone of a more florid type than that usually seen in straightforward ankylosing spondylitis.

patients with psoriasis. All stages may be seen from asymptomatic sacroiliitis to widespread intervertebral fusion (Figs. 13.17 & 13.18). Radiologically, psoriatic spondylitis and Reiter's spondylitis may be distinguished from ankylosing spondylitis because there is asymmetry of involvement, more florid paraspinal ossification and new bone formation further away from the disc space than in ankylosing spondylitis (Fig. 13.19).

Pathology

In general terms the pathological distinction between psoriatic and rheumatoid arthritis is much less apparent than the clinical difference. The histological features of the synovitis strongly resemble those seen in rheumatoid disease although it has been suggested that psoriatics show increased fibrosis of joint tissues. There are more bony changes in psoriasis with periostitis and increased osteolysis. There are no systemic manifestations of psoriatic arthritis apart from the skin disease.

Radiology

Radiographs of peripheral joints often help distinguish psoriatic arthritis from other inflammatory arthropathies. The radiological differences reflect the clinical and pathological changes. There is greater asymmetry of joint distribution than in rheumatoid disease (Fig. 13.20). Associated osteolysis leads to 'pencil-in-cup' deformities (Fig. 13.21). Fluffy periosteal new bone around the involved joints is typical (Fig. 13.22). Bony fusion in the extremities occurs more often than in rheumatoid arthritis.

Fig. 13.20 Hand radiograph showing the typical changes of psoriatic arthritis.

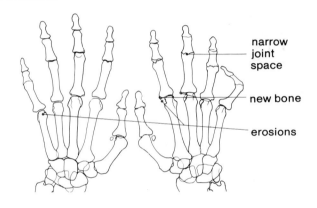

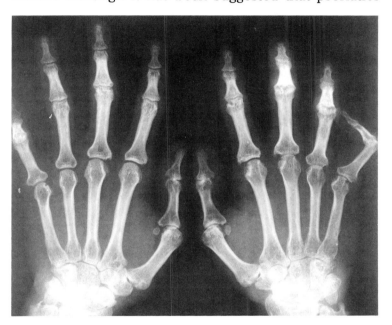

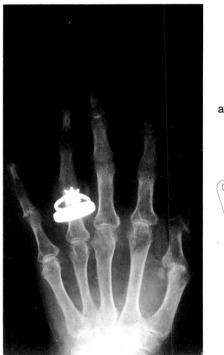
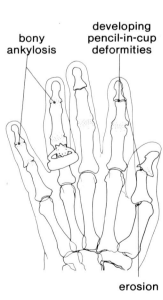

Fig. 13.21 Hand radiograph in established psoriatic arthritis showing joint fusion and developing pencil-in-cup deformity.

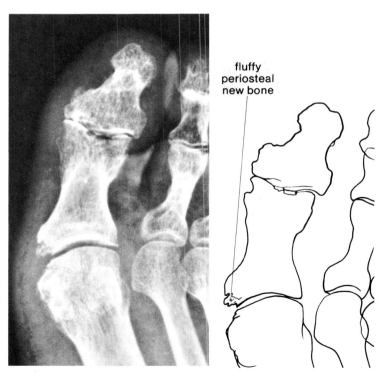

Fig. 13.22 Radiograph of the great toe showing fluffy periosteal new bone.

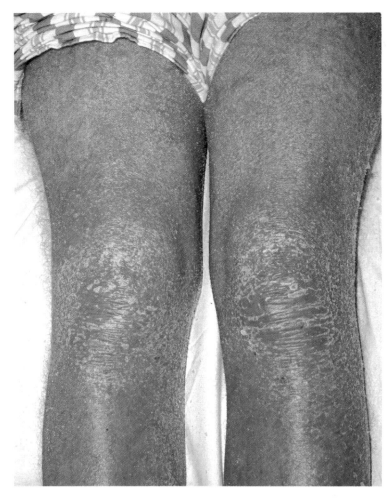

Fig. 13.23 A patient with severe psoriasis showing an arthritis of the right knee with a small effusion.

Association Between Skin and Joint Changes

A coincident skin or nail lesion over an involved joint simplifies the diagnosis (Fig. 13.23). Psoriatic nail dystrophy is obvious, but may be limited to small numbers of pits in a few nails (Fig. 13.24). When faced with an arthritis of unknown etiology a careful search must be made for psoriatic skin lesions over the common sites including the knees, elbows, hairline, umbilicus and natal cleft (Fig. 13.25).

There is very little relationship between skin and joint disease. Either may appear first. Severe or prolonged arthritis may coexist with minimal skin disease and vice versa. A few patients with a strong family history of seronegative spondarthritis develop an arthritis typical of the psoriatic type but without any skin disease. A few patients find skin and joints worsen in parallel whereas others find they have an inverse relationship with the skin improving if the joints worsen. In many cases there is no relationship at all between the skin and joint manifestations.

REITER'S DISEASE

The triad of urethritis, conjunctivitis and arthritis is known as Reiter's disease despite its earlier description by Benjamin Brodie. The disease may follow sexual intercourse or infectious diarrhoea (Fig. 13.26).

The disease is much commoner in men than women. Urethritis usually appears first even if the disease follows a bowel infection. It occurs up to three weeks after the initial infection and lasts about ten days. This is followed rapidly by conjunctivitis, with arthritis predominantly

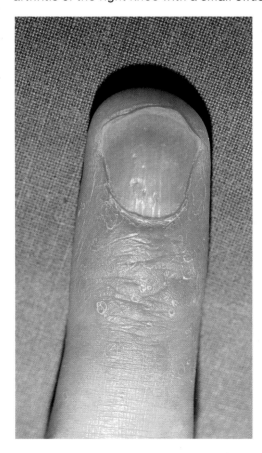

Fig. 13.24 A few nail pits in a single nail.

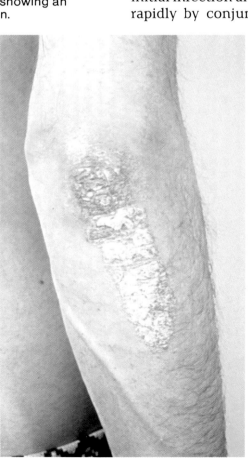

Fig. 13.25 Psoriasis over one elbow (left) and in the umbilicus which had

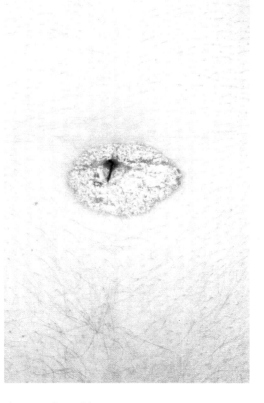

been missed by an orthopedic surgeon (right).

involving large joints of the lower limbs, especially the knees (Fig. 13.27). These may be so grossly distended that pain arises from capsular distension. Insertional lesions may also occur, principally in the lower limbs, presenting especially as plantar fasciitis or Achilles tendinitis ('lover's heel') (Figs. 13.28 & 13.29). There may also be clinical evidence of sacroiliitis early in the disease with associated local tenderness.

FEATURES OF REITERS DISEASE

Urethritis

Conjunctivitis

Arthritis

Enthesopathy

Sacroiliitis

Keratoderma blenorrhagica

Mouth ulcers

Circinate balanitis

Cervicitis

Iritis

Fig. 13.26 Table listing the features of Reiter's disease.

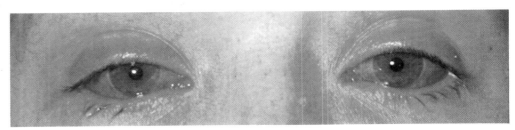
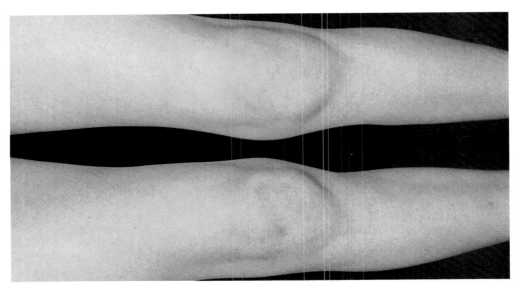

Fig. 13.27 Involvement of the knee (lower) and conjunctivitis (upper) in Reiter's disease. Courtesy of Professor H. Lambert.

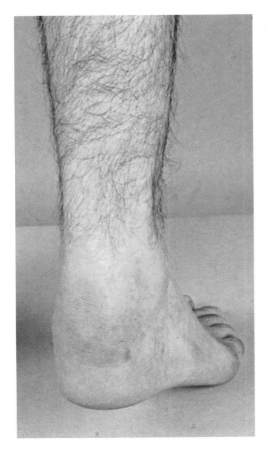

Fig. 13.28 Achilles tendinitis in Reiter's disease.

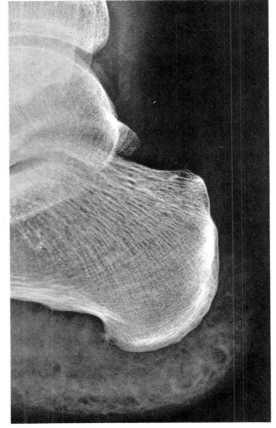
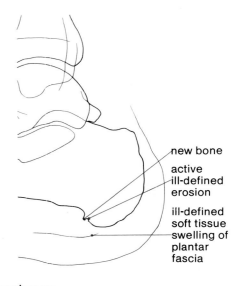

new bone

active ill-defined erosion

ill-defined soft tissue swelling of plantar fascia

Fig. 13.29 Lateral radiograph of the heel showing an eroded plantar spur with adjacent new bone formation.

Several other lesions of skin and mucous membranes may occur in Reiter's disease. These include keratoderma blenorrhagica, a pustular skin disease of the soles of the feet, characteristic of Reiter's disease but pathologically indistinguishable from pustular psoriasis (Fig. 13.30). Large but painless ulcers of mucous membranes, particularly occurring in the mouth and on the tongue and pharynx, are easily missed during clinical examination. Circinate balanitis is characteristic (Fig. 13.31) and cervicitis may occur in women. Iritis as well as conjunctivitis may develop although this is usually at a later stage of the condition.

The initial attack of Reiter's disease usually lasts about a month but may take much longer to settle completely and often has minor exacerbations and remissions. There is a very high recurrence rate with any, or all of the members of the triad recurring in varying degrees of severity. Eighty percent of patients suffer such recurrences and may become disabled by the chronic disease. Patients with the tissue type HLA-B27 are more likely to develop Reiter's disease when challenged by a urethral or intestinal infective agent and are more likely to have severe recurrent disease. This applies particularly when spondylitis follows Reiter's disease, the end result of

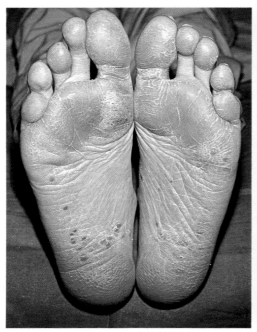 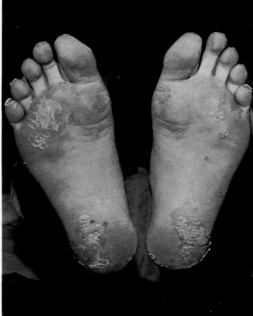 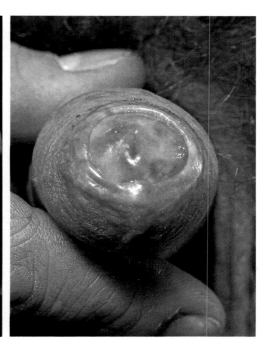

Fig. 13.30 Mild (left) and advanced (right) keratoderma blenorrhagica.

Fig. 13.31 Circinate balanitis.

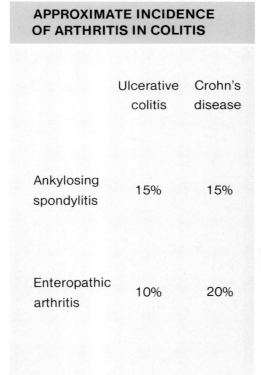

APPROXIMATE INCIDENCE OF ARTHRITIS IN COLITIS

	Ulcerative colitis	Crohn's disease
Ankylosing spondylitis	15%	15%
Enteropathic arthritis	10%	20%

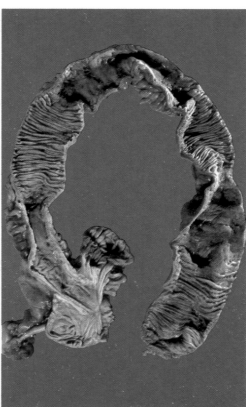

Fig. 13.32 Table showing the approximate incidence of arthritis in inflammatory bowel disease and the gross appearance of the colon in Crohn's disease (courtesy of Dr. A.B. Price).

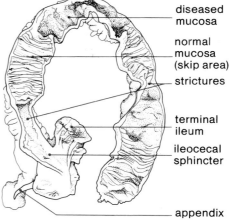

diseased mucosa

normal mucosa (skip area)

strictures

terminal ileum

ileocecal sphincter

appendix

which may be clinically indistinguishable from anky-losing spondylitis. Severe joint disease may develop in the lower limbs. Recurrent attacks of conjunctivitis and/or iritis may lead to visual problems. Urethral strictures occasionally develop. Recurrences of the disease may occur in the absence of any obvious triggering factor.

ARTHRITIS AND INFLAMMATORY BOWEL DISEASE
Both ulcerative colitis and Crohn's disease may be complicated by a peripheral arthritis (enteropathic arthritis) or by ankylosing spondylitis (Fig. 13.32).

Enteropathic Arthritis
This is a mono- or polyarthritis of limited duration, usually affecting large joints of the lower limbs. The most commonly affected joint is the knee. Attacks of synovitis are self-limiting and associated with episodes of active inflammation of the bowel. Other systemic manifestations such as erythema nodosum may also be present. Occasionally the patients present with joint disease; thus the rheumatologist must be aware of the need to take a full gastrointestinal history and initiate the appropriate investigations such as sigmoidoscopy with biopsy and barium studies (Figs. 13.33 & 13.34).

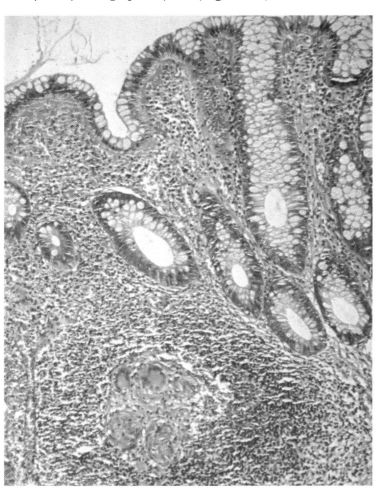

Fig. 13.33 Rectal mucosa in Crohn's disease. The giant cell granuloma established the diagnosis. H & E stain, x 240. Courtesy of Dr. A.B. Price.

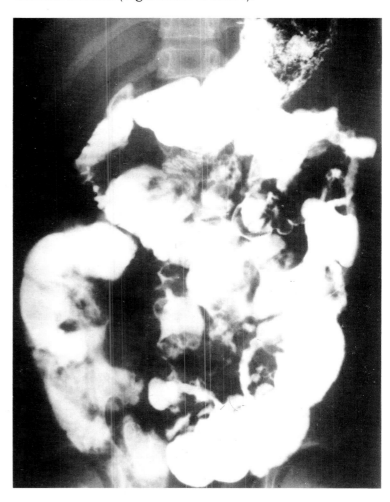

Fig. 13.34 Barium follow through demonstrating multiple strictures of Crohn's disease. The intervening loops of bowel are dilated.

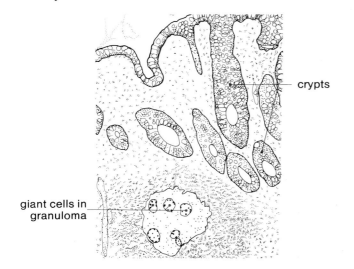

crypts

giant cells in granuloma

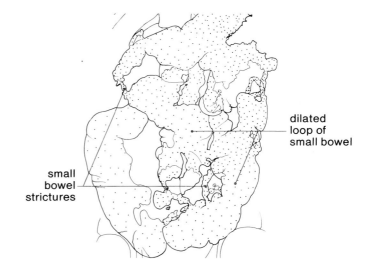

dilated loop of small bowel

small bowel strictures

Ankylosing Spondylitis

Radiological or clinical evidence of ankylosing spondylitis occurs in about 15% of patients with inflammatory bowel disease and appears to be equally distributed between the sexes. The diagnosis is easily overlooked (Fig. 13.35). Patients may be told either that their back pain is referred from their inflamed bowel, or that they have mechanical low back pain. Two-thirds of patients with spondylitis carry the HLA-B27 antigen. There is a familial aggregation of ankylosing spondylitis in the families of patients with inflammatory bowel disease. The condition is clinically and radiologically indistinguishable from idiopathic ankylosing spondylitis.

REACTIVE ARTHRITIS

This condition is now recognized much more frequently. It presents with a predominantly lower limb arthritis of the knees and ankles, often with an associated enthesopathy. It occurs within weeks of an infection, either of the gastrointestinal tract (enteropathic reactive arthritis) or of the urogenital tract (sexually acquired reactive arthritis). The clinical features are identical to those of acute Reiter's disease or enteropathic arthritis. However, skin and mucous membrane lesions are less common. The initial attack is normally short-lived, but recurrence is common. Severe disability may result in the long term especially in two-thirds of patients who possess the HLA-B27 antigen.

JUVENILE CHRONIC ARTHRITIS

Ankylosing spondylitis, psoriatic arthropathy and reactive arthritis all occur in children. The pauciarticular form of juvenile chronic arthritis occurring in older boys may be a prelude to ankylosing spondylitis in later life (Fig. 13.36). This condition should probably be grouped with the other seronegative spondarthritides.

WHIPPLE'S DISEASE AND BEHCET'S DISEASE

Some physicians have classified these two rare diseases in the seronegative spondarthritis group (Figs. 13.37 & 13.38). Others argue that the synovitis of Whipple's disease is due to the organism found in the involved bowel and that Behçet's disease is a distinct entity with a different epidemiological and familial clustering from that of the seronegative spondarthritides.

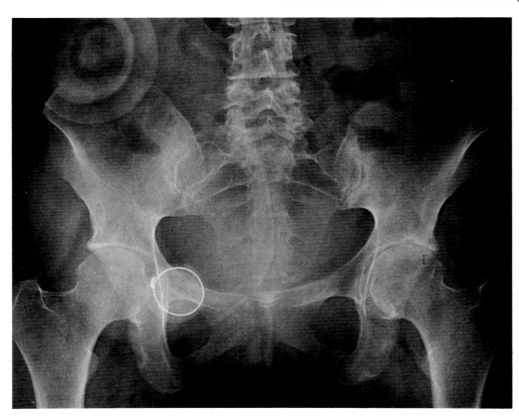

Fig. 13.35 Pelvic radiograph in a patient with Crohn's disease showing sacroiliitis and an ileostomy bag. The patient previously had a colectomy.

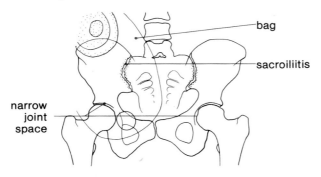

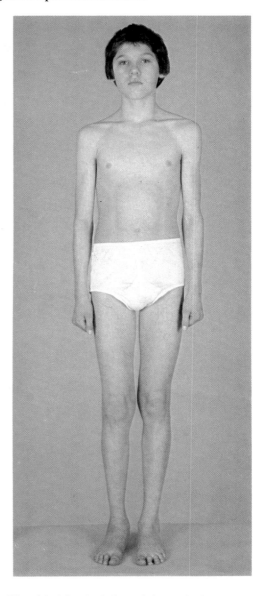

Fig. 13.36 Arthritis of the right knee and ankle in a boy who went on to develop ankylosing spondylitis.

FEATURES OF WHIPPLE'S DISEASE

Malabsorption

Arthritis

Fever

Lymphadenopathy

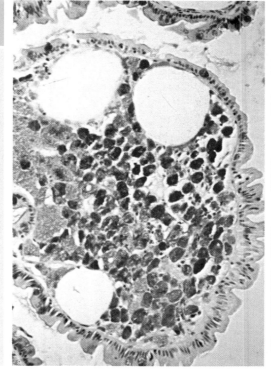
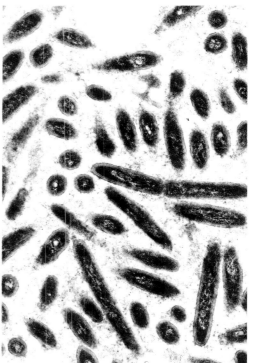

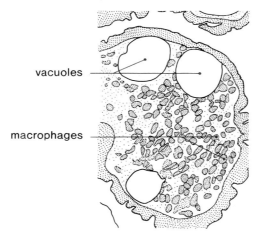

vacuoles

macrophages

Fig. 13.37 Table showing the major features of Whipple's disease (left), the typical mucosal appearance with large vacuoles and macrophages filled with periodic acid-Schiff reagent (x 180, middle), and an electron micrograph showing the rod-shaped organisms which lie free in the lamina propria (x 17,000, right). Courtesy of Dr. A.B. Price.

CLINICAL FEATURES OF BEHCETS DISEASE

Buccal ulceration	99%
Genital ulceration	80%
Uveitis	66%
Cutaneous vasculitis	66%
Synovitis	55%
Meningoencephalitis	20%

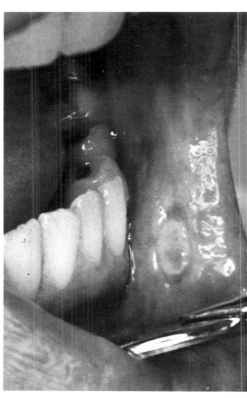

Fig. 13.38 Table showing the approximate frequency of the six major clinical features of Behçet's disease (left) and the characteristic buccal ulceration (right).

FAMILIAL AGGREGATION, HLA-B27 AND THE SERONEGATIVE SPONDARTHRITIDES

The familial aggregation and clinical overlap of this group of diseases raises important and interesting questions about their etiology and pathogenesis. The finding of a very high incidence of HLA-B27 in ankylosing spondylitis and an increased prevalence of the same antigen in other members of this group of diseases has stimulated extensive research (Fig. 13.39). Many different theories have been put forward to account for these associations. It has been suggested that HLA-B27 shares antigenic properties with some bowel commensal organisms such as *Klebsiella*. Also 'molecular mimicry' of HLA-B27 could lead to altered recognition of viral and other antigens, or to changes in immunological defence mechanisms. Another theory suggests that it is the genes close to that coding for HLA-B27 which are important, rather than the antigen itself.

The frequency of the seronegative spondarthritides appears to be increasing but this may be related to more frequent diagnosis. They certainly present a common and challenging group of potentially disabling disorders of young people for both the clinician and the research worker to explore.

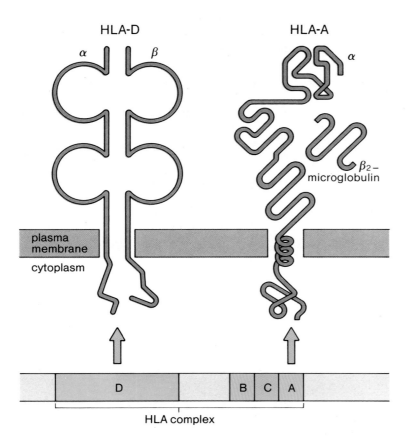

Fig. 13.39 Diagram showing a genetic map of the human major histocompatibility complex (HLA) and a representation of the HLA-B and HLA-D antigens encoded by the genes in this complex. The antigens consist of α and β chains and are shown here embedded in the plasma membrane.

14
Arthritis in Children

Arthralgia and arthritis are not uncommon in children, and have many possible causes. Discomfort arising in or around the joints is often mild, transient and unimportant, and can be caused by trauma, general ill-health or psychogenic factors (eg. attention seeking), as well as by joint disease. With the recent decline in the incidence of rheumatic fever, it is the viral infections, Henoch-Schönlein purpura and juvenile chronic arthritis (JCA) that have become the commonest causes of a true arthritis. However, blood dyscrasias (eg. leukemia), neoplasia (eg. neuroblastoma), connective tissue diseases, osteomyelitis and several other rare conditions can also

present with joint disease in childhood. The clinical presentation is variable and depends on age. Older children may complain of pain, but this is rare under the age of 5, and a limp, reluctance to use a limb, repeated falls or general malaise may be the main features. Rashes, fevers and other systemic signs may be present, aiding the diagnosis. The main subdivisions of juvenile chronic arthritis and some of the other important causes of arthritis in childhood will be illustrated here. Viral arthritis, infections, and arthritis due to systemic diseases which can occur in children are mentioned elsewhere.

JUVENILE CHRONIC ARTHRITIS

General abbreviations: J.C.A. in Europe
                        J.R.A. in U.S.

Features:

1. Onset under 16 years
2. Persistent arthritis in one or more joints
3. Duration:
   : three months or longer (Europe)
   : six weeks or longer (U.S.)
4. Other defined causes of arthritis in childhood excluded

Fig. 14.1 Diagnostic criteria of juvenile arthritis. Juvenile chronic arthritis (JCA or juvenile rheumatoid arthritis) is defined as a persistent arthritis of one or more joints in children under the age of 16 in whom other defined disorders can be excluded.

SUBGROUPS OF JUVENILE CHRONIC ARTHRITIS

Systemic onset:	fever and at least one other systemic feature
Pauciarticular	four or less joints involved in first six months of disease
Polyarticular	seronegative polyarthritis

Fig. 14.2 Subgroups of juvenile chronic arthritis. There are three main types of onset: systemic, pauciarticular and polyarticular.

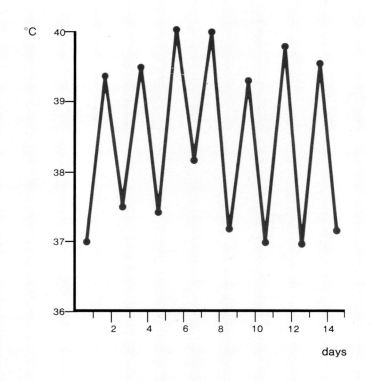

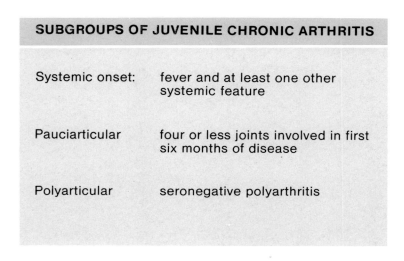

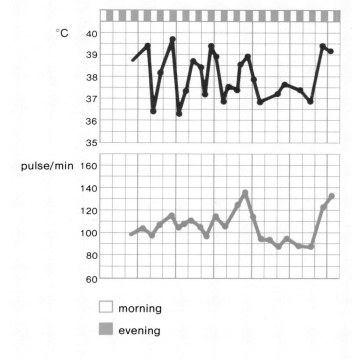

☐ morning

▨ evening

Fig. 14.3 Typical fever chart in a young girl with systemic JCA (left). Temperature chart in a 27 year old man with adult onset Still's disease (right). Note the high swinging pyrexia, peaking in the evening, and the associated tachycardia.

Juvenile Chronic Arthritis

About 70% of childhood arthritis is due to JCA, which has a prevalence of about 0.05% in schoolchildren. The criteria for making this diagnosis are shown in figure 14.1. The condition is further subdivided into three distinct types according to onset, which may be systemic, polyarticular or pauciarticular (Fig. 14.2).

1 Systemic Onset

This type of onset has an equal sex incidence, and is commonest in 2-3 year olds; it is a distinct disease, which occasionally occurs in adults, and is similar to that described by Dr. George Still in 1897 (hence the now out-dated term Still's disease, and 'adult-onset Still's disease'). The condition is a serious systemic illness which may have a dramatic acute onset and carries a significant mortality.

The main features are a swinging pyrexia (Fig. 14.3) and a typical rash which is present in about 50% of cases (Fig. 14.4). Lymphadenopathy and hepatosplenomegaly are common, and pericarditis may occur (Figs. 14.5 and 14.6).

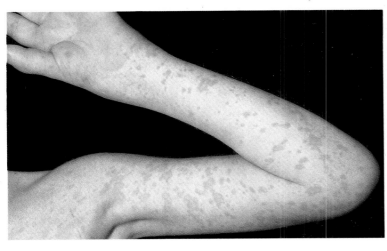

Fig. 14.4 The typical rash of systemic onset JCA (Still's rash) is an evanescent maculopapular eruption, often seen on the trunk, and most marked during febrile episodes or after a hot bath. The rashes shown are on the arm (left) and trunk (right) of a young girl with JCA.

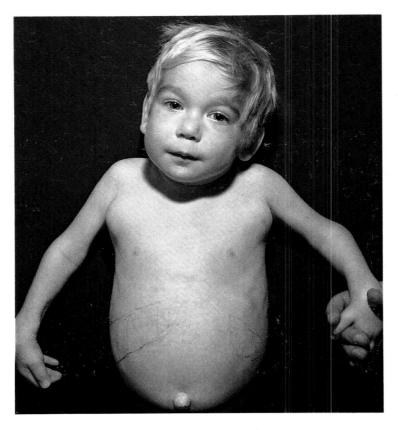

Fig. 14.5 Hepatosplenomegaly in a young boy with systemic onset JCA. Note the axillary lymphadenopathy.

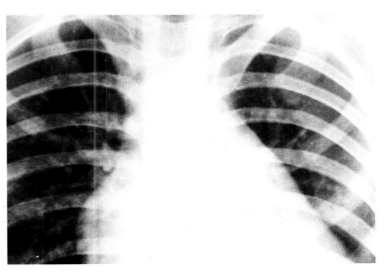

Fig. 14.6 Chest radiograph of a patient with systemic onset JCA showing a pericardial effusion. Note the large globular configuration of the heart and the sharply defined straight border on the left. The outline of the effusion extends up to the aorta.

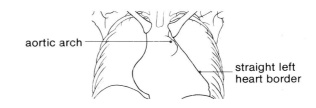

aortic arch

straight left heart border

14.3

If the condition occurs in an adult (which is very rare), the clinical findings are similar. The polyarticular, large joint episodic arthritis may be late in onset but persistent. The systemic features usually remit in 1-2 years, but early death can be caused by myocarditis, liver failure or overwhelming infection (to which the children are especially susceptible); late fatality is related to the development of amyloidosis (Fig. 14.7). Growth is impaired and may be further retarded by the use of steroids (Fig. 14.8).

2 Polyarticular Onset

Polyarticular JCA may be seronegative or seropositive (ie. with or without a positive test for IgM rheumatoid factors). Most are seronegative and girls predominate (Fig. 14.9).

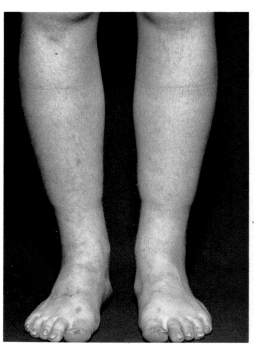

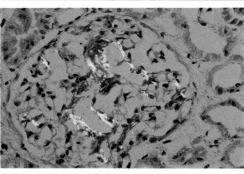

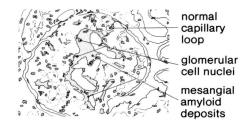

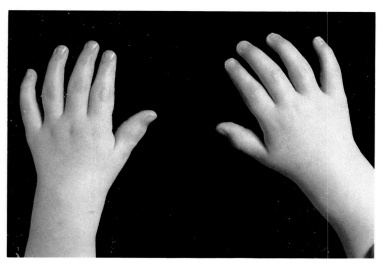

Fig. 14.7 Swelling of the legs in a child with juvenile chronic polyarthritis who presented with proteinuria and edema secondary to amyloidosis (left). Renal biopsy shows amyloid infiltration (right): high power view of a glomerulus stained by Sirius red showing early amyloid deposition restricted to the mesangium (upper) and the characteristic orange birefringence under polarized light (lower).

normal capillary loop

glomerular cell nuclei

mesangial amyloid deposits

Fig. 14.8 A young girl with systemic onset juvenile chronic arthritis who has been treated with steroids, with consequent Cushingoid appearance and growth failure. Courtesy of Dr. J.T. Scott.

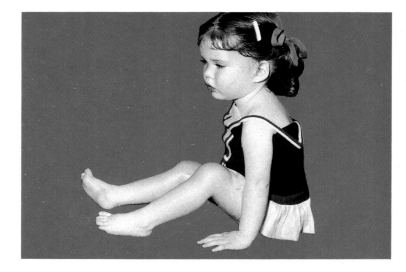

Fig. 14.9 A three year old girl with polyarticular JCA. She has many painful swollen joints, flexion deformities of the knees and difficulty with walking.

Fig. 14.10 Early polyarticular JCA showing wrist synovitis after only a few weeks of disease.

Seronegative polyarticular JCA often begins in the wrists, knees and elbows. Carpal and interphalangeal joint involvement is characteristic and flexion deformities of the proximal interphalangeal joints may appear early (Figs. 14.10 & 14.11). Typical deformities of the lower limbs may also develop (Fig. 14.12). Hip involvement is common, often resulting in fixed flexion deformity (Fig. 14.13). Late stage hip destruction may be a major cause of disability, and requires surgical management (Fig. 14.14). The neck is often involved: early loss of extension may be followed by bony fusion. Associated disease of the temporomandibular joint may cause abnormal mandibular growth, resulting in micrognathia and the typical bird-like facies (Fig. 14.15). Premature

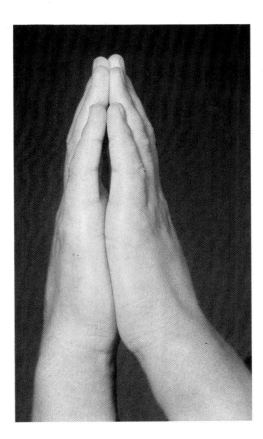

Fig. 14.11 The hands 2½ years after the polyarticular onset of JCA in a young boy. Early flexion deformities of the fingers are developing.

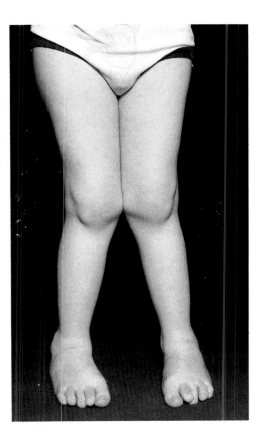

Fig. 14.12 Lower limb involvement in polyarticular JCA showing valgus deformity of the knees and varus deformity of the ankles with a consequent knock-kneed gait.

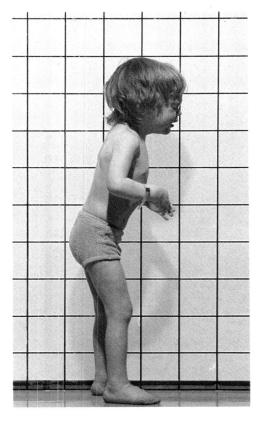

Fig. 14.13 Loss of hip extension in a little girl who is walking, bent forwards, due to flexion deformity.

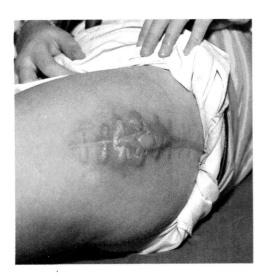

Fig. 14.14 Exuberant new bone formation in a case where osteophytic overgrowth is extending to the subcutaneous tissues around the site of operation.

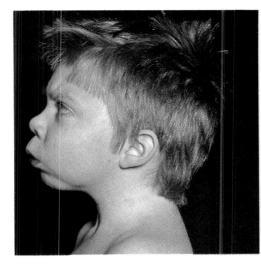

Fig. 14.15 Early loss of neck extension. Note also the micrognathia due to involvement of the

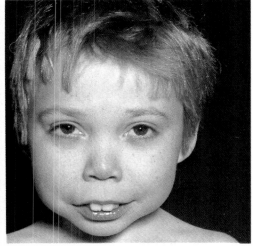

temporomandibular joints and failure of growth of the mandible, producing the typical bird-like facies.

14.5

closure or overgrowth of epiphyses occurs elsewhere, causing inequalities of growth with shortening (especially in upper limbs) or lengthening (especially in lower limbs) (Figs. 14.16 & 14.17). The radiological changes include early soft tissue swelling, periarticular osteoporosis and often periosteal new bone formation

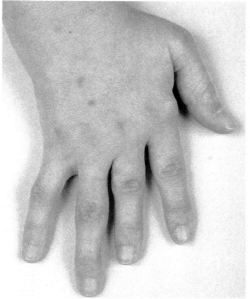

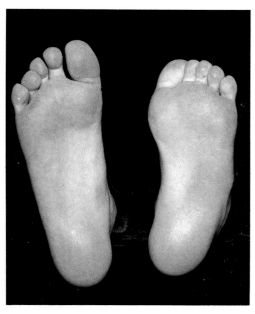

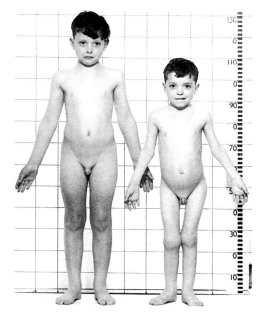

Fig. 14.16 Differential epiphyseal growth due to JCA resulting in inequality in the length of the fingers (left), and foot (right).

Fig. 14.17 Retardation of growth in JCA. The twin on the right has JCA; note the valgus deformity of the knees, inequality of leg length and much shorter stature compared with the twin on the left.

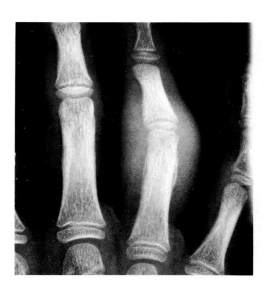

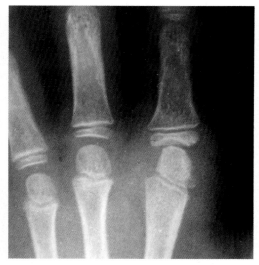

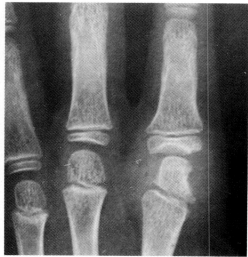

Fig. 14.18 Radiograph of the hand in early JCA. There is soft tissue swelling around the proximal interphalangeal joint of the ring finger, periarticular osteoporosis and periosteal new bone along the proximal phalanx. There is slight loss of articular cartilage, and a flexion deformity has developed.

Fig. 14.19 Progressive radiographic changes at an MCP. The radiograph on the left was taken nine months before that on the right. Initially there is soft tissue swelling around the joint and

mild joint space narrowing. There is progressive erosion of the epiphysis of the metacarpal, and to a lesser extent of the base of the proximal phalanx (right).

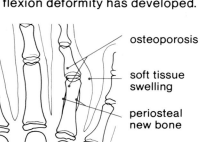

osteoporosis

soft tissue swelling

periosteal new bone

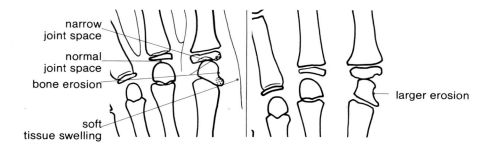

narrow joint space

normal joint space

bone erosion

soft tissue swelling

larger erosion

(Fig. 14.18). The articular cartilage of children is thicker and more resistant to damage than that of adults, but may become thinned resulting in joint space narrowing (Figs. 14.18 & 14.19). Erosions of epiphyses may occur (Fig. 14.19). As the disease progresses, growth abnormalities due to early epiphyseal fusion may develop, as may joint ankylosis (Fig. 14.20). In a small number of patients severe progressive joint disease results in gross radiographic changes (Fig. 14.21). Characteristic radiological changes of late JCA also develop in the hips (Fig. 14.22) and neck (Fig. 14.23). Early fusion, particularly at the C2/3 level, may occur (Fig. 14.23).

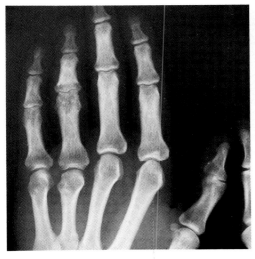
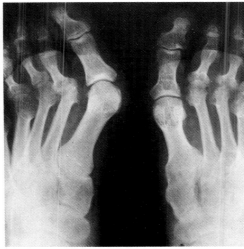
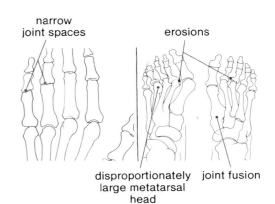

Fig. 14.20 Radiographic evidence of growth abnormalities due to JCA. The hand (left) has a short ring finger metacarpal, an enlarged proximal phalanx and narrowed interphalangeal joints, but no erosions. The feet (right) of the same patient have erosions of several metatarsophalangeal (MTP) joints, a short great toe on the right, and overgrowth of the heads of several metatarsals. The cuneiform-metatarsal joint is fused on the right.

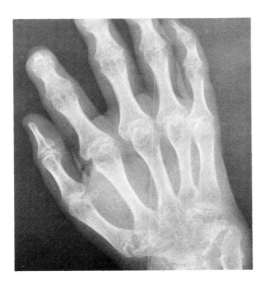
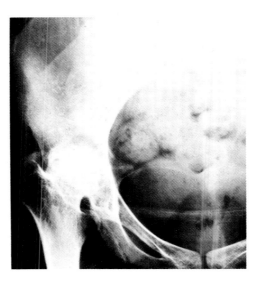
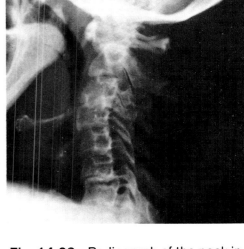

Fig. 14.21 Hand radiograph in severe polyarticular JCA showing small short bones which have large ends due to premature epiphyseal fusion. There are old surface erosions of the interphalangeal joints and areas of periarticular osteoporosis.

Fig. 14.22 Pelvic radiograph of old JCA. Chronic disease in childhood has resulted in relative underdevelopment of the iliac wing, short femoral neck and overgrowth of the greater trochanter. There are numerous old surface erosions of the hip joint.

Fig. 14.23 Radiograph of the neck in JCA. The odontoid peg is eroded, with atlantoaxial subluxation. There is old discitis at the C3/4 level and 'stepladdering' subluxation of the lower cervical vertebrae.

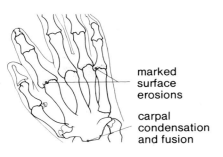
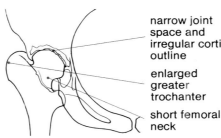

14.7

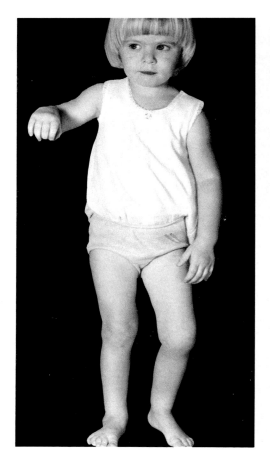

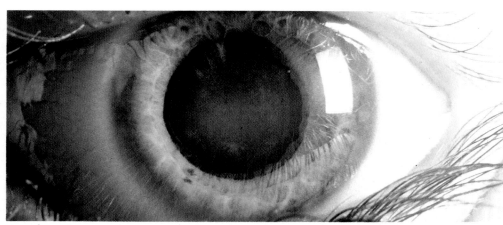

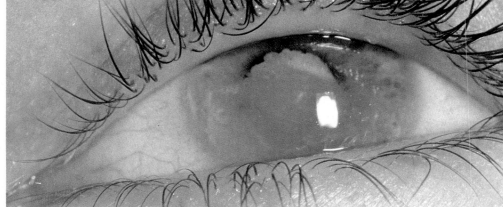

Fig. 14.24 Pauciarticular JCA in a young girl showing involvement of one knee, an elbow and an ankle.

Fig. 14.25 Iridocyclitis in a young girl with pauciarticular JCA and a positive antinuclear factor: early stage showing clouding of the anterior chamber of the eye (upper) and the late chronic stage

showing severe scarring of the eye which has led to almost complete blindness, and secondary cataract formation (lower).

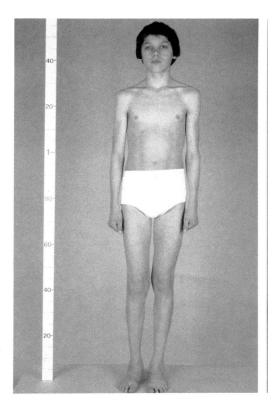

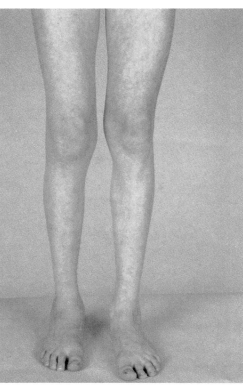

Fig. 14.26 Pauciarticular onset of JCA in a teenage boy. His right knee and ankle are the only joints affected.

Fig. 14.27 Loss of hip and lumbar spine flexion in a boy with pauciarticular JCA developing sacroiliitis and spondylitis. He is HLA-B27 positive.

3 Pauciarticular Onset

An onset involving four or less joints in the first 6 months of disease is quite common. It commonly occurs in girls aged 2-5 years and often affects the knees, elbows and ankles (Fig. 14.24). Eighty per cent of cases have a positive antinuclear factor test. This is strongly associated with the insidious development of chronic asymptomatic iridocyclitis (Fig. 14.25). This type of onset is also seen in older boys, many of whom develop sacroiliitis or frank ankylosing spondylitis about 5 years after onset (Figs. 14.26 & 14.27). These boys are generally HLA-B27 positive, and may also suffer acute attacks of iritis. Pauciarticular JCA is sometimes persistent and occasionally converts into a progressive destructive disease (Fig. 14.28). The radiographs show changes similar to those of polyarticular JCA, but confined to the few involved joints (Fig. 14.29).

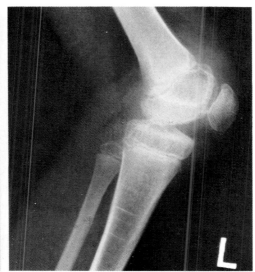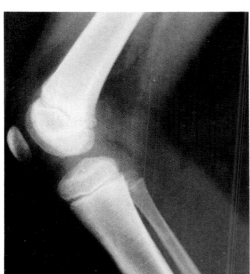

Fig. 14.28 Persistent knee synovitis in JCA. There is also inequality of finger growth due to previous involvement of the metacarpophalangeal (MCP) joints.

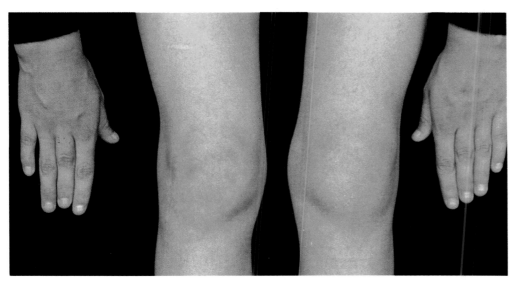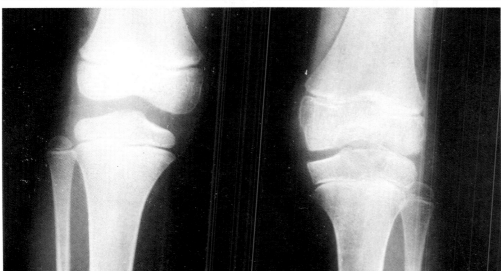

Fig. 14.29 Radiograph of the knees of a 13 year old with pauciarticular JCA. The right knee is normal. The left knee shows slight synovial thickening and decreased bone density. The epiphyses are enlarged and have a square configuration. The patella is enlarged. There is hyaline cartilage attrition and irregularity of the bony cortical margin, but no erosions.

normal femoral epiphysis   enlarged femoral epiphysis   surface irregularity   synovial thickening

normal joint space   slight synovial thickening   narrow joint space   'squared' outline of enlarged epiphyses

The overall prognosis of JCA is good: 70-80% of children recover completely. Growth abnormalities may remain, and joint fusion (especially in the knee, wrist or neck) or deformity may persist (Figs. 14.30-14.32). Prognosis depends on age of onset (the younger the onset, the worse the outlook), duration of active disease and the presence or absence of eye disease or amyloidosis; however the majority of children recover, and many return to normal (Fig. 14.33).

Other Forms of Arthritis in Children

A large number of diseases account for the remaining 30% of cases of arthritis in childhood. Some of the more important are illustrated.

Seropositive rheumatoid arthritis is a very rare disease in children, but when it occurs is similar to that seen in adults. Nodules and other extra-articular features occur (Fig. 14.34) and severe destructive radiological changes may develop.

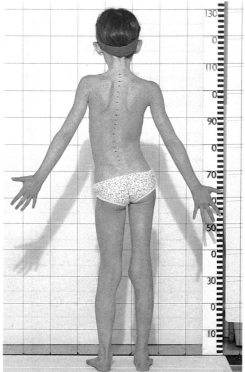

Fig. 14.30 Inequality of leg length secondary to JCA. A marked pelvic tilt and secondary scoliosis of the lumbar spine is also apparent.

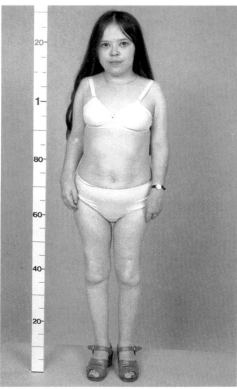

Fig. 14.31 A 32 year old lady who suffered growth retardation due to JCA and steroid therapy. There is a pelvic tilt as well as a very short stature, flexion deformities of the elbows, and destructive changes in the knees and hands; she is also mildly Cushingoid.

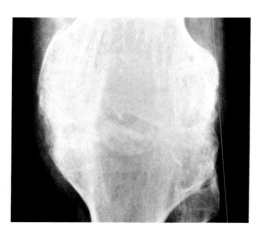

Fig. 14.32 Radiograph of a knee of a patient with old inactive JCA. The joint has become 'squared off', and there is bony fusion, with continuity of trabeculae right across the joint space. Note also bony ankylosis at the proximal tibio-fibular joint.

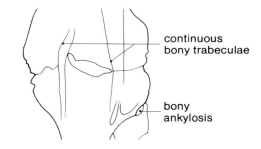

continuous
bony trabeculae

bony
ankylosis

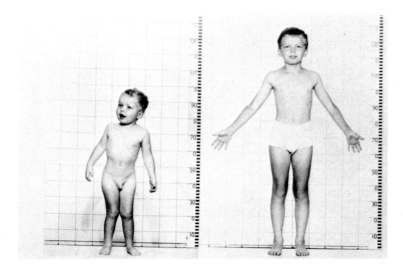

Fig. 14.33 This young boy presented with quite severe JCA: the hips, knees and ankles are characteristically deformed (left). Five years later the disease has burnt out and he is perfectly normal (right).

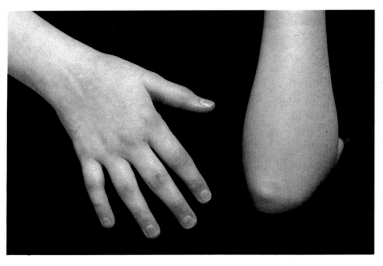

Fig. 14.34 Seropositive juvenile chronic polyarthritis. The proximal interphalangeal joints are swollen and there is a rheumatoid nodule over the elbow.

Although psoriasis is common in children, psoriatic arthropathy is not. It only occurs in older children (usually girls), and the patterns described are similar to those in adults (Figs. 14.35 & 14.36). In about half of the cases psoriasis comes first, but in the others arthritis precedes the rash. Severe clinical or radiological evidence of joint damage can occur (Fig. 14.37). It should also be noted that a few children with poly- or pauci-articular onset of JCA later develop psoriasis and features of psoriatic arthritis, although the diagnosis may not be possible until they are well into adulthood.

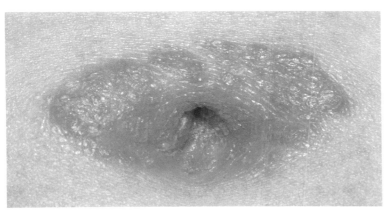
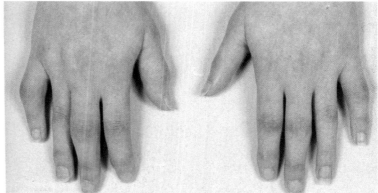

Fig. 14.35 Psoriatic arthropathy in a 10 year old child showing the typical rash around the umbilicus (left) and the asymmetrical arthropathy involving the hands (right).

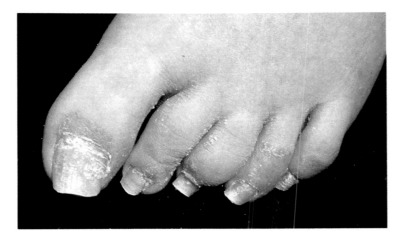

Fig. 14.36 Psoriatic arthropathy in a 16 year old – the interphalangeal joints of one foot are involved and there is a rash around the nail bed and nail dystrophy.

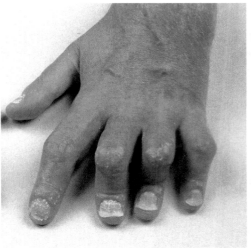
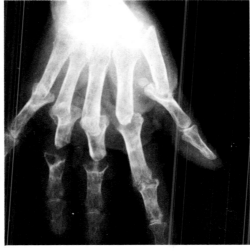
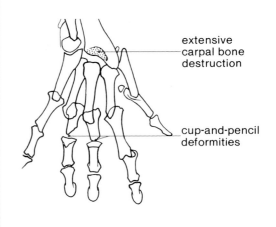

extensive carpal bone destruction

cup-and-pencil deformities

Fig. 14.37 Psoriatic arthropathy in an adult. The disease began at the age of 12 and has led to Boutonniere deformities of the fingers (left). The radiograph shows arthritis mutilans in a different patient with juvenile onset psoriatic arthropathy. Note particularly the complete destruction of the carpal bones and the well-marked cup-and-pencil deformities at many joints (right).

RHEUMATIC FEVER

School child: sore throat three weeks previously

fever

flitting arthritis

erythema marginatum

nodules

carditis

Fig. 14.38 The features of rheumatic fever.

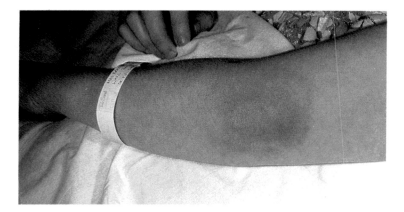

Fig. 14.39 Redness over the joint in rheumatic fever. This patient presented with a flitting arthritis involving the wrists, elbows, ankles and knees with transient redness over each of the involved joints.

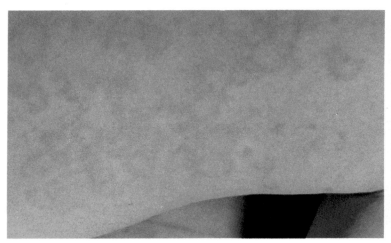

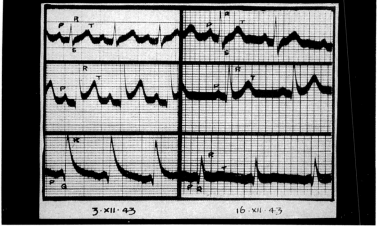

Fig. 14.40 Rheumatic fever. The typical erythema marginatum rash (left) and an ECG (right, courtesy of Professor E. Bywaters) in lead II showing a tachycardia with elevation of the S-T segment with a 'scooped-out' pattern. The second ECG two weeks later shows resolution of the changes.

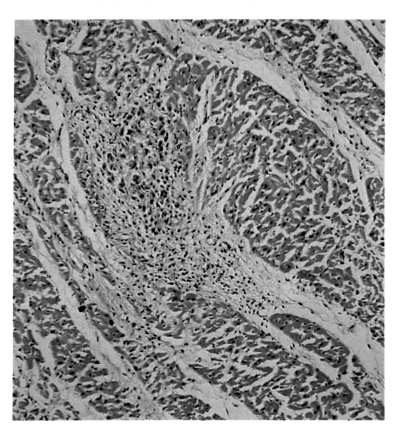

Fig. 14.41 Cardiac pathology in rheumatic fever showing the Aschoff body, composed of plump macrophages with a mantle of lymphocytes and central fibrin. H&E stain, x 75.

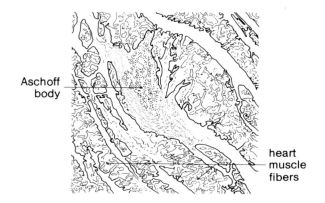

Aschoff body

heart muscle fibers

As with psoriasis, inflammatory bowel disease in children is occasionally associated with arthritis of the type seen in adults; similarly, the bowel inflammation may only develop after the arthritis. Reiter's syndrome has also been described after bowel infections in children.

The post-streptococcal disease rheumatic fever is declining in incidence in advanced countries. It is characterized by arthritis and carditis, and may cause a rash (erythema marginatum) subcutaneous nodules and chorea (Fig. 14.38). The arthritis is usually a migratory, acute condition of large joints, with redness of the overlying skin (Fig. 14.39). The rash and fever may aid diagnosis and the carditis is characteristic (Figs. 14.40 & 14.41).

Henoch-Schönlein purpura is a relatively common widespread vasculitis in children, affecting the skin, joints, gastrointestinal tract and kidney. Features include a rash, a mild flitting arthritis of the kness and ankles, abdominal pain and a focal glomerulonephritis causing hematuria and proteinuria (Fig. 14.42).

Connective tissue diseases are uncommon in children, although systemic lupus erythematosus (SLE), dermatomyositis and scleroderma together account for about 15% of arthritic diseases in childhood.

Systemic lupus erythematosus in children is most common in adolescent girls; the condition is similar to that in adults, with arthritis (which may mimic JCA), fever and rashes being the commonest presenting features (Fig. 14.43). Variants, such as mixed connective tissue disease, also occur (Fig. 14.44).

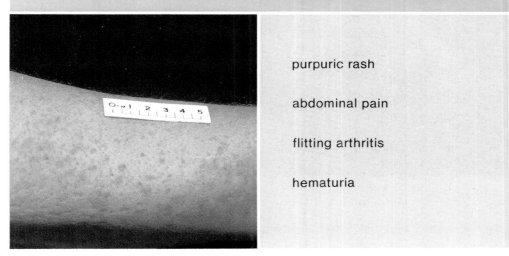

SOME CLINICAL FEATURES OF HENOCH-SCHÖNLEIN PURPURA

purpuric rash

abdominal pain

flitting arthritis

hematuria

Fig. 14.42 Henoch-Schonlein purpura. The purpuric rash on the leg of a schoolchild who presented with abdominal pain (left), and the main features of the disease (right).

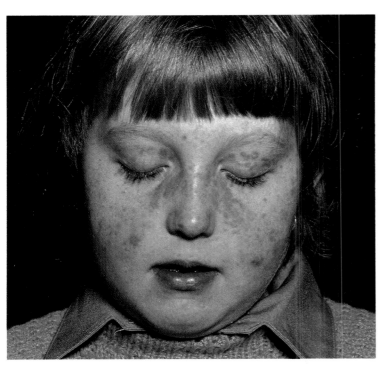

Fig. 14.43 The typical facial ('butterfly') rash of SLE in a young girl.

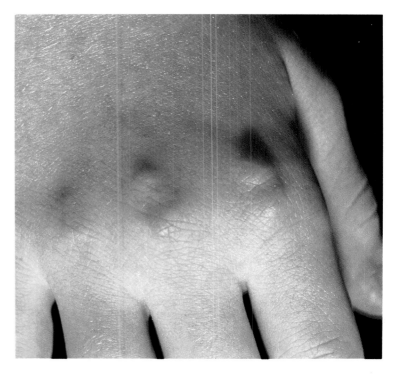

Fig. 14.44 Subcutaneous nodules, redness of the overlying skin and mild arthritis in a child with mixed connective tissue disease.

Dermatomyositis is the one connective tissue disease that occurs more frequently in children than in adults. It usually presents with muscle weakness, falls and fatigue. There is a characteristic hand and facial rash with periorbital edema. Neurological examination reveals weakness of proximal limbs, paraspinal and abdominal muscles (Fig. 14.45). Severe cases may progress unremittingly, although nowadays the prognosis has improved considerably and most children now recover. Late calcinosis of muscle and subcutaneous tissues is common and may be extensive (Fig. 14.46). Dermatomyositis of childhood, unlike the adult form, is not associated with malignancy. Scleroderma can also occur in children and is usually confined to localized skin involvement (morphea), but is occasionally widespread and progressive (Figs. 14.47 & 14.48). Systemic sclerosis is very rare.

Miscellaneous Conditions

A variety of other conditions can present as arthritis in children. A reactive arthritis may follow infections such as rubella, although less commonly than in adults. In children polyarteritis is extremely rare, but can follow

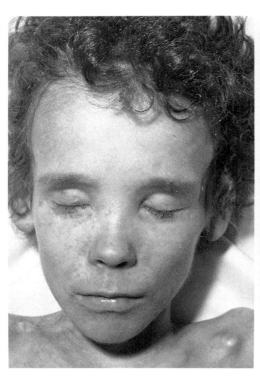

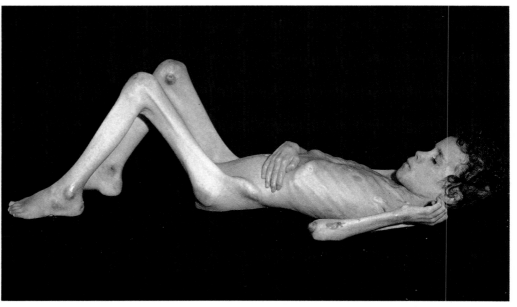

Fig. 14.45 Severe dermatomyositis in a young boy showing a heliotrope rash over the eyelids and muscle wasting in the neck (left), with severe weight loss, muscle wasting elsewhere and flexion deformities (right).

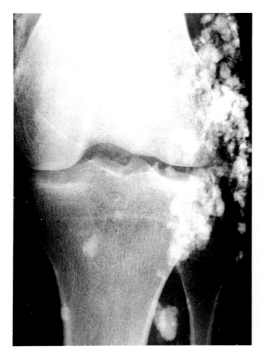

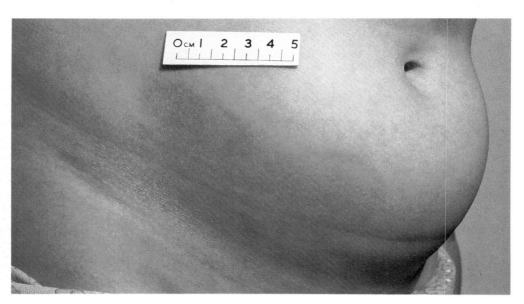

Fig. 14.46 Radiograph showing extensive calcinosis of the muscles and subcutaneous tissue around the knee secondary to dermatomyositis in childhood.

Fig. 14.47 Morphea on the trunk in a young girl who first presented with limb pain.

upper respiratory tract infections. It may mimic other arthritides, such as that of Henoch-Schönlein purpura, in the early stages.

Septic arthritis is uncommon, and may be due to spread from metaphyseal bone of osteomyelitis. Bone sepsis may also mimic arthritis and produce a sympathetic effusion, although the presence of bony tenderness aids the clinical differentiation. Redness or sinuses of the overlying skin may develop (Fig. 14.49). Radiographs are normal for the first few days, but characteristic changes may develop rapidly (Fig. 14.50).

Nearly all the childhood malignancies can cause musculo-skeletal symptoms mimicking arthritis. Leukemia may present in this way, pain arising from periarticular infiltration of tissues with leukemic cells. Radiographs may show metaphyseal osteoporosis, osteolytic lesions or periostitis (Fig. 14.51) but can be normal. If systemic features are present the condition may mimic systemic onset JCA. Other malignancies such as neuroblastomas may cause severe joint and bone pain due to widespread secondary deposits.

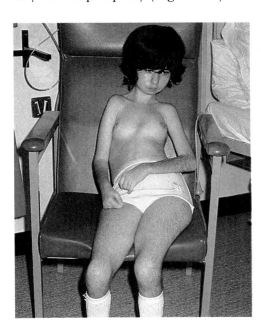

Fig. 14.48 Severe scleroderma in a 14 year old girl showing abnormal and severe wasting. Deformities are due to a combination of myositis and skin involvement.

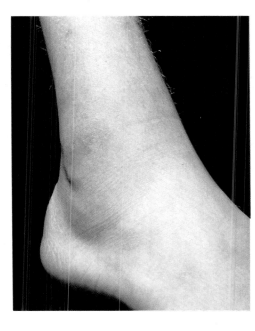

Fig. 14.49 Osteomyelitis of the lower end of the fibula. This boy presented with a diagnosis of erythema nodosum. Severe bone tenderness adjacent to the joint is usually the clue to osteomyelitis in children.

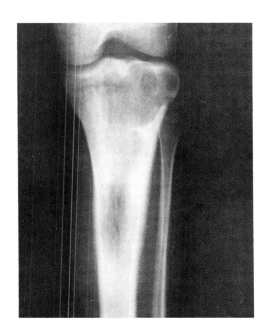

Fig. 14.50 Radiograph of acute on chronic osteomyelitis of the tibia. The large cystic areas in the bone are due to chronic multifocal osteomyelitis. The central area has fluffy periosteal changes, hazy trabeculae and is actively infected, with extension into soft tissue.

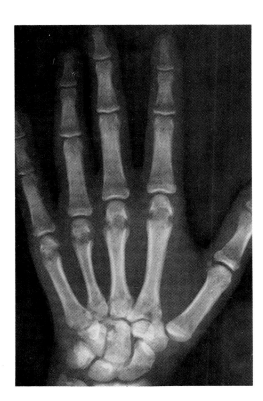

Fig. 14.51 Radiograph of the hand in a child with leukemia showing extensive metaphyseal destruction and periosteal new bone formation.

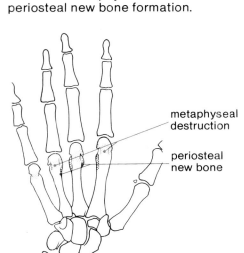

metaphyseal destruction

periosteal new bone

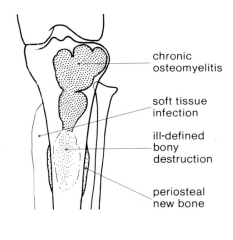

chronic osteomyelitis

soft tissue infection

ill-defined bony destruction

periosteal new bone

A variety of miscellaneous genetic and congenital malformations and diseases of bone may also mimic childhood arthritis. Common amongst these are the avascular necrosis syndromes, calcific discitis, chondromalacia patellae, neurodystrophy, Osgood-Schlatter disease and other osteochondritides (Figs. 14.52-55).

There are, therefore, a multitude of causes of joint pain in children; most are benign although a few herald the onset of serious arthritic or other diseases. The prognosis in most cases is good, but early diagnosis and careful management are of paramount importance.

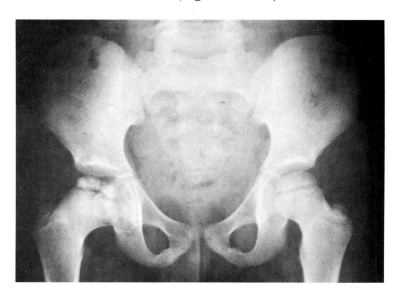

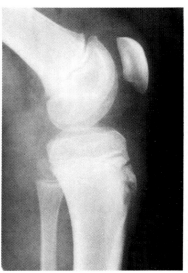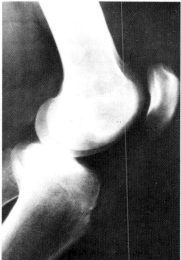

Fig. 14.52 Radiograph in Perthes' disease. The whole head of the femur is involved with fragmentation and loss of height of the epiphysis and irregularity of the metaphysis compared with the normal, left hip.

Fig. 14.53 Osgood-Schlatter's disease. In childhood (left) there is fragmentation of the tibial tubercle, soft tissue swelling and mild patella alta. The late, adult appearance (right) includes old irregularity and reossification of the tubercle, and an elongated inferior pole of the patella due to previous Sinding Larsen disease.

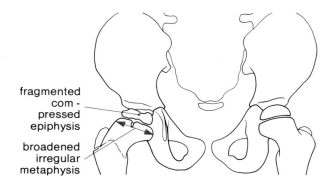

fragmented com-pressed epiphysis

broadened irregular metaphysis

patella alta

fragmented tibial tubercle

soft tissue swelling

elongated inferior pole of patella

irregular ossification of tibial tubercle

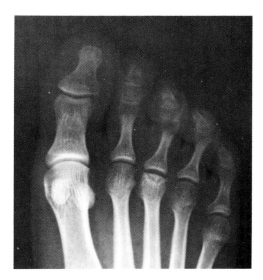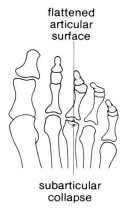

flattened articular surface

subarticular collapse

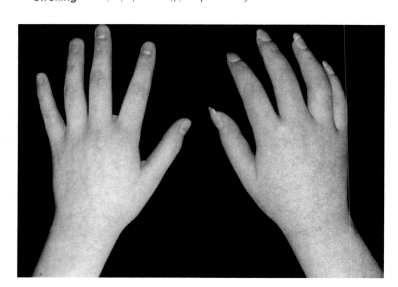

Fig. 14.54 Freiberg's disease. The infarction of the third metatarsal has caused a subarticular radiolucency into which the surface has collapsed, resulting in a flat head of the bone.

Fig. 14.55 Algoneurodystrophy showing the puffy swelling of the hand. The bones were tender, and the radiograph showed multiple areas of osteoporosis.

15
Osteoarthritis

The term osteoarthritis is one of a number of synonyms used to describe a group of conditions affecting the synovial joints. These are characterized by loss of articular cartilage with overgrowth and remodelling of the underlying bone.

Osteoarthritis (OA) affects many different species and there is skeletal evidence that it has been present since the earliest history of the human race. It is an extremely common disease. Radiological surveys suggest that about 10% of all adults have moderate or severe disease. The incidence increases with age although not all of those with radiological changes have symptoms. Nevertheless, about three quarters of those people classified as disabled from arthritis are said to have OA

and about 30% of sickness incapacity in the working age group from rheumatic disease is attributed to this disease. The natural history is one of slow progression and the lives of many middle aged and elderly people are made miserable by osteoarthritis.

Osteoarthritis affects both spinal and peripheral joints and the pathological, radiological and clinical features of osteoarthritis affecting the peripheral joints will be illustrated (spinal disease is covered separately). The condition can be subdivided into a number of subsets on the basis of known mechanical, inflammatory or metabolic factors influencing its pathogenesis. Some examples of these subsets will also be shown.

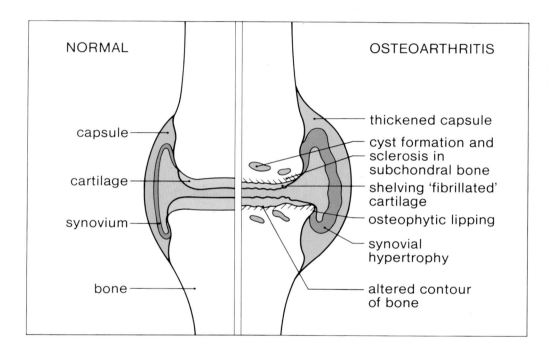

Fig. 15.1 Diagrammatic cross-section of a joint affected by OA. Note the loss of cartilage, sclerosis and cyst formation in the underlying bone, osteophytic lipping at the margin and soft tissue reaction.

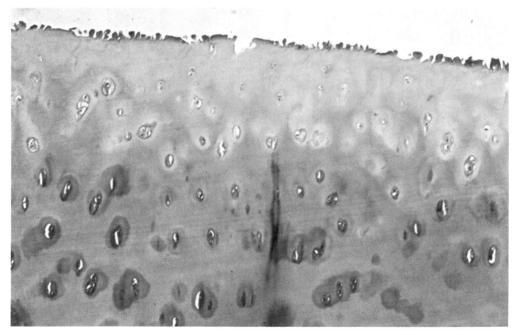

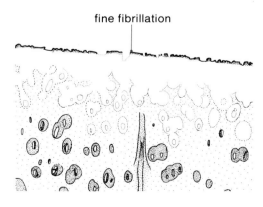

Fig. 15.2 Histology of cartilage in early OA showing fine fibrillation. H & E stain, x 80.

The Pathology of Osteoarthritis

All tissues of the joints are affected by osteoarthritis. The most striking features are:
(1) destruction of articular cartilage
(2) sclerosis and remodelling of the subchrondral bone. There is also a variable degree of synovial inflammation, hypertrophy, and thickening and fibrosis of the capsule (Fig. 15.1).

Articular Cartilage: Biochemical changes of early osteoarthritis probably include an increase in water content, alteration in the proteoglycans and an increase in cellular activity of the articular chondrocytes. The earliest change seen microscopically is fibrillation of the surface of the cartilage (Fig. 15.2). Chondrocytes form clusters of two or three known as 'brood-nests'. Not all fibrillation progresses to cartilage destruction. However, in progressive lesions, a decrease in proteoglycan staining of cartilage is seen first. Loss of thickness of the cartilage with more obvious surface defects then becomes apparent (Fig. 15.3). As the condition progresses the cartilage may be lost exposing the underlying subchondral bone (Fig. 15.4).

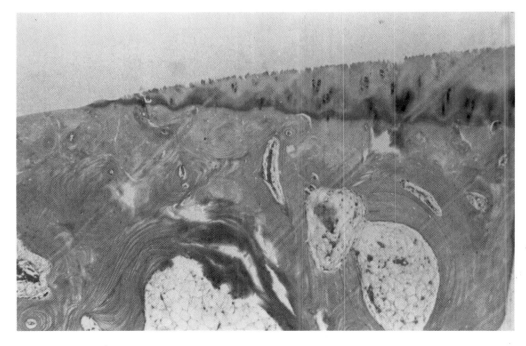

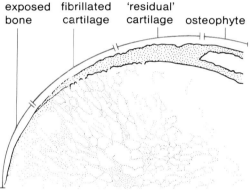

Fig. 15.3 Histological section from an osteoarthritic femoral head showing four regions: exposed bone (with sclerosis and marrow fibrosis); shelving 'fibrillated' cartilage; 'residual cartilage', and an osteophyte. H & E stain, x 4.

exposed bone   fibrillated cartilage   'residual' cartilage   osteophyte

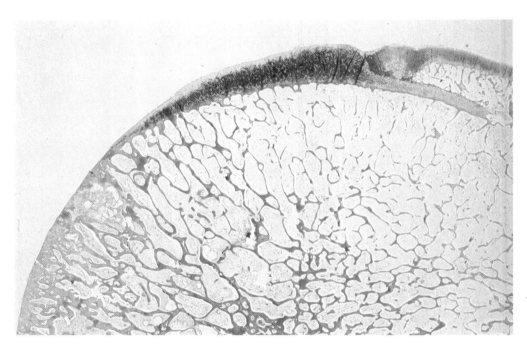

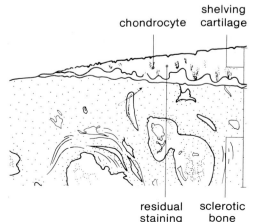

Fig. 15.4 Histology of cartilage and underlying bone in gross OA showing shelving finely fibrillated cartilage, reduced staining, small clumps of chondrocytes and bone sclerosis (little alteration in marrow). H & E stain, x 40.

chondrocyte   shelving cartilage

residual staining   sclerotic bone

Bone Changes: Subchondral bone shows increased vascularity, increased cellular activity and sclerosis in osteoarthritis (Fig. 15.5). This is also associated with the growth of marginal osteophytes which usually arise from periarticular fibrocartilage and later fuse with bone. The formation of necrotic cystic areas in the bone – 'bone cysts' – also occurs.

Soft Tissues: A variable degree of synovial reaction is seen in osteoarthritis (Fig. 15.6). The changes are often patchy and may include hyperemia, which can be observed arthroscopically, and the formation of small grape-like villi with a patchy cellular infiltrate and slight increase in lining cell activity. In a few cases, patchy areas of synovium show much more extensive cellular infiltration and may include lymphocytes, plasma cells and giant cells (Fig. 15.7). The capsule often becomes grossly thickened and fibrosed particularly in advanced disease.

Osteoarthritic synovial fluid is usually fairly viscous and has a relatively low cell count (0.2 – 2 cells x 10^9 per litre). Cartilage and bone fragments with or without calcium phosphate crystals are often present (Fig. 15.7).

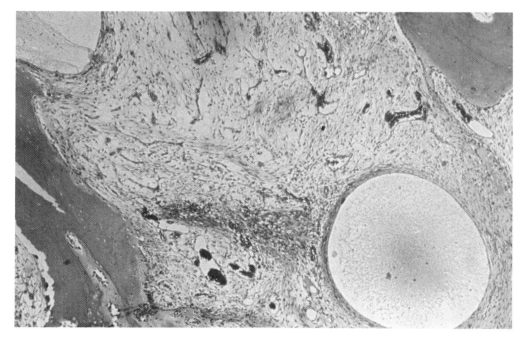

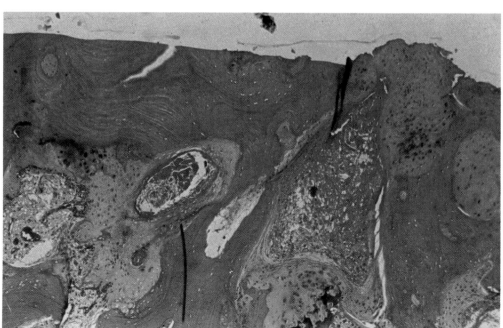

Fig. 15.5 Histology of superficial portion of exposed bone showing resorbing surface (with osteoclasts), fibrotic marrow with congested blood vessels and developing mucoid degeneration, active osteoblasts, newly formed bone, and cysts (upper). The reaction further into the bone shows fibrocartilage in marrow spaces with small cysts, sclerotic bone which is locally necrotic (with empty osteocyte lacunae), and bone resorption (other surfaces now inactive) (lower).
H & E stain, x 40.

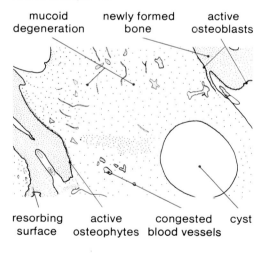

mucoid degeneration   newly formed bone   active osteoblasts

resorbing surface   active osteophytes   congested blood vessels   cyst

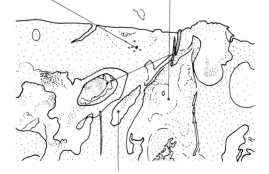

sclerotic and necrotic bone   fibrocartilage in marrow space with small cysts

bone resorption

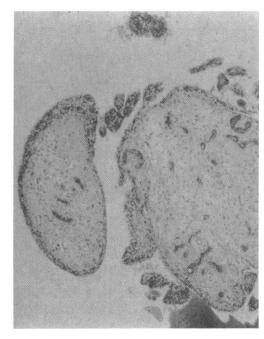
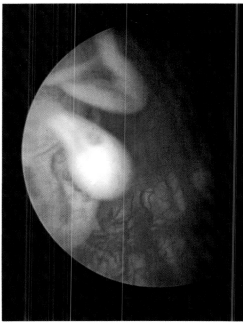
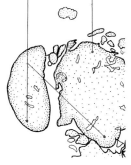
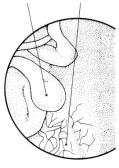

Fig. 15.6 Histology of synovium in advanced OA showing the grape-like villi of synovium with variable hypertrophy of the lining cells (left). H & E stain, x 80. Arthroscopic view of the synovium showing some background hyperemia and small grape-like villous extension of the synovial lining (right).

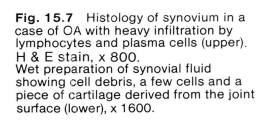

enlarged villi   surface cells proliferating   synovial villus   vascular hyperemia

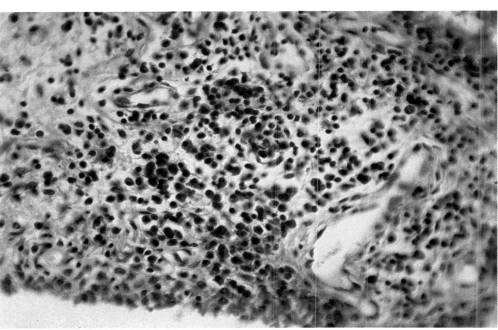

Fig. 15.7 Histology of synovium in a case of OA with heavy infiltration by lymphocytes and plasma cells (upper). H & E stain, x 800.
Wet preparation of synovial fluid showing cell debris, a few cells and a piece of cartilage derived from the joint surface (lower), x 1600.

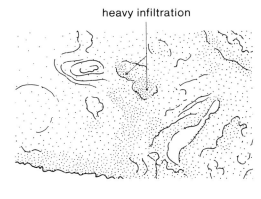

heavy infiltration

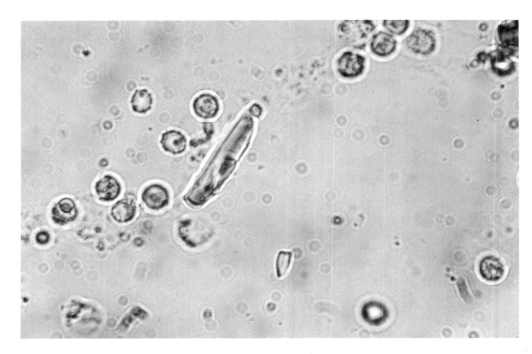
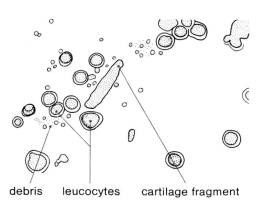

debris   leucocytes   cartilage fragment

RADIOLOGICAL FEATURES OF OA

Narrowing of joint space

Osteophytosis

Altered bone contour

Bone sclerosis and cysts

Periarticular calcification

Soft tissue swelling

Fig. 15.8 The main radiological features of OA.

The Radiology of Osteoarthritis

The pathological features of osteoarthritis described in the preceding section are associated with a predictable set of radiological features. These include narrowing of the joint space due to loss of articular cartilage, sclerosis and cyst formation in the underlying subchondral bone, marginal osteophytes and sometimes evidence of articular or periarticular mineral deposition (Fig. 15.8).

The correlations between the gross morphology and radiology of osteoarthritis is well illustrated by comparing the naked eye appearance of early and late osteoarthritic femoral heads and slab radiographs taken from the same samples resected at operation for hip replacement (Figs. 15.9 & 15.10).

The Clinical Features of Osteoarthritis

Not everyone with pathological or radiological evidence of osteoarthritis suffers from any clinical problem. Although there is a reasonable correlation between

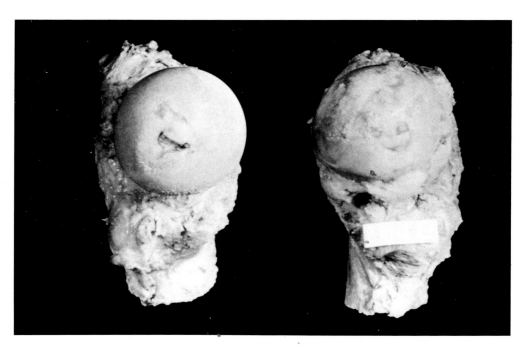

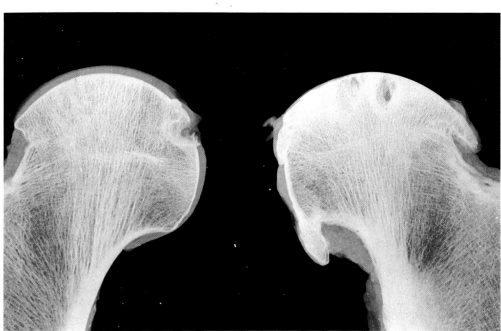

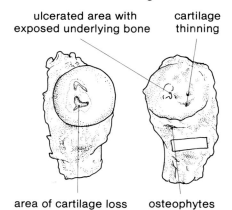

Fig. 15.9 Resected femoral heads taken at the time of operation for OA of the hip. The head on the left shows early osteoarthritic changes with an area of cartilage loss in the center. More advanced changes with extensive cartilage loss and exposed underlying bone are shown on the right.

ulcerated area with exposed underlying bone

cartilage thinning

area of cartilage loss

osteophytes

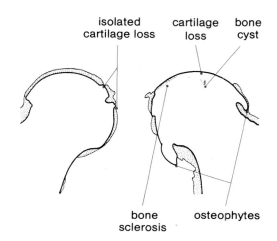

Fig. 15.10 Slab x-rays of the two femoral heads illustrated in the previous figure. On the left the isolated area of cartilage loss is shown and on the right the extensive loss of cartilage, sclerosis of underlying bone, bone cysts and osteophytosis are all clearly apparent.

isolated cartilage loss

cartilage loss

bone cyst

bone sclerosis

osteophytes

radiological changes and symptoms at the knee joint this is not so obvious at other sites. In the back, hip and hand for example, gross radiological changes may be asymptomatic whereas other people with relatively minor x-ray abnormalities can suffer severe pain. The origin of symptoms in osteoarthritis is not yet clear and the poor correlation between pathology and symptoms seen in some cases remains to be explained.

The condition usually starts around the age of 50 but may begin in early adulthood or old age. Women outnumber men by three to one and OA is usually slowly progressive. Occasional cases improve spontaneously, or progress rapidly. It is often a polyarticular disease although a clear mechanical cause can result in osteoarthritis at one site alone. The most commonly involved sites are the knees, hands, hips and feet in that order.

The main symptoms are pain, stiffness and loss of movement (Fig. 15.11). Pain is usually worse on use of the joint and at the end of the day. Stiffness is mild and short lasting in the mornings but may be quite severe after prolonged inactivity. Creaking of the joints (crepitus) is common and may be audible or palpable. Mild bony or soft tissue swelling is usual and tenderness is often present. This may be over the joint line itself but quite commonly in osteoarthritis tenderness is isolated to a few points either over the osteophytes, insertion of capsules or ligaments, or in other periarticular sites. Active and passive movement of the joint is usually painful and limited.

The Etiology and Pathogenesis of Osteoarthritis

Osteoarthritis can be thought of as an end stage condition, or 'joint failure' synonymous with heart failure. Several different pathogenic mechanisms may be involved and the same end result can arise from many factors affecting synovial joints (Fig. 15.12).

Genetic factors are important and there are racial differences in expression of the disease. For example, OA of the hand is common in Caucasian women and OA of the knee rare in Chinese. Genetic factors are particularly obvious in subsets of OA such as the generalized 'nodal' form in which a polygenic inheritance is postulated, and middle aged women are usually affected. It commonly starts around the time of the menopause and there is often an obvious inflammatory element with red, inflamed distal interphalangeal joints (DIPs) (Fig. 15.13).

SYMPTOMS AND SIGNS OF OA
Pain – worse on use of joint
Stiffness-mild in morning, severe after immobility
Loss of movement
Pain on movement / restricted range
Tenderness (articular or periarticular)
Bony swelling
Soft tissue swelling
Joint crepitus

Fig. 15.11 The main signs and symptoms of OA.

MULTIFACTORIAL ETIOLOGY OF OA
Joint instability
Age
Hormonal factors
Trauma
Altered biochemistry
Inflammation
Genetic predisposition
? Others

Fig. 15.12 The multifactorial etiology of osteoarthritis. OA can be regarded as joint failure and may be the product of several different etiological factors.

Fig. 15.13 Tender, swollen, red DIPs in a case of generalized inflammatory OA affecting a middle aged female.

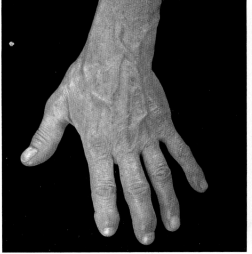
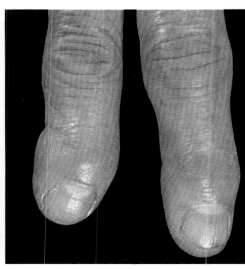

Mechanical factors are also very important in the pathogenesis of this disease. Meniscectomy of the knee joint results in significant osteoarthritis in about 40% of cases if followed up 15 years later (Fig. 15.14). Similarly, severe trauma to a joint, an abnormality in joint congruity (for example of the hip) or hypermobility (Fig. 15.15) can result in severe premature OA of that site alone. Similarly, employment affects the distribution of disease, it being common in the hips and backs of miners and in the hands and necks of cotton workers. A few obvious occupational forms of OA exist including wicket keepers' thumb, Zulu dancers' hip and pica thumpers' thumb (OA of the carpometacarpal joint (CMC) in print setters who spent their time flicking letters across the tray with their thumbs). Some metabolic abnormalities predispose to OA, a well known example being ochronosis in which the accumulation of an abnormal amino acid derivative in the cartilage causes premature severe degenerative changes with pigment deposition and mineral formation (Fig. 15.16). Other examples of metabolic diseases that result in OA include acromegaly, gout and Kashin-Beck disease.

Abnormal joint mechanics can result from congenital or acquired diseases, and may cause premature osteoarthritis. Examples include rare forms of epiphyseal dysplasia (Fig. 15.17) and congenital dislocation of the hip (Fig. 15.18). Osteoarthritis of the hip is a common

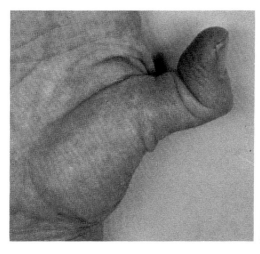

Fig. 15.14 Knee radiograph of a patient, who had a medial meniscectomy several years previously, showing joint space narrowing and osteophyte formation predominantly on the medial side.

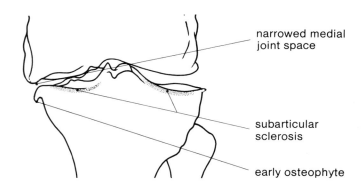

narrowed medial joint space

subarticular sclerosis

early osteophyte

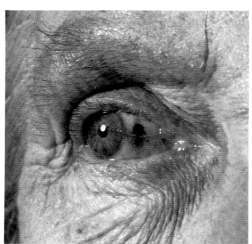
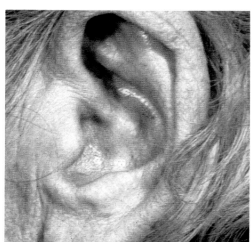

Fig. 15.15 A patient with hypermobility at the base of the thumb demonstrating her ability to dislocate the joint at will (left). This patient developed OA of the CMCs of the thumb only. OA of the CMC associated with overuse (pica thumpers' thumb) is shown radiologically (right). Note the similarity to sepsis.

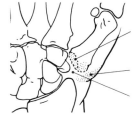

irregular bone resorption without sclerosis or osteophytes

soft tissue swelling

widened joint space

Fig. 15.16 Discolouration of the sclera and cartilage of the ear in a case of ochronosis. Deposition of products of amino acid metabolism in the cartilage in ochronosis can lead to severe premature OA in the spine and peripheral joints.

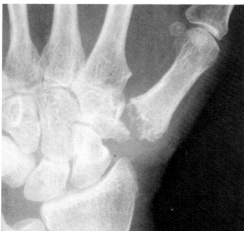

disease, and some predisposing factor that causes an altered shape of the femoral head or acetabulum can often be found.

Inflammatory diseases of the joint can also result in OA. Late rheumatoid disease can sometimes present a radiological and pathological picture that is virtually indistinguishable from advanced OA although there is a tendency for less bone sclerosis and less formation of osteophytic outgrowth than in uncomplicated OA (Fig. 15.19). An early inflammatory element is often apparent in OA without there being any evidence of another underlying arthropathy. The presence of synovial inflammation and of early inflammation around the DIPs in generalized OA of middle aged women have already been mentioned. Inflammatory features also contribute to the symptoms of OA as is apparent from their response to anti-inflammatory therapy.

Patients with osteoarthritis sometimes have a clear dominant etiological factor. In most cases this is not obvious however, and multifactorial pathogenesis can be postulated with a combination of genetic predisposition, mechanical factors and inflammatory changes contributing to the destruction of cartilage and remodelling of the underlying bone.

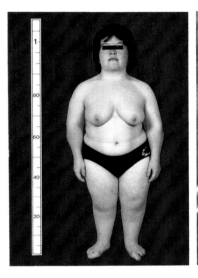
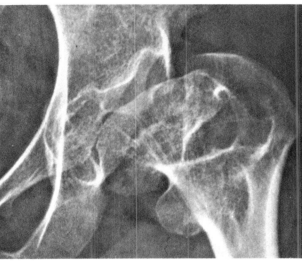

Fig. 15.17 A 24 year old lady with multiple epiphyseal dysplasia who is developing premature OA of the hips (left) and a hip radiograph from another patient with epiphyseal dysplasia showing severe deformation of the acetabulum and femoral head (right).

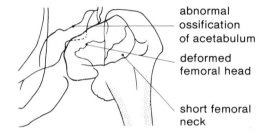

abnormal ossification of acetabulum

deformed femoral head

short femoral neck

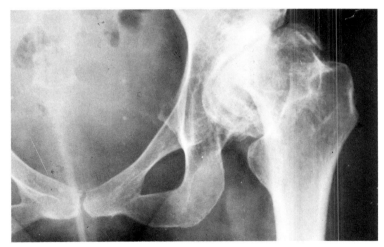

Fig. 15.18 Hip radiograph from a patient who suffered congenital hip dislocation and is developing premature OA in early adulthood. Note the deformation and flattening of the femoral head, bone sclerosis and osteophytic lipping of the secondary OA.

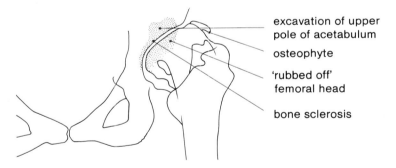

excavation of upper pole of acetabulum

osteophyte

'rubbed off' femoral head

bone sclerosis

Fig. 15.19 Hip osteoarthritis secondary to rheumatoid disease showing protrusio acetabuli and relative lack of osteophyte formation. These are features of old rheumatoid disease which do not generally occur in primary OA.

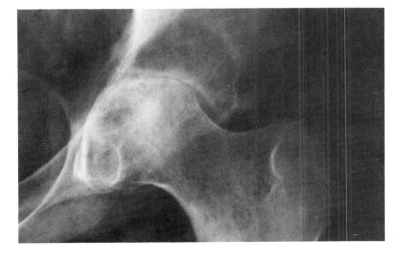

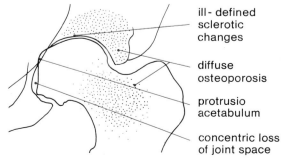

ill-defined sclerotic changes

diffuse osteoporosis

protrusio acetabulum

concentric loss of joint space

Regional Illustrations of Osteoarthritis

The Hip: Osteoarthritis of the hip results in pain that is usually felt in the groin and the front of the thigh. It may be referred to the knee causing diagnostic confusion. Early on, painful loss of internal rotation is the main sign.

In more advanced disease, complete loss of rotation, external rotation deformity, flexion deformities, loss of abduction and shortening of the leg can all occur (Figs. 15.20 & 15.21). These may be extremely disabling, preventing the patient from walking far, from climbing

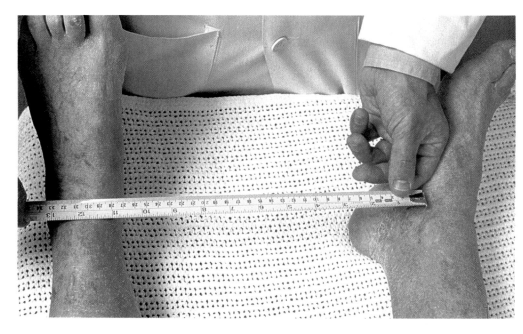

Fig. 15.20 OA of the hip. The intermalleolar distance is being measured and is reduced due to loss of abduction of the hips. External rotation deformity is also present on the right.

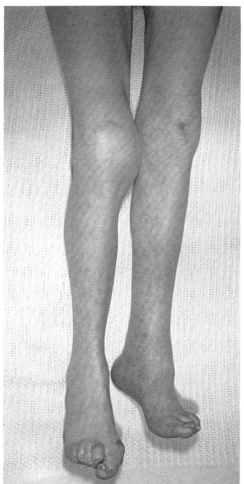

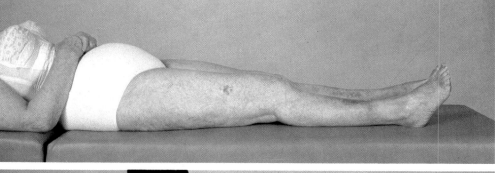

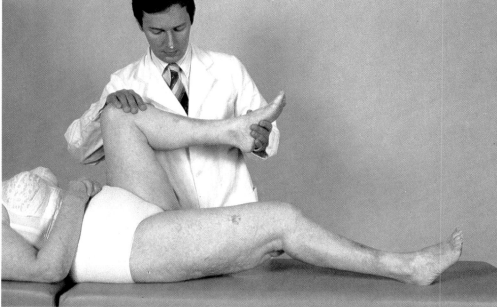

Fig. 15.21 Advanced OA of the hip showing shortening of the affected leg and fixed external rotation deformity. Note also the knee swelling on the opposite side ('long-leg arthropathy').

Fig. 15.22 Thomas' test. The patient has OA of the right hip which lacks extension (a fixed flexion deformity). The patient is able to lie flat on the couch due to a compensatory lumbar lordosis (upper).

When the normal, left hip is fully flexed by the examiner the lumbar lordosis is overcome by pelvic rotation and the fixed flexion deformity is unmasked, the right leg then lifting from the couch (lower).

stairs or getting on buses, inhibiting sexual activity, and resulting in severe night pain. The characteristic gait involves a downwards tilt of the pelvis when weight is taken off the affected side (Figs. 15.22 & 15.23). On x-ray, gross OA of the affected hip is clearly apparent (Fig 15.24) and can only be treated successfully by resection of the femoral head and insertion of a total hip prosthesis.

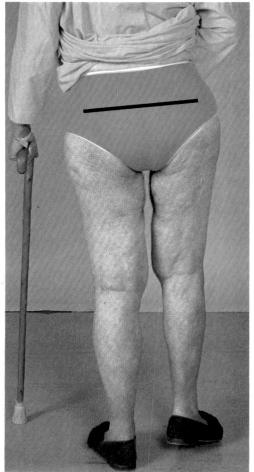
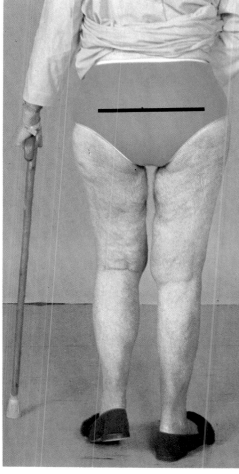

Fig. 15.23 Trendelenburg's sign. This patient has OA of the right hip. She uses a stick held in the left hand to reduce weight-bearing across the diseased hip. When asked to stand on the normal, left leg the right hemipelvis lifts in the normal way (left). When she tries to stand on the affected, right leg the left hemipelvis tilts downwards (right).

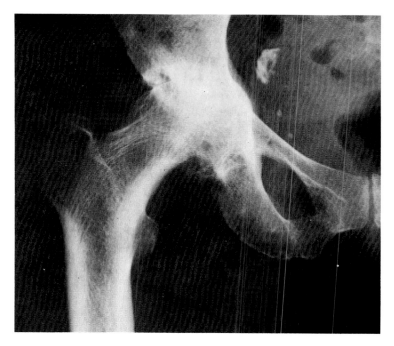

Fig. 15.24 Hip osteoarthritis showing the typical radiological changes.

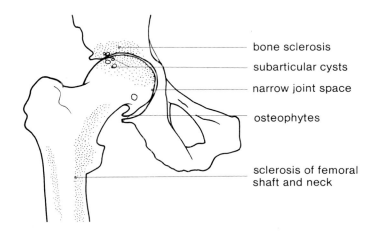

- bone sclerosis
- subarticular cysts
- narrow joint space
- osteophytes
- sclerosis of femoral shaft and neck

Radiological changes of the hip joint vary considerably, and careful X-ray assessment may give many clues to the etiology of the condition. Three different types of distribution have been described. In many cases the main joint space narrowing and bone changes are in the upper pole of the hip (Fig. 15.25). In other cases the main changes are either on the medial pole (Fig. 15.26) or there is a concentric loss of joint space (Fig. 15.27). Bilateral changes or concentric abnormalities are commonly associated with generalized disease affecting the hands as well as other joints. Upper pole disease is more common in working men and often associated with changes of the spine, or with isolated disease of the hip only.

Osteoarthritis of the hip is often a result of a structural abnormality of the neck or head of the femur or acetabula. Congenital dislocation of the hip predisposes to premature OA (see Fig. 15.18) as does Perthe's disease or any form of epiphyseal dysplasia affecting the joint. Tilt abnormalities of the femoral neck or head can result in OA and minor changes of this sort are thought by some authors to be discernable in the majority of cases (Fig. 15.28). Another form of OA that may be detected radio-

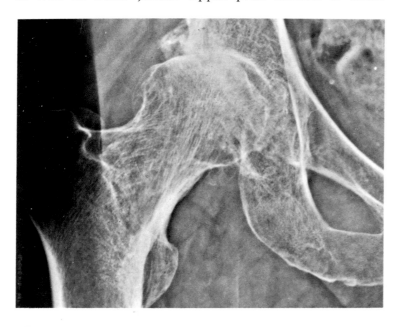

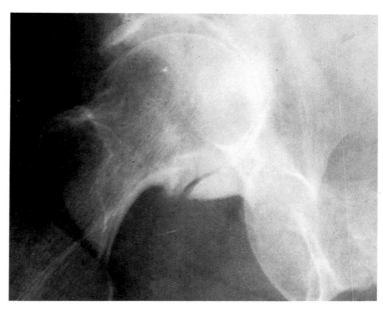

Fig. 15.25 Upper pole OA of the hip. Note the greater joint space narrowing in the upper pole, sclerosis, and cyst formation.

Fig. 15.26 Medial pole OA of the hip. This oblique view clearly shows the joint space narrowing occurring predominantly on the medial side with underlying bone sclerosis and 'jet stream' osteophytes at the lower pole.

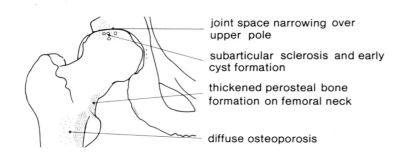

joint space narrowing over upper pole

subarticular sclerosis and early cyst formation

thickened perosteal bone formation on femoral neck

diffuse osteoporosis

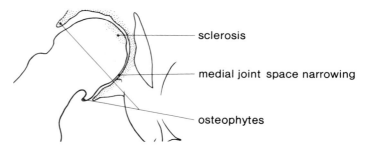

sclerosis

medial joint space narrowing

osteophytes

Fig. 15.27 Concentric joint space loss in OA. The cartilage is narrowing equally around the hip joint and the femoral head is enlarged and deformed (coxa magna).

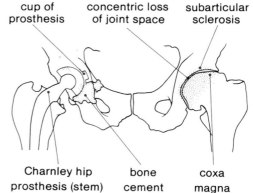

cup of prosthesis

concentric loss of joint space

subarticular sclerosis

Charnley hip prosthesis (stem)

bone cement

coxa magna

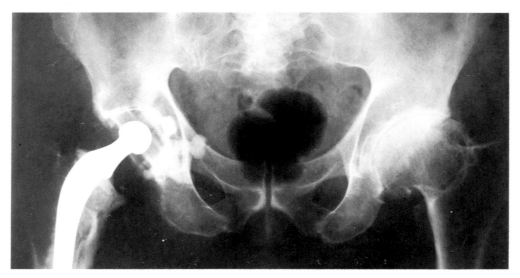

logically is that which occurs in association with Forestier's disease (idiopathic skeletal hyperostosis). Massive osteophytic outgrowths are seen in this condition (Fig. 15.29). In advanced osteoarthritis the upper pole of the femoral head may collapse, and migrate laterally. This tendency for the femoral head to move laterally and be buttressed by osteophytes of the upper pole is illustrated in figure 15.30.

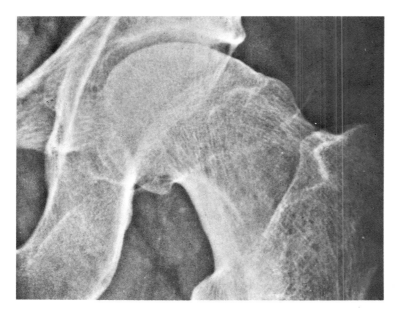

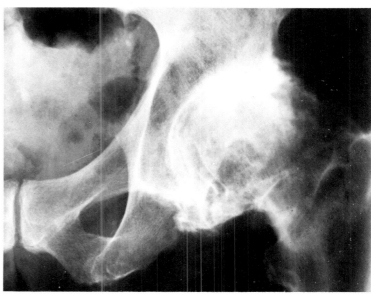

Fig. 15.28 Coxa magna: early OA of the hip in conjunction with a tilt deformity of the femoral head. Many cases of hip OA are thought to be due to minor abnormalities of the femoral head as in the case illustrated here.

Fig. 15.29 Advanced OA of the hip showing massive body reactions with large cyst formations and exuberant osteophytosis. These changes often occur in conjunction with vertebral hyperostosis.

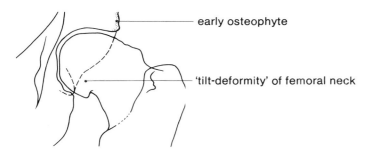

early osteophyte

'tilt-deformity' of femoral neck

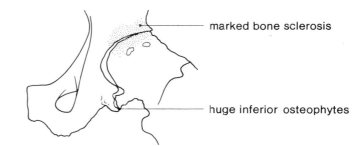

marked bone sclerosis

huge inferior osteophytes

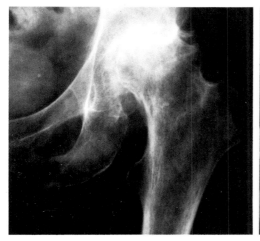

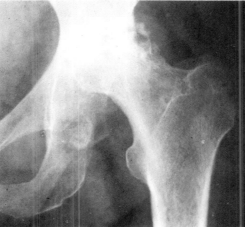

Fig. 15.30 Osteoarthritic hip with flattening and collapse of the upper pole. Lateral movement of the femoral head (left). Advanced avascular necrosis of the femoral head in association with osteoarthritic changes showing femoral head bone destruction and collapse into cyst formation (right).

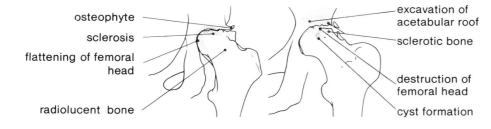

osteophyte
sclerosis
flattening of femoral head
radiolucent bone

excavation of acetabular roof
sclerotic bone
destruction of femoral head
cyst formation

The Knee: The knee is the other main weight-bearing joint affected by OA and is the commonest site of the disease. Pain is the dominant symptom and may arise from the joint itself; but often tenderness of the peri-articular tissue, particularly the insertion of the capsule and collateral ligaments is a major source of symptoms (Fig. 15.31). Bony and soft tissue swelling can normally be palpated, and small effusions, warmth over the joint and Baker's cysts are all quite common (Figs. 15.32 & 15.33).

In advanced OA of the knee joint instability can occur and varus or valgus deformities may arise due to disease predominantly affecting the medial or lateral compartments respectively (Figs. 15.34 & 15.35).

'Long-leg arthropathy' is a special form of OA of the knee, in which there is inequality of leg length which may be apparent from a pelvic tilt and lumbar scoliosis, and in which OA predominantly affects the knee of the longer leg. A common set of deformities involves spinal scoliosis and pain, OA of one hip with consequent shortening and OA of the contralateral knee (see Fig. 15.21).

Patello-femoral joint disease is sometimes dominant resulting in pain on climbing stairs, or on compression of the patella against the femur.

These clinical features are also characteristic of chondromalacia patellae in young adults in which there is softening and fibrillation of the articular cartilage on the patella (Fig. 15.36). The condition is often self-limiting although some patients progress to develop typical OA and in others symptoms become severe enough to warrant surgery (Fig. 15.37). The relationship of chondromalacia patellae to OA is disputed.

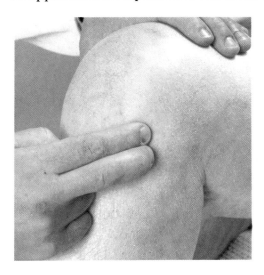

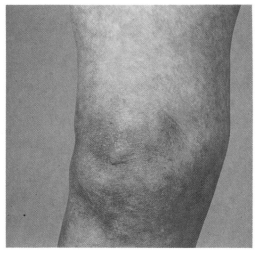

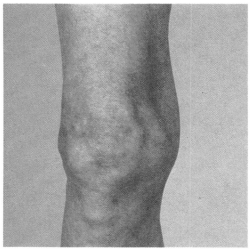

Fig. 15.31 Periarticular tissue tenderness in an osteoarthritic knee. The examiner is palpating the areas of insertion of the capsule and collateral ligaments where there is often isolated tenderness. They may be the only or main source of symptoms.

Fig. 15.32 Swelling of osteoarthritic knees may be due to osteophytic lipping and bony outgrowths; to hypertrophy of the capsule and soft tissues; or an effusion into the knee joint (left). Knobbly-knees: a case of osteoarthritis

illustrating bony swellings around the knee and secondary wasting of the vastus medialis, a common feature in OA of the knee often leading to instability (right).

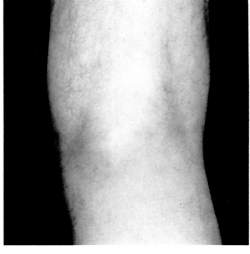

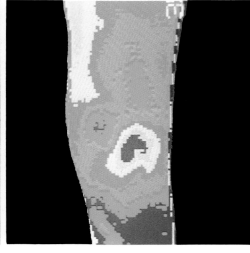

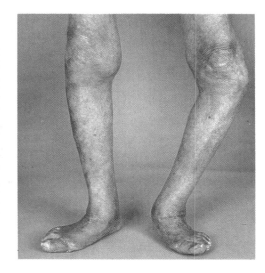

Fig. 15.33 A Baker's cyst in OA illustrating soft tissue swelling at the back of the knee due to cyst formation (left). These may rupture as in rheumatoid disease. Abnormal thermographic images occur in about a third of

cases of OA affecting the knee. The area of increased temperature is shown in red (right). Courtesy of Mr E.F.J. Ring, Royal National Hospital for Rheumatic Diseases.

Fig. 15.34 Genu varum in OA due to collapse of the medial compartment of the knee and rupture of the lateral collateral ligament. Note quadriceps wasting and secondary valgus deformity of the ankle.

15.14

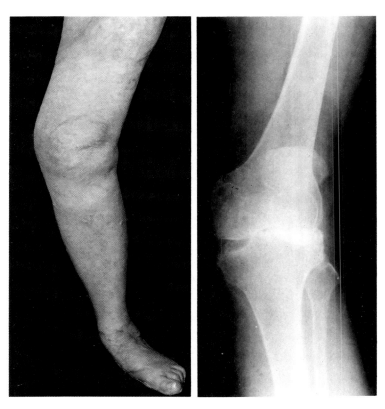

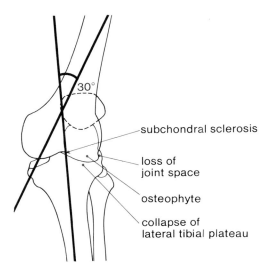

Fig. 15.35 Genu valgum. There is collapse of the lateral compartment of the knee joint (left). The weight-bearing x-ray illustrates the collapse of the lateral tibial plateau with obliteration of the joint space (right). Lines drawn through the long axes of the femur and tibia allow the angle of the deformity to be measured. A non weight-bearing x-ray may show no deformity.

30°

subchondral sclerosis

loss of joint space

osteophyte

collapse of lateral tibial plateau

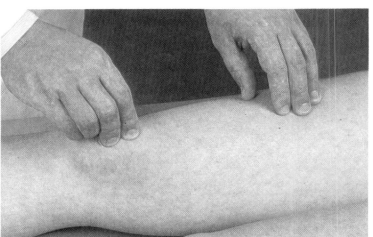

Fig. 15.36 Testing for patello-femoral pain in chondromalacia patellae. The patient contracts the quadriceps apparatus while the examiner presses down on the patella. Crepitus of the patello-femoral joint may be palpated and the symptoms are reproduced.

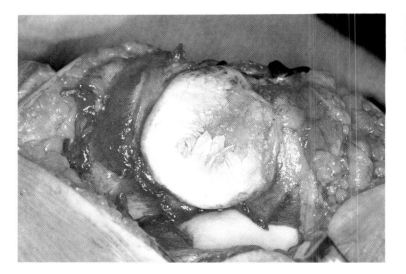

Fig. 15.37 Operative picture of advanced chondromalacia patellae showing severe fibrillation, surface softening and loss of cartilage at the back of the patella. Courtesy of Mr. J. Browett.

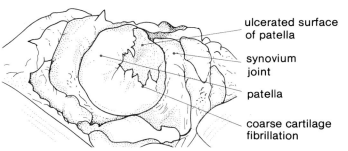

ulcerated surface of patella

synovium joint

patella

coarse cartilage fibrillation

The radiological assessment of knee osteoarthritis is important. Early changes include narrowing of the joint space, which may occur predominantly in the medial or lateral compartment of the patello-femoral joint, spiking of the tibial spines, sclerosis and marginal osteophytes (Figs. 15.38-41). As the disease progresses the joint space may become obliterated. Large 'tear-drop' osteophytes may occur particularly if vertebral hyperostosis or chondrocalcinosis are present. Collapse of the tibial plateau may occur in advanced disease in association with a varus or valgus deformity (Fig. 15.42). The radiograph may indicate etiological factors such as meniscectomy in which case the condition may be markedly asymmetrical and chiefly affecting one compartment of the joint (see Fig. 15.14). Chondromalacia patellae is sometimes best visualized by special views of the joint; skyline views of the patella or arthrography show up the deformities of the cartilage on the back of the patella (see Figs. 15.36 & 15.37).

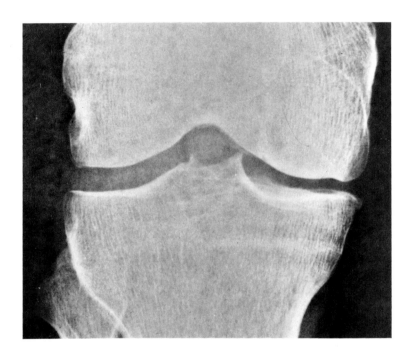

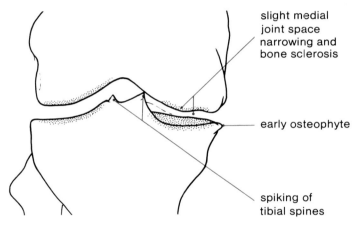

Fig. 15.38 Radiological changes in early OA of the knee. There is joint space narrowing, early osteophyte formation in the medial compartment, and spiking of the tibial spines. The medial compartment is often involved in OA.

slight medial joint space narrowing and bone sclerosis

early osteophyte

spiking of tibial spines

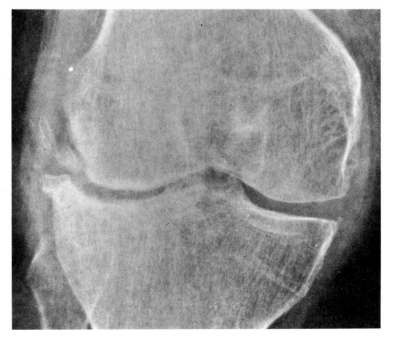

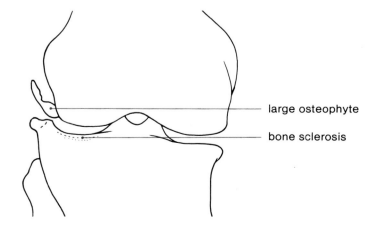

Fig. 15.39 Radiograph of severe OA of the lateral compartment of the knee joint. Joint space narrowing is not apparent in this non weight-bearing radiograph.

large osteophyte

bone sclerosis

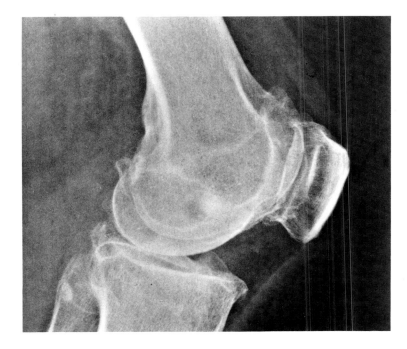

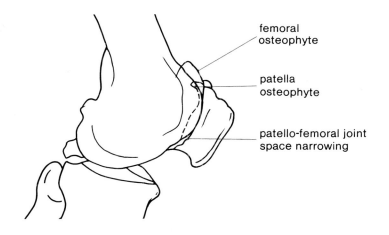

Fig. 15.40 Lateral radiograph of the knee joint in OA showing joint space narrowing and osteophyte formation at the patello-femoral joint.

femoral osteophyte

patella osteophyte

patello-femoral joint space narrowing

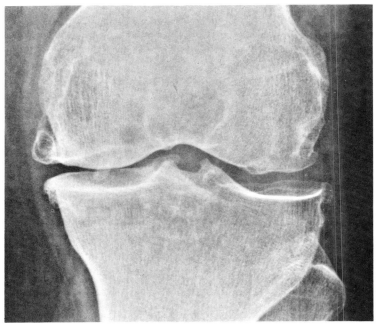

Fig. 15.41 Radiograph of knee in moderate OA showing joint space narrowing and sclerosis around the margin of the bone. The characteristic 'tear-drop' osteophytes are also apparent.

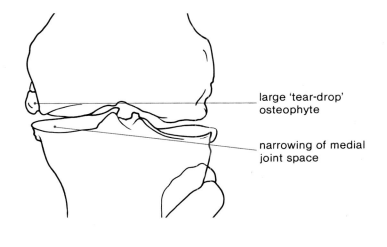

large 'tear-drop' osteophyte

narrowing of medial joint space

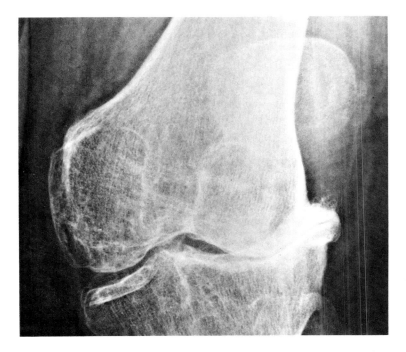

Fig. 15.42 A weight-bearing radiograph of the knee in advanced OA showing extensive collapse of the lateral compartment, resulting in a marked angulation deformity (a gross tibia valga).

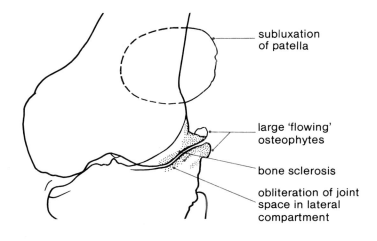

subluxation of patella

large 'flowing' osteophytes

bone sclerosis

obliteration of joint space in lateral compartment

15.17

The Hands: The hand is the second commonest site of involvement of OA and the distribution of changes is characteristic, chiefly affecting the CMC in the thumb and the DIPs. A characteristic clinical feature is the so called Heberden's node: firm swelling over the dorsum of the DIPs commonly found on the index fingers (Fig. 15.43). Although the swellings are firm early in disease, radiology shows that the soft tissues and not bone are swollen. However, as the disease advances, osteophytic outgrowths form true bony protuberances at the joint margins. As well as being seen radiologically, disease of the DIPs is apparent on a technetium labelled disphos-

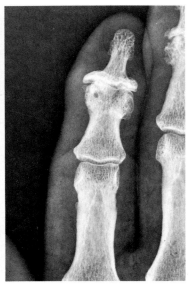

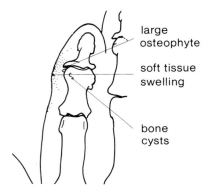

Fig. 15.43 Osteoarthritis at the DIP. The characteristic clinical finding is hard swelling either side of the dorsum of the DIP (Heberden's nodes) (left). The characteristic radiological changes include the osteophytic lipping, sclerosis and joint space narrowing (right). The index finger is usually involved and nodes may form as a part of generalized OA or as an isolated post-traumatic event.

large osteophyte

soft tissue swelling

bone cysts

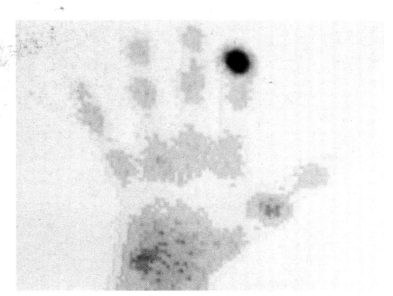

Fig. 15.44 A delayed technetium labelled diphosphonate scan in OA showing isolated uptake of the isotope (black) at the involved DIP.

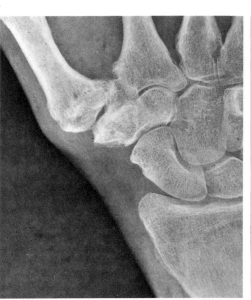

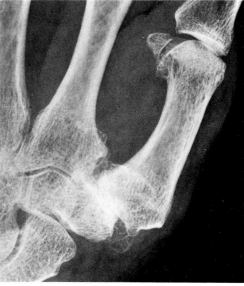

Fig. 15.45 Radiological changes in OA at the CMC of the thumb. Relatively mild changes with joint space narrowing (left); more advanced changes with considerable bony sclerosis and osteophyte formation (right).

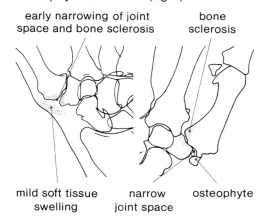

early narrowing of joint space and bone sclerosis

bone sclerosis

mild soft tissue swelling

narrow joint space

osteophyte

phanate scan of the joints, which demonstrates a well defined hot area over the involved articulation (Fig. 15.44). The other commonly involved joint is the trapezio metacarpal joint (the CMC of the thumb). The described radiological changes of early and late disease are illustrated (Fig. 15.45) and joint scanning may show hot uptake in this area (Fig. 15.46). The combination of nodal changes of the DIPs and deformity of the CMC results in the so-called 'square hand' of OA, common in middle aged and elderly women (Fig. 15.47). Severe changes in the DIPs sometimes occur leading to angulation deformities which are occasionally quite gross (Fig. 15.48).

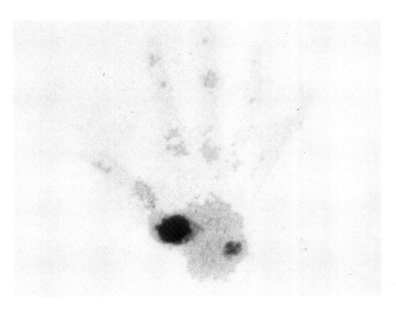

Fig. 15.46 A delayed diphosphonate bone scan showing uptake at the CMC of the thumb (black).

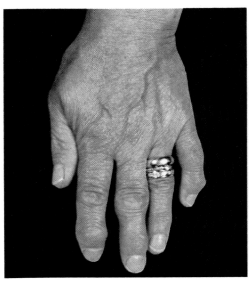

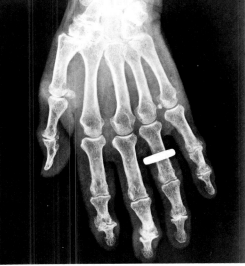

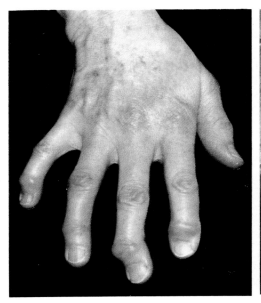

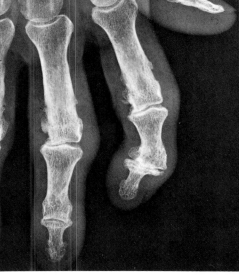

Fig. 15.47 Square hand in OA. A combination of CMC disease and Heberden's nodes leads to a squaring off of the hand which can be seen both clinically and radiologically.

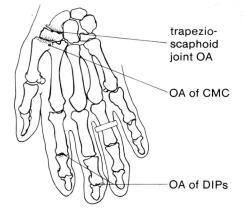

trapezio-scaphoid joint OA

OA of CMC

OA of DIPs

Fig. 15.48 In advanced OA of the DIPs angulation deformities often occur which can be seen clinically and radiologically.

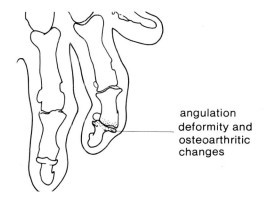

angulation deformity and osteoarthritic changes

The disease may affect the proximal interphalangeal joints (PIPs) and less commonly the metacarpophalangeal joints (MCPs). In some cases the PIP is the dominant joint, the firm swellings analogous to the Heberden's nodes being known as Bouchard's nodes (Fig. 15.49). A single interphalangeal joint may be involved, particularly where trauma has predisposed to the condition. Heberden's and Bouchard's nodes are sometimes subdivided into (a) the idiopathic type which are usually multiple, occur predominantly in middle aged women and may be associated with periarticular inflammation, and (b) the post-traumatic type: commonest in the index finger and often associated with an angulation deformity. Other changes that may be seen in the hand with OA include the formation of synovial cysts over the DIPs. If punctured, thick jelly-like material consisting mainly of hyaluronate can be squeezed out (Fig. 15.50). Formation of small periarticular ossicles is often apparent radiologically (Fig. 15.51).

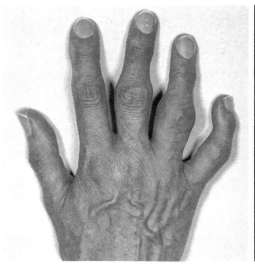 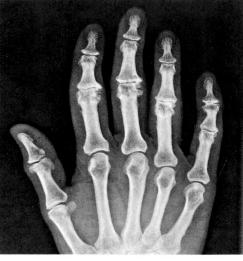 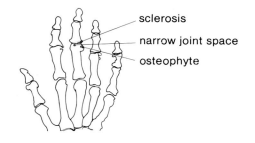

Fig. 15.49 Osteoarthritis at the PIP. OA sometimes predominantly affects the PIPs rather than the DIPs. Firm swellings which are seen clinically (left) are sometimes referred to as Bouchard's nodes. A radiograph showing OA predominantly affecting the PIPs (right).

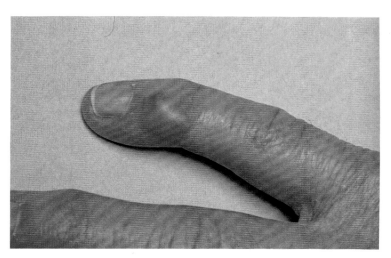 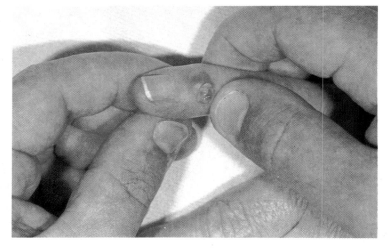

Fig. 15.50 Soft tissue cysts may form in the area adjacent to involved DIPs (left). If these are punctured a small amount of thick gelatinous material mainly containing hyaluronate can be squeezed out (right).

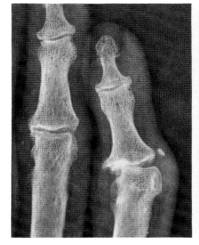 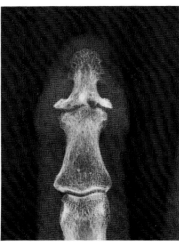

Fig. 15.51 Other radiological changes occurring in interphalangeal osteoarthritis include ossicle formation (periarticular calcification). The index finger PIP joint is involved and a small calcific deposit can be seen in the periarticular area (left). Note the angulation deformity from old collateral ligament injury. Erosions on the articular surface occasionally occur in OA. Quite extensive soft tissue swelling can also be seen around this joint. (right).

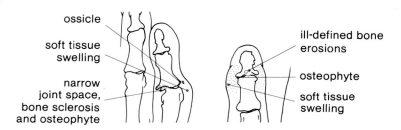

15.20

The Feet: The first metatarsophalangeal joint (MTP) of the great toe is the commonest site of OA in the feet. The condition results in two main deformities: hallux rigidus, in which there is marked restriction of movement of the joint, or hallux valgus deformity. This often results in the formation of inflamed subcutaneous bursae over the joint, ie. the formation of 'bunions' or 'poor man's gout' (Fig. 15.52). Radiological changes of hallux rigidus and hallux valgus are characteristic (Figs. 15.53 & 15.54). The other MTPs are sometimes involved in OA, though the mid- and hindfoot are less commonly affected.

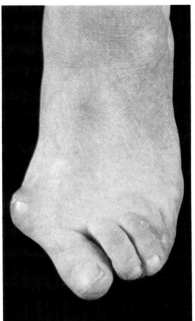
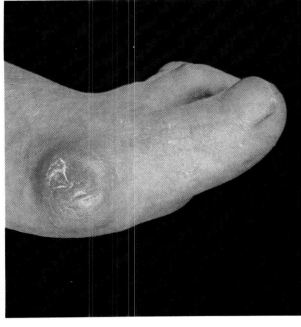

Fig. 15.52 Severe hallux valgus with bunion formation. The angulation deformity of the hallux is clearly shown (left) and soft tissue swelling formation over the bony prominence can be seen (right).

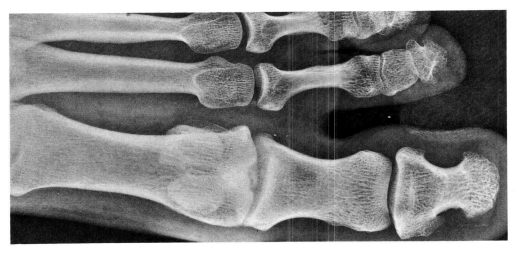

Fig. 15.53 The early radiological lesion of hallux valgus showing the area of central bone loss in the MTP.

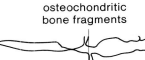

osteochondritic bone fragments

bone defect and sclerosis

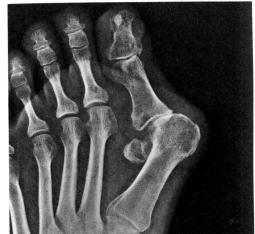
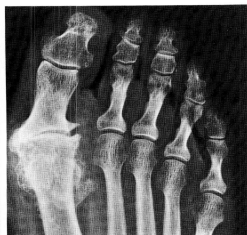

Fig. 15.54 Radiological changes of advanced hallux valgus and hallux rigidus. Angulation deformity and subluxation (left); bone overgrowth and osteophytic formation immobilising the joint in hallux rigidus (right).

metatarsus varus   hallux valgus   osteophytes

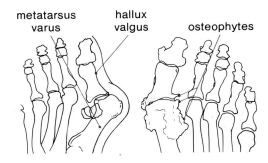

15.21

Other Joints: Any other peripheral synovial joints may be affected with OA, particularly if there is a special occupational insult, traumatic incident or mechanical factor creating damage at a certain site. Shoulders, elbows (Fig. 15.55) and ankles are all sometimes involved and other joints that may be affected include the sterno-clavicular and acromio-clavicular joints (Fig. 15.56). Wrist involvement may also occur following trauma such as Colle's fracture and is relatively common in association with chondrocalcinosis (Fig. 15.57).

The diverse sites of involvement and the wide spectrum in severity and associated symptoms, results in a wide range of clinical presentations.

Conclusions

Osteoarthritis of peripheral synovial joints is a common multifactorial disease with genetic, mechanical, metabolic and inflammatory features contributing to its pathogenesis and clinical consequences. It has a characteristic distribution, and the wide variety of clinical and radiological findings help to differentiate subsets of this fascinating, but all too common disabling disease.

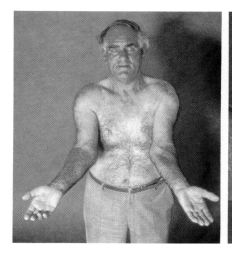
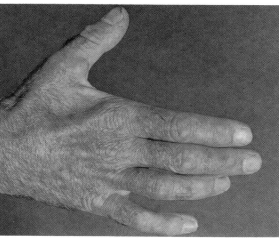

Fig. 15.55 Osteoarthritis of the elbow resulting in flexion deformities and ulnar nerve entrapment. There is a marked inability to straighten the arms (left) and small muscle wasting of the hand due to ulnar nerve damage (right). Courtesy of Mr. J. Browett.

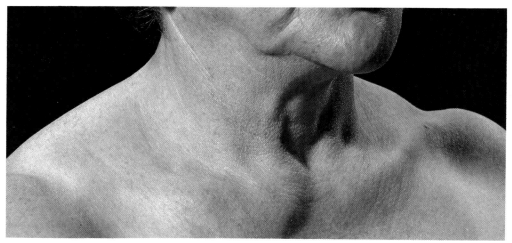

Fig. 15.56 Swelling of the sterno-clavicular joint in OA provides an example of one of the less frequently involved peripheral joints.

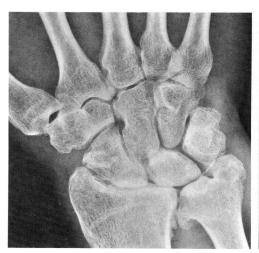
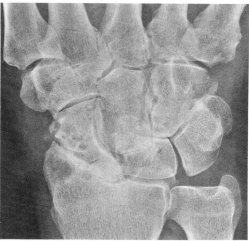

Fig. 15.57 Radiological OA of the wrist showing osteophytosis around the inferior radio-ulnar joint (left) and cystic changes in the radio-carpal joints (right).

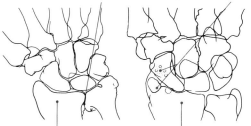

osteophytes and joint space narrowing of inferior radio-ulnar joint   bone cysts

subarticular sclerosis   excavation of bone

Infective Arthritis

with Drs. W. Carson Dick
and Philip N. Platt

A wide variety of infectious agents may provoke disease of bone and joints by a number of possible mechanisms (Fig. 16.1). Despite this diversity, response to these agents by the host is limited and hence the symptoms and signs of an infective arthritis are relatively stereo-typed (Fig. 16.2). Where differences do occur they are in emphasis rather than in basic pathophysiology.

TYPES OF INFECTION AND JOINT DISEASE

INFECTION	CHARACTERISTICS	EXAMPLES
1. Direct Infection	Multiplication of organisms in joint	Acute pyogenic infection Tuberculosis
2. Post Infective	Presence of microbial antigen in joint	Hepatitis B Post meningococcal
3. Cross-Reactive	No evidence of organism or antigen in joint	Rheumatic fever Yersiniosis
4. Inductive 'Self + X'	Modification of host cells by external agent	? Rheumatoid arthritis ? Seronegative spondarthritis

Fig. 16.1 Mechanisms of joint disease induced by infectious agents.

SIGNS AND SYMPTOMS OF INFECTIVE ARTHRITIS

Pain

Warmth

Swelling

Redness

Loss of function

Constitutional symptoms (fever)

Fig. 16.2 Signs and symptoms of infective arthritis.

Acute Pyogenic Arthritis

The incidence of pyogenic arthritis has fallen during the past 30 years and there has been a change in the age distribution. Whereas acute pyogenic arthritis was once characteristically a disease of childhood, the incidence is now shifting towards an older age group and to patients with other, underlying diseases.

A red hot joint (Fig. 16.3) is a medical emergency and demands prompt aspiration. The major differential diag-noses are sepsis or a crystal-induced synovitis and the only certain method to pursue this is examination of synovial fluid. In the case of septic arthritis thick pus, requiring a wide-bore needle for aspiration, is often obtained (Fig. 16.4), and Gram stain and culture of the pus confirms the diagnosis (Fig. 16.5).

The agent responsible for most of acute pyogenic arthritis seen in Britain is *Staphylococcus aureus*, although its dominant position is being eroded by an ever widening range of alternative infecting organisms. These include hemolytic *Streptococcus, E.coli, Salmonella spp., Pseudomonas,* pneumococcus, *Hemophilus influenzae, H. bacteroides* and others. Both *Staphylococcus spp.* and *Salmonella spp.* show a predilection for the hip and this is probably related to the peculiarities in blood supply to that joint.

Despite the variety of organisms involved the histo-logical appearances of an acute pyogenic arthritis are relatively consistent, with a pronounced polymorpho-nuclear leucocyte infiltrate, edema and necrosis (Fig. 16.6). Infection can reach a joint by hematogenous

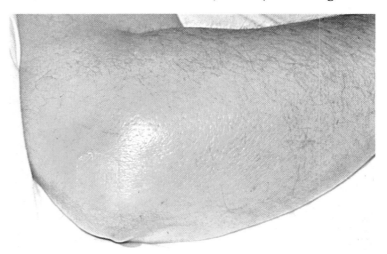

Fig. 16.3 Septic arthritis of the elbow joint showing swelling with overlying edema and redness of the skin.

Fig. 16.4 Aspiration of pus from a knee joint. Note the use of a wide bore needle to obtain the thick exudate.

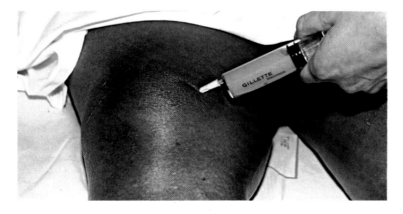

spread, by local extension from pre-existing infection in soft tissue or bone and occasionally via accidental or therapeutic direct puncture. If the diagnosis is delayed or treatment inadequate or inappropriate, very severe tissue destruction can occur (Fig. 16.7), and the morbidity and even mortality rise in proportion to the time taken to institute effective treatment (Fig. 16.8).

Radiological changes in the acute stage are confined to soft tissue swelling and osteoporosis unless there is pre-existing damage. However, destruction of articular cartilage and changes in underlying bone may become apparent after two or more weeks. The changes which should alert the physician to possible infection include areas of ill-defined bone loss, intense osteoporosis

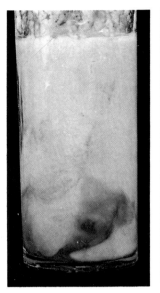
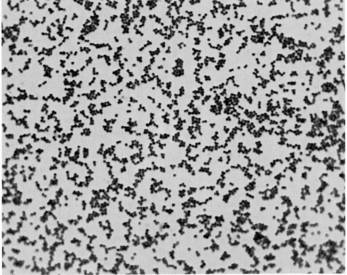

Fig. 16.5 Synovial fluid from an infected joint (left). A Gram stain showed the presence of gram-positive cocci (right, courtesy of Dr. D. Seal). The organism was confirmed as a *Staphylococcus aureus* on culture.

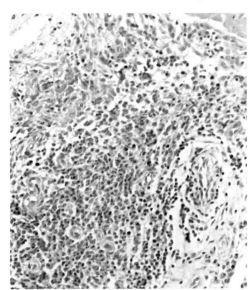

Fig. 16.6 A histological section of the synovium in acute pyogenic arthritis showing infiltration by polymorphonuclear leucocytes and fibrinous exudate. H&E stain, x 560.

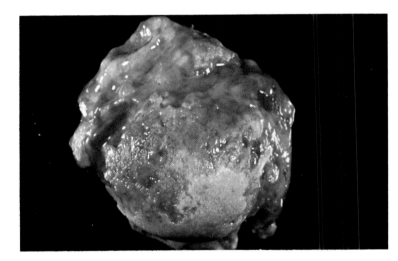

Fig. 16.7 Severe destruction of the head of the humerus due to septic arthritis. There is loss of articular cartilage and erosion of the underlying bone.

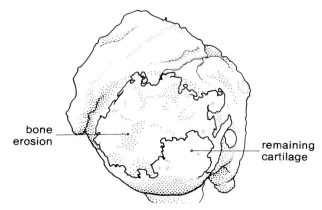

bone erosion — remaining cartilage

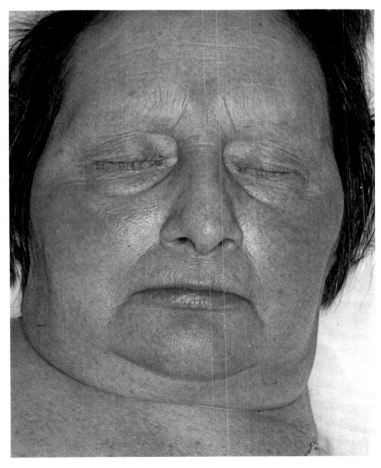

Fig. 16.8 A patient admitted to hospital four days after the onset of septic arthritis secondary to rheumatoid disease. She was severely dehydrated, comatose and close to death.

confined to one area of the joint and reactive periosteal changes (Fig. 16.9). Chronic infection may produce gross joint destruction (Figs. 16.10 & 16.11).

These destructive consequences of infection can be particularly obvious in children because of damage to the epiphysis with subsequent deformity (Fig. 16.12). Acute pyogenic arthritis may occur in joints with pre-existing disease, in particular, rheumatoid arthritis (Fig. 16.13), and may be mistaken for an exacerbation of the underlying disorder. Patients with immunosuppression

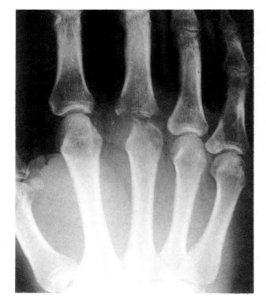

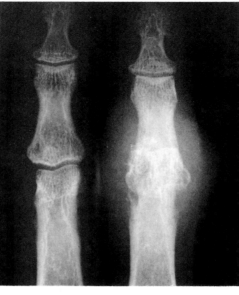

Fig. 16.9 Radiograph in acute septic arthritis of the third metacarpo-phalangeal joint (MCP) showing soft tissue swelling, osteoporosis, narrowing of the joint space and bone destruction.

Fig. 16.10 Radiographs in chronic septic arthritis showing interphalangeal joint destruction. There is soft tissue swelling and new bone formation (left) and bone fragmentation (right).

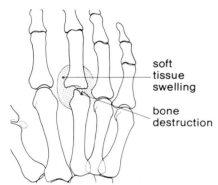

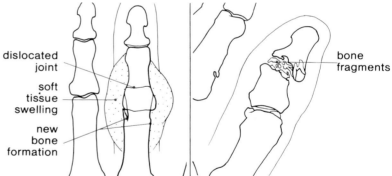

Fig. 16.11 Gross destruction of the knee joint due to old septic arthritis.

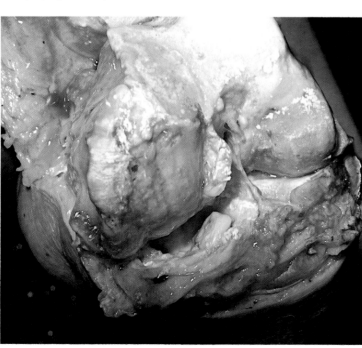

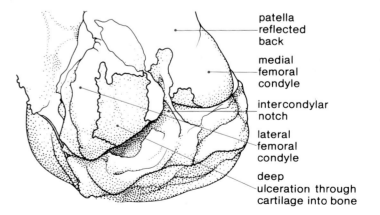

due to disease or treatment are also liable to develop pyogenic arthritis which may be due to unusual organisms such as the gram-negative or normally saprophytic organisms (Fig. 16.14). The physical signs normally associated with the presence of sepsis may be masked by immunosuppression or by disease, leading to late recognition of the problem and hence to severe damage (Fig. 16.15).

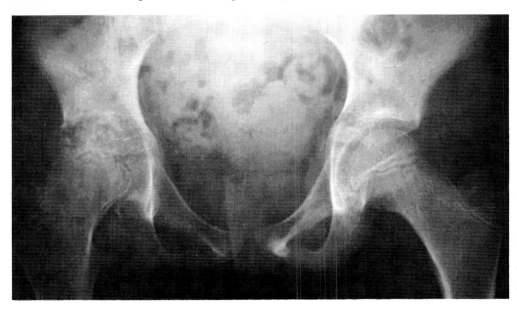

Fig. 16.12 Pelvic radiograph of a child with a two-week-history of hip pain showing severe destructive changes at the right hip joint due to septic arthritis.

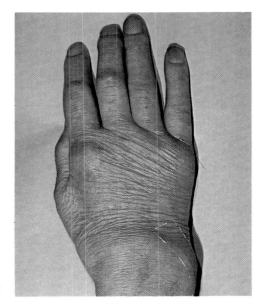

Fig. 16.13 Septic arthritis of the index finger MCP in a patient with pre-existing RA. The wrist deformity is due to the rheumatoid disease; the swollen MCP developed acutely in association with fever and malaise.

Fig. 16.14 Radiograph of a patient with a septic arthritis of the hip due to *Pseudomonas spp.* showing osteoporosis and a lytic lesion in the acetabulum.

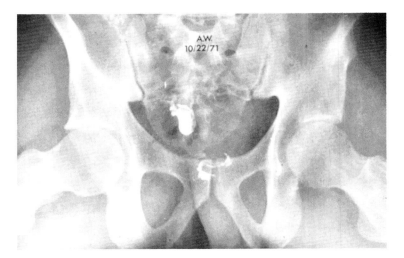

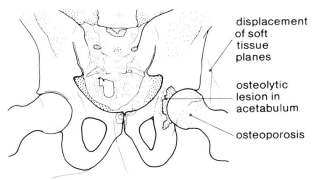

displacement of soft tissue planes

osteolytic lesion in acetabulum

osteoporosis

Fig. 16.15 Post mortem specimen of an infected joint from a patient with pre-existing joint disease. The cause of death was not apparent until the joint was opened at post mortem.

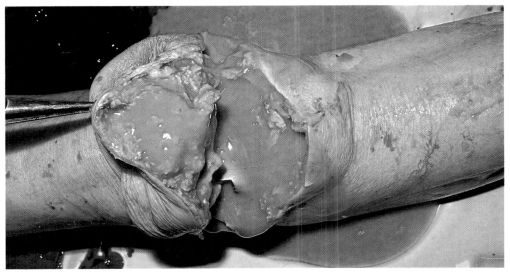

Patients who have undergone prosthetic bone or joint surgery are at risk from a variety of organisms (Fig. 16.16). Infection may lead to failure of the prosthesis due to loosening of the cement and the prosthesis may have to be removed before the infection can be controlled. Prosthetic infection may become apparent soon after operation or, alternatively, may emerge only many years later. Nevertheless, in these 'late' infections it may be shown that the organisms were introduced at the original operation. Scintigraphy may help diagnosis (Fig. 16.17 & 16.18).

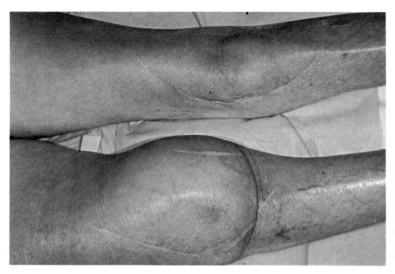
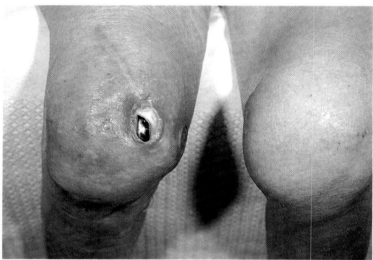

Fig. 16.16 Joint swelling (left) and fistula formation (right) in patients who have had previous prosthetic surgery for rheumatoid arthritis of the knee joints. In each case the prosthesis was infected by different organisms.

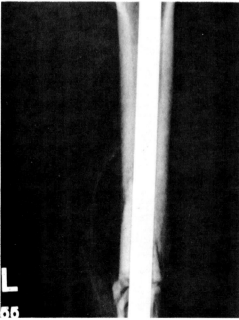

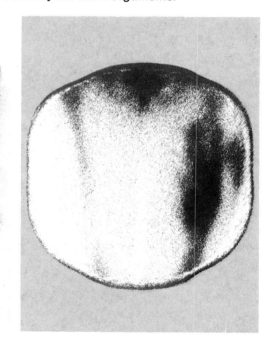

Fig. 16.17 Radiograph showing a K nail inserted into the femur for a fracture. There is a soft tissue mass with cortical destruction and new bone formation around the fracture site. Scintigraphy revealed evidence of infection confirmed at re-operation.

Fig. 16.18 Technetium labelled diphosphonate (left) and gallium (right) scans in the patient whose plain radiograph is shown in Fig. 16.17. The diphosphonate scan shows increased uptake due to increased bone turnover around the fracture and a hotter area due to unsuspected osteomyelitis. The gallium scan also showed evidence of osteomyelitis as well as the soft tissue abscess.

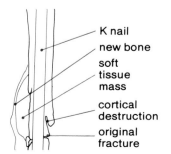

K nail
new bone
soft tissue mass
cortical destruction
original fracture

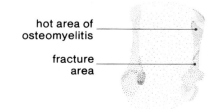
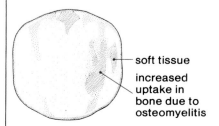

hot area of osteomyelitis
fracture area

soft tissue
increased uptake in bone due to osteomyelitis

Persistent infection can lead to the formation of a fistula which may prove difficult to eradicate despite vigorous antibiotic treatment (Figs. 16.19 & 16.20).

Axial joints (Fig. 16.21) and sacroiliac joints (Fig. 16.22) may also be infected by *Staphylococcus aureus*. Staphylococcal discitis is an uncommon cause of severe back pain, associated with fever and constitutional symptoms. It may be difficult to diagnose, although soft tissue swelling may be seen on the radiograph, and needle biopsy or scanning techniques may aid investigation.

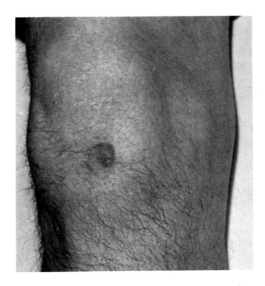

Fig. 16.19 Sinus formation at the site of a chronic infection of the knee joint.

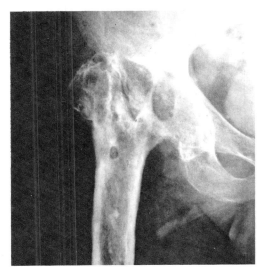

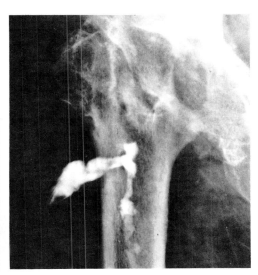

Fig. 16.20 Plain radiograph (left) and arthrogram (right) at the site of a hip prosthesis that had to be removed because of infection.

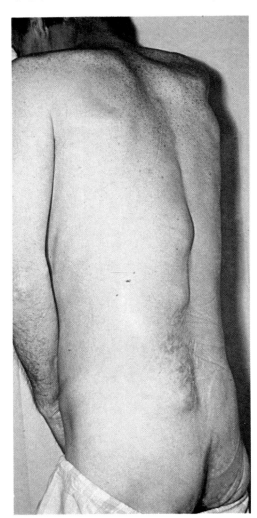

Fig. 16.21 Staphylococcal abscesses pointing around the spine of a patient with chronic discitis.

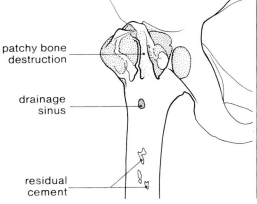

patchy bone destruction

drainage sinus

residual cement

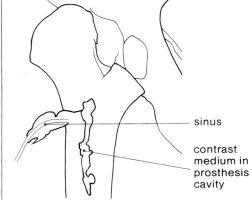

sinus

contrast medium in prosthesis cavity

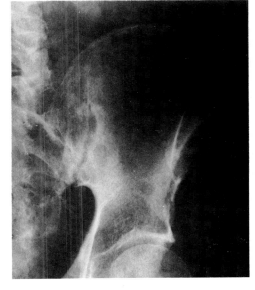

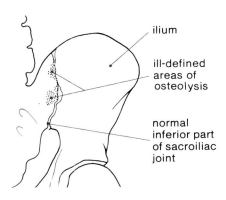

ilium

ill-defined areas of osteolysis

normal inferior part of sacroiliac joint

Fig. 16.22 Pelvic radiograph showing joint destruction caused by *S. aureus*. This 55-year-old man had recently been immunosuppressed following transplant surgery. He developed back pain and sacroiliac tenderness. Courtesy of Dr. M. Corbett.

The disc space is later destroyed (Figs. 16.23 & 16.24). The sternoclavicular joint is another axial joint which may become septic (Fig. 16.25).

Osteomyelitis

Osteomyelitis may occur in association with pyogenic arthritis by direct spread from an infected joint or vice versa. Severe bone involvement is common in patients with infected prostheses, or other metal inserted in bone, and may lead to extensive bone damage and reactive periostitis. Radioisotope scanning may aid diagnosis. Agents such as technetium-labelled diphosphonate show increased blood flow, and Gallium 67 has some specificity for pus (Fig. 16.18).

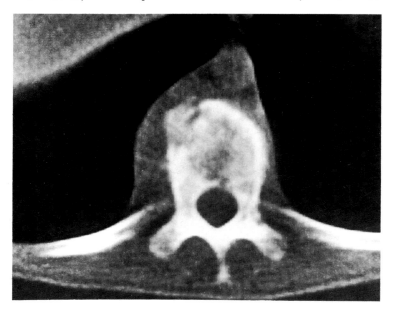

Fig. 16.23 CT scan of a thoracic vertebra showing osteomyelitis due to staphylococcal infection.

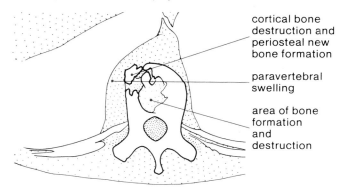

cortical bone destruction and periosteal new bone formation

paravertebral swelling

area of bone formation and destruction

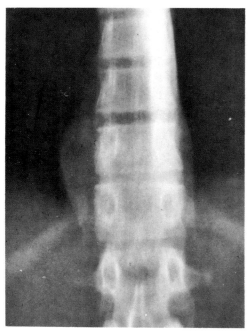

Fig. 16.24 Tomogram of the thoracic spine showing a soft tissue mass around an infected disc space.

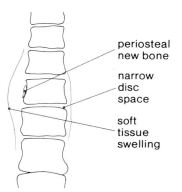

periosteal new bone

narrow disc space

soft tissue swelling

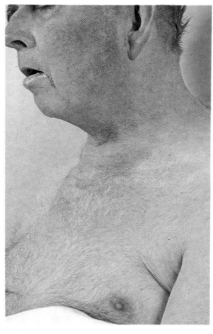

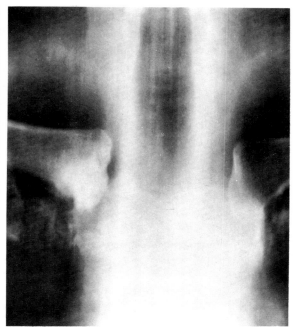

Fig. 16.25 Sternoclavicular joint infection. The patient (left) presented with atypical chest pain. Plain radiographs appeared normal, but the tomogram (right) revealed destructive changes typical of condensing osteitis. Coexistent infection was confirmed by open biopsy.

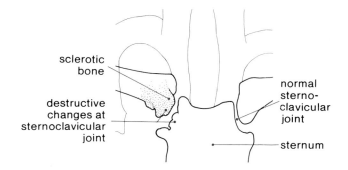

sclerotic bone

destructive changes at sternoclavicular joint

normal sterno-clavicular joint

sternum

Primary osteomyelitis is commoner in children than in adults. It may result in sympathetic joint effusion (Fig. 16.26). As in the case of pyogenic arthritis radiographs are initially unremarkable and scintigraphy may aid diagnosis. As the disease progresses typical bone damage and periostitis develop and later cystic changes in bone may appear (Figs. 16.27 & 16.28).

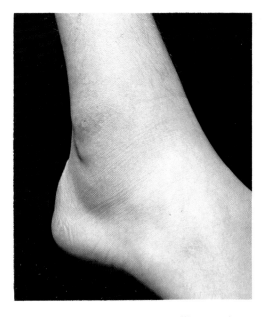

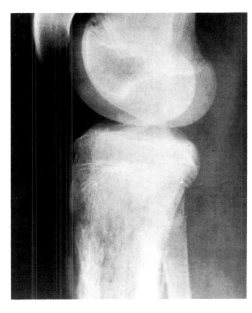

Fig. 16.26 Soft tissue swelling and erythema around an area of osteomyelitis in the fibula of a 14-year-old child.

Fig. 16.27 Plain radiograph in acute osteomyelitis of the tibia showing diffuse bone destruction extending to the epiphysis and new bone formation.

epiphysis

ill-defined bone destruction

new bone

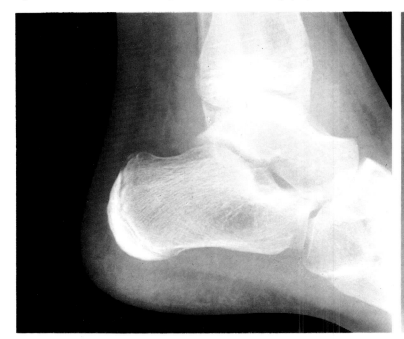

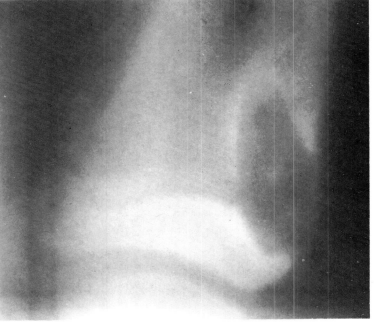

Fig. 16.28 Chronic osteomyelitis of the tibia. The plain radiograph (left) shows soft tissue swelling and a 'Brodie's abscess'. The tomogram (right) shows sclerosis around the abscess and sequestrum in its centre. Note the extension across the metaphyseal plate.

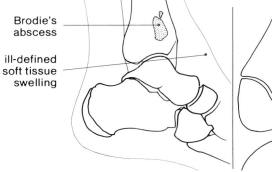

Brodie's abscess

ill-defined soft tissue swelling

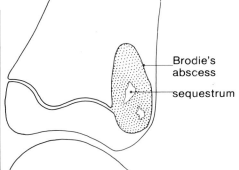

Brodie's abscess

sequestrum

Gonococcal Infections

The incidence of gonococcal arthritis has risen with the increased incidence of gonococcal infections in the population, although the increase in Britain has been much less marked than in the USA. The disease is more common in females than males, as females are the major reservoir of untreated gonococcal infection. There are two mechanisms by which gonococcal infections produce joint involvement – firstly, a direct type 1 acute purulent arthritis and secondly, a type 3 reactive arthritis.

The clinical picture of polyarthralgia, tenosynovitis, fever and skin lesions is characteristic. The joints most commonly involved are the knee, wrist and small joints of the hand, with polyarticular involvement being more common (Fig. 16.29). The skin lesions usually begin as red papules that either disappear or proceed through vesicular and pustular stages to develop a grey necrotic centre (Fig. 16.30).

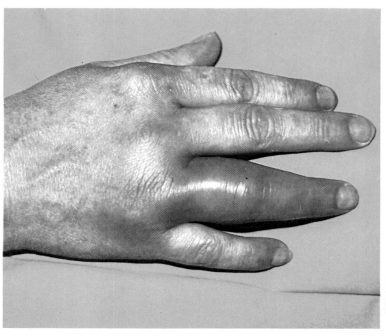
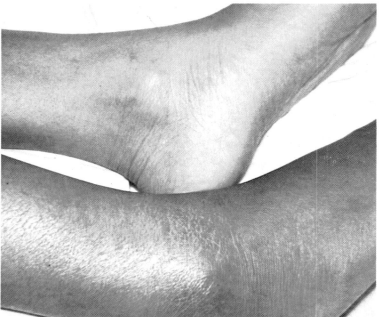

Fig. 16.29 Gonococcal arthritis: dactylitis of the ring finger due to tenosynovitis (left, courtesy of Dr. S.E. Thompson) and septic arthritis of the ankle (right, courtesy of Dr. T.F. Sellers Jr.) in a 24-year-old woman.

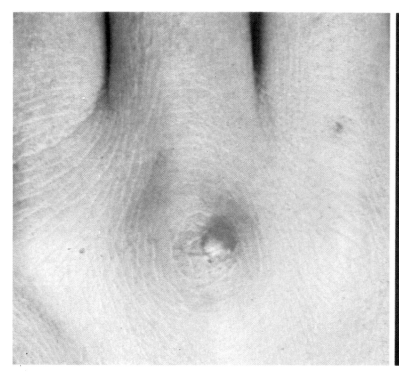
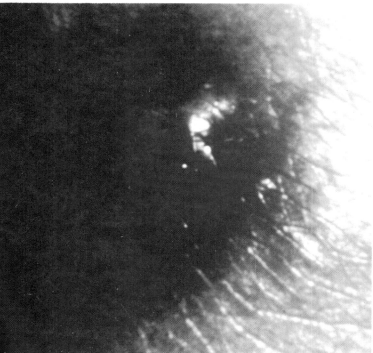

Fig. 16.30 Gonococcal skin lesions. A typical pustule on the back of the hand (left, courtesy of Dr. T.F. Sellers Jr.) and a hemorrhagic lesion (right, courtesy of Dr. S.E. Thompson).

Confirmation of the diagnosis of gonococcal arthritis may be difficult. Quick transport of warm specimens to the bacteriology laboratory, using special transport media (eg. Thayer-Martin medium), followed by immediate culture on chocolate agar or other special growth plates may increase the yield of positive bacteriology from skin, genital or joint lesions (Fig. 16.31). The condition usually responds quickly to treatment with penicillin.

Brucella Infections

As the incidence of brucella infection has fallen, bone and joint involvement has become uncommon. Various patterns of infection can occur including a monoarthritis and a bursitis (particularly pre-tibial bursitis, Fig. 16.32). The most characteristic lesion is spondylitis. This may develop weeks or months after infection and may present as severe back pain. Radiology shows a destructive lesion with narrowing of the disc space, and characteristically there is exuberant osteophyte formation (Fig. 16.33).

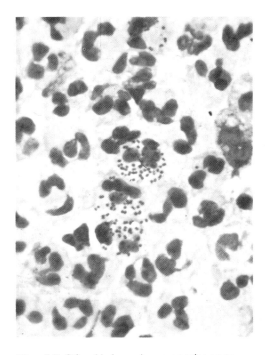

Fig. 16.31 *Neisseria gonorrhoeae*: Gram stain of urethral exudate in gonorrhoea showing intracellular gram-negative reniform diplococci. Courtesy of Dr. S.E. Thompson.

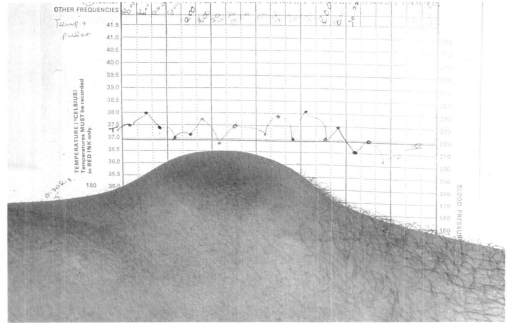

Fig. 16.32 Pre-tibial bursitis due to infection by brucella. The red swollen bursa with the 'undulating' fever chart are illustrated.

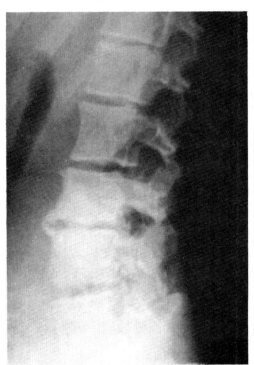

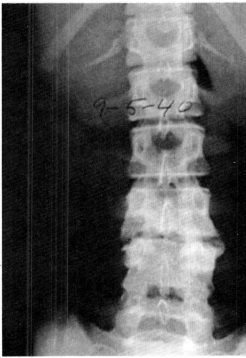

Fig. 16.33 Plain radiograph in brucella infection of the spine showing narrowing of the joint space, bony sclerosis and new bone formation with large osteophytes.

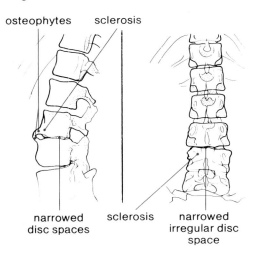

osteophytes   sclerosis

narrowed disc spaces   sclerosis   narrowed irregular disc space

Tuberculosis

The incidence of tuberculosis involving bones and joints has fallen under the triple onslaught of better general conditions of hygiene and nutrition, preventative measures and effective chemotherapy. Despite this it still occurs, particularly in some immigrant groups, and may be missed through failure to include it as a possible differential diagnosis.

The most commonly affected site is the thoracic spine, where involvement of a vertebral body leads to production of a cavity filled with caseous material. Extension frequently occurs to the intervertebral disc, which is characteristically destroyed, and to other vertebrae (Figs. 16.34 & 16.35). Severe destruction may produce a marked angulation, or gibbus deformity (Fig. 16.36). Paravertebral abscesses may form secondary to vertebral

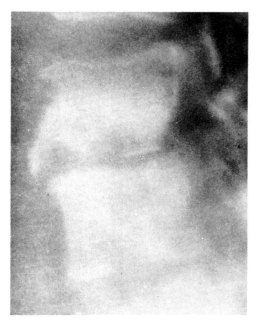

Fig. 16.34 Tomogram in spinal tuberculosis showing disc space narrowing, destruction of both end plates and bony sclerosis.

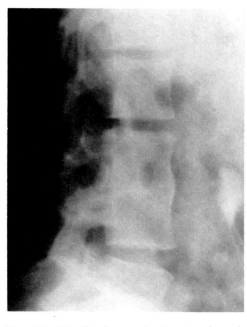

Fig. 16.35 Radiograph showing fused 'block' vertebrae from old tuberculosis.

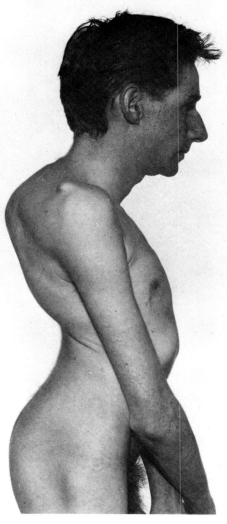

Fig. 16.36 Tubercular spinal gibbus.

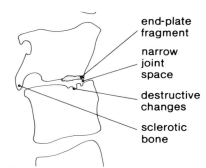

end-plate fragment
narrow joint space
destructive changes
sclerotic bone

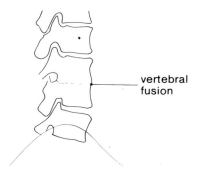

vertebral fusion

Fig. 16.37 Intravenous urogram showing a perinephric abscess. The kidneys are of normal size but on the right there is a perirenal gas halo due to the abscess; the psoas shadow is obliterated on that side. Courtesy of Professor A.W. Asscher.

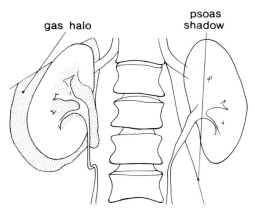

gas halo
psoas shadow

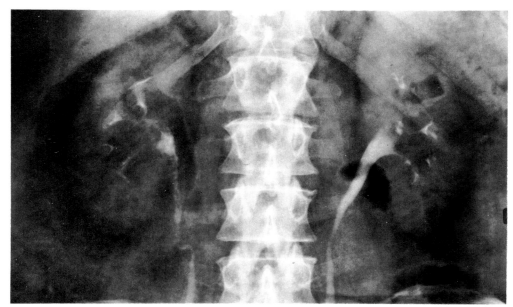

involvement and may track along tissue planes to produce for instance the classical psoas abscess (Fig. 16.37). Sacroiliac joint involvement occurs and should be considered particularly when the sacroiliitis is unilateral (Fig. 16.38). The appendicular skeleton may also be affected by tuberculosis. Children rarely develop a dactylitis (Fig. 16.39), which may be associated with tenosynovitis.

Any large joint can be affected by tuberculosis, the hip and knee being most frequently involved with symptoms of gradual loss of movement, swelling, stiffness and pain. Tuberculous synovitis may require a formal open biopsy before a diagnosis can be made on the basis of the characteristic histological findings of caseating granulomata (Fig. 16.40).

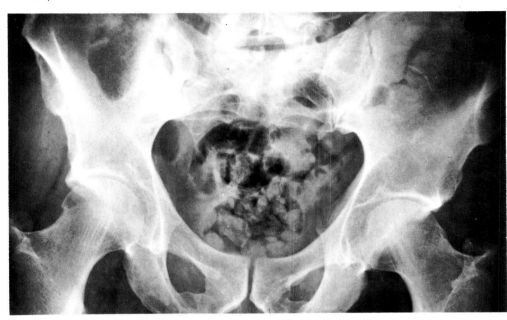

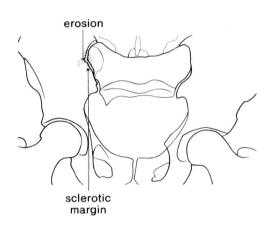

Fig. 16.38 Radiograph showing unilateral sacroiliitis due to tuberculosis. Note the widened eroded joint space.

erosion

sclerotic margin

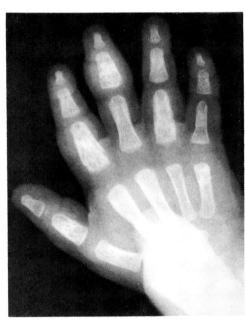

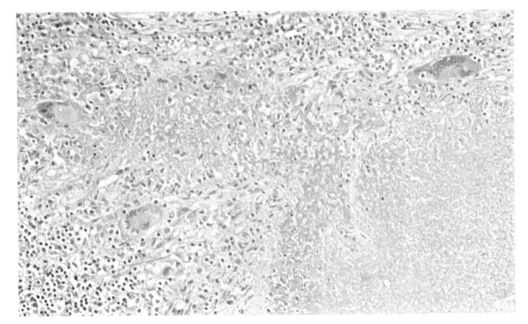

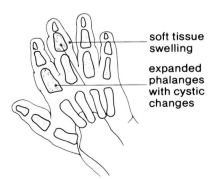

Fig. 16.39 Tuberculous dacytlitis. Courtesy of Professor H.P. Lambert.

Fig. 16.40 Histological section of tuberculous synovium showing necrosis and giant cell formation. H&E stain, x 1000.

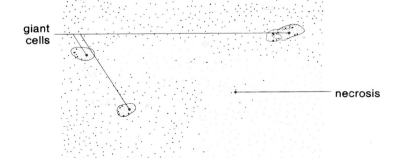

soft tissue swelling

expanded phalanges with cystic changes

giant cells

necrosis

The typical radiological changes of tuberculous arthritis include erosive damage on both sides of the joint line (Figs. 16.41 & 16.42).

Syphilitic Infections

Bone and joint involvement may occur in both congenital and acquired forms. In the congenital form osteochrondritis, periostitis, joint effusions and, rarely, dactylitis occur. Acquired forms produce a variety of lesions: periostitis, gummata and, in the tertiary stages of neurosyphilis, neuropathic or Charcot's joints (Figs. 16.43 & 16.44). Charcot's joints may yield synovial fluid containing free and ingested crystals of calcium pyrophosphate dihydrate and hydroxyapatite raising the question "Does the crystal cause the destruction or does the destruction favour crystal nucleation?"

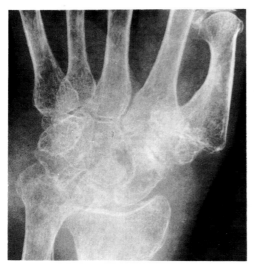

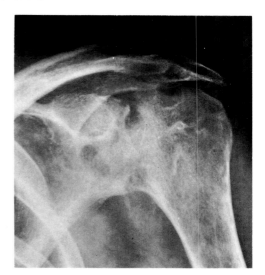

Fig. 16.41 Radiographs of the wrist in tuberculosis: early erosive changes (left) can lead to severe joint destruction (right).

Fig. 16.42 Shoulder radiograph in tuberculosis showing the classical 'caries sicca' changes with large corticated erosions and disuse osteoporosis.

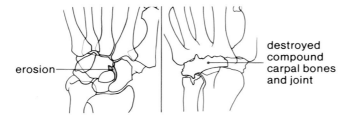

erosion

destroyed compound carpal bones and joint

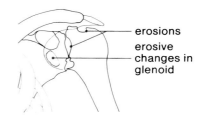

erosions

erosive changes in glenoid

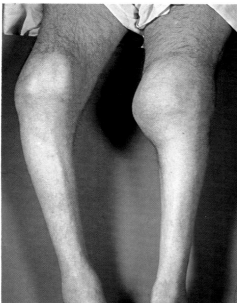

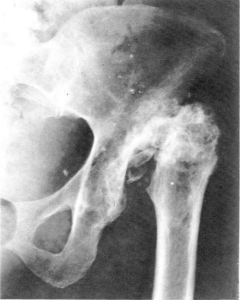

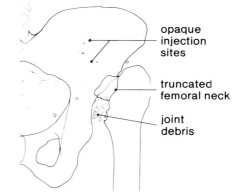

opaque injection sites

truncated femoral neck

joint debris

Fig. 16.43 Syphilitic Charcot knee joints showing gross destructive changes.

Fig. 16.44 Radiograph of a Charcot hip joint. The joint is subluxed supero-laterally due to destruction of both the femoral head and acetabular roof. Note the joint debris and multiple opacities in the buttock due to previous bismuth injections. The patient had had syphilis.

Rheumatic Fever

Acute rheumatic fever is now very rare in the developed countries but still occurs frequently in the third world. The clinical features of carditis, flitting polyarthritis, nodules, chorea and erythema marginatum are well known. The joints are warm and swollen with erythema particularly over the smaller joints (Fig. 16.45). Erythema marginatum, although diagnostic, only occurs in a small proportion of active cases and then only fleetingly. The characteristic feature is the sharply demarcated spreading edge of the lesion (Fig. 16.46). The cardiac lesions are characteristic and cause long-term problems. Late joint abnormalities are rare, although non-correctable ulnar deviation of the fingers, without radiological evidence of destruction (Jaccoud's arthritis, Fig. 16.47) can occur.

Viral Arthritis

Self-limiting polyarthritides are increasingly being recognized in association with common viral infections such as rubella and infectious mononucleosis. Joint symptoms occur in only a small proportion of cases in these infections; however a much higher frequency is reported in the mosquito-borne viral diseases such as chikungunya and o'nyong-nyong.

Of a more controversial nature is the role of viruses in the induction of chronic destructive inflammatory arthritides such as rheumatoid arthritis where one outcome of interaction between viral nucleic acid and host DNA may lead to modification of the host cells (Fig. 16.48). Certainly there has been a resurgence of interest in the last decade in the interaction of exogenous infection with an immunogenetically predisposed host.

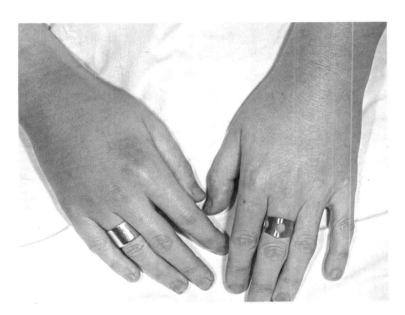

Fig. 16.45 The typical redness over the involved joints in rheumatic fever.

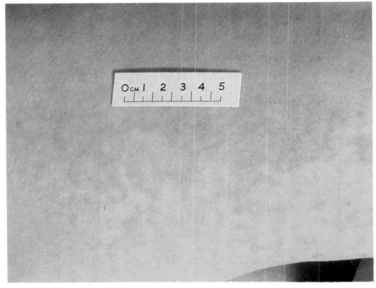

Fig. 16.46 Erythema marginatum in rheumatic fever.

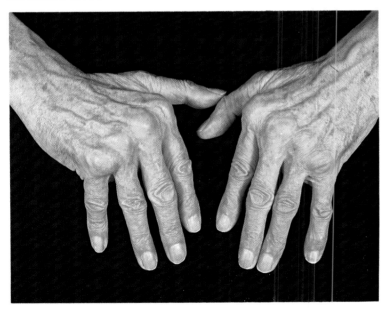

Fig. 16.47 Jaccoud's arthritis. Ulnar deviation has occurred as a result of fibrosis around joints previously affected by rheumatic fever.

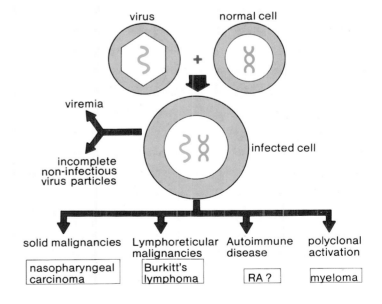

Fig. 16.48 Modification of the host cell by viruses: when viral nucleic acid interacts with a host cell there are a number of possible outcomes. In the example of Epstein Barr virus some of these outcomes are well established (eg. lymphoreticular malignancy) and others, such as autoimmune disease in the form of rheumatoid arthritis, are speculative.

16.15

Soft Tissue Infections

Acute soft tissue infections can produce secondary bone and joint damage (Fig. 16.49). Chronic dactylitis can occur in tuberculosis and with fungal and other chronic infections; biopsy may be required to make the diagnosis (Fig. 16.50). Soft tissue infections are also common in diabetes, and can result in chronic changes in the underlying bone and joints (Fig. 16.51).

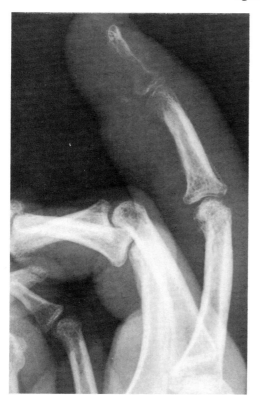

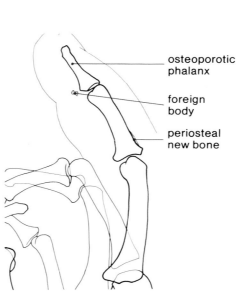

Fig. 16.49 Radiograph showing soft tissue infection in the hand. The foreign body caused infection and swelling of the soft tissue with secondary periostitis and bone damage.

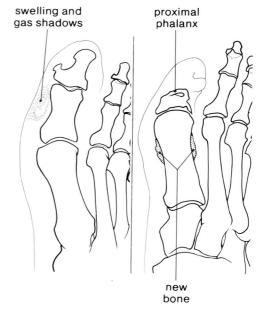

Fig. 16.50 Chronic dactylitis. There is soft tissue swelling of the whole finger and redness of the overlying skin.

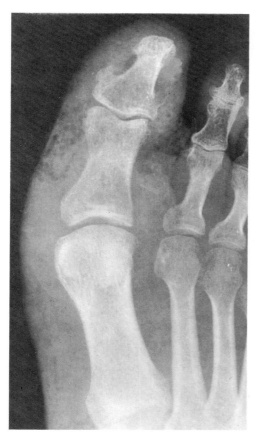

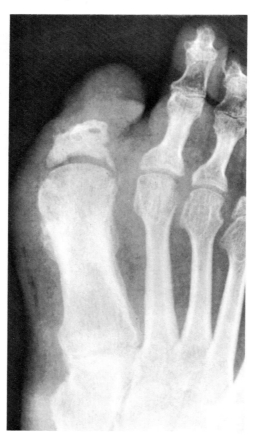

Fig. 16.51 Radiographs of the right foot of a diabetic patient. The earlier radiograph (left) shows soft tissue swelling and gas shadows due to gas gangrene, the later picture (right) shows subsequent destructive bony changes and periosteal new bone formation (the terminal phalanx has been removed).

17

Spinal Diseases and Back Pain

with Professor Malcolm I.V. Jayson

The vertebral column consists of 24 vertebrae linked to each other, to the base of the skull above, and to the sacrum and pelvis below. The column is linked by the intervertebral discs and apophyseal joints together with a series of longitudinal ligaments and muscles (Figs. 17.1 & 17.2). A wide variety of disorders may affect this complex structure and cause back symptoms.

Back pain may result from disorders arising within the spine and associated structures, or be referred from abdominal and pelvic viscera (Fig. 17.3). By far the most common are structural or mechanical problems (Fig. 17.4). These include prolapse of an intervertebral disc, lumbar spondylosis, Scheuermann's osteochondritis, fractures, spinal stenosis and spondylolisthesis. 'Non-specific back pain' is a term which describes a large number of patients whose pain seems to be of mechanical origin yet in whom it is difficult to define the precise source of the symptoms.

Assessment of the Back Pain Patient

The clinical history and examination include not only full details of the development, evolution and current status of the back pain syndrome but also a general system enquiry and examination for other features which may point to some generalized disorder causing the clinical problem. Routine investigations, particularly for patients developing back pain for the first time, may include a blood sedimentation rate (or plasma viscosity), blood count, routine biochemical screening including calcium, phosphate and alkaline phosphatase, the acid phosphatase in males and, if there is any possibility of myelomatosis, protein electrophoresis. Routine radiographs are not required for every patient as the majority of back pain attacks are transient mechanical problems and resolve rapidly. Radiographs should be reserved for those patients in whom grounds for suspicion of a non-structural cause arise from the history or blood examinations, and for the patient who has a persistent and severe back problem.

The physical examination should include observation of spinal movements in flexion, extension, lateral rotation and lateral flexion in both directions. Measurements of these movements, particularly flexion and extension, may be made using the spirit level goniometer (Fig. 17.5), or with a tape measure by the Schober technique (Fig. 17.6).

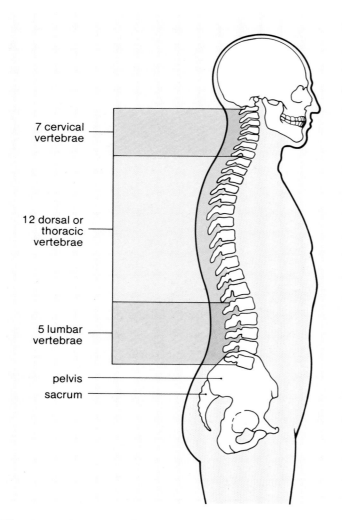

Fig. 17.1 Diagram of the vertebral column showing the 7 cervical, 12 thoracic and 5 lumbar vertebrae articulating with the sacrum and pelvis.

7 cervical vertebrae

12 dorsal or thoracic vertebrae

5 lumbar vertebrae

pelvis

sacrum

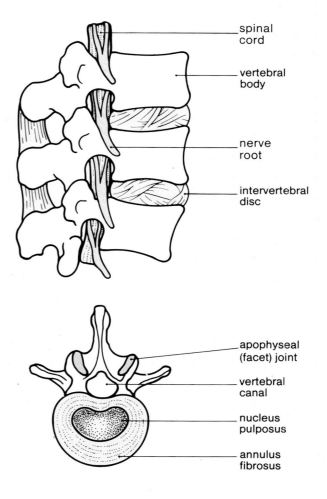

spinal cord

vertebral body

nerve root

intervertebral disc

apophyseal (facet) joint

vertebral canal

nucleus pulposus

annulus fibrosus

Fig. 17.2 Diagram showing the vertebral structure. The vertebral bodies are joined by the intervertebral disc anteriorly and the apophyseal (facet) joints posteriorly. Each disc consists of a central nucleus pulposus surrounded by the oblique fibres of the annulus fibrosis. The spinal cord and nerve roots pass down through the vertebral canal and the roots emerge through the intervertebral foramina.

CAUSES OF BACK PAIN	STRUCTURAL OR MECHANICAL CAUSES OF BACK PAIN

CAUSES OF BACK PAIN

1. In the spine

   Structural/Mechanical

   Inflammatory

   Metabolic

   Neoplasms/Reticuloses

2. Referred from abdominal

   or visceral disease

STRUCTURAL OR MECHANICAL CAUSES OF BACK PAIN

Prolapsed intervertebral disc

Lumbar spondylosis

Spondylolisthesis

Fractures

Scheuermann's osteochondritis

Diffuse idiopathic skeletal hyperostosis

Spinal stenosis

Non-specific

Fig. 17.3 Classification of the causes of back pain.

Fig. 17.4 Classification of the structural or mechanical problems causing back pain.

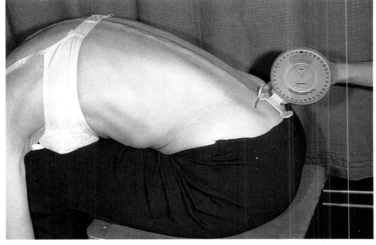

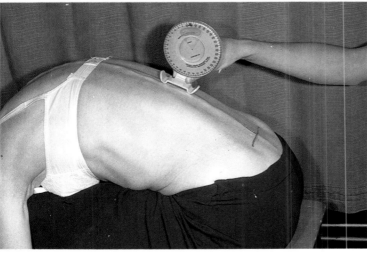

Fig. 17.5 Measurement of spinal movement using the spirit level goniometer. The goniometer is placed at the dorsolumbar and lumbosacral junctions so that the curvature of the spine may be measured. By repeating this test in the upright and fully flexed positions the amount of flexion can be determined.

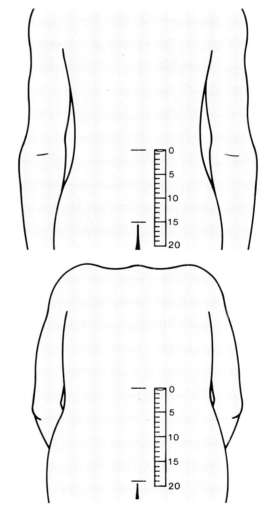

Fig. 17.6 Measurement of forward flexion of the lumbar spine using a modified Schober technique. Two marks, 15cm apart with the 10cm mark at the level of the Dimples of Venus, are drawn over the lumbar spine with the patient standing upright. Forward flexion results in a movement of 4cm.

The straight leg raising test (Fig. 17.7) gives a guide to dural sheath compression and neurological examination will provide a guide to nerve root damage (Figs. 17.8 & 17.9). In addition to observation and palpation of the spine and paravertebral structures, leg length should be measured, the patient's posture and gait noted, and a general physical examination carried out.

Prolapsed Intervertebral Disc

Prolapse of an intervertebral disc most commonly affects the L4/5 and L5/S1 discs but may occur at other levels. Although prolapse of the lumbar discs usually follows some excessive load on the spine, it seems very likely that it develops in previously damaged discs. Excessive load on a normal disc readily produces end-plate fractures with Schmörl's nodes (Figs. 17.10 & 17.11) rather than posterior or posterolateral prolapse.

The patient with an acute posterior disc prolapse develops acute back pain, sometimes with pain referred down the leg in a non-root distribution. A posterolateral prolapse, causing nerve root compression, provokes pain and parasthesiae in the affected root and the acute back pain often eases leaving only the root compression pain. On examination a scoliosis induced by protective spasm in the paraspinal muscles is often seen. Flexion and extension are limited and painful, although lateral flexion may be preserved. Straight leg raising and neurological abnormalities corresponding to the root involvement may be found.

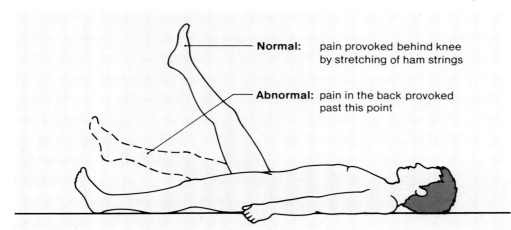

Normal: pain provoked behind knee by stretching of ham strings

Abnormal: pain in the back provoked past this point

Fig. 17.7 The straight leg raising test is used as an index of dural compression.

LUMBAR ROOT LESIONS

Dermatome distribution Anterior / Posterior	Root	Muscle weakness/ movement affected	Tendon reflex decreased
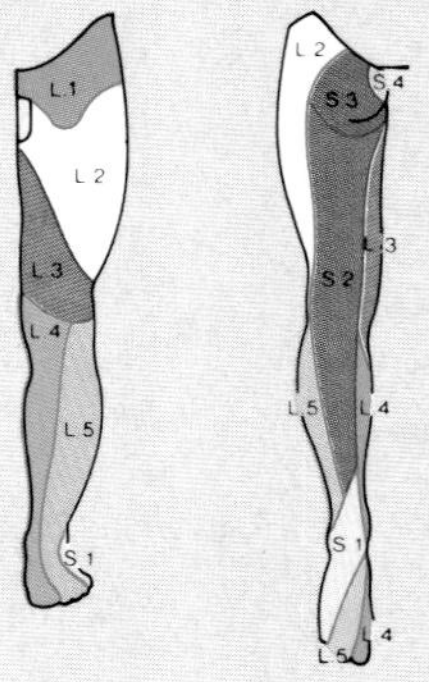	L.2	Hip flexion/adduction	
	L.3	Hip adduction Knee extension	Knee jerk
	L.4	Knee extension Foot inversion/dorsiflexion	Knee jerk
	L.5	Hip extension/abduction Knee flexion Foot/toe dorsiflexion	
	S.1	Knee flexion Foot/toe plantar flexion Foot eversion	Ankle jerk

Fig. 17.8 Table showing the principal features used in identifying lumbar nerve root lesions. This does not list the total distribution of each nerve root.

CERVICAL ROOT LESIONS

Dermatome distribution Anterior / Posterior	Root	Muscle weakness/ movement affected	Tendon reflex decreased
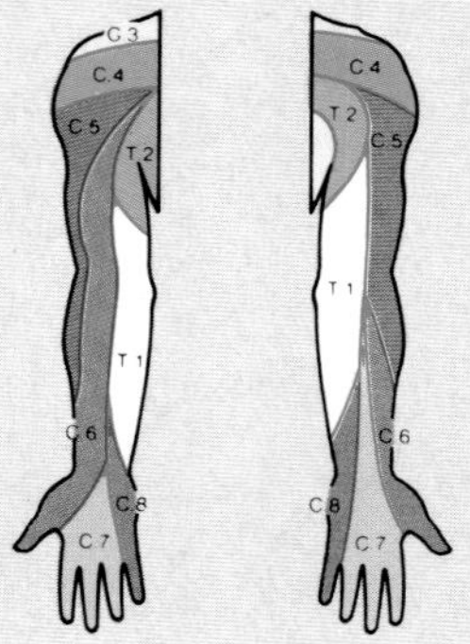	C.5	Shoulder abduction Elbow flexion	Biceps jerk
	C.6	Wrist extension/pronation	Supinator jerk
	C.7	Elbow/finger extension	Triceps jerk
	C.8	Wrist/finger flexion	Finger jerk
	T.1	Finger abduction Thumb adduction/ opposition	

Fig. 17.9 Table showing the principal features used for identifying the sites of cervical nerve root lesions. This table does not list the total distribution of each nerve root.

Radiographs of the lumbar spine are usually normal except perhaps for the scoliosis, but may show slight narrowing of the disc space. In later years disc space narrowing, osteophyte formation and changes in the facet joints develop. Radiculography using a water soluble radio-opaque dye, will outline the nerve roots which show poor filling at the site of a prolapse (Fig. 17.12).

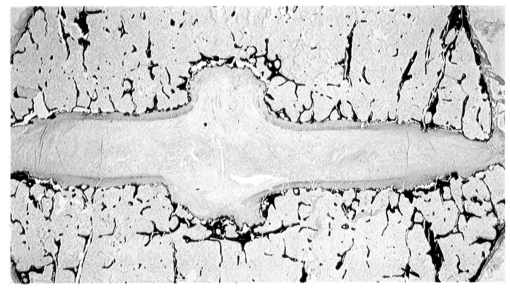

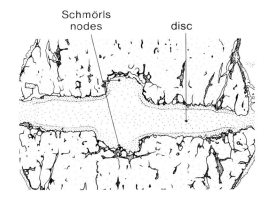

Fig. 17.10 Section of a disc affected by Schmorl's nodes. The bone, which has been stained black by the von Kossa technique, has formed a shell around the extruded material. Courtesy of Professor B. Vernon-Roberts.

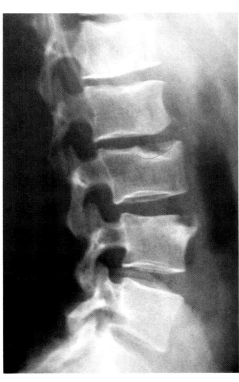

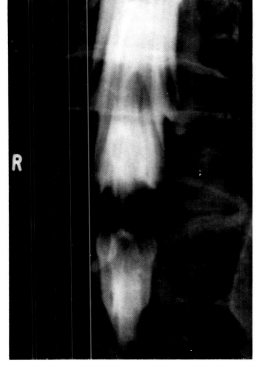

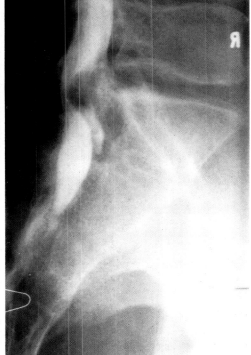

Fig. 17.11 Lumbar radiograph showing extensive anterior Schmörl's nodes with surrounding sclerotic reaction.

Fig. 17.12 Water soluble radiculogram demonstrating a large protrusion of the L5/S1 disc. The AP view (left) shows an obstruction to the column of dye and

the left sided nerve root sheath does not fill. The lateral film (right) shows the nerve roots stretched around the bulging disc.

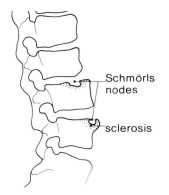

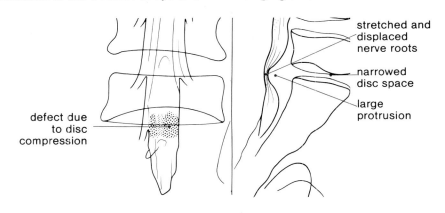

High resolution computerized tomography may also reveal such lesions (Fig. 17.13). Discograms are obtained by direct injection of dye into the nucleus of the intervertebral disc. Not only can disc damage be seen (Fig. 17.14) but the injection may reproduce the patient's symptoms helping to define their precise origin. Although actual disc prolapse is less common elsewhere in the spine, a thoracic disc prolapse may produce signs and symptoms referred to the legs. Many prolapsed thoracic discs calcify (Fig. 17.15).

Lumbar Spondylosis

This term refers strictly to degenerative changes in the intervertebral disc. Initially there is disorganization of disc structure (Figs. 17.16 & 17.17) followed by loss of disc substance, sclerosis of the disc margins and osteophyte formation (Fig. 17.18). The term, however, usually includes osteoarthritic changes in the apophyseal joints (Fig. 17.19).

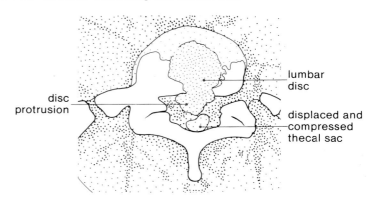

Fig. 17.13 CT scan at L5/S1 demonstrating a large central disc protrusion indenting the thecal sac.

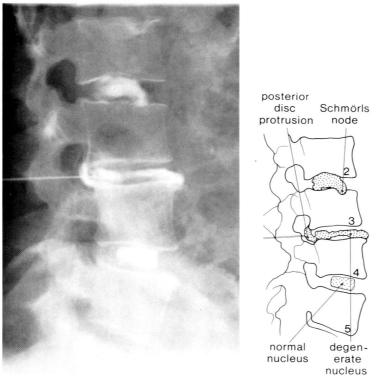

Fig. 17.14 Lumbar discography at multiple levels. The L4/5 disc is normal. At L3/4 the disc shows degenerative changes with posterior herniation of the nuclear substance. At L2/3 there is a Schmörl's node with extension of the nuclear material into the vertebral body.

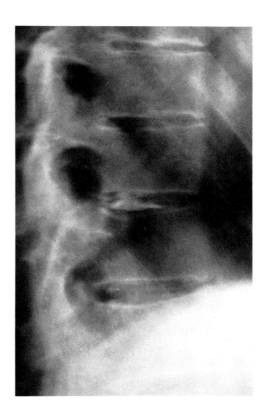
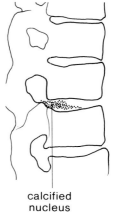

Fig. 17.15 Thoracic radiograph showing calcification of the nucleus of a disc. Note the extension of the calcified material into the neural canal.

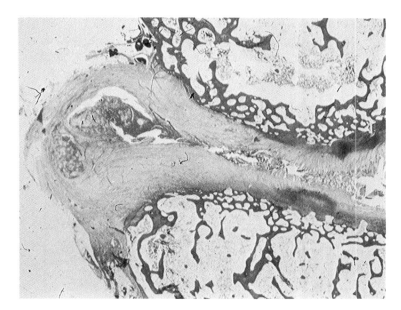

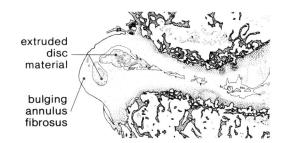

Fig. 17.16 Early degenerative changes in the disc with pigmentation of the nucleus and early fissure formation. Courtesy of Professor B. Vernon-Roberts.

extruded
disc
material

bulging
annulus
fibrosus

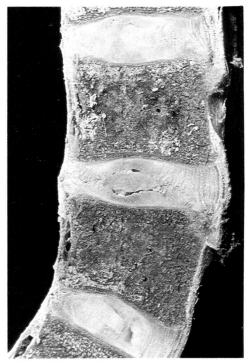

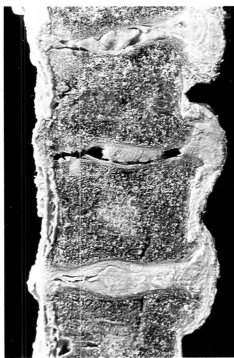

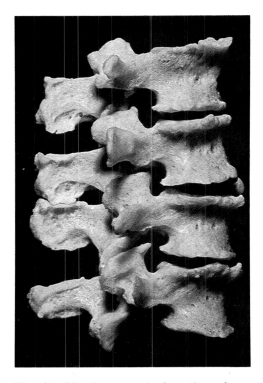

Fig. 17.17 A section through a protruded disc showing nuclear material contained within a bulging section of the annulus fibrosus. Courtesy of Professor B. Vernon-Roberts.

Fig. 17.18 Advanced disc degeneration with marked cleft formation throughout the posterior annulus. The nucleus is sequestrated. The anterior annulus is bulging and marked anterior osteophyte formation is present. Courtesy of Professor. B. Vernon Roberts.

Fig. 17.19 A macerated portion of lumbar spine in spondylosis showing narrowing of the intervertebral spaces with marginal osteophyte formation, osteoarthritis of the apophyseal joints with osteophytes extending into the intervertebral foramina and pseudarthrosis between the spines of the vertebrae.

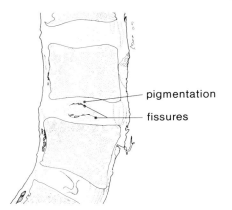

pigmentation

fissures

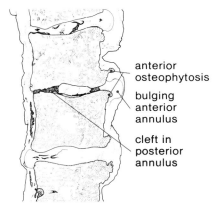

anterior
osteophytosis

bulging
anterior
annulus

cleft in
posterior
annulus

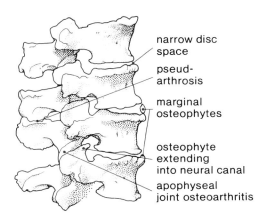

narrow disc
space

pseud-
arthrosis

marginal
osteophytes

osteophyte
extending
into neural canal

apophyseal
joint osteoarthritis

The radiological changes of spondylosis are common and indeed almost universal from middle age onwards (Fig. 17.20). The relationship between radiological changes in spondylosis and back pain is extremely poor: back pain is almost as prevalent in those with normal or virtually normal radiographs as in those with advanced degenerative changes. The finding of radiographic changes in a patient with back pain does not necessarily mean that these are the source of the symptoms and it is easy to be misled.

Scheuermann's Osteochondritis

This is an ill-understood condition in which there is irregular ossification of vertebral end-plates, principally in the dorsal but also in the upper lumbar spine (Fig. 17.21). It predominantly affects adolescent males, who develop a smooth dorsal kyphosis with round shoulders and a flat chest. Radiographs show the narrow disc spaces and wedged vertebrae which are narrower anteriorly. Secondary spondylotic change is common in later years.

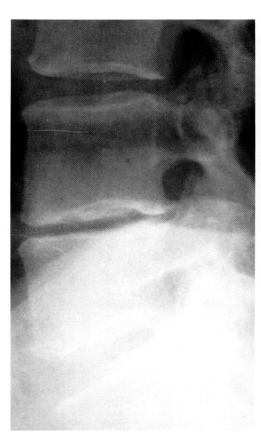

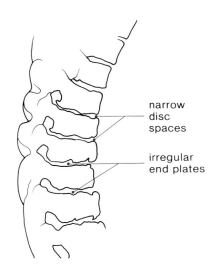

Fig. 17.20 Lumbar radiographs showing degenerative spondylosis at L4/5. A lateral radiograph (left) shows marked degenerative spondylosis. The disc space height is reduced with end-plate sclerosis and small posterior osteophytes.

A frontal view (right) demonstrates more widespread features of degenerative spondylosis with typical osteophyte formation.

Fig. 17.21 Spinal radiograph showing extensive features of Scheuermann's disease including disc space narrowing, end-plate irregularities due to Schmörl's nodes and thoracic kyphosis.

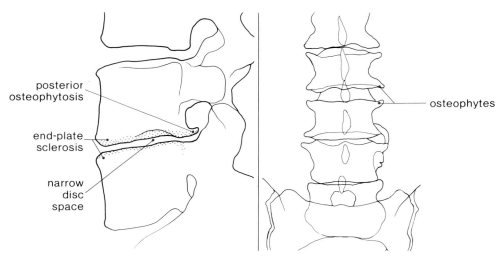

Diffuse Idiopathic Skeletal Hyperostosis (DISH)

This condition, also known as Forestier's disease or ankylosing hyperostosis, is a condition of exuberant new bone formation particularly at the margins of joints and bones. It is most obvious in the spine and bears a superficial resemblance to lumbar spondylosis except that the disc spaces are frequently preserved. New bone forms in the spine, particularly around the margins of the discs, producing huge osteophytes which may meet and even fuse (Fig. 17.22). Macerated specimens of vertebrae may show the excess of new bone which is particularly marked on the right-hand side of the vertebral column and may form the appearance of dripping candle wax (Fig. 17.23). Radiographs again reveal marked osteophyte formation particularly anteriorly and to the right side with relative preservation of the disc spaces (Fig. 17.24). Despite these florid pathological and radiological changes, it is doubtful whether this condition causes symptoms other than a progressive stiffening of spinal movements.

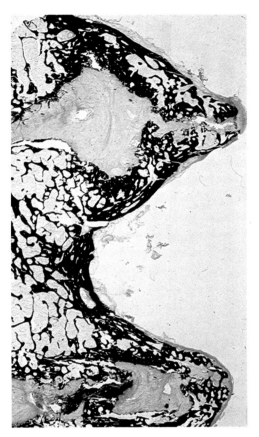

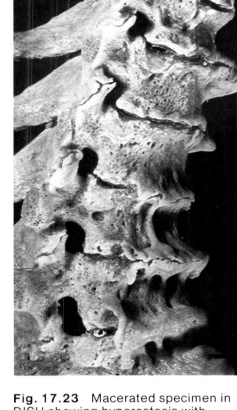

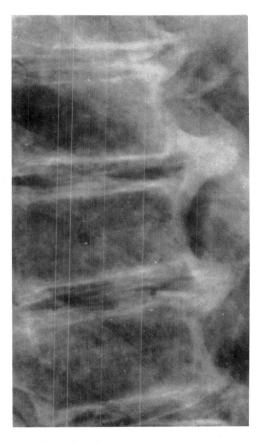

Fig. 17.22 Vertebral section in DISH showing osteophyte (stained black) surrounding herniated disc material (stained orange). Von Kossa's stain. Courtesy of Professor B. Vernon-Roberts.

Fig. 17.23 Macerated specimen in DISH showing hyperostosis with marked new bone formation along the length of the longitudinal ligaments and the formation of the appearance of 'candle-wax osteophytes'.

Fig. 17.24 Thoracic spine radiograph in DISH demonstrating large osteophytes fusing the disc spaces anteriorly. Disc space height is preserved.

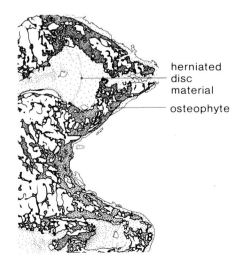

herniated disc material

osteophyte

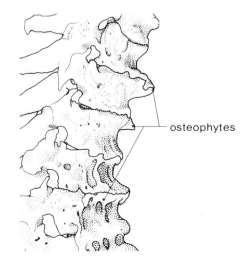

osteophytes

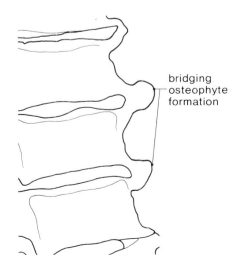

bridging osteophyte formation

Spinal Stenosis

There is considerable variation in the shape of the vertebral canal. In particular it may have a trefoil shape with extremely shallow lateral recesses through which the nerve roots emerge (Fig. 17.25). Degenerative changes, particularly in association with the trefoil canal, may give rise to the spinal stenosis syndrome. Other, rarer, causes include Paget's disease and new bone formation following previous surgery. The patient presents with back and lower limb root pain aggravated by exercise and relieved by rest; it can closely resemble intermittent claudication. There is evidence that the spinal canals of patients with sciatica due to a straightforward prolapsed disc are smaller than normal; thus even a small prolapse may produce significant nerve root compression and damage.

Assessment of vertebral canal size and shape is difficult from conventional radiographs. A contrast study may show the limited dimensions of the dural sac and any encroachment upon it (Fig. 17.26). Computerized axial tomography seems the best method for demonstrating spinal stenosis and may be combined with myelography (Figs. 17.27 & 17.28). An ultrasonic method has been developed by which an ultrasonic beam is aimed antero-medially from behind the laminae, thus providing a guide to the vertebral canal dimensions (Fig. 17.29). The cervical canal may also be developmentally shallow so that long tract signs and symptoms develop with minimal degenerative changes in later life (Fig. 17.30).

Spondylolysis and Spondylolisthesis

A spondylolysis is a defect in the posterior element of a vertebra and may be visualized on a lateral (Fig. 17.31) or oblique radiograph.

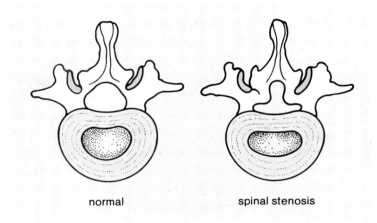

normal   spinal stenosis

Fig. 17.25 Diagram showing vertebral canal shapes, comparing a normal open canal to the trefoil canal of developmental spinal stenosis.

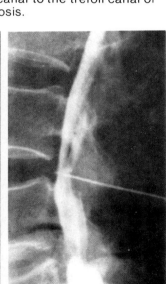
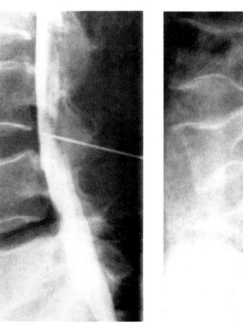
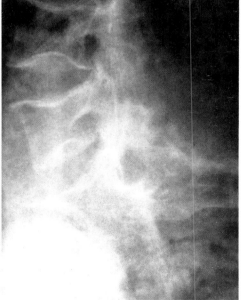

Fig. 17.26 Radiculograms in acquired spinal stenosis demonstrating the virtual occlusion of the neural canal on back extension and its relief on back flexion. Maximum stenosis is at L4/5, the level below the lumbar puncture needle.

Fig. 17.27 Radiograph at the lumbo-sacral level showing the typical severe developmental spinal stenosis in achondroplasia. This lateral radiograph demonstrates a severely narrowed neural canal and horizontally placed sacrum.

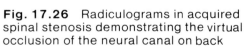
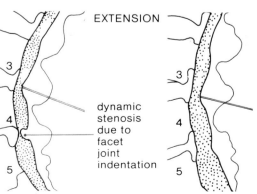

EXTENSION   NEUTRAL   FLEXION

dynamic stenosis due to facet joint indentation

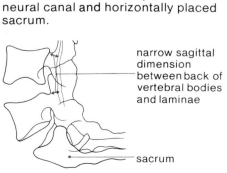

narrow sagittal dimension between back of vertebral bodies and laminae

sacrum

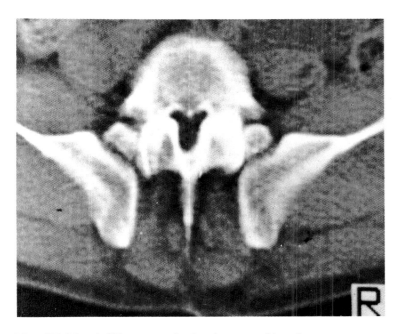

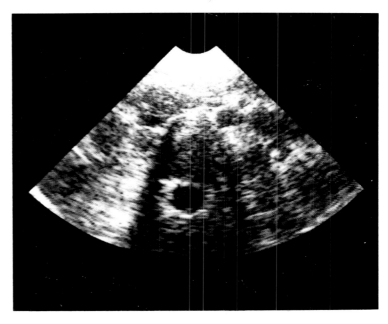

Fig. 17.28 A CT scan at the lumbo-sacral level demonstrating a grossly stenotic trefoil-shaped canal in achondroplasia.

Fig. 17.29 Real time transverse ultrasound scan at the level of L1–2 showing the pancreas anteriorly, apposed to the anterior body of L1. The neural canal is shown. Courtesy of Dr. H. Andrews.

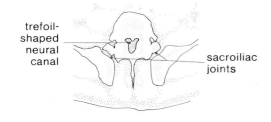

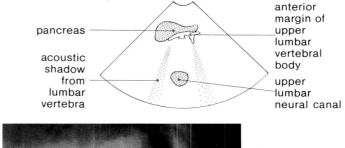

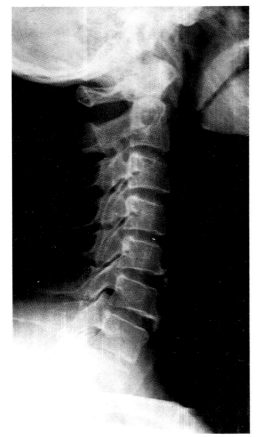

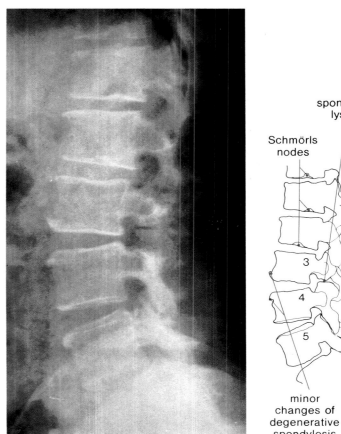

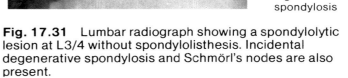

Fig. 17.30 Cervical radiograph showing modest degenerative spondylosis. The neural canal is developmentally shallow in this patient with spinal stenosis who complained of arm pain.

Fig. 17.31 Lumbar radiograph showing a spondylolytic lesion at L3/4 without spondylolisthesis. Incidental degenerative spondylosis and Schmörl's nodes are also present.

17.11

The defect itself does not produce symptoms but it may allow one vertebra to slip forwards on to that below – spondylolisthesis (Fig. 17.32). It can also develop in association with degeneration of the intervertebral disc (degenerative spondylolisthesis, Fig. 17.33) but frequently it is not clear whether the instability produces the damage to the disc or vice versa. In spondylolisthesis the subject may suffer from low back pain and, in severe cases, pain in the lower limbs due to compression of the nerve roots.

Arachnoiditis

Chronic inflammation with thickening of the nerve root sheaths within the vertebral canal is known as arachnoiditis. Most commonly it follows some invasive procedure such as myelography using an oil-based medium, or previous spinal surgery. Rarely, it is a consequence of previous meningitis. It causes chronic and sometimes severe back pain and sciatica. The radiculogram will show distortion of the dural sac with poor or absent filling of the nerve root sheaths (Fig. 17.34).

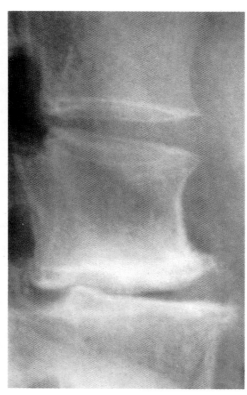

Fig. 17.32 Lumbar radiograph in spondylolytic spondylolisthesis. A defect in the posterior elements at L4/5 has allowed the L4 vertebra to slip forwards on the L5 segment.

Fig. 17.33 Lumbar radiograph in degenerative spondylolisthesis. The slip between the vertebrae is associated with degenerative disease in the intervertebral disc. In this example the upper vertebra has slipped dorsally on that below causing a reverse spondylolisthesis. Gas is present within the degnerative L4/5 disc, the so-called 'vacuum sign'.

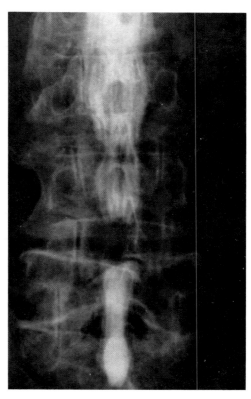

Fig. 17.34 A radiculogram in arachnoiditis demonstrating gross irregularity of the outline of the dural sac due to adhesive arachnoiditis, in this case secondary to a previous myelogram using an oil-based contrast medium. Disc compression has obliterated the intrathecal space. The neural canal is also markedly narrowed at L4/5 due to recurrent disc protrusion and the nerve root sheaths do not fill.

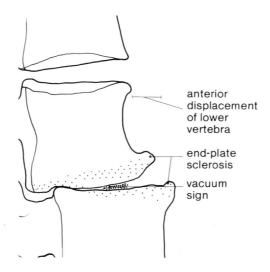

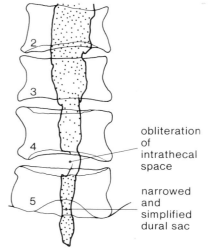

INFLAMMATORY CAUSES OF BACK PAIN
Ankylosing Spondylitis

This disorder most commonly occurs in young males but may develop in females and other age groups. It is characterized by low back pain and stiffness aggravated by rest and relieved by physical activity. There is progressive loss of motion of the spine which may be complicated by synovitis, particularly in the lower limbs. Inflammatory features may occur elsewhere. In advanced disease the characteristic posture is loss of the lumbar lordosis with a straight lumbar spine, a smooth dorsal kyphosis and a protruded neck resulting from the effort to look forwards. The hips are frequently held slightly flexed with flexion in the knees to compensate (Fig. 17.35). In less severe cases the posture may be reasonably preserved but with loss of movement of the lumbar spine in all directions. In many patients however, the lumbar spine movement may appear normal and the loss of movement only occurs as the disease progresses.

The early radiological features are sacroiliitis (Fig. 17.36) which may progress in more severe cases to fusion of the

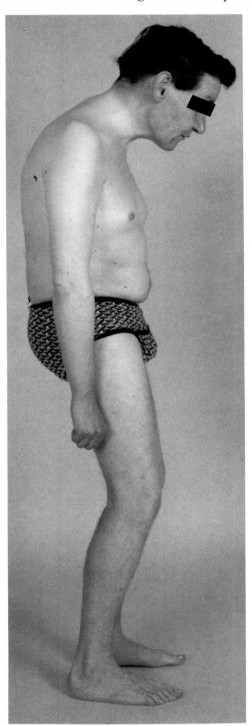

Fig. 17.35 The typical posture in ankylosing spondylitis with the loss of lumbar lordosis, smooth thoracic kyphosis and a hyper-extended protruded neck. The hips and knees are slightly flexed.

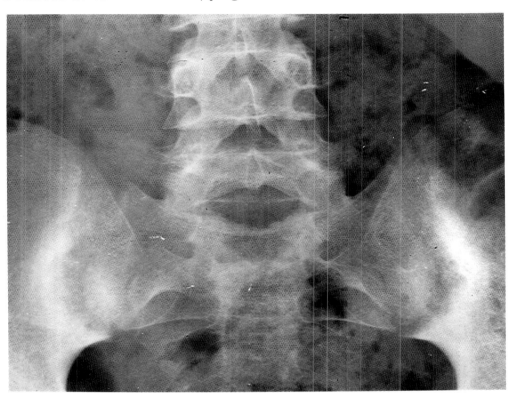

Fig. 17.36 Pelvic radiograph showing bilateral erosive sacroiliitis. There is widening and erosion of both sacroiliac joints. Sclerosis is present adjacent to these erosions, particularly on the iliac aspects.

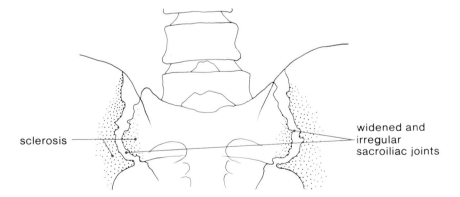

sclerosis

widened and irregular sacroiliac joints

sacroiliac joints (Fig. 17.37) and ossification of the longitudinal ligament of the spine (Figs. 17.38 & 17.39). In some patients with advanced disease one mobile segment may remain where all movement is concentrated and severe degenerative changes with pain may occur at this level (Fig. 17.40). Diagnosis from radiographs is difficult in the early stage but this is the time when a gamma scan using bone-seeking isotopes is most helpful (Fig. 17.41). In advanced disease when there is fusion of damaged joints the bone scan may return to normal. Fusion of peripheral joints also occurs, but is much less common. Usually a large joint is afflicted with a 'frozen joint' appearance (Fig. 17.42).

Infection

Infections in the spine can produce severe pain. Most commonly there are destructive changes in the intervertebal disc and the surrounding vertebrae (Figs. 17.43 & 17.44). The most common organism causing acute infection is *Staphylococcus aureus* but *Streptococcus, Pseudomonas, E. coli* and other microorganisms can be responsible. Tuberculous infection and brucellosis may be found and can cause severe destructive changes before being recognized.

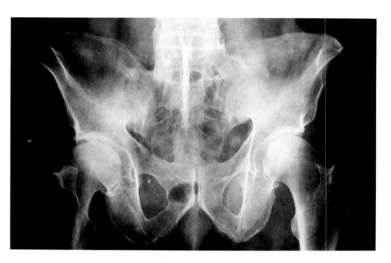

Fig. 17.37 Pelvic radiograph in advanced ankylosing spondylitis showing bony fusion of the sacroiliac joints.

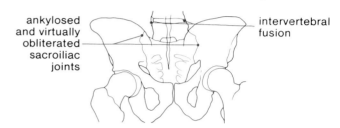

ankylosed and virtually obliterated sacroiliac joints — intervertebral fusion

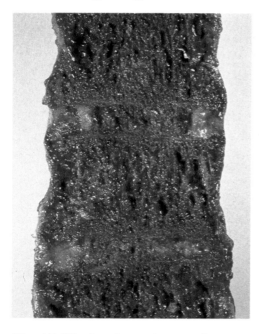

Fig. 17.38 Lumbar spine specimen demonstrating bony bridging in established ankylosing spondylitis. Courtesy of Professor B. Vernon Roberts.

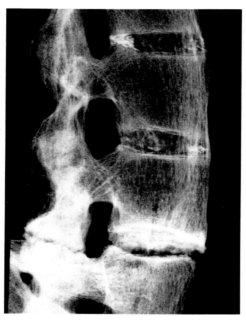

Fig. 17.39 Post mortem lumbar radiograph demonstrating discrete intervertebral fusion. There is also a spondylodiscitis with pseudoarthritis involving disc and facet joints at the lower segment.

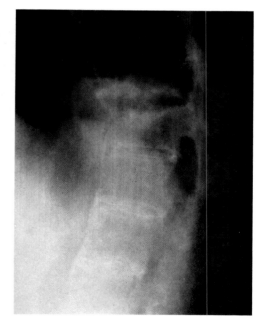

Fig. 17.40 Thoracic spine radiograph in spondylodiscitis. The segments above and below this are completely fused, causing abnormal movement at this level: marked destructive and degenerative changes have occurred and caused extreme pain.

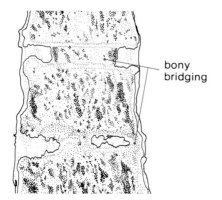

bony bridging

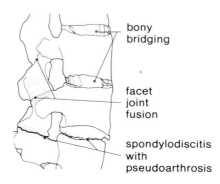

bony bridging

facet joint fusion

spondylodiscitis with pseudoarthrosis

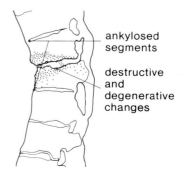

ankylosed segments

destructive and degenerative changes

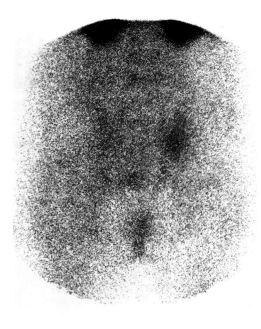
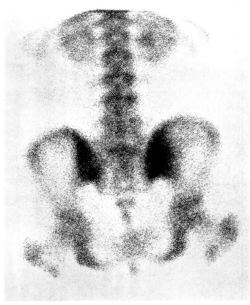

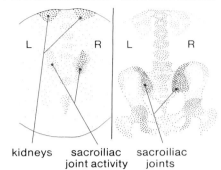

Fig. 17.41   99m Technetium MDP bone-scans in asymmetrical inflammatory sacroiliitis. There is increased perfusion on the right (these are posterior views). It is also increased on the delayed image. The abnormal activity is easier to appreciate on the perfusion scans.

PERFUSION IMAGE   DELAYED IMAGE

kidneys   sacroiliac   sacroiliac
          joint activity   joints

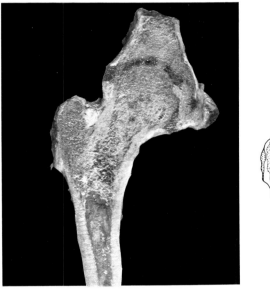
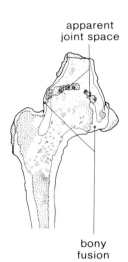

apparent joint space

bony fusion

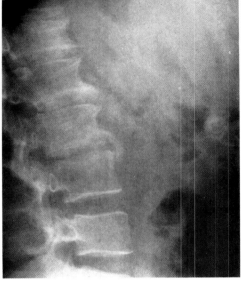
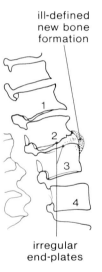

ill-defined new bone formation

irregular end-plates

Fig. 17.42   Hip joint specimen illustrating large joint fusion in ankylosing spondylitis. Ossification surrounds the apparently preserved joint space. Courtesy of Professor B. Vernon Roberts.

Fig. 17.43   Lumbar radiograph showing infective discitis at L2/3. Osteoporosis and destructive changes are present at the margins of this disc together with ill-defined new bone anteriorly. Note that this disc and the one more proximally are degenerate.

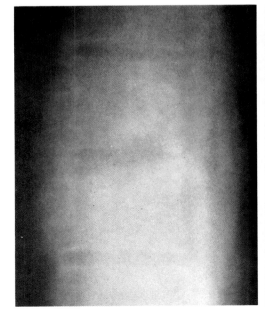
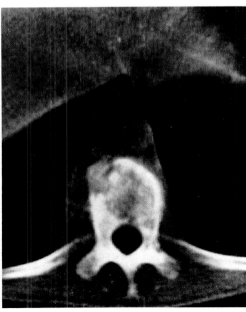

Fig. 17.44   An antero-posterior tomogram showing infective discitis at T8/9 with narrowing of the disc space, erosion of the end-plate and soft tissue swelling adjacent to the vertebrae due to a paraspinal abscess (left). These features are also well-demonstrated on the CT scan (right). The infective organism was staphylococcus.

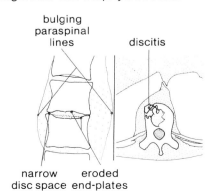

bulging paraspinal lines

discitis

narrow disc space   eroded end-plates

Metabolic Bone Disease

Disorders such as osteoporosis and osteomalacia are painless unless there is vertebral collapse, which causes acute episodes of pain. These will usually subside within a few days or weeks with rest. In more advanced cases, deformity and particularly a dorsal kyphosis may result (Fig. 17.45). Diagnosis may be made from radiographs. The commonest causes of osteoporosis are post-menopausal osteoporosis, steroid therapy (Fig. 17.46) particularly in rheumatoid patients, and other endocrine disorders.

Paget's disease may occur in the spine and can be extremely painful. The recent development of pain in a longstanding case of Paget's disease does raise the possibility of malignant change.

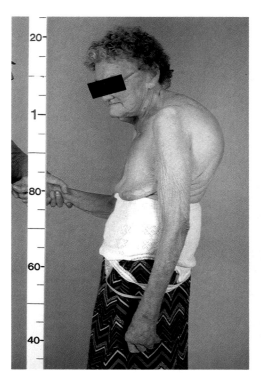

Fig. 17.45 An elderly female patient with a thoracic kyphosis due to idiopathic osteoporosis – the so-called 'Dowager's hump'.

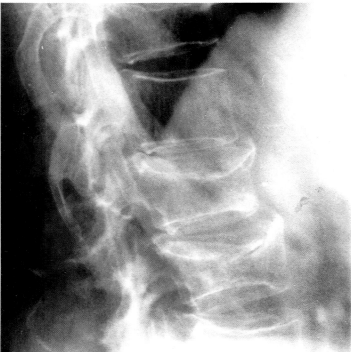

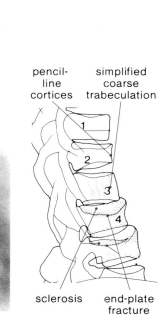

Fig. 17.46 Lumbar radiograph in steroid induced osteoporosis showing a generalized reduction in bone density with a pencil-line cortex and a simplified trabecular pattern. Note the preservation of disc space height with end-plate fractures in the bodies of L3 and L4. The presence of sclerosis adjacent to these end-plates suggests steroid therapy as a cause of this condition.

Fig. 17.47 Thoracic spine radiographs showing vertebral destruction with loss of vertebral height (left) and ablation of the left pedicle of T12 (right) due to metastasis from carcinoma of the breast.

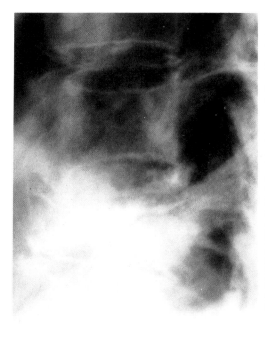

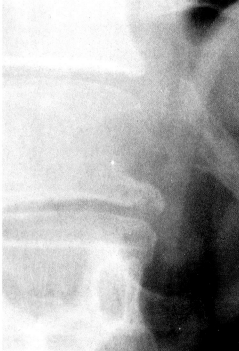

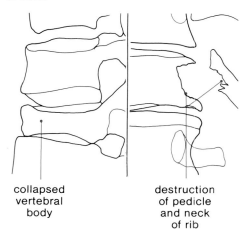

Tumors, Reticuloses and Myelomatosis

Although primary malignancies may develop in the spine they are extremely rare. Deposits are most commonly due to metastases from carcinoma of the prostate, bronchus, breast, thyroid or kidney. They may present with vertebral collapse (Fig. 17.47). Carcinoma of the prostate may produce osteosclerotic as well as osteolytic deposits, whereas the others are usually osteolytic. The progressive development of back pain, perhaps with gradual evolution of neurological changes due to nerve root damage, raises the possibility of malignancy. Pain due to malignant disease is often worse at night.

Reticuloses occasionally develop within the spine and may produce spinal cord and nerve root syndromes. Myelomatosis can produce back pain particularly due to vertebral collapse; it may be recognized radiologically (Fig. 17.48) and by the characteristic biochemical changes. On occasions primary intrathecal tumors, both benign and malignant (Figs. 17.49 & 17.50) may present as apparently simple back pain or sciatica.

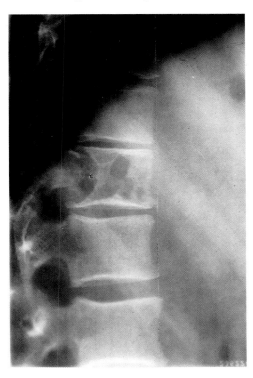

Fig. 17.48 Typical spinal involvement with myeloma. In addition to the generalized reduction in bone density, similar to that seen in osteoporosis (the appearances may be identical), focal bony destruction is demonstrated.

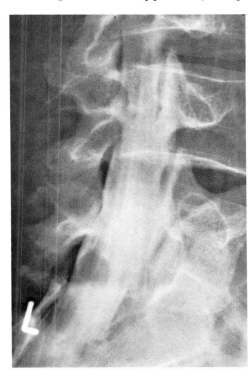

Fig. 17.49 Water-soluble radiculogram demonstrating a neurofibroma associated with a lower lumbar nerve root.

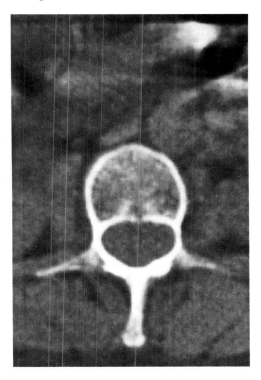

Fig. 17.50 CT scan in a patient with an ependymoma of the conus showing considerable expansion of the neural canal and pedicular thinning.

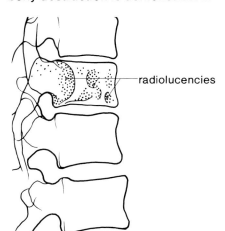

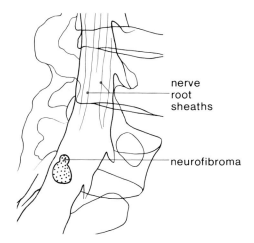

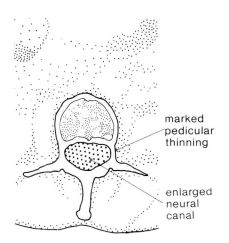

Osteoid osteoma is a benign tumor which may occur in the spine. Pain is characteristically well localized and a bone scan may show a very small focus of increased uptake (Fig. 17.51).

Miscellaneous

Numerous unusual causes of low back pain may present, including developmental anomalies both bony (Fig. 17.52) or more complex with cord/root involvement (Fig. 17.53).

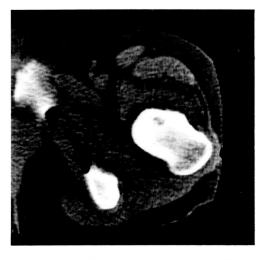
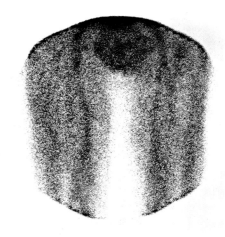
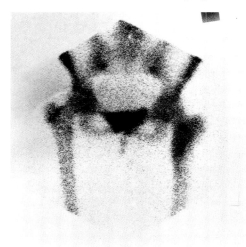

Fig. 17.51 Osteoid osteoma. The CT scan (left) shows a radiolucent nidus of tumor. The early phase bone scan (middle) shows a discrete focus of increased activity consistent with the vascular nidus, and the late scan (right) a more localized focus within the abnormal area – the 'double density sign'.

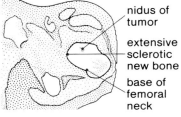

- nidus of tumor
- extensive sclerotic new bone
- base of femoral neck

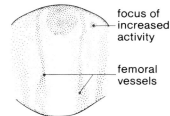

- focus of increased activity
- femoral vessels

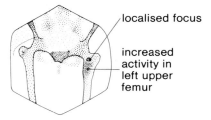

- localised focus
- increased activity in left upper femur

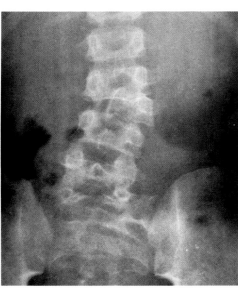
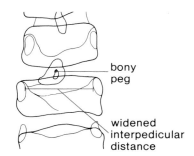
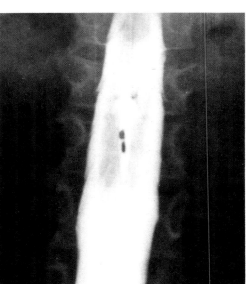

Fig. 17.52 Lumbar radiograph showing hemivertebra and a localized scoliosis at the same level.

Fig. 17.53 Diastematomyelia. The plain film (left) demonstrates a widened neural canal with a bony peg within it. A myelogram (right) shows the cord split into two hemicords wrapped around the diastematomyelic head.

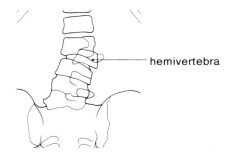

- hemivertebra

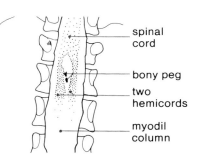

- bony peg
- widened interpedicular distance

- spinal cord
- bony peg
- two hemicords
- myodil column

18
Gout

Excellent descriptions of gout can be found in the earliest medical writings. The aphorisms of Hippocrates (c. 400 BC) documented the fact that gout is predominantly a disease of adult men and only appears in women after the menopause. Sydenham (sometimes called the 'English Hippocrates') was himself a gout sufferer and his vivid descriptions of the disease, written in 1683, can still make the big toe itch! Gout was extremely common in Georgian England, and many of the best known figures in English political and cultural life suffered from the disease; the extreme pain of acute attacks of gout has been responsible for anger, frustration, and misjudged decisions in the highest political circles (eg. Pitt and the Boston Tea Party).

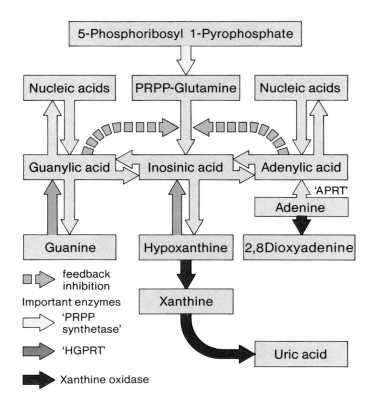

Fig. 18.1 Simplified diagram of some of the metabolic steps involved in the production of uric acid from the nucleic acid bases adenine and guanine.

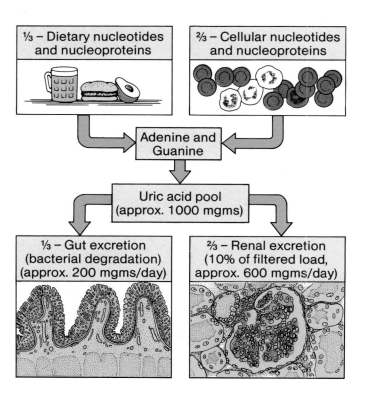

Fig. 18.2 Input and output of the total pool of uric acid in the body.

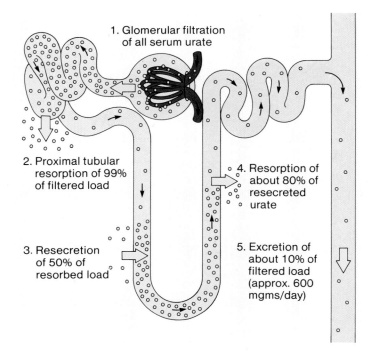

Fig. 18.3 A simplified diagram of the pathways probably involved in the excretion of uric acid from the kidney.

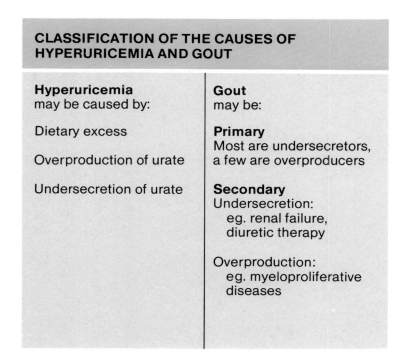

Fig. 18.4 Classification of the causes of hyperuricemia and gout.

CLASSIFICATION OF THE CAUSES OF HYPERURICEMIA AND GOUT

Hyperuricemia may be caused by:	Gout may be:
Dietary excess	**Primary** Most are undersecretors, a few are overproducers
Overproduction of urate	
Undersecretion of urate	**Secondary** Undersecretion: eg. renal failure, diuretic therapy
	Overproduction: eg. myeloproliferative diseases

Gout is now recognized as a crystal deposition disease. Its clinical and pathological manifestations are due to the presence of crystalline salts of urate within the connective tissues. Since Sir Alfred Baring Garrod first described hyperuricemia in 1848 and suggested that crystals caused the disease, modern research has focussed on the production of excess urate, its crystallization, and the ways in which the crystals can induce the disease.

Uric Acid, Hyperuricemia and Crystals

Urate is a breakdown product of the purine residues of nucleic acid, namely guanine and adenine.

The pathways of *de novo* synthesis of the nucleic acid residues are now well established and proceed throughout the body via the key compounds 5-phosphoribosyl 1-pyrophosphate, and inosinic acid. Inosinic acid can either be converted into the bases for inclusion into nucleic acid, or broken down through hypoxanthine and xanthine to form uric acid. The whole pathway is controlled by feedback inhibition, and salvage pathways exist that allow intermediate breakdown products to be reincorporated into nucleic acids (Fig. 18.1).

In a normal person the total pool of body uric acid is about 1 gram and serum uric acid levels range from 0.1-0.4 mmols/litre (Fig. 18.2). Serum levels are slightly higher in men than in women, reaching a peak in men at the age of 20 and rising in women after the menopause. Two thirds of excreted uric acid is lost via the kidney and one third via the gut. The renal handling of urate seems to involve a four component system which includes filtration through the glomerulus, almost total reabsorption through the proximal tubule and partial resecretion and reabsorption in the distal part of the nephron (Fig. 18.3). Hyperuricemia can result from excess dietary purines, from overproduction of uric acid, from under-secretion in the kidney or from a combination of all these factors (Fig. 18.4).

In most cases of gout, no causative disease can be found; the disease is then termed primary gout. In these patients dietary factors including alcohol can be implicated in 50% of patients, about 30% have a tendency to be natural overproducers and some 70% are undersecretors. It follows that a combination of factors is operating in many of these patients.

In a minority, another disease is the cause of hyperuricemia (secondary gout). The most common diseases resulting in gout are the myeloproliferative disorders (such as polycythemia rubra vera) or renal failure. Diuretic therapy and other drugs can interfere with the renal handling of urate and are becoming common in the genesis of gout, particularly in the aged.

The solubility of monosodium urate in physiological conditions is about 0.4 mmols/litre (6.8 mg/dL). As this figure lies at the upper end of the normal range of serum uric acid, hyperuricemia will therefore result in supersaturation of the body fluids. However, much higher levels are needed for spontaneous crystallization to occur; thus hyperuricemic individuals are metastable for uric acid but another factor is necessary in order to nucleate the crystals. Nucleation proceeds more easily at low temperatures which may help to explain the peripheral distribution of gout. It may be aided by interaction with connective tissue components such as proteoglycans or collagen, although the formation of crystals *in vivo* is not yet fully understood. The gout culprit is the crystal of monosodium urate monohydrate. It can form either amorphous precipitates or needle-shaped crystals which are relatively insoluble in water (Fig. 18.5). The urate needles vary in length from about 0.2 – 2μm; they are only deposited in connective tissue, and have a predilection for peripheral synovial joints.

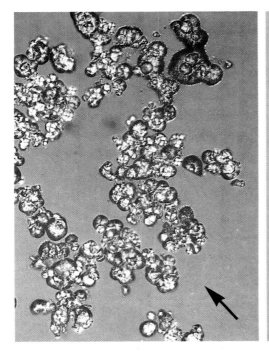 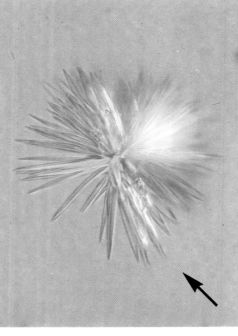

Fig. 18.5 The sodium salt of uric acid. It can crystallize as amorphous particles or 'spherulites' (left), or as crystals of monosodium urate monohydrate (right). These crystals are usually needle-shaped (acicular) and vary in length from 0.2 to 20 μm. Polarized light micrographs with first order red compensator, x 1200.

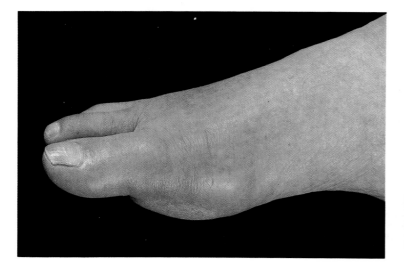

Fig. 18.6 The swollen, red, shiny appearance of the toe in early acute gout.

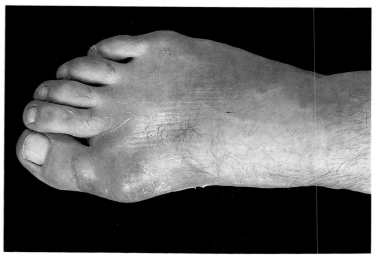

Fig. 18.7 Acute gout of the first MTP joint. As the attack progresses the skin over the inflamed joint may desquamate.

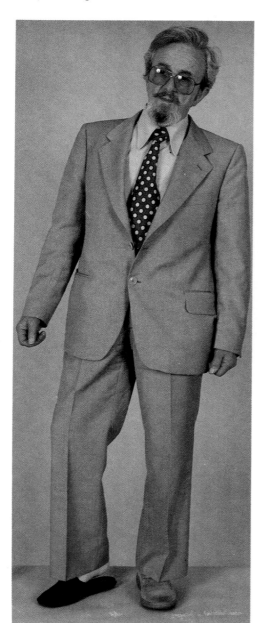

Fig. 18.8 The sight of a middle-aged man hopping into the office with a slipper on one foot may be typical of gout.

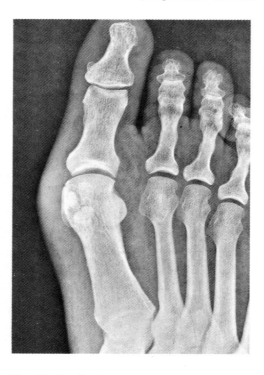

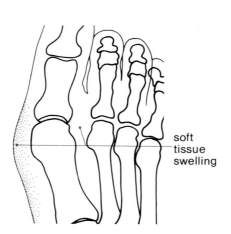

Fig. 18.9 Radiograph of the great toe in a case of acute gout. Ill-defined soft tissue swelling around the first MTP is the only abnormality.

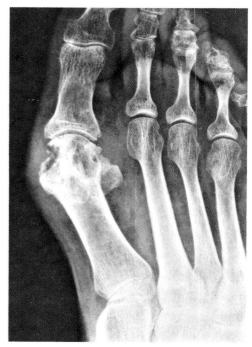

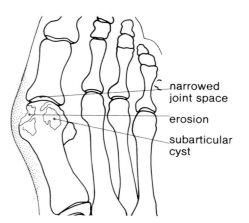

Fig. 18.10 Radiograph of the great toe in a case of chronic gout. In this patient several previous attacks have occurred and chronic changes of gout including a characteristic 'punched-out', well-defined erosion, subarticular cysts, and narrowing of the joint space is shown.

soft tissue swelling

narrowed joint space

erosion

subarticular cyst

Clinical Features

Gout is sometimes described as having four clinical phases:
(1) asymptomatic hyperuricemia, (2) acute attacks, (3) inter-critical gout (between attacks), and (4) chronic tophaceous gout. The most dramatic and clinically obvious manifestation of this disease is the acute attack.

Acute Gout

Seventy per cent of all acute attacks occur in the first metatarsophalangeal joint (MTP). The patient usually has no warning although prodromal symptoms are occasionally described. The attack may be precipitated by trauma, alcoholic excess, or intercurrent illness. The pain often starts at night and usually becomes extremely severe within a few hours of onset. It is associated with joint swelling and red shiny skin (Figs. 18.6 & 18.7). At its height the acute attack is excruciatingly painful but it will subside spontaneously, often with desquamation of the skin, the toe finally returning to a completely normal state after a few days or weeks (Fig. 18.8). The radiograph in acute gout only shows soft tissue swelling around the toes (Fig. 18.9). However, in a chronic case, or if there have been many previous attacks, some of the characteristic changes of chronic gout may also be seen (Fig. 18.10).

Gout is also common in the hand, wrist, ankle and knee. Attacks are sometimes polyarticular involving two, three or more individual sites (Figs. 18.11 – 18.13). The signs are

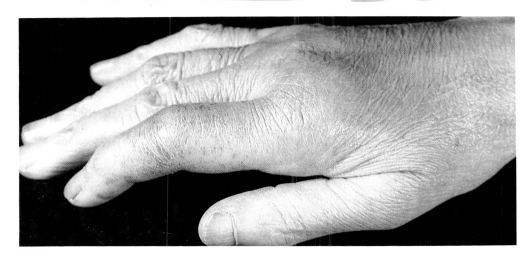

Fig. 18.11 Swelling of the metacarpophalangeal joints (MCPs) and redness of the overlying skin. This redness is caused by inflammation of periarticular tissues as well as of the joint.

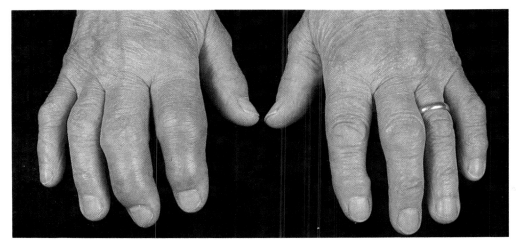

Fig. 18.12 Swollen fingers in a patient with asymmetrical polyarticular acute gout.

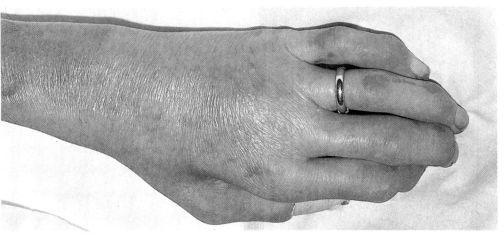

Fig. 18.13 A polyarticular attack of gout affecting the wrist and fingers.

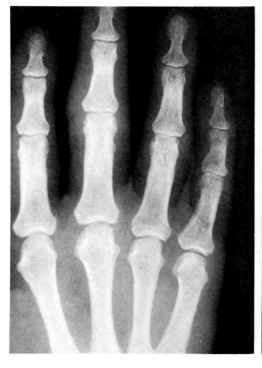

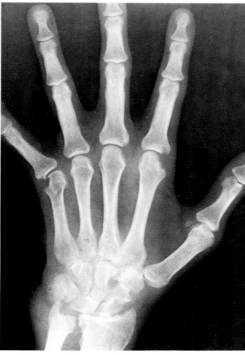

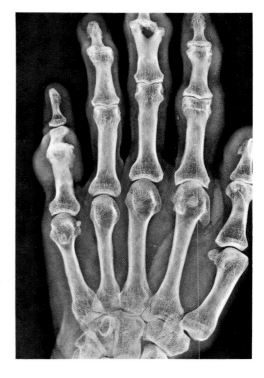

Fig. 18.14 Radiographs of the hand and wrist in acute gout. Asymmetrical, ill-defined, soft tissue swelling can be seen around the proximal interphalangeal joint (PIP) of the middle finger (left) and adjacent to the wrist joint (right). The wrist, intercarpal and inferior radio-ulnar joints have chronic gouty erosions, and there are some secondary osteophytes.

Fig. 18.15 Radiograph of the hand in chronic gout showing large asymmetrical soft tissue swellings, joint space narrowing and a large subarticular cyst. There is a flexion deformity of the little finger and a large osteophyte of the index MCP.

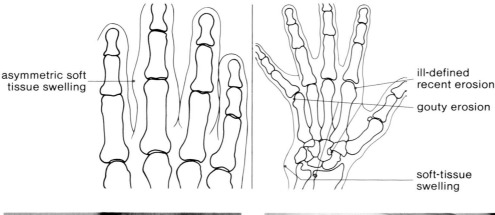

asymmetric soft tissue swelling

ill-defined recent erosion

gouty erosion

soft-tissue swelling

subarticular cyst

soft tissue swelling

joint space narrowing

osteophyte

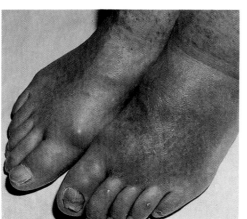

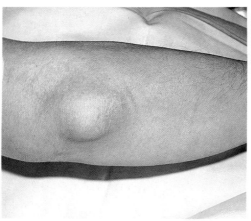

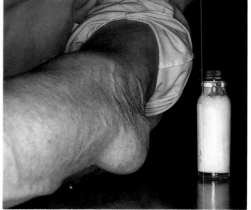

Fig. 18.16 Gouty cellulitis. Urate crystal-induced inflammation occasionally occurs primarily in the soft tissue of periarticular areas causing an appearance similar to that of streptococcal cellulitis.

Fig. 18.17 Bursitis in gout. The olecranon bursa is a common site of involvement of gout; acute attacks may cause a large fluid swelling (left). In chronic gout large crystal deposits may form, resulting in a knobbly swelling which may have characteristic white tophaceous patches on it. The fluid aspirated from these areas is rich in urate, and may look like toothpaste (right).

similar to those found in the foot or elsewhere and radiographs show soft tissue swelling with or without evidence of chronic gouty changes in the bones (Figs. 18.14 & 18.15).

There is usually redness of the overlying skin in acute attacks of gout implying that the inflammation has spread to periarticular tissue. Sometimes the inflammation is confined to these areas and resembles cellulitis (Fig. 18.16). Bursae or tendon sheaths may also be involved resulting in, for example, olecranon bursitis (Fig. 18.17). These soft tissue inflammatory changes occasionally cause diagnostic confusion and a combination of olecranon bursitis and tophi of the elbow may lead to an erroneous diagnosis of rheumatoid arthritis (Fig. 18.18).

Chronic Tophaceous Gout

In chronic tophaceous gout the total body pool of uric acid may be raised to 20 or even 50 times normal. It only occurs after prolonged severe hyperuricemia and is now rarely seen, as acute gout and hyperuricemia can be effectively treated by modern therapy. Large urate deposits accumulate in the periarticular and subcutaneous tissues. The sheets of urate crystals are interspersed with a protein matrix containing immunoglobulin and may be surrounded by fibrosis and chronic inflammatory cells. However, inflammation is usually mild or absent and tophi are generally asymptomatic unless large enough to cause mechanical problems. The commonly involved sites are over the first MTP (Fig. 18.19), the ear (Fig. 18.20), elbow and achilles tendon. Tophi occasionally occur in other sites (Fig. 18.21). When present there is often

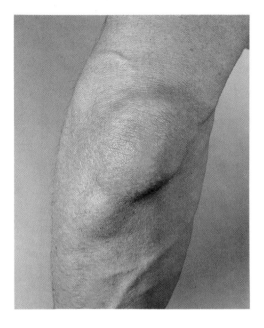

Fig. 18.18 A combination of olecranon bursitis and a tophus near the elbow may simulate chronic nodular rheumatoid disease.

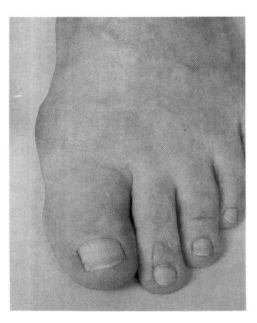

Fig. 18.19 A swollen first MTP in chronic tophaceous gout.

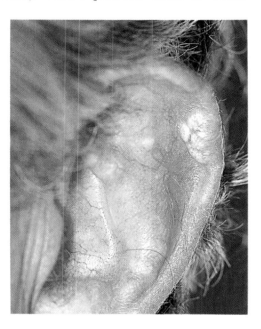

Fig. 18.20 Characteristic tophi on the helix of the ear, a common site of urate deposits in chronic tophaceous gout.

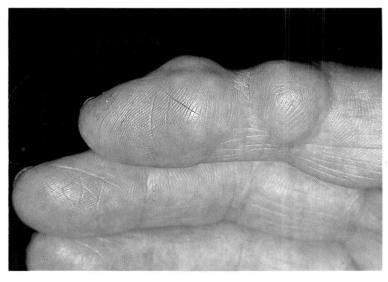

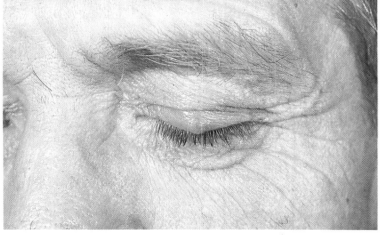

Fig. 18.21 Tophi on the finger (left) and eyelid (right) in chronic tophaceous gout.

advanced joint disease leading to characteristic asymmetrical deformities of the hands associated with large swellings (Fig. 18.22). Tophi often have a white shiny surface and may ulcerate through the skin exuding a chalky or toothpaste-like material (Fig. 18.23).

In the chronic tophaceous stage the radiology is characteristic. There is loss of joint space and some osteoarthritic change secondary to repeated inflammation, and urate deposits are present. More diagnostic is the finding of erosive changes and tophi (Figs. 18.24 &

18.25). The erosions tend to be a little way down the shaft of the bones, adjacent to the involved joint. They are often large and may have a rim of sclerotic bone surrounding them, sometimes forming hooks which are never seen around rheumatoid erosions. The tophi, if they only contain uric acid, are relatively radiolucent, but in advanced disease flecks of calcific material may be seen and occasionally tophi calcify due to associated hydroxyapatite deposition (Fig. 18.26).

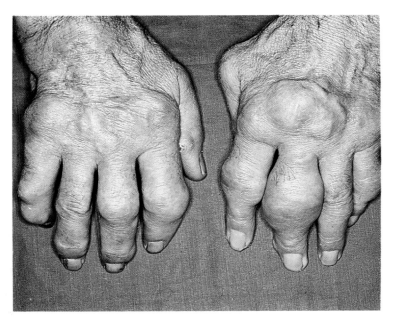

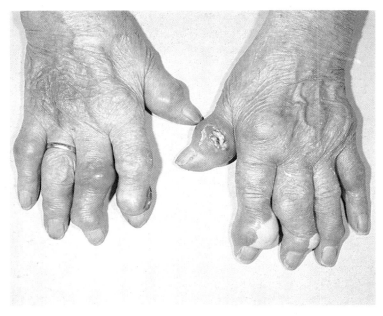

Fig. 18.22 Severe hand deformities in a case of chronic gout in which a combination of tophaceous and chronic deforming joint disease leads to the striking abnormalities.

Fig. 18.23 Finger tophi. Shiny white deposits of urate are clearly visible through the skin. They may ulcerate as on the thumb, and 'chalky' or toothpaste-like material may exude. This patient developed tophi after being given diuretics; the exuding 'pus' was treated with antibiotics, but the condition only began to resolve when the diuretic was stopped.

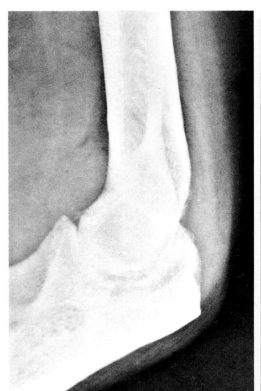

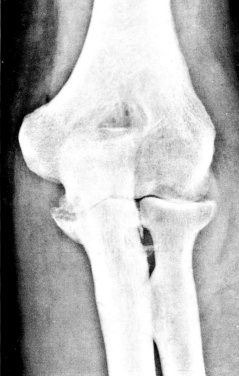

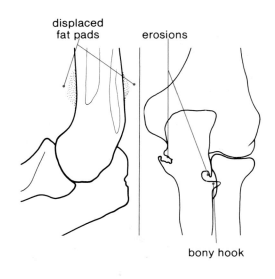

Fig. 18.24 Anteroposterior and lateral radiographs of the elbow in chronic tophaceous gout. The displaced fat pads caused by a joint effusion are seen on the lateral view. The AP view shows gouty erosions with a characteristic bony hook or overhanging margin of bone.

displaced fat pads   erosions

bony hook

The Diagnosis of Gout

Many people have mild hyperuricemia but only a minority of them will ever suffer gout: serum uric acid levels are a relatively poor guide to gout. Although the chances of having the disease increase as the level of urate in the serum rises, sufferers occasionally have normal levels.

The only way to make a definitive diagnosis of gout is to visualize the crystals. Where there is diagnostic doubt the involved joints should be aspirated (Fig. 18.27).

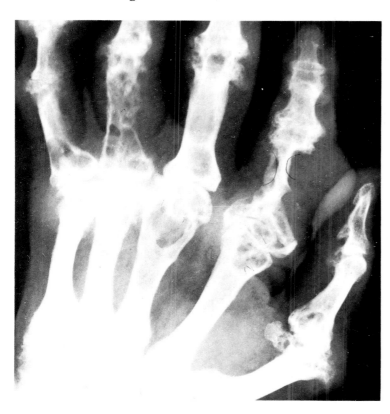

Fig. 18.25 Hand radiograph in advanced chronic tophaceous gout. There are numerous erosions with joint destruction and cyst formation. Bone loss on the shaft of the index proximal phalanx is caused by pressure from the tophus. (The wrist was ankylosed.)

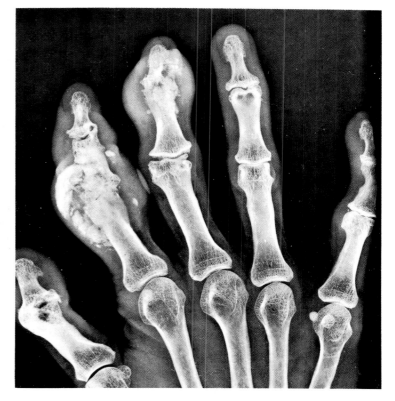

Fig. 18.26 Radiograph showing tophi in chronic gout. There are flecks of calcium and larger deposits of calcified material due to hydroxyapatite deposition in association with the urate.

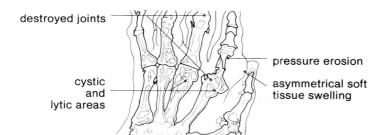

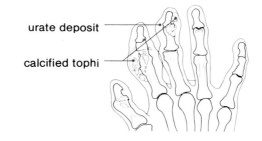

Fig. 18.27 Aspirating the first MTP to obtain synovial fluid to be examined under polarized light microscopy in order to confirm the diagnosis of gout.

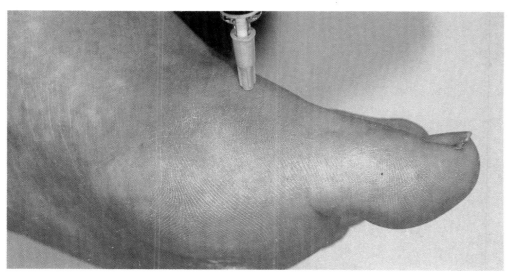

18.9

A small drop of fluid is sufficient to examine either as a wet preparation or a dry smear on a microscope slide. Identification is made using the polarized light microscope. This makes use of the property of birefringence of urate crystals, which means that plane polarized light rays in parallel with the optical axis of the crystal will be split into two divergent components, producing an effective alteration in the vector of the emergent ray (Fig. 18.28). If crossed polars are placed in the microscope above and below the stage no light can pass through to the observer. However, the alteration in vector induced by the crystals will make them shine out as bright objects against the dark background (Fig. 18.29).

Insertion of a first order red compensator into the system produces a red background and allows the sign of birefringence to be estimated. This compensator is a quartz crystal of uniform thickness, and is inserted into the microscope with its optical axis at 45° to the plane of the polarizer and analyser. It absorbs certain wavelengths of the visible spectrum resulting in a red background. Birefringent crystals aligned with their optical axes parallel to the axis of the compensator will cause a small shift in the resulting wavelengths of absorbed light. This is seen as a color shift towards the yellow (negative) or blue (positive) end of the visible spectrum of light. The morphological and optical axis of a crystal are usually the same, so in practice the specimen stage of the microscope is revolved until the crystal lies with its long axis in

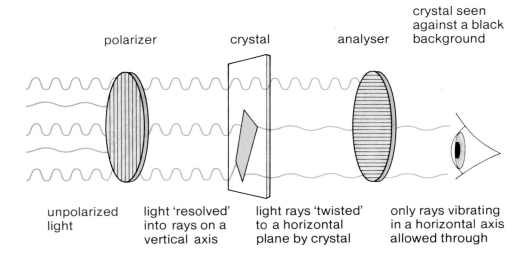

polarizer   crystal   analyser   crystal seen against a black background

unpolarized light   light 'resolved' into rays on a vertical axis   light rays 'twisted' to a horizontal plane by crystal   only rays vibrating in a horizontal axis allowed through

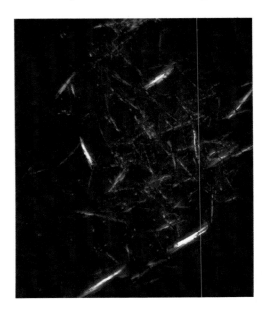

Fig. 18.28 Simplified scheme of the principles behind the use of polarized light microscopy, showing a birefringent crystal altering the vector of plane polarized light, allowing it to pass through the analyser and be seen at the microscope eye piece.

Fig. 18.29 Urate crystals viewed in the polarized light microscope. They are seen between crossed polars and stand out as bright needles against a dark background. High power micrograph.

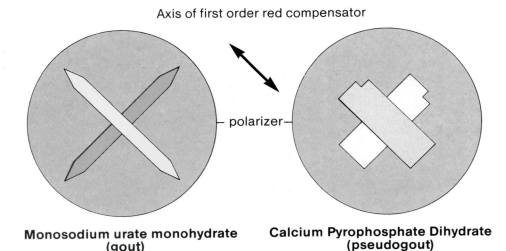

Axis of first order red compensator

polarizer

Monosodium urate monohydrate (gout)

Calcium Pyrophosphate Dihydrate (pseudogout)

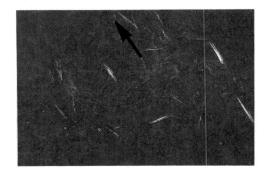

Fig. 18.31 Urate crystals from a gouty joint identified in the polarized light microscope after insertion of the first order red compensator. This dry smear was formed from a minute amount of fluid expressed from the needle end after an apparently unsuccessful aspiration of an MTP. Crystals in parallel with the axis of the compensator are yellow and those at right angles to it are blue (negative birefringence). Polarized light micrograph, x 800.

Fig. 18.30 Diagram to show the different morphology, and sign of birefringence of urate and pyrophosphate crystals. Birefringence can be detected by a color shift to blue (positive) or yellow (negative) when the long axis of the crystal is aligned with the optical axis of a first order red compensator.

the same direction as the axis marked on the compensator and its color noted (Fig. 18.30).

Monosodium urate monohydrate needles are strongly negatively birefringent. This means that when their optical axis lies parallel to that of the first order red compensator, they appear yellow, and when the optical axes are crossed they will appear blue (Fig. 18.31).

In acute gout, synovial fluid usually contains large numbers of these characteristic needle-shaped crystals. Many of them can be observed attached to, or within, the polymorphonuclear leucocytes that predominate in the fluid (Fig. 18.32, left). This can often be seen quite clearly in wet preparations; cell clefts produced by intracellular crystals can also be observed in histological preparations

from synovial fluid pellets containing the polymorphonuclear cells (Fig. 18.32, right).

Sometimes tophaceous material is more readily available for the diagnosis of gout than is synovial fluid. A small piece of material squeezed out of, or extracted from, a tophus can be examined under a polarized light microscope to confirm a diagnosis of gout. The crystals tend to be slightly larger and lie tightly packed in sheets interspersed with a protein matrix (Fig. 18.33). They may be surrounded with a low grade inflammatory infiltrate and a fibrous capsule.

The crystalline deposits may also be visualized arthroscopically and can be seen lying on the surface of cartilage or within the synovium (Fig. 18.34). Histological

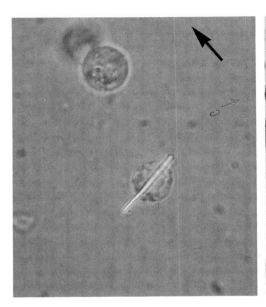
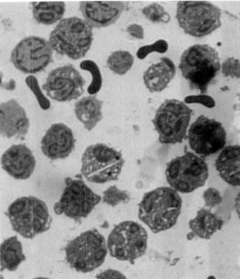

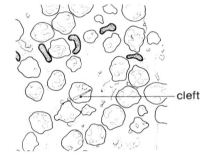

Fig. 18.32 Synovial fluid phagocytosis of urate crystals seen under polarized light (left) and in a sectioned cell pellet (right, uridine stain). On histological sections crystals may be dissolved out by processing and appear as clefts in the cells. Note the characteristic acicular morphology of the crystals, x 1200.

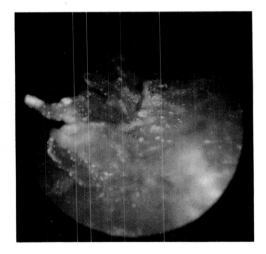
cleft

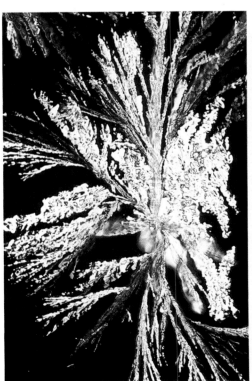
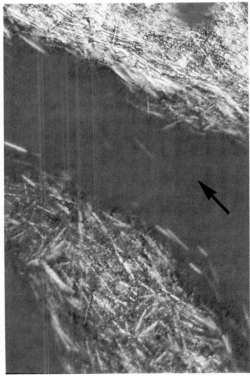

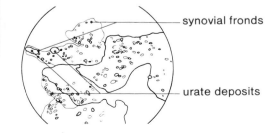

Fig. 18.34 Arthroscopic view of large deposits of urate crystals in the synovium in a case of chronic tophaceous gout. Courtesy of Dr. D. Yates.

Fig. 18.33 Urate crystals extracted from a tophus form clumps of larger sized crystals than those seen in synovial fluid: separate tophaceous deposits viewed between crossed polars (left) and after insertion of a first order red compensator (right). Polarized light micrographs, x 720.

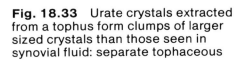
synovial fronds

urate deposits

sections will show the areas of crystal deposition surrounded by inflammatory cells (Fig. 18.35). Acid fixatives and stains tend to dissolve the urate deposits but other neutral staining techniques can be used. In chronic gout the joint pathology may include widespread, characteristic, bony lesions infiltrated by the crystals as well as cartilage and synovial deposits.

The Associations of Gout

The associations of gout have been called 'the associations of plenty'. In general, hyperuricemic individuals are affluent, overweight, drink more alcohol than others, are hypertensive, hyperlipidemic and prone to cardiovascular disease. The interrelationship of all these factors is not clearly understood, although a reducing diet, or limiting alcohol intake, are often sufficient to abolish hyperuricemia without resorting to other therapy.

About ninety per cent of gout sufferers are men who are obese and may have a characteristic heavy-jowled appearance (Fig. 18.36). The increasing use of diuretics in elderly people is increasing the number of female sufferers. They are older than the men and have less severe disease with less risk of renal involvement.

When gout is very severe or occurs in a young person, or if there is evidence of overproduction of urate, a specific enzyme defect leading to hyperuricemia should be suspected. The best known example is hypoxanthine guanine phosphoribosyl transferase (HGPRT) deficiency. Complete deficiency leads to the character-

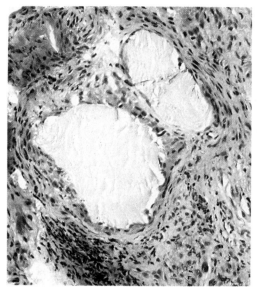
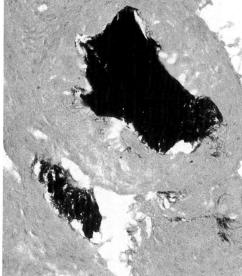
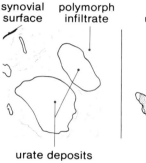
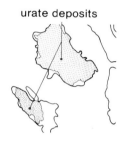

Fig. 18.35 Histological section of the synovium in chronic tophaceous gout. Sections have been fixed in alcohol and stained with hematoxylin and eosin (left) and Gomori's stain (right). The area of crystalline deposits can be seen and is surrounded by a low grade inflammatory cell reaction. High power.

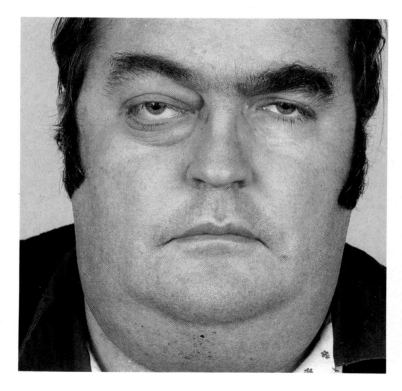

Fig. 18.36 A typical gout sufferer. He is obese, hypertensive, hyperlipidemic and a beer drinker. Note the round ruddy complexion and heavy-jowled appearance.

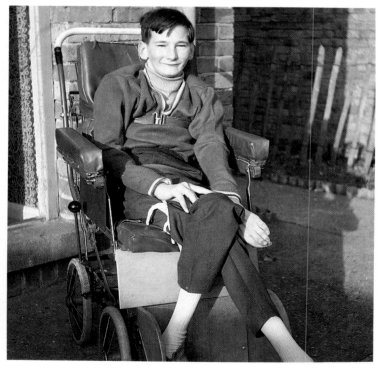

Fig. 18.37 A boy suffering from the Lesch-Nyhan syndrome. He is confined to a wheelchair because of mental retardation and tendency to self mutilation as well as problems arising from the gout.

istic Lesch-Nyhan syndrome, a rare disease of children who are mentally deficient and prone to self mutilation; they also have severe gout and may have renal disease due to urate deposition (Figs. 18.37 & 18.38). Partial deficiency may lead to massive overproduction of urate and severe gout in young adults. Several other rare enzyme defects have recently been described.

The Pathogenesis of Gout

Several factors are involved in the pathogenesis of gout. Various causes of hyperuricemia have already been outlined. However, hyperuricemia per se is not a sufficient cause, and other factors must be present to allow the crystals to nucleate and grow. As has already been said, the connective tissues in general, and the articular cartilage of peripheral synovial joints in particular, are susceptible to urate deposition (as they are to deposition of other crystals).

The crystal deposits probably grow slowly and form primarily in articular cartilage or synovium (Fig. 18.39). It is unlikely that other areas of the joint are sites of crystallization.

An acute attack of gout could result either from acute crystallization of urate, or from crystal shedding of preformed deposits. The weight of present evidence favors crystal shedding as a mechanism of initiation of inflammation. Once sufficient numbers of crystals are present in a fluid-filled space such as the synovial sac, they are available for interaction with the proteins and cells present (Fig. 18.40). It is likely that protein coating

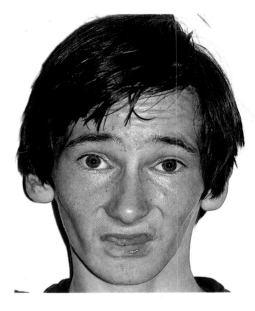
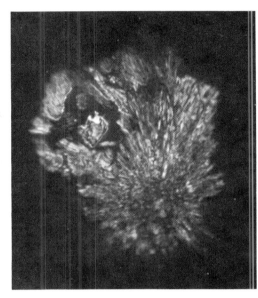

Fig. 18.38 Facial appearance of a boy with Lesch-Nyhan syndrome showing the lip deformity due to repeated lip-biting (left). A frozen section of the kidney, stained with hematoxylin and eosin, from another patient with HGPRT deficiency, shows crystal deposits in the damaged renal tissue (right, courtesy of Dr. J. Pincott and Professor T.M. Barratt).

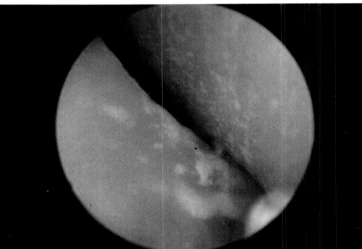

Fig. 18.39 Arthroscopic view of large articular cartilage urate deposits in chronic gout.

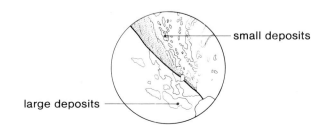

small deposits

large deposits

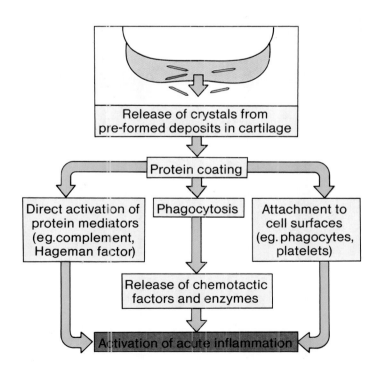

Fig. 18.40 Some of the pathways probably involved in crystal-induced inflammation.

is inevitable and IgG in particular has a high affinity for the surface of crystals, which themselves possess a high negative charge. This coating can be observed on electron micrographs (Fig. 18.41). Other proteins that can interact with the surface of the crystal include complement components. Urate and other crystals are capable of direct activation of the complement cascade. Crystal phagocytosis is another central feature of acute inflammation. Once within cells, the crystals can be seen to be surrounded by invaginated cell membrane which may then fuse with intracellular lysosomes to form a phagolysosome (Fig. 18.42). Cells ingesting urate crystals excrete a number of destructive enzymes and the crystal surface itself is also membranolytic; many of the

phagocytes die after ingesting crystals. This leads to release of more proteolytic enzymes and inflammatory mediators.

These complex processes lead to massive hyperemia of involved joints and to influx of large numbers of poly-morphonuclear leucocytes. The synovial fluid is often very rich in polymorphs and may look like infected pus. The phlogistic potential of the crystals can be shown by injecting a small quantity intradermally in human volunteers (Fig. 18.43).

The pathogenesis of chronic tophaceous gout is less clear. The slow accumulation of crystals in a tightly packed matrix probably makes them unavailable for protein coating and phagocytosis, and this may explain

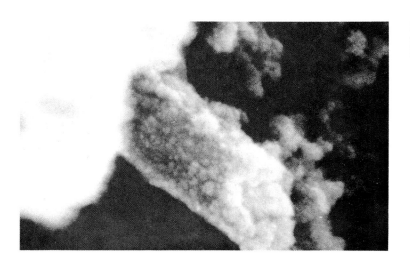

Fig. 18.41 Electron micrograph of a urate crystal being phagocytosed by a synovial fluid polymorphonuclear cell. Note the granular surface coating on the crystal. x 240,000.

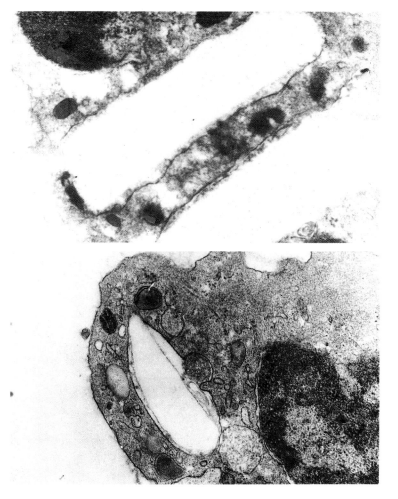

Fig. 18.42 Synovial fluid crystals ingested within phagocytic cells seen under electron microscopy. The crystals have fallen out of the spaces within the cells during processing leaving clefts, but the membrane surrounding the phagolysosome (upper, x 3,600,000) and the lysosomal attachment to the cell wall surrounding the crystal (lower, x 800,000) can be seen.

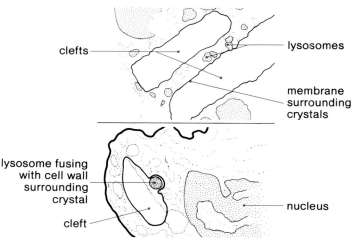

why the inflammatory reaction of tophi is minimal. However, why continuing accumulation should lead to the defects in the bone and joint is not yet known.

Gout and the Kidney

The complex renal tubular handling of urate has already been mentioned (Fig. 18.3). Many gout sufferers are undersecretors of urate and also have a defect of ammonia secretion so that they form a more acid urine. Gout and renal disease are interrelated in a number of other ways (Fig. 18.44).

(1) The filtration and proximal tubule reabsorption of urate are dependent upon the number of functioning nephrons. Therefore, renal failure is associated with hyperuricemia (although the creatinine clearance needs to fall below about 20 ml/minute before significant hyperuricemia occurs).

(2) Because urate is principally secreted by the kidney, this organ is also prone to the deposition of urate salts. Interstitial renal disease can arise from the formation of monosodium urate monohydrate crystals in the substance of the kidney itself.

(3) Uric acid may be precipitated in the tubules forming renal calculi (Figs. 18.45 & 18.46). The acid urine predisposes to crystallization of uric acid itself rather than of monosodium urate which is the naturally occurring precipitate in the tissue. Some stones in patients with gout contain calcium salts rather than uric acid, as hyperuricemia is also associated with an increased incidence of calcium urolithiasis.

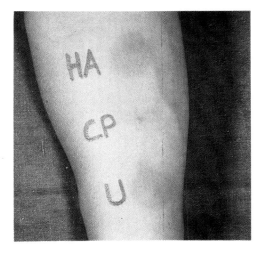

Fig. 18.43 Inflammatory reaction to injection of 5mg of hydroxyapatite (upper lesion), pyrophosphate (middle lesion), and urate (lower lesion) crystals. This photograph was taken 24 hours after injection of sterile crystals in sterile saline. The resulting inflammation can be measured thermographically or as the diameter or redness and degree of induration of the skin.

GOUT AND THE KIDNEY: INTERRELATIONSHIPS

Renal failure causes hyperuricemia

Hyperuricemia may cause crystal deposition in the renal parenchyma

Hyperuricosuria can result in uric acid calculi

Hyperuricemia and hypertension are associated

Familial gout with severe renal disease occasionally occurs

Calculi of 2,8 dioxyadenine occasionally form

Fig. 18.44 Interrelationships between gout and renal disease.

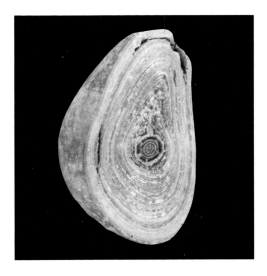

Fig. 18.45 Section across a urate stone in a case of calculus disease of the kidney in association with chronic hyperuricosuria. Note the laminated structure. Courtesy of Dr. E. Sanders.

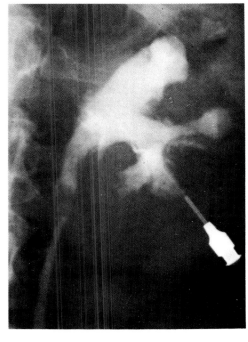

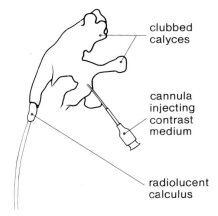

Fig. 18.46 An antegrade pyelogram showing a blockage at the upper end of the ureter due to a large radiolucent urate stone. Note also the clubbed calyces secondary to obstructive uropathy. Courtesy of Professor A.W. Asscher.

clubbed calyces

cannula injecting contrast medium

radiolucent calculus

(4) Due to the association between hypertension and hyperuricemia, vascular changes are often seen in the kidneys of patients with gout, caused by the high blood pressure rather than gout (Fig. 18.47).

(5) Recently, rare familial cases of hyperuricemia associated with premature renal disease have been described (Fig. 18.47).

(6) Finally, patients with calculus disease have occasionally been identified as crystallizers of 2,8 dioxyadenine which is a different metabolite of the purine pathways (Fig. 18.48).

Recent surveys suggest that there is some reduction of renal function in patients with gout but only a minority suffer significant renal impairment. Calculi form in some 10-20% of patients with primary gout.

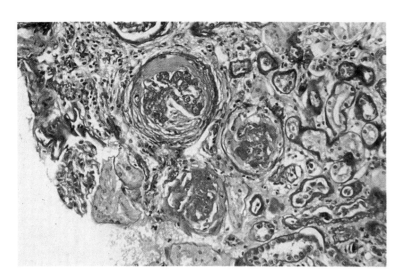

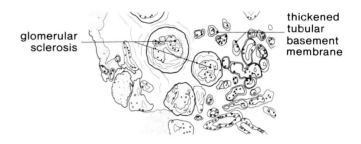

Fig. 18.47 Section of the kidney from a 14 year old girl with familial gout and renal failure, showing glomerular sclerosis with thickened tubular basement membranes and scarring, spreading throughout the kidney, with associated cellular infiltration. These changes, predominantly affecting renal interstitium, are identical to those seen in middle-aged men with gout and hypertension. Alcan blue PAS, x 80. Courtesy of Dr D. Fairbrother.

glomerular sclerosis

thickened tubular basement membrane

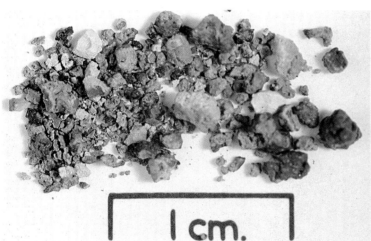

Fig. 18.48 Urinary stones recovered from a young child. These stones contain 2,8 dioxyadenine and not urate. Courtesy of Dr. A. Simmonds.

19

Chondrocalcinosis:
Calcium Pyrophosphate Dihydrate Crystal Deposition and Associated Arthropathies

Calcification of articular and periarticular cartilage is a common and important pathological process, affecting fibrous as well as synovial joints. During growth, hyaline cartilage is the precursor of bone and it is therefore not surprising that calcification with bone mineral (hydroxyapatite) can occur in the adult. However, pathological chondrocalcinosis occurs more commonly in fibrocartilage than in hyaline cartilage and the salt is more often calcium pyrophosphate dihydrate than hydroxyapatite.

The Crystals and their Sites of Deposition

The term chondrocalcinosis means calcification of cartilage. The three types of joint cartilage affected are intra-articular fibrocartilage, articular hyaline cartilage, and the cartilage of tendon and ligamentous attachments to bone (the enthesis) (Fig. 19.1). The four common joint sites are the knee menisci, the triangular ligament of the wrist, the pubic symphysis and the intervertebral discs. Large joints such as the knee, hip and shoulder are more often affected than the small joints of the hands and feet, but almost any site can be involved. X-ray diffraction studies of crystal deposits within postmortem knee menisci have identified three main salts. Calcium pyrophosphate dihydrate ($Ca_2P_2O_7$.

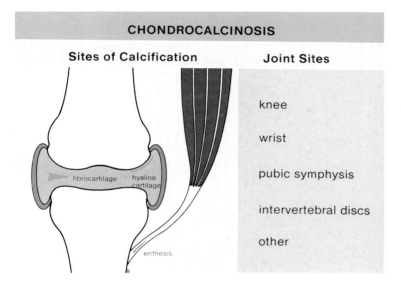

Fig. 19.1 Diagram of a knee joint showing the three types of cartilage prone to calcification: articular hyaline cartilage, articular fibrocartilage, and the enthesis and periarticular tendons and ligaments. The common joint sites are listed.

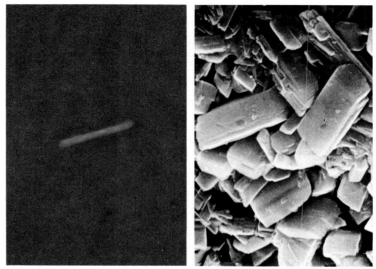

Fig. 19.2 Calcium pyrophosphate dihydrate: polarized light micrograph of a triclinic crystal (left, x 800) and a scanning electron micrograph of a clump of pyrophosphate crystals from a cartilage deposit (right, x 5,000).

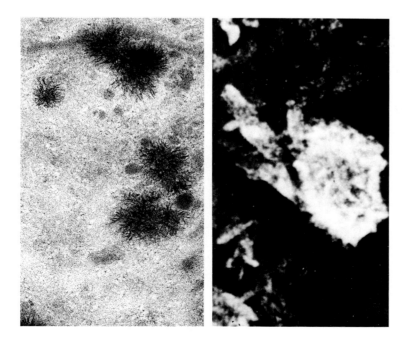

Fig. 19.3 Electron micrographs of clumps of hydroxyapatite crystals: typical cartilage nodules consisting of clumps of microcrystals (left, x 160,000, courtesy of Dr. Y. Ali) and a similar aggregate of crystals identified in osteoarthritic synovial fluid under scanning electron microscopy (right, x 80,000). The nodules vary from 0.05 to 0.5 μm in diameter.

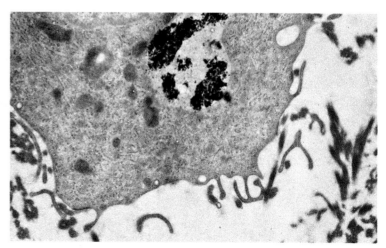

Fig. 19.4 Aggregates of hydroxyapatite crystal within phagolysosomes of synovial fluid leucocytes. Individual crystals are about 50 nm long. x 60,000.

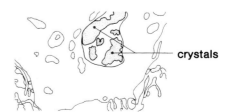

$2H_2O$) is the commonest: its triclinic form is always seen, with or without monoclinic crystals (Fig. 19.2). Hydroxyapatite ($Ca_{10}(PO_4)_6(OH)_2$) may be found in the cartilage matrix, or in vascular calcification of the small vessels penetrating the bone end plate (Figs. 19.3 & 19.4). More rarely, calcium hydrogen phosphate dihydrate ($CaHPO_4$. $2H_2O$ − brushite) is deposited (Fig. 19.5). Recent work suggests that other calcium phosphates occasionally occur, and that other salts may be precursors of the common pyrophosphate and hydroxyapatite crystals. Within the cartilage, deposits are usually seen in the midzone. Sections of knee or wrist menisci, or of pubic symphysis, reveal macroscopic deposits in a line deep within the tissue (Fig. 19.6). Microscopic examination also shows discrete crystals near chondrocytes and on the surface of the cartilage, as well as in the synovium and capsule (Fig. 19.7). The smallest crystals are often identified in the perichondrocyte lacunae, which may be the initial site of deposition, the crystals then migrating through the cartilage and into synovium via the synovial fluid. The pyrophosphate crystals that form the predominant mineral phase in cartilage in most cases show variable morphology on electron microscopy (Fig. 19.8).

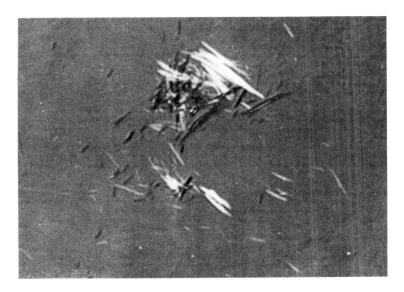

Fig. 19.5 Low power polarized light micrograph of brushite crystals. They are usually larger than most urate or pyrophosphate crystals (10–25 μm long), positively birefringent, and may have 'arrow-head' tips. Note that brushite may precipitate out of synovial fluid *after* aspiration.

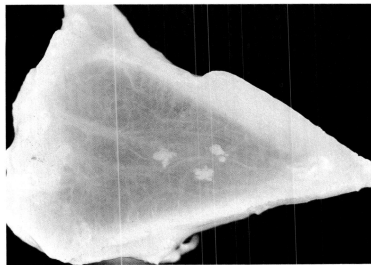

Fig. 19.6 Cross-section of knee meniscus showing large deposits of calcified material in the middle of the fibrocartilage.

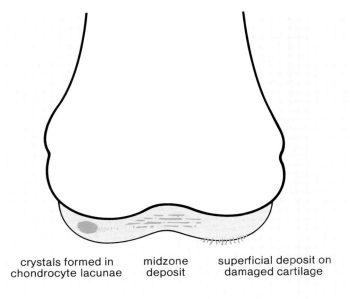

crystals formed in   midzone   superficial deposit on
chondrocyte lacunae   deposit   damaged cartilage

Fig. 19.7 Diagram showing the three sites within cartilage in which crystal deposits are found: the pericellular region of chondrocytes, the midzone, and the superficial layers. The deposits are usually heaviest in the midzone and form a line through the cartilage.

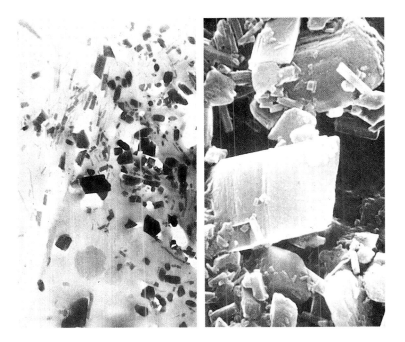

Fig. 19.8 Electron micrographs of pyrophosphate crystals extracted from the midzone of articular cartilage showing the variation in size and shape of crystals: transmission (left, x 10,000) and scanning (right, x 20,000).

Estimates of the prevalence of chondrocalcinosis vary. Radiological surveys range from a 2% to 35% incidence, the higher figures being due to better techniques and examination of older age groups. Pathological studies have led to estimates of an overall prevalence of about 5% of the adult population. The age association is striking; chondrocalcinosis is very rare below the age of 45, but present in nearly 50% of people over 90. The age of the population affected may explain the slight female preponderance found in most surveys (Fig. 19.9).

People with chondrocalcinosis do not necessarily have any overt evidence of calcification. There are three common manifestations of the pathological process: radiological chondrocalcinosis, synovial fluid crystals, and a characteristic arthropathy. However, these three phenomena can occur singly or in any combination (Fig. 19.10).

The remainder of this review will outline the radiological features, synovial fluid findings, and associated arthropathy of chondrocalcinosis. In nearly all cases calcium

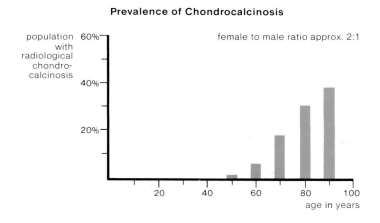

Prevalence of Chondrocalcinosis

Fig. 19.9 Histogram showing the approximate prevalence of radiological chondrocalcinosis in different age groups.

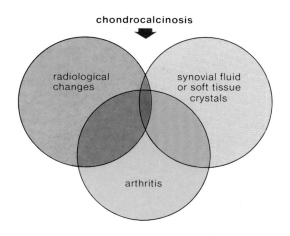

Fig. 19.10 The effects of chondrocalcinosis. The presence of crystal deposits in the articular cartilage may result in radiological changes (if the deposit is large enough), crystals in synovial fluid or soft tissues (if they are shed from the cartilage) and a characteristic arthritis. Each of these phenomena may occur alone or in any combination.

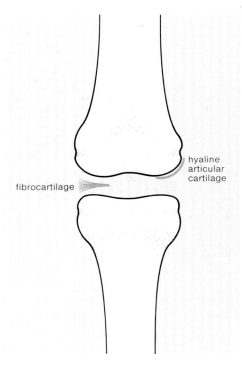

Fig. 19.11 Diagram showing the two main sites of radiological chondrocalcinosis: fibrocartilage (usually containing the denser, more obvious deposits), and hyaline articular cartilage (deposits here show up as a faint thin line).

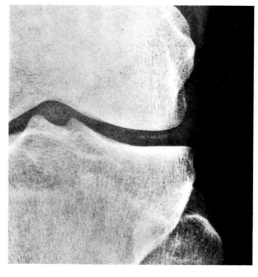
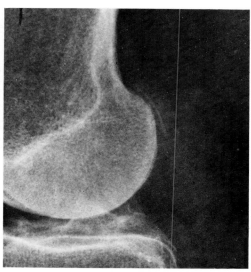

Fig. 19.12 Anteroposterior radiograph showing faint cartilage calcification which could easily be overlooked (left).

The calcification is more obvious on the lateral film (right).

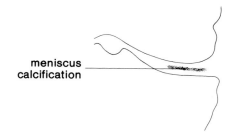
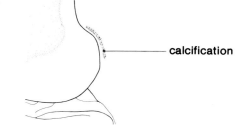

pyrophosphate dihydrate is the salt deposited (with or without small amounts of hydroxyapatite) and the descriptions therefore apply to 'pyrophosphate arthropathy' (synonym: calcium pyrophosphate dihydrate deposition disease).

Radiological Features

A radiological diagnosis of chrondrocalcinosis is based on the presence of linear deposits of calcific density in the characteristic sites (Fig. 19.11). These deposits often have a granular appearance but vary in density (Figs. 19.12 & 19.13). The knee, wrist and pubic symphysis are most likely to be affected, and should always be X-rayed if the diagnosis is suspected (Figs. 19.12 – 19.15). The fine thin lines closely applied to bone indicating calcification of hyaline articular cartilage are less often seen than fibrocartilage deposits and are easy to overlook (Fig. 19.16). Radiological evidence of an associated arthropathy may or may not be present.

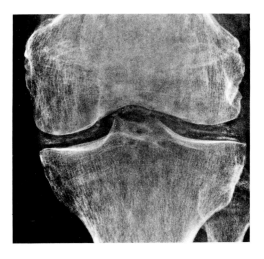
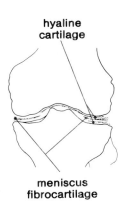

Fig. 19.13 Knee radiograph showing extensive chondrocalcinosis. There is heavy calcification of both hyaline and fibrocartilage illustrating the linear distribution and typical spotty appearance of deposits. Note that in spite of heavy calcification the joint space is well preserved. (There was no significant arthropathy clinically.)

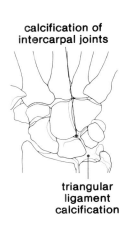

Fig. 19.14 Wrist radiograph showing triangular ligament calcification at the ulno-carpal joint without any associated arthropathy. There is also some calcification in the intercarpal joints. This illustrates the fact that chondrocalcinosis can occur in otherwise normal joints, especially in the elderly.

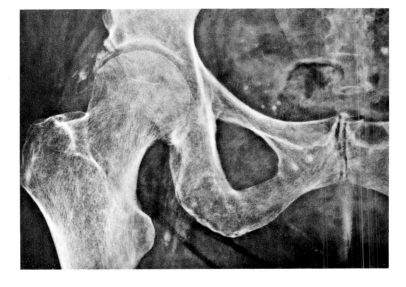

Fig. 19.15 Pelvic radiograph showing calcification of the pubic symphysis, the hip joint and the tendon of the psoas muscle.

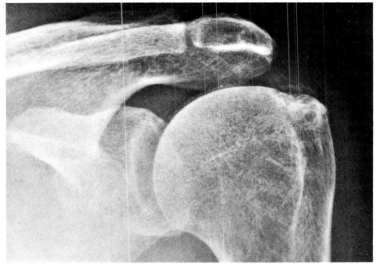

Fig. 19.16 Shoulder radiograph showing a thin line of calcification of the hyaline cartilage of the humeral head.

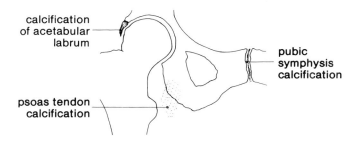

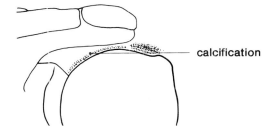

Synovial Fluid Crystals

Synovial fluid analysis by polarized light microscopy is the standard technique used to identify crystals of calcium pyrophosphate dihydrate. The crystals are usually between 0.5 μm and 10 μm long, and triclinic or monoclinic in morphology. They usually exhibit weak positive birefringence; using the standard first order red compensator, crystals appear blue when lined with their long axis in the direction of the optical axis of the compensator (Fig. 19.17). This may be difficult to establish, particularly if there are only a few small crystals attached to cells of fibrin (Fig. 19.18), and the apparent sign of birefringence

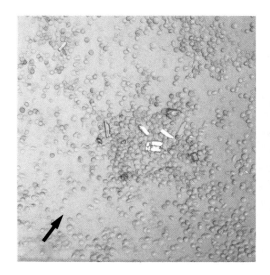

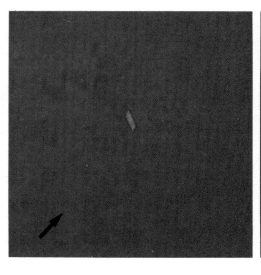

Fig. 19.17 Polarized light micrograph of a clump of pyrophosphate crystals in blood-stained synovial fluid illustrating the positive sign of birefringence. First order red compensator (arrow), x 450.

Fig. 19.18 High power polarized light micrographs of pyrophosphate crystals: in a clump of fibrin strands (left) and within a synovial fluid leucocyte (right). First order red compensator (arrow).

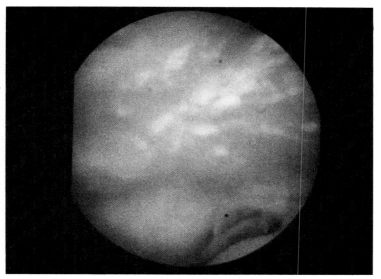

Fig. 19.19 High power polarized light micrograph of synovial fluid pyrophosphate crystals showing crystal twinning and apparent negative as well as positive birefringence. This occasionally happens and illustrates the difficulty in identification. First order red compensator (arrow).

Fig. 19.20 Arthroscopic appearance of deposits of pyrophosphate crystals within synovium.

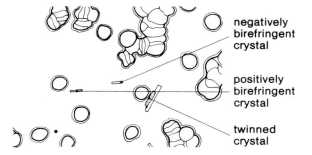

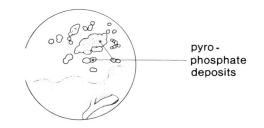

is not invariably positive (Fig. 19.19). Pyrophosphate crystals are much more difficult to identify than urate crystals.

Pyrophosphate deposition can also be diagnosed at arthroscopy or arthrotomy, when the tiny white deposits of crystals may be seen on the surface of cartilage or synovium (Figs. 19.20 & 19.21). Confirmation of the diagnosis is then made by examination of the fluid or of biopsy samples in the polarized light or electron microscope (Figs. 19.22 & 19.23).

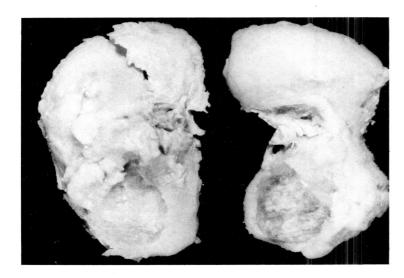

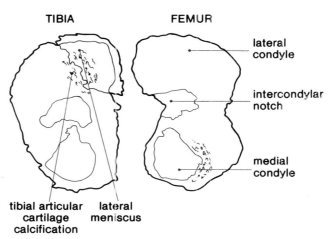

Fig. 19.21 Post-mortem appearance of a knee joint affected by pyrophosphate arthropathy showing cartilage destruction and crystal deposits. On the femur there is an area of ulcerated necrotic bone on the medial condyle and relatively well-preserved cartilage on the lateral condyle. On the tibia the medial condyle is ulcerated and there is chondrocalcinosis of the tibial articular cartilage and the residual part of the lateral meniscus.

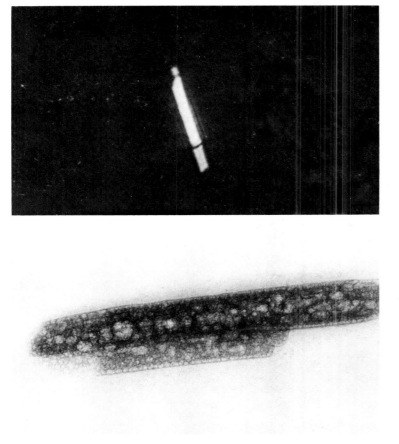

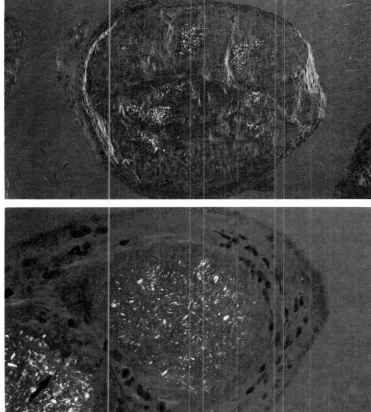

Fig. 19.22 A single calcium pyrophosphate dihydrate crystal extracted from a joint: high power polarized light micrograph showing positive birefringence and crystal twinning (upper), and a scanning transmission electron micrograph showing the foamy changes caused by damage from the electron beam (lower, x 20,000).

Fig. 19.23 Polarized light micrographs of a synovial biopsy showing a heavy deposit of pyrophosphate crystals within the synovial membrane: crossed polars (upper, x 50), and with the first order red compensator (lower, x 300).

Clinical Features

Chondrocalcinosis is often asymptomatic, but in common with other crystal deposition diseases it is associated with both acute self-limiting attacks of synovitis and a chronic destructive arthropathy.

The Acute Disease

The acute arthritis affects the knee joint in the majority of cases and is sometimes known as pseudogout (Figs. 19.24 – 19.30). However, the attacks usually take a little longer to develop and are less intense than the typical gouty arthritis. Most cases are monoarticular, although an initial attack in one joint may be followed by synovitis in several others (cluster attacks). In a few cases a poly-articular acute arthritis occurs and causes diagnostic confusion as it may simulate acute rheumatoid arthritis (Fig. 19.29). Minor trauma or surgery may initiate attacks, probably by causing crystal shedding from cartilage deposits. The synovial fluid may look like pus (Fig. 19.30), and is often blood-stained (Fig. 19.24); a diagnosis of traumatic hemarthrosis may be made. Patients with pyro-phosphate arthropathy tend to fall into two groups: elderly ladies (mean age about 75), and slightly younger men (mean age about 65). The male group have more acute attacks, and more often have this as the only clinical manifestation of chondrocalcinosis. Large lower limb joints are usually affected; small joints of the hands and feet are less often involved (Fig. 19.27).

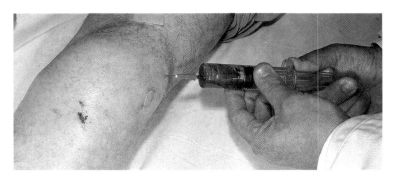

Fig. 19.24 Blood-stained synovial fluid being withdrawn from an acutely inflamed knee joint in an attack of pseudogout exacerbated by minor trauma.

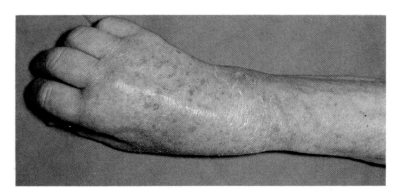

Fig. 19.25 Acute inflammation of the wrist joint due to pseudogout. This attack began shortly after a minor abdominal operation.

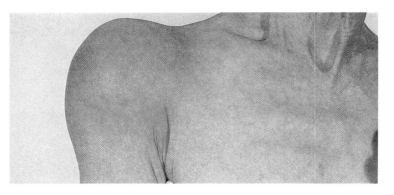

Fig. 19.26 Acute inflammation of the shoulder due to pseudogout following minor trauma.

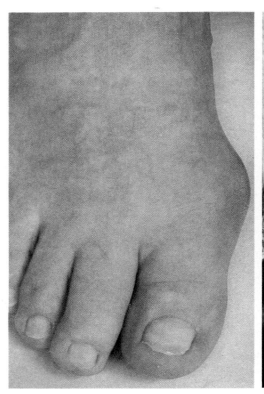

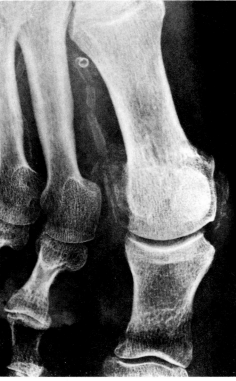

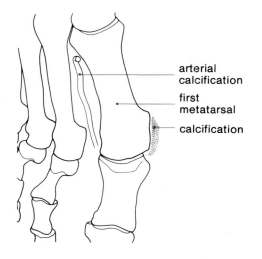

Fig. 19.27 Acute inflammation of the first metatarsophalangeal joint (pseudo-podagra) (left) associated with radio-logical chondrocalcinosis (right). Note the coincidental arterial calcification.

arterial calcification

first metatarsal

calcification

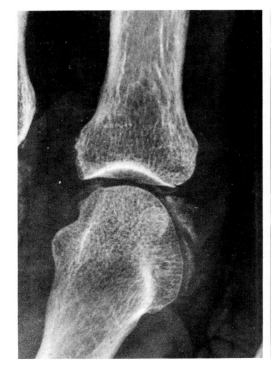
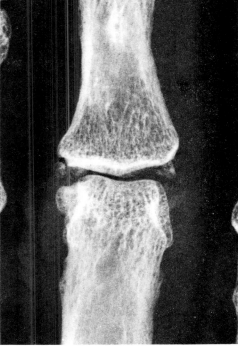

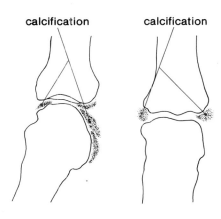

Fig. 19.28 Chondrocalcinosis in a patient who developed acute inflammation of a single proximal interphalangeal joint after a hernia operation: metacarpophlangeal joint (left) and proximal interphalangeal joint (right). Pyrophosphate crystals were found in the synovial fluid.

calcification   calcification

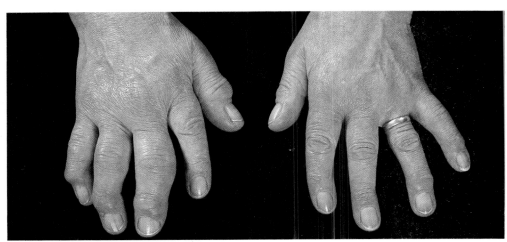

Fig. 19.29 Polyarticular inflammation in the hand in association with chondrocalcinosis. This patient was initially misdiagnosed as having acute rheumatoid arthritis.

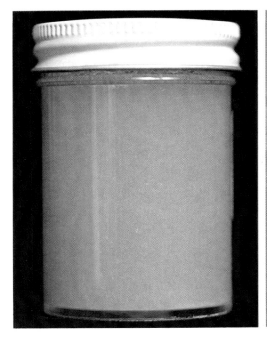
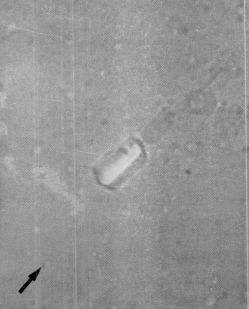
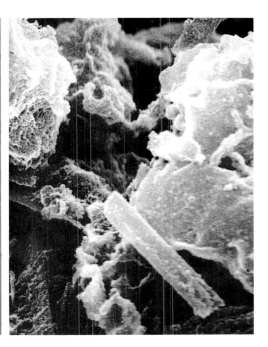

Fig. 19.30 Pus removed from an acutely inflamed knee joint (left). The patient had a mild fever and was diagnosed as having septic arthritis. The fluid culture was sterile, but numerous pyrophosphate crystals were found in the fluid: crystals under high power polarized light microscopy (middle), and scanning electron microscopy (right, x 50,000).

Radiographs usually show chondrocalcinosis and a joint effusion (Fig. 19.31).

The Chronic Disease

Chronic pyrophosphate arthropathy principally affects the knee joint. However, wrists, elbows, shoulders and hips, and, less commonly, the small joints of the hands and feet may also be involved (Figs. 19.32 & 19.33). The condition occurs mainly in elderly women, and is characterized by a progressive destructive arthritis with associated mild inflammation, punctuated by acute attacks of synovitis in some cases.

Chondrocalcinosis is common in the elderly, and its frequent association with generalized or localized osteoarthritis may occur by chance (Fig. 19.34). The evidence that chronic pyrophosphate arthropathy is a distinctive,

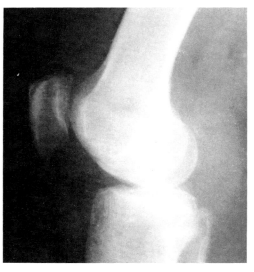
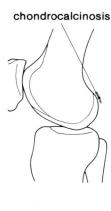

Fig. 19.31 Radiograph in acute pseudogout of the knee showing the area of chondrocalcinosis.

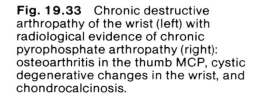

Fig. 19.32 Chronic destructive pyrophosphate arthropathy affecting the knees and wrists.

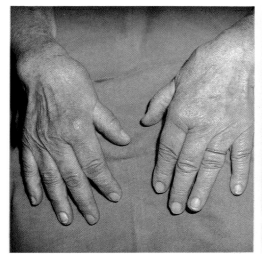
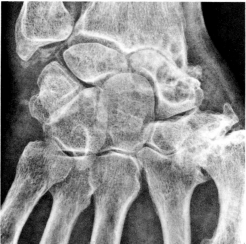

Fig. 19.33 Chronic destructive arthropathy of the wrist (left) with radiological evidence of chronic pyrophosphate arthropathy (right): osteoarthritis in the thumb MCP, cystic degenerative changes in the wrist, and chondrocalcinosis.

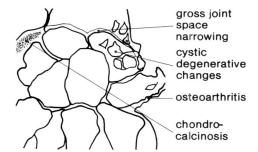

gross joint space narrowing

cystic degenerative changes

osteoarthritis

chondro-calcinosis

Fig. 19.34 Typical clinical appearance of generalized osteoarthritis (left) in a patient with radiological evidence of chondrocalcinosis in the triangular ligament, as well as radiological generalized osteoarthritis (right).

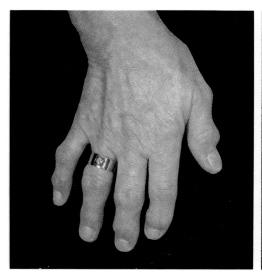
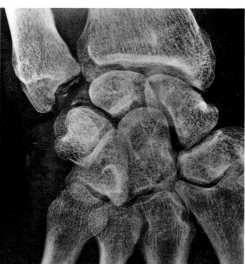
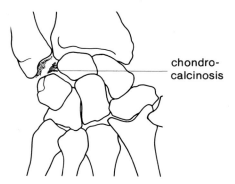

chondro-calcinosis

separate disease entity is based on its distribution, severity and radiological features (Fig. 19.35). Wrist and shoulder involvement are common in pyrophosphate arthropathy and rare in osteoarthritis; rapidly progressive, very severe destructive changes are sometimes seen. Radiological features are similar to those of osteoarthritis, but marked cyst formation with relatively minor osteophytosis, and extensive new bone formation are common (Figs. 19.36–19.41). The destructive changes in cartilage and bone may lead to a loss of obvious radiological chondrocalcinosis (Fig. 19.36). Changes in the patello-femoral joints are often florid and characteristic (Fig. 19.37), and enthesis calcification may be seen (Fig. 19.40).

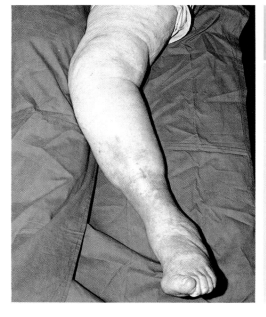

FEATURES OF CHRONIC PYROPHOSPHATE ARTHROPATHY DISTINGUISHING IT FROM OA

distribution
eg. wrists, shoulders and ankles

radiology
eg. patello-femoral disease with new bone formation, cysts and large osteophytes

severity
eg. formation of 'Charcot-like' destructive changes in some cases

Fig. 19.35 Severe chronic destructive arthritis of the knee joint in association with pyrophosphate arthropathy (left). The angulation deformity is due to tibial plateau collapse and subchondral fracture. Distinctive features of chronic pyrophosphate arthropathy are listed (right).

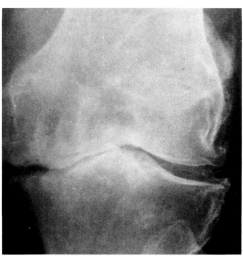

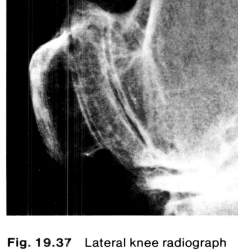

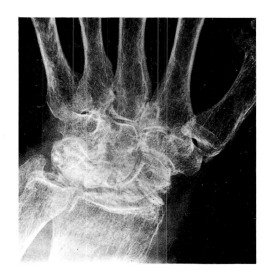

Fig. 19.36 Knee radiograph showing chondrocalcinosis associated with a destructive arthritis. The cartilage damage and loss of joint space is severe in the medial compartment; the chondrocalcinosis is no longer visible.

Fig. 19.37 Lateral knee radiograph showing the typical changes of chondrocalcinosis and marked new bone formation.

Fig. 19.38 Wrist radiograph showing chrondrocalcinosis with extensive changes of pyrophosphate arthropathy. There is attrition of the proximal row of the carpal bones with scapho-lunate diastasis and cystic changes.

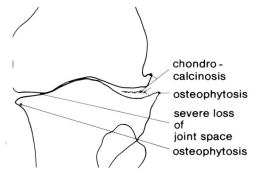

chondro-calcinosis
osteophytosis
severe loss of joint space
osteophytosis

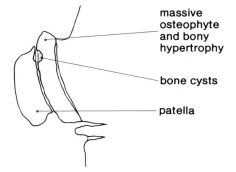

massive osteophyte and bony hypertrophy
bone cysts
patella

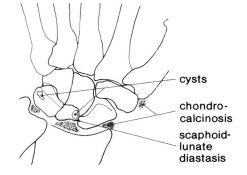

cysts
chondro-calcinosis
scaphoid-lunate diastasis

Pyrophosphate deposition has been found in Charcot joints caused by syphilis or syringomyelia. The very severe destructive changes seen in some cases of chronic pyrophosphate arthropathy lead to a similar clinical picture ('pseudo-neurotrophic arthropathy') (Fig. 19.42).

The Causes and Associations of Chondrocalcinosis

Inorganic pyrophosphate ($P_2O_7^{4-}$) is a natural breakdown product of energy-producing cellular reactions. Most of the large amount of pyrophosphate generated is broken down to phosphate by pyrophosphatases and alkaline phosphatase (Fig. 19.43). In both chondrocalcinotic and osteoarthritic joints, increased amounts of inorganic pyrophosphate are found within the synovial fluid, and present evidence indicates that chondrocytes are the likely source. Perichondrocyte lacunae are also the probable sites of initial crystallization, although primary deposition at other sites cannot be ruled out. Deposition of calcium pyrophosphate dihydrate is a complex physicochemical process also influenced by the physical matrix of the cartilage, its pH, and concentrations of calcium, magnesium and iron. However, it is not yet known why calcification occurs in some elderly people and not in others. Cases of chondrocalcinosis can be classified as familial, metabolic, secondary, sporadic or age-associated (Fig. 19.44).

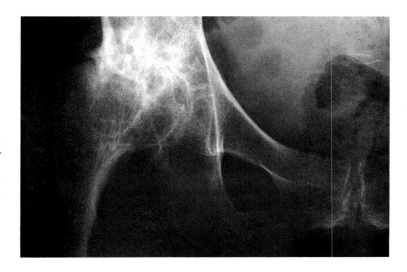

Fig. 19.39 Pelvic radiograph showing pubic symphysis chondrocalcinosis. There are very severe cystic and degenerative changes in the hip joint. Although chondrocalcinosis is not visible in the hip at operation it was found to be extensively affected by pyrophosphate deposition.

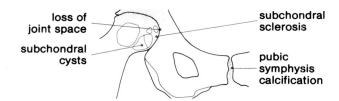

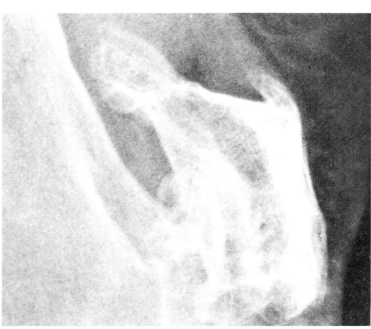

Fig. 19.40 Lateral knee radiograph showing enthesis ossification at the insertion of the quadriceps tendon, as well as patello-femoral joint disease with marked osteophytosis.

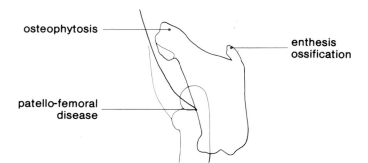

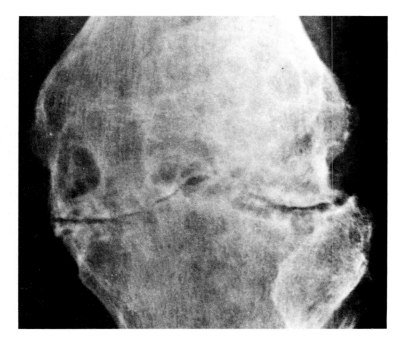

Fig. 19.41 Knee radiograph showing severe degenerative changes and subarticular cysts. Destruction may become so severe as to simulate a Charcot joint.

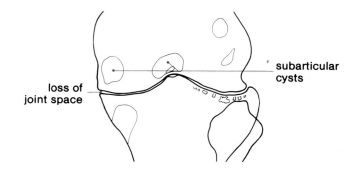

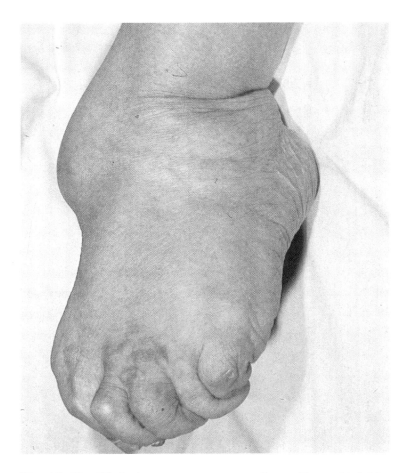

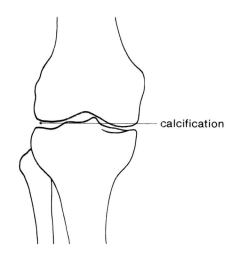

Fig. 19.42 Clinical appearance suggesting a Charcot joint in a patient with hypermobility and pyrophosphate deposition. No neurological abnormality was present.

Fig. 19.43 Simplified scheme of some of the pathways involved in the metabolism of pyrophosphate. Energy producing reactions such as the breakdown of ATP result in intracellular $P_2O_7^{4-}$. This is normally degraded to orthophosphate (PO_4^{2-}). It may complex with cations; magnesium complexes are soluble but the calcium salts are relatively insoluble.

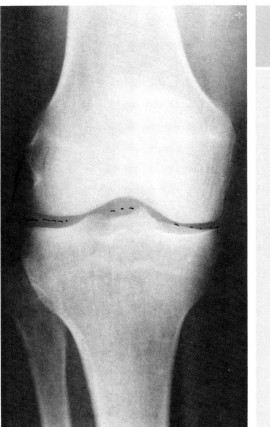

CLASSIFICATION OF THE CAUSES OF PYROPHOSPHATE DEPOSITION

familial

metabolic

secondary

sporadic

age-associated

Fig. 19.44 Classification of the causes of pyrophosphate deposition. The knee radiograph showing a linear calcification represents the typical appearance of chondrocalcinosis.

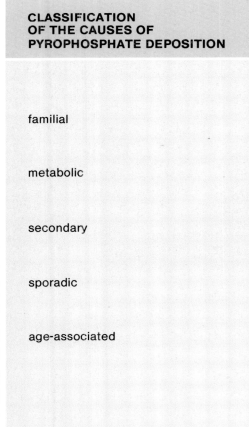

A number of familial cases have been described from different parts of the world. Among the best documented are a series of families in Czechoslovakia. Careful radiological studies of these cases have demonstrated the accumulation of mineral deposits within the cartilage prior to the development of chronic destructive arthritis, strongly suggesting that chondrocalcinosis can be a direct cause of joint damage. Familial cases are rare and characterized by premature chondrocalcinosis appearing in the second, third and fourth decade, rather than in the seventh or eighth decade as is usual in sporadic cases.

In a few cases a clear-cut metabolic abnormality is apparent. Hyperparathyroidism and hemochromatosis are well-described associations (Figs. 19.45 & 19.46). Hypophosphatasia or hypomagnesemia occur rarely. Other probably metabolic associations include gout, ochronosis, Wilson's disease and hypothryoidism (Fig. 19.47). However, because chondrocalcinosis is a

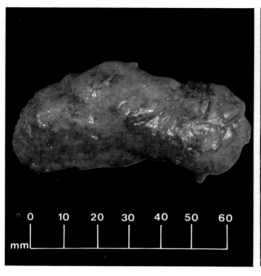
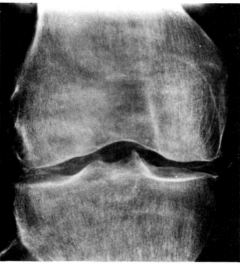
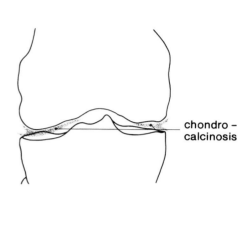

Fig. 19.45 Parathyroid adenoma removed from a patient with hyperparathyroidism (left, courtesy of Dr. R. Corrall) and a knee radiograph showing widespread chondrocalcinosis (right). The degree of chondrocalcinosis is generally related to the duration and severity of the hyperparathyroidism.

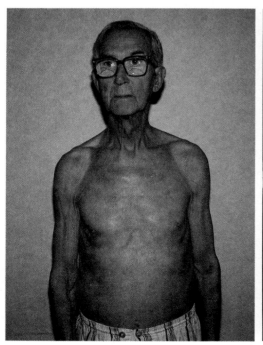
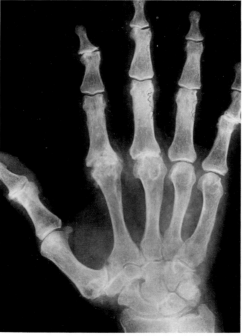
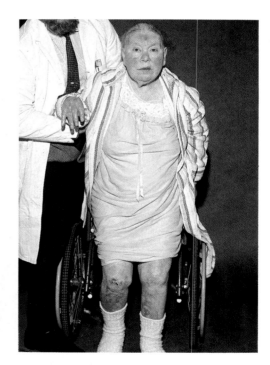
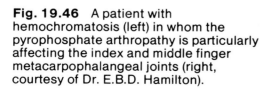

Fig. 19.46 A patient with hemochromatosis (left) in whom the pyrophosphate arthropathy is particularly affecting the index and middle finger metacarpophalangeal joints (right, courtesy of Dr. E.B.D. Hamilton).

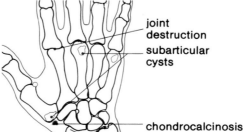

joint destruction

subarticular cysts

chondrocalcinosis

Fig. 19.47 A patient with myxedema and chronic pyrophosphate arthropathy. She is having difficulty getting out of the chair because of destructive changes in the knee joint and associated weakness of the quadriceps muscles.

common phenomenon, and because few controlled studies of its disease associations have been carried out, it is difficult to be certain about metabolic causes. Patients with chondrocalcinosis, particularly if under 60, should be screened for hypercalcemia or hypothryoidism as these associations may be asymptomatic and not clinically obvious.

Some cases occur in previously damaged joints. It is not uncommon, for example, to find chondrocalcinosis confined to a single knee joint which has undergone meniscectomy many years before (Fig. 19.48). More generalized chondrocalcinosis has also been associated with widespread joint hypermobility or instability (Fig. 19.49).

In a great majority of cases no familial or metabolic abnormality is apparent. There is however, a clear association with age in the so-called sporadic cases, which occur predominantly in the sixth, seventh and eighth decades of life. Surveys of elderly people show a high incidence of unsuspected, asymptomatic chondrocalcinosis although those joints with crystal deposits have a higher incidence of symptomatic disease than others. Surveys of patients with pyrophosphate arthropathy (ie. joint disease plus evidence of pyrophosphate deposition) show a 3:1 female predominance and a high mean age (about 70 years or over). Metabolic abnormalities or familial associations are found in a minority (5–10%), and there is a high incidence of co-existing joint damage, including pre-existing instability.

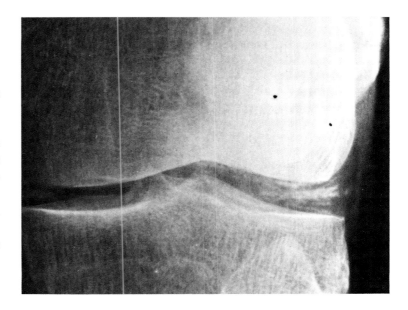

Fig. 19.48 AP radiograph of the knee joint of a middle-aged man who had a medial meniscectomy twenty years previously, showing calcinosis in the lateral compartment. There was no evidence of chondrocalcinosis anywhere else in the body.

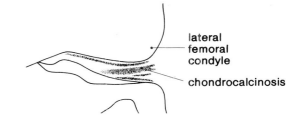

lateral femoral condyle

chondrocalcinosis

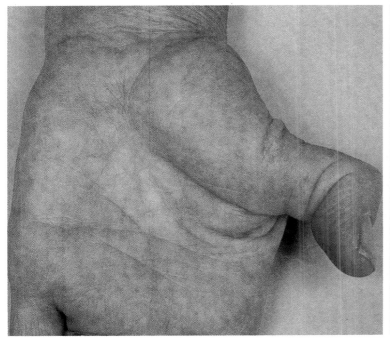

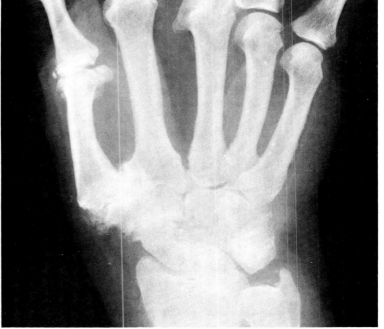

Fig. 19.49 Hypermobility of an unstable thumb (left). Radiologically there is exaggerated osteophytosis, subluxation and degenerative changes between the scaphoid and trapezium, typical of pyrophosphate arthropathy. Chondrocalcinosis is present at the wrist joint (right).

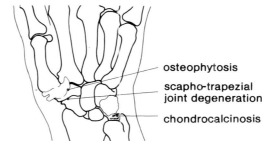

osteophytosis

scapho-trapezial joint degeneration

chondrocalcinosis

Conclusions

Chondrocalcinosis is a common, age-associated pathological reaction of joints. It is usually due to the deposition of calcium pyrophosphate dihydrate crystals in the mid-zone of articular fibrocartilage or, less commonly, hyaline cartilage. The cause of this deposition remains unknown.

Chondrocalcinosis is occasionally familial, or due to a metabolic disease. More commonly age, or pre-existing damage are the only associations. It may be asymptomatic, but characteristic attacks of acute synovitis (pseudogout), and an unusual form of destructive arthritis (chronic pyrophosphate arthropathy) occur in the presence of these crystals.

It has therefore been proposed that chondrocalcinosis is one of the reactions a joint may undergo on insult. If mineral deposits occur in a damaged joint, they may cause inflammation and mechanical destruction of the joint, thus increasing the destruction. Chondrocalcinosis is seen as an amplification loop pathway in chronic rheumatic diseases (Fig. 19.50).

Hydroxyapatite crystals frequently coexist with pyrophosphate, and probably have a similar significance. In addition, periarticular and articular hydroxyapatite is associated with separate types of arthropathy (see 'Non-articular Rheumatism').

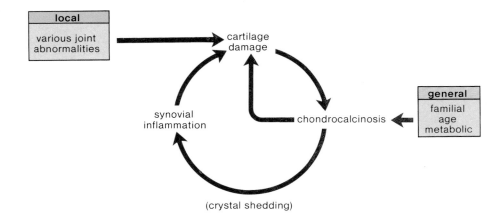

Fig. 19.50 Proposed relationships between the apparent causes and effects of chondrocalcinosis. Aging, metabolic diseases (eg. hyper-parathyroidism) and familial abnormalities may cause generalized chondrocalcinosis. A variety of local joint abnormalities may also predispose to calcification of cartilage (eg. instability). Deposits may remain asymptomatic. However, the crystals can cause further joint damage by direct mechanical or other effects on the cartilage, or via inflammatory pathways if they are shed from the site of deposition. Cartilage damage can cause further crystal shedding. Thus an amplification loop of accelerated joint damage may operate. This might help explain the severe progressive damage seen in some cases.

20
Non-articular Rheumatism

with Dr. Thomas L. Vischer

The majority of rheumatic symptoms do not arise from the joints themselves, but from periarticular structures. These include ligaments and tendons and their bony insertions (the entheses), tendon sheaths, bursae, and muscles (Fig. 20.1). There are three principal causes of pain and inflammation (Fig. 20.2):

MECHANICAL Pain may be due to trauma, either acute or chronic, with subsequent inflammation inducing secondary abnormal movements and further strain. This is the mechanism in some of the enthesopathies and in certain forms of tenosynovitis or bursitis, where the structures become mechanically irritated.

INFLAMMATORY Similar symptoms may be caused by inflammation due to one of the classical rheumatic diseases. The seronegative spondarthritides induce enthesopathies whereas all inflammatory rheumatic diseases which cause synovitis can involve both tendon sheaths and bursae. The pain of osteoarthritis often arises from periarticular structures.

CRYSTAL DEPOSITION Calcium crystal deposition is common in periarticular tissue, and can play a major role in disease, inducing intermittent inflammatory reactions. These crystals can have a similar phlogistic effect to urate crystals in gout, although periarticular deposits are often symptomless.

In this discussion some of the more common and important localized periarticular soft tissue lesions are considered under the following four headings:

Calcific periarthritis
Enthesopathies
Tenosynovitis
Bursitis

Calcific Periarthritis

Calcific periarthritis is characterized by the deposition of aggregates of calcium-containing crystals around joints. They usually consist of hydroxyapatite, although calcium pyrophosphate dihydrate crystals are sometimes situated in tendons near their insertions. The deposits may be diffuse but can form small aggregates, seen radiologically as dense opacities. The common sites of involvement (Fig. 20.3) include the supraspinatus tendon near the shoulder joint (Fig. 20.4), the distal interphalangeal joint (Fig. 20.5) and the hip joint, either in the rectus femoris tendon, or near the greater trochanter of the femur (Fig. 20.6). In any one patient, a single, isolated deposit may be present. However multiple involvement should be sought using appropriate radiographs (Fig. 20.7).

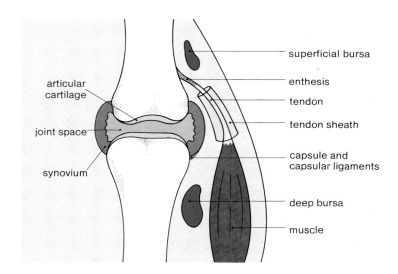

Fig. 20.1 Diagrammatic cross-section of a synovial joint showing the common sites of origin of periarticular symptoms.

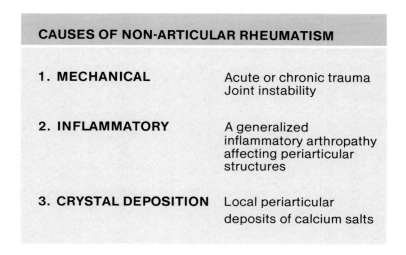

Fig. 20.2 The main causes of non-articular rheumatism.

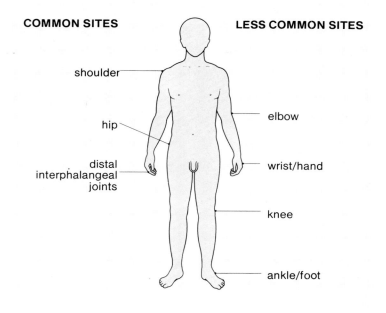

Fig. 20.3 Diagram to show the most common sites of involvement of calcific periarthritis.

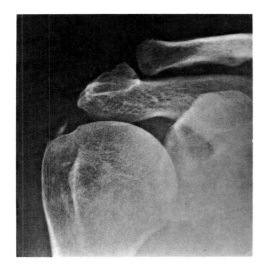
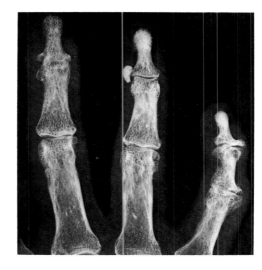
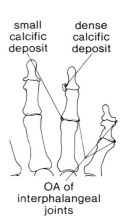

Fig. 20.4 Radiograph of the shoulder joint showing a small dense calcific deposit which probably lies in the supraspinatus tendon. This is the most common site of deposition of periarticular hydroxyapatite.

Fig. 20.5 Hand radiograph showing a dense calcific deposit adjacent to the ring finger DIP. There is a smaller deposit in the ring finger PIP. Such small deposits are frequent in generalized OA and features of this disease are also present here. Larger deposits (eg. at the DIP) are less common.

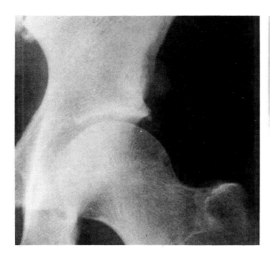
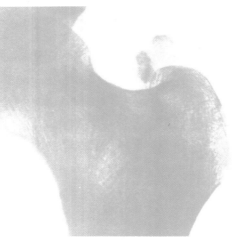
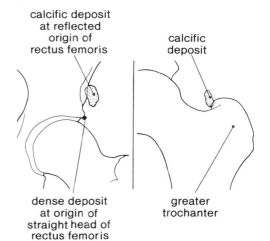

Fig. 20.6 Calcific periarthritis around the hip joint: radiograph showing an area of calcification at the insertion of the rectus femoris muscle (left) and xeroradiograph showing calcification near the greater trochanter (right).

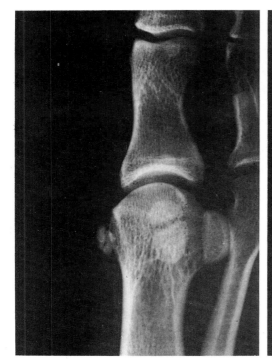
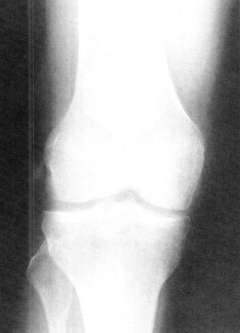
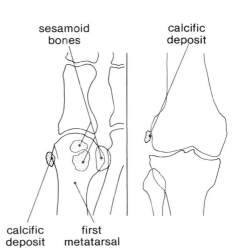

Fig. 20.7 Calcific periarthritis around the first MTP (left). This was found on radiological screening of a patient with calcific periarthritis of the shoulder. An area of calcification of the lateral aspect of the knee joint following trauma (the Pellegrini-Stieda syndrome) (right).

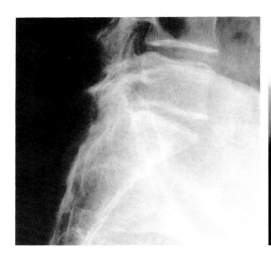
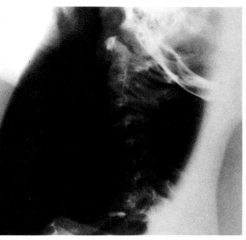
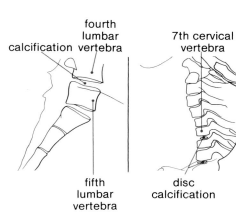

fourth
lumbar
calcification vertebra

7th cervical
vertebra

fifth
lumbar
vertebra

disc
calcification

Fig. 20.8 Lateral radiograph of the spine showing areas of calcific density in the nucleus pulposus of the intervertebral disc. This is a common site of deposition of both hydroxyapatite and pyrophosphate salts, particularly in adults (left). It occasionally occurs in children (right) and may cause a severe, transient, painful disorder followed by disappearance of the calcification.

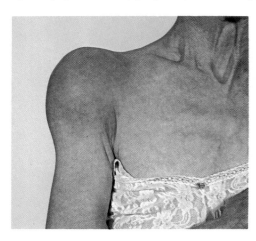

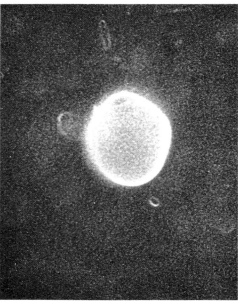

Fig. 20.9 An inflamed shoulder with a large, red painful swelling caused by calcific periarthritis and acute inflammation induced by hydroxyapatite crystals.

Fig. 20.10 Electron micrograph of hydroxyapatite extracted from a deposit in calcific periarthritis. The tiny hydroxyapatite crystals often aggregate together to form round bodies approximately 0.5 microns in diameter. They are identified either by analytical electron microscopy or by other techniques if sufficient material is obtained.

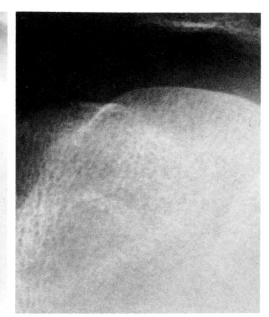

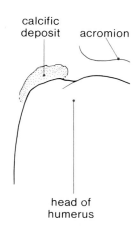

calcific
deposit

acromion

head of
humerus

Fig. 20.11 Radiographs of a shoulder joint before and after an attack of acute calcific periarthritis of the shoulder. Before the attack (left) a large area of calcification is seen in the region of the subdeltoid bursa. Following the acute attack the dispersal of crystals which caused the inflammation has resulted in loss of the calcific density (right).

20.4

The spine can also be involved: the calcification may then be found in the nucleus pulposus of the intervertebral discs (Fig. 20.8) or seen on the lateral radiograph as small opacities at the anterior corners of the vertebrae.

Clinically, these calcifications are often asymptomatic. However, acute severe pain and inflammation can occur, which subsides spontaneously after several days. The most typical example is acute calcific periarthritis of the shoulder, which can be so painful that examination of the joint becomes impossible (Fig. 20.9). This occurs when the calcium deposits penetrate into the neighboring bursa and the crystal masses induce an acute synovitis. If the bursa is drained, the extracted chalk-like material can be identified as hydroxyapatite (Fig. 20.10). If not drained, the calcific material is resorbed and disappears from the radiographs (Fig. 20.11).

Calcific periarthritis is not uncommon, and often easy to diagnose around the shoulders or hips. Other less common sites of involvement may cause confusion (Fig. 20.12). Calcific attacks might also explain some transient painful vertebral syndromes, periarthritis at other sites, and some cases of arthritis of small joints.

Enthesopathies

Enthesopathies are characterized by localized tenderness and inflammation at tendon and ligament insertions. They are due either to traumatic strain as in most cases of epicondylitis or epitrochleitis, or to an underlying rheumatic inflammation as in the seronegative spondarthritides. Calcification of the tendons does not occur, although there may be ossification at their bony insertions. The most frequent example of an enthesopathy is 'tennis elbow', or lateral epicondylitis. It is characterized by acute or chronic pain at the site of insertion of the epicondylic muscles which are responsible for extension of the fingers and hand and for supination (Fig. 20.13).

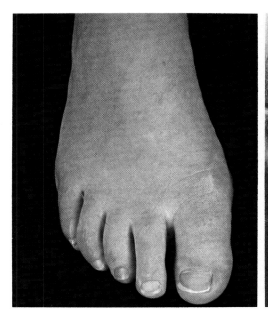
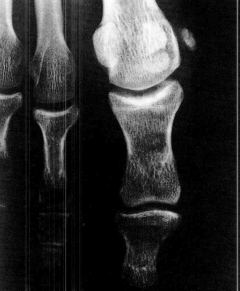
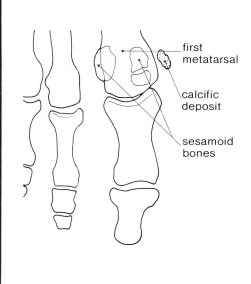

first metatarsal

calcific deposit

sesamoid bones

Fig. 20.12 Acute calcific periarthritis of the first MTP. The clinical picture on the left shows an inflamed joint with red shiny skin which caused the clinical diagnosis of gout to be made. The radiograph on the right shows the calcific deposit due to deposition of hydroxyapatite. The pseudo-gouty inflammatory attack was caused by the hydroxyapatite crystals and not by urate crystals.

Fig. 20.13 Diagram showing the common extensor origin of muscles of the forearm. This is the site of inflammation in the enthesopathy lateral epicondylitis (tennis elbow).

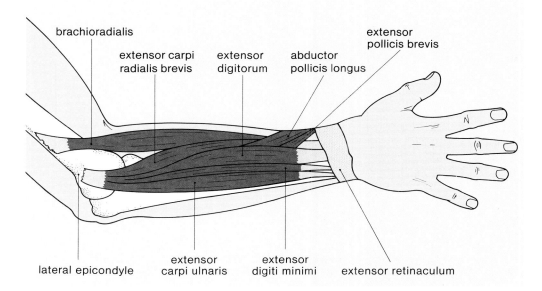

brachioradialis

extensor carpi radialis brevis

extensor digitorum

abductor pollicis longus

extensor pollicis brevis

lateral epicondyle

extensor carpi ulnaris

extensor digiti minimi

extensor retinaculum

The pain, elicited by palpation of the epicondylar region, often radiates to the forearm or hand and more rarely towards the shoulder. Movements which put strain on the muscles exacerbate the symptoms (Fig. 20.14). Epicondylitis is due to 'wear and tear' damage. It is often caused by acute over-exertion, as in the occasional tennis player or the 'weekend amateur craftsman'. If repeated insult is not avoided chronic problems may develop. Epicondylitis can also be one of the signs of the 'fibrositis syndrome' in which local periarticular pain occurs at many sites and where psychological elements are sometimes important.

Medial epicondylitis or epitrochleitis is very similar but affects the insertions of the flexors of the hand and the fingers and some of the muscles responsible for pronation (Fig. 20.15). It is often called 'golfer's elbow', indicating one of the more frequent causes, although as with tennis elbow no etiological factor may be apparent.

An enthesopathy can also cause periarthritis of the hip when the insertion of the gluteus muscle at the greater trochanter is irritated (Fig. 20.16). The symptoms are similar to those of calcific periarthritis of the hip, with local tenderness on palpation above the greater trochanter. The muscle involved is an abductor of the hip which stabilizes the pelvis when the weight is put on one leg; abduction of the hip against resistance therefore exacerbates the pain (Fig. 20.17). Periarthritis of the hips can be due to calcific periarthritis, an enthesopathy or a bursitis, as several synovial bursae are also present between the muscles and around their insertions and the trochanteric bursa is frequently inflamed (Fig. 20.18). All these are frequently misdiagnosed as 'hip pain' even though the hip radiograph is normal.

A similar situation is present around the knee. Tendinitis of the pes anserinus is due to strain on the common insertion of the sartorius, gracilis and semitendinous muscles at the medial part of the proximal end of the tibia (Fig. 20.19). However, several bursae are also present and it is often impossible to tell which of all these anatomical structures is involved or whether the pain comes from the medial ligament insertion. Clinically, pes anserinus tendinitis is characterized by pain on palpation, often with some swelling and redness; symptoms are felt mainly on walking or going downstairs.

Painful heels, exacerbated by standing and walking, are a frequent problem, and there are several possible sites of origin of the symptoms (Fig. 20.20).

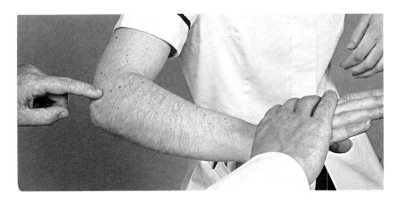

Fig. 20.14 Examination of the elbow to elicit signs of lateral epicondylitis. Palpation over the common muscle origin will elicit pain which may radiate up or down the arm. Straining the muscles by resisted extension of the wrist exacerbates the symptoms.

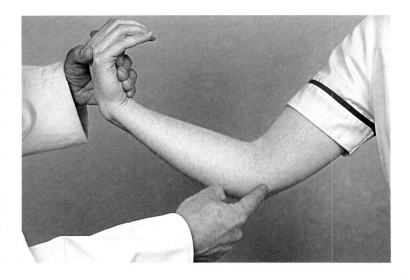

Fig. 20.15 Clinical examination to elicit the signs of medial epicondylitis (golfer's elbow). Localized pressure over the medial epicondyle (the common origin of the forearm plexus) will elicit pain. Symptoms are also exacerbated by a resisted flexion of the wrist joint and fingers.

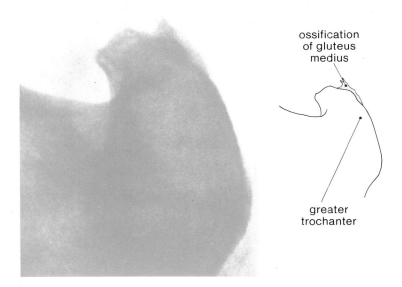

ossification
of gluteus
medius

greater
trochanter

Fig. 20.16 Xeroradiograph of the greater trochanter of the hip showing ossification of the insertion of the gluteus medius muscle. The patient had a chronic enthesopathy of this tendon insertion point with secondary ossification.

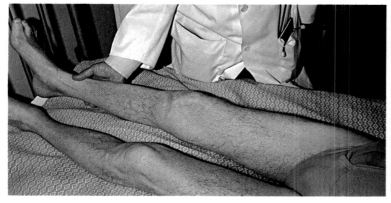

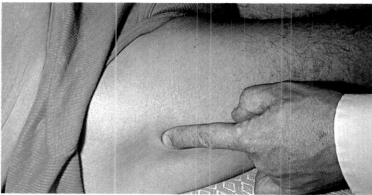

Fig. 20.17 Clinical examination of the hip to elicit signs of enthesopathy of the gluteus medius muscle or trochanteric bursitis. Resisted abduction of the hip (upper) caused pain of the lateral aspect of the joint. There was also localized tenderness over the greater trochanter (lower), the patient having an enthesopathy of gluteus medius. Trochanteric bursitis only causes local tenderness over the trochanter.

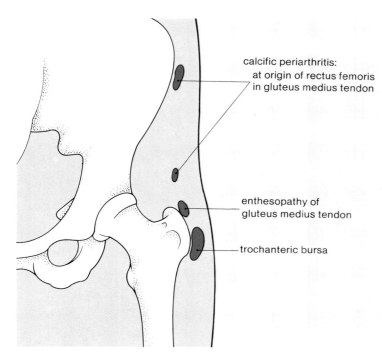

calcific periarthritis:
at origin of rectus femoris
in gluteus medius tendon

enthesopathy of
gluteus medius tendon

trochanteric bursa

Fig. 20.18 Three common causes of periarticular pain and tenderness around the hip joint. These are calcific periarthritis occurring in the tendons around the joint, enthesopathy of the gluteus medius tendon insertion and inflammation of the trochanteric bursa.

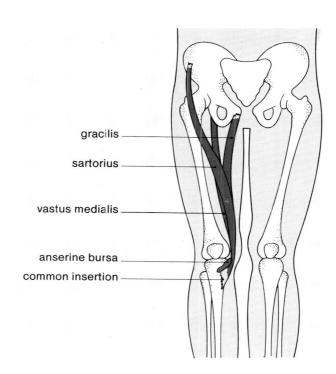

gracilis

sartorius

vastus medialis

anserine bursa

common insertion

Fig. 20.19 The anatomy of the pes anserinus. The common insertion of the sartorius and semitendinosus muscles is on the medial anterior side of the tibia and is a common site of an enthesopathy. The nearby anserine bursa may become inflamed giving rise to similar signs and symptoms.

Fig. 20.20 The common sites of origin of periarticular symptoms around the heel. The Achilles tendon or its insertion may be involved and the nearby bursa may become inflamed. Symptoms may also arise from the insertion of the plantar fascia into the calcaneum.

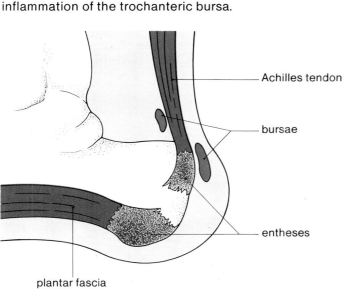

Achilles tendon

bursae

entheses

plantar fascia

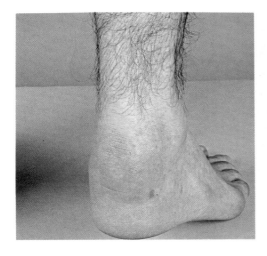

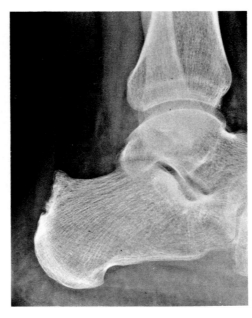

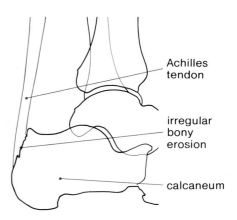

Achilles
tendon

irregular
bony
erosion

calcaneum

Fig. 20.21 Inflammatory swelling at the insertion of the Achilles tendon in a patient with Reiter's syndrome and an inflammatory enthesopathy.

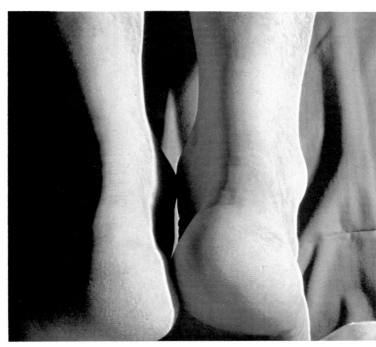

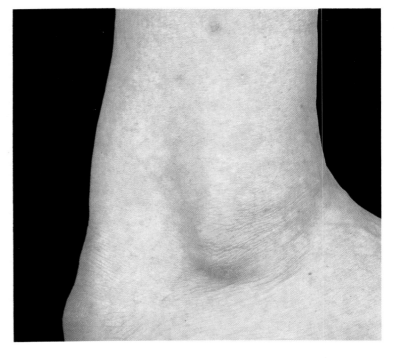

Fig. 20.23 Thickening of the Achilles tendon due to tuberculous peri-tendinitis. Diagnosis was confirmed by biopsy. The patient also has tuberculosis of the right knee.

Fig. 20.24 Thickening of the Achilles tendon due to repetitive microtrauma associated with sport.

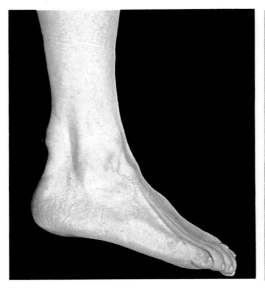

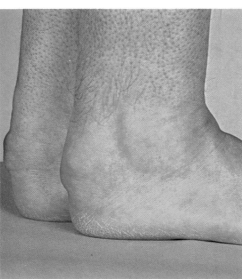

Fig. 20.25 Nodules on the Achilles tendon. Rheumatoid arthritis and lipid deposits cause similar-looking nodules in the Achilles tendon which may cause diagnostic confusion with an enthesopathy or traumatic Achilles tendinitis. Diagnoses in these cases were rheumatoid arthritis (left) and xanthomata due to type 4 hyperlipidemia (right).

The Achilles tendon insertion is a common site for an enthesopathy. In addition to local pain and tenderness, a diffuse, palpable swelling may be present, particularly if the condition is due to Reiter's syndrome or ankylosing spondylitis (Fig. 20.21). It is then often accompanied by bony changes (Fig. 20.22). Rarely, Achilles tendinitis is tuberculous (Fig. 20.23). Small tears due to microtrauma in the tendon can cause nodular Achilles tendinitis which has a degenerative base (Fig. 20.24). Xanthomata and rheumatoid nodules can imitate such nodules (Fig. 20.25) and bursitis can also cause pain near the insertion of the Achilles tendon.

The plantar fascia is commonly inflamed in the seronegative spondarthritides, with formation of bony spurs (Fig. 20.26). The footpad may be enlarged and is painful and tender (Fig. 20.27).

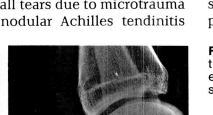

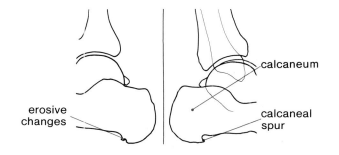

Fig. 20.26 Radiographs of the heel showing a bony spur at the insertion of the plantar fascia (left) and some irregular erosive changes due to inflammation (right) in a case of a seronegative spondarthritis.

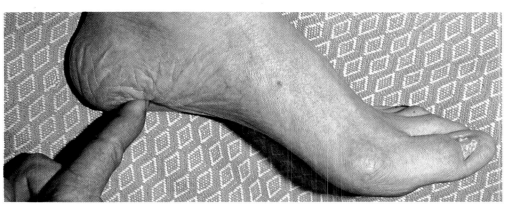

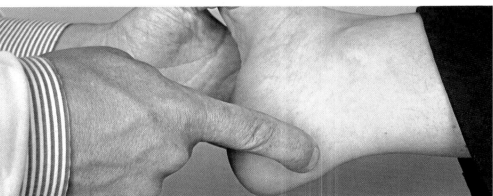

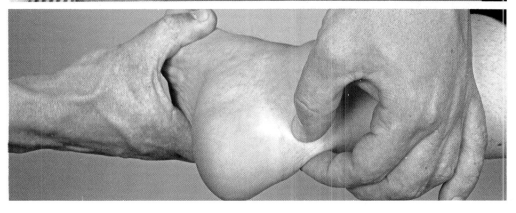

Fig. 20.27 Palpating the heel to elicit tenderness at the insertion of the plantar fascia into the calcaneum (upper) the insertion of the Achilles tendon (middle) and the body of the Achilles tendon (lower).

Osteoarthritic spurs of the plantar face of the calcaneum are usually painless but, even if present, other causes of heel pain have to be excluded (Fig. 20.28). Plantar fasciitis is often traumatic, occurring in people who stand for long periods (hence 'policeman's heel'), particularly if the longitudinal arch is flattened, straining the insertion of the fascia into the calcaneum.

Tenosynovitis

Tenosynovitis differs from enthesopathy. In enthesopathies, tendon and ligament insertions are irritated, whereas in tenosynovitis, the synovial tendon sheaths are inflamed. Therefore tenosynovitis can be a part of a generalized synovitis and is common in rheumatoid disease. It can also result from localized mechanical strain but is frequently idiopathic. Tenosynovitis occurs most frequently in the hands. Both the extensor and the flexor tendons can be involved. Trigger finger is due to a small nodule on a flexor tendon becoming caught in a fibrotic area of the tendon sheath at the level of the MCP (Fig. 20.29). When the finger is flexed, the nodule is caught and the patient can only straighten it by force (Fig. 20.30). A click is then felt.

In de Quervain's tenosynovitis, the tendons of the abductor pollicis longus and the extensor pollicis brevis have difficulty in sliding through their inflamed sheaths at the sites where they pass over the styloid process of the radius (Figs. 20.30 – 20.32). It is usually due to over-exertion ('diaper wrist'). Crepitus is felt when the tendon slides through the inflamed sheath and palpation is painful. There is often some swelling, heat and redness.

Another very frequent tenosynovitis involves the long head of M. biceps brachii. It occurs at the site where the tendon has to change direction below its origin and slide in its sheath around a bony prominence (Fig. 20.33). The pain is felt in the anterior part of the shoulder and

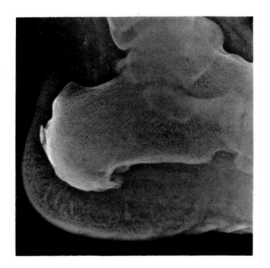
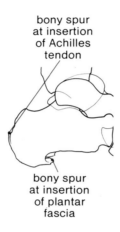

Fig. 20.28 Radiograph of the heel showing an osteoarthritic spur at the insertion of the plantar fascia. These spurs are often symptomless.

bony spur at insertion of Achilles tendon

bony spur at insertion of plantar fascia

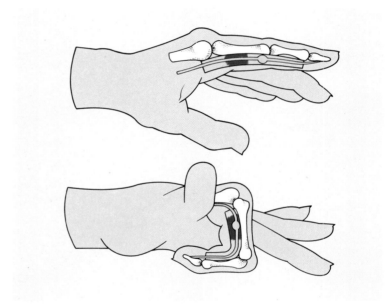

Fig. 20.29 Trigger finger. The flexor tendon becomes caught in a fibrotic area of the tendon sheath at the level of the MCP.

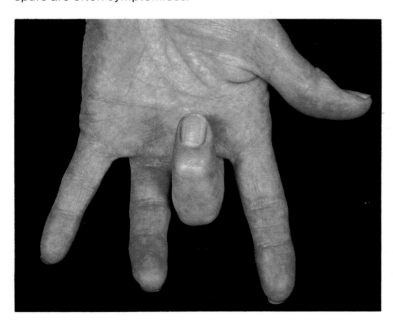

Fig. 20.30 Trigger finger showing the ring finger caught in flexion. The patient was able to straighten the finger with force and an audible click could be felt.

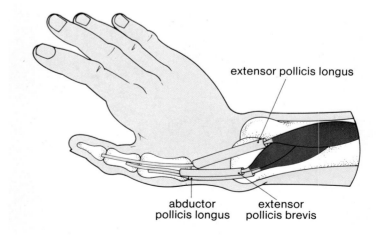

extensor pollicis longus

abductor pollicis longus

extensor pollicis brevis

Fig. 20.31 Diagram of the tendons involved in de Quervain's tenosynovitis.

the arm and might radiate upwards and downwards. Palpation elicits the typical pain with its radiation as does contracting the long head of the biceps muscle. Superior to the gleno-humeral joint lies the rotator cuff, comprised of the tendons of the supraspinatus, infra-spinatus and subscapularis. They are responsible for rotation and for the first 40° of abduction of the arm. Wear and tear damage is frequent under the acromion as the head of the humerus is pressed against it during abduction and elevation of the arm (Fig. 20.34), and a

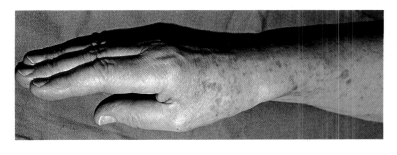

Fig. 20.32 A patient with de Quervain's tenosynovitis showing characteristic swelling of the tendon sheath of abductor pollicis longus and extensor pollicis brevis over the styloid process of the radius (left). There was palpable

crepitus of the tendons. The signs and symptoms resolved following injection of hydrocortisone into the tendon sheath (right).

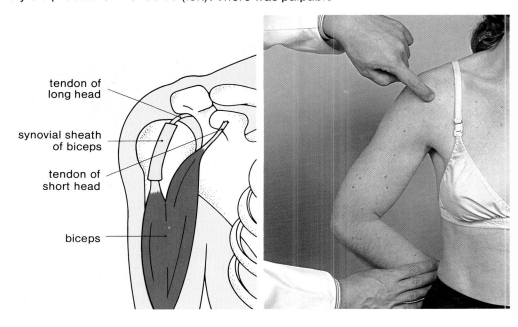

tendon of long head

synovial sheath of biceps

tendon of short head

biceps

Fig. 20.33 Bicipital tendinitis. The diagram shows the anatomy of the tendon and the site that becomes inflamed over the head of the humerus (left). The examiner is palpating the tendon in its groove for evidence of local tenderness (right).

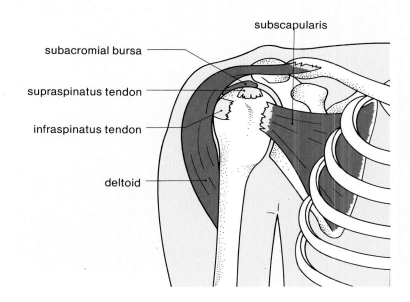

subscapularis

subacromial bursa

supraspinatus tendon

infraspinatus tendon

deltoid

subacromial bursa   acromio-clavicular joint

deltoid

infraspinatus tendon

subscapularis

Fig. 20.34 The rotator cuff apparatus. The tendons of supraspinatus, infraspinatus and subscapularis pass between the top of the head of the humerus and the acromio-clavicular joint. The subacromial bursa is also found in this region (left).

Abduction of the arm causes compression of the tendons and bursae and increases pain when the structures are inflamed (right).

20.11

'painful arc' may occur (Fig. 20.35). This is a frequent cause of periarthritis of the shoulder, especially in the elderly. Pain is often felt at night as well. Most characteristic is pain in the subacromial region, radiating upwards and downwards over the lateral aspect of the arm. It is increased on resisted abduction or rotation according to which of the tendons is involved (Figs. 20.36 – 20.38). Tears of the tendon can occur and power of the relevant movement is then diminished, independently of pain. This is best recognized by comparing power and move-

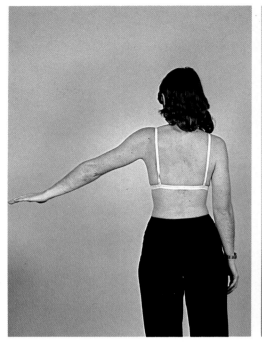
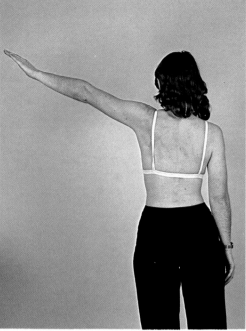
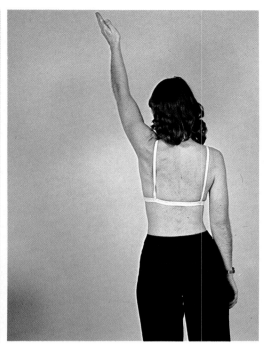

Fig. 20.35 Inflammation of the subacromial bursa or rotator cuff tendons may cause a 'painful arc' during abduction of the shoulder. The initial movement (from the deltoid) is painless (left), but the next 90° of movement cause pain (middle). When the arm reaches full abduction (right) the pain ceases as the pressure is taken off the rotator cuff apparatus.

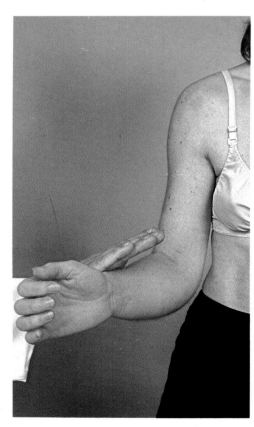
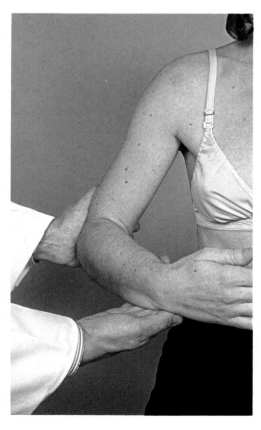
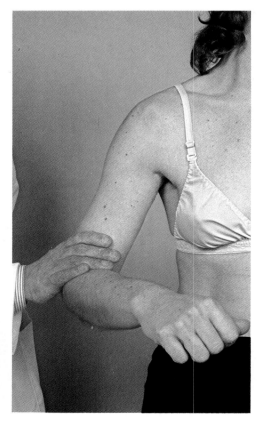

Fig. 20.36 Testing for inflammation of the infraspinatus tendon. Resisted external rotation of the shoulder causes pain.

Fig. 20.37 Testing for inflammation of the subscapularis tendon. Resisted internal rotation of the shoulder exacerbates the pain in the subacromial region.

Fig. 20.38 Testing for inflammation of the supraspinatus tendon. Resisted abduction increases the pain felt in the subacromial region.

ment of both shoulders. Complete rupture occurs occasionally and then no active movement is possible (the 'pseudoparalytic shoulder'). Radiologically, upward subluxation of the humerus is seen, especially in slight abduction, due to loss of the tendons interposed between the humerus and the acromion (Figs. 20.39 & 20.40).

Bursitis

Synovial bursae can become inflamed and painful in a systemic synovial inflammatory disease such as rheuma-toid arthritis. They often become damaged by trauma over bony prominences such as the patella or the olecranon at the elbow (Fig. 20.41). Pre-patellar bursitis of the knee for example, is often called 'housemaid's knee', from the times when kneeling down to scrub floors was a frequent cause. At the elbow, olecranon bursitis is frequent. Localized swelling, heat, redness and pain are the main symptoms and the underlying joints are not affected (Figs. 20.42 & 20.43). These bursae easily become infected as well and sepsis must be considered

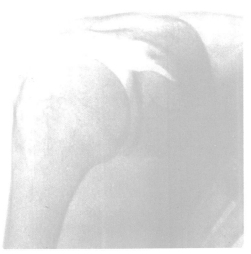

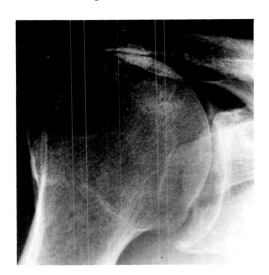

Fig. 20.39 Xeroradiograph showing a partial rupture of the rotator cuff. The head of the humerus subluxes upwards during abduction of the shoulder joint.

Fig. 20.40 Radiograph of the shoulder joint showing complete rupture of the rotator cuff. The head of the humerus has subluxed upwards and there is a compression lesion at the head of the acromion.

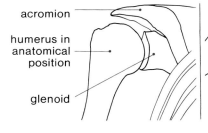

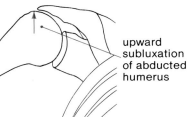

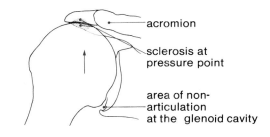

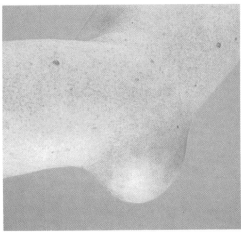

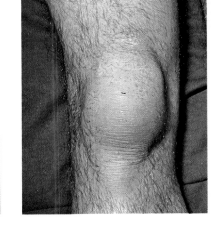

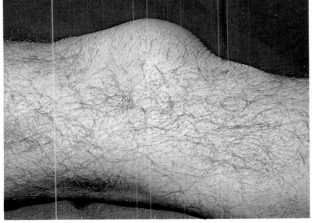

Fig. 20.41 Olecranon bursitis. Bursal swelling can be caused by trauma and is frequently found in association with rheumatoid arthritis.

Fig. 20.42 Pre-patellar bursitis: anterior (left) and lateral (right) view of a red, swollen, painful pre-patellar bursa.

in each individual case. Both gout and pseudogout can also cause crystal-induced inflammation in bursae. Aspiration and analysis of the fluid for organisms and crystals is therefore mandatory (Fig. 20.44). Bursitis can also be a cause of periarthritis of the hip (see Enthesopathies), shoulder (subacromial bursitis) or of heel pain. The Achilles, subacromial and other bursae become inflamed in the course of a generalized inflammatory arthritis or after trauma. Localized non-articular rheumatism is frequent. A careful history and examination usually allows a precise anatomical and etiological diagnosis to be made, and the appropriate local treatment is then obvious and easy. The examples cited above are among many sites of involvement.

Generalized musculoskeletal pain and stiffness, in the absence of joint disease, also occurs. There are many possible causes (Fig. 20.45). The fibrositis syndrome is a common example and is characterized by widespread pain, aching and exhaustion, multiple tender spots, and sleep disturbance (Fig. 20.46).

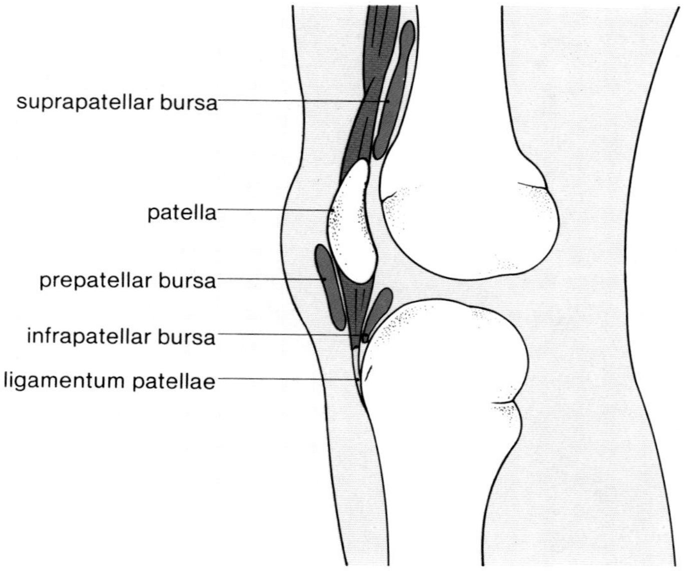

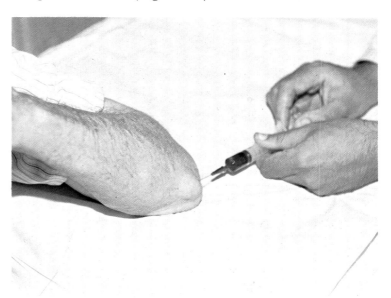

Fig. 20.44 Aspiration of a bursa. The fluid is analysed for crystals and evidence of infection.

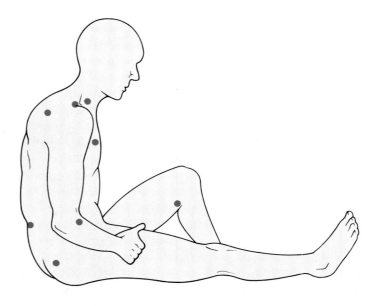

Fig. 20.43 Diagram showing the bursae at the front of the knee joint which may become inflamed.

- suprapatellar bursa
- patella
- prepatellar bursa
- infrapatellar bursa
- ligamentum patellae

COMMON CAUSES OF GENERALIZED MUSCULOSKELETAL PAIN

Prodromal phase of a rheumatic disease (eg. RA)

Polymyalgia rheumatica

Depression

Viral (influenza) and other infections

Parkinson's disease
Hypothyroidism
Malignant disease
Paraproteinemias
Hypermobility
Osteomalacia
Hypokalemia

Contraceptive pill, barbiturates, steroid withdrawal

Fig. 20.45 A list of some common causes of generalized musculoskeletal pain.

Fig. 20.46 Frequent sites of localized spot tenderness in the fibrositis syndrome. This condition is characterized by sleep disturbance and tenderness at multiple periarticular sites as shown.

21

Arthritis of Systemic Diseases

Many rheumatic complaints are secondary to disease of another system. Musculoskeletal symptoms or signs sometimes pre-date the diagnosis of the underlying illness, although in other cases the bones and joints are only affected as a late complication, when diagnosis of the primary disease is obvious. Rheumatological

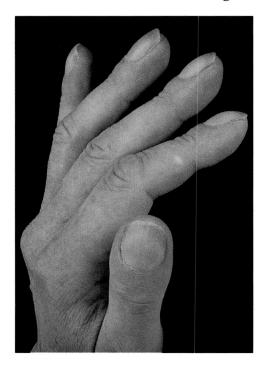

Fig. 21.3 Hypertrophic osteoarthropathy. This patient with a bronchial carcinoma has finger clubbing.

RHEUMATOLOGICAL PRESENTATION OF SYSTEMIC DISEASES

Polyarthritis
  viruses
  bacterial endocarditis/septicemia
  malignancy
  myxedema
  sarcoidosis

Oligoarthritis
  bleeding diatheses
  hyperlipidemia

Neuropathic arthritis
  syphilis
  diabetes

Bone involvement
  secondary deposits
  hyperparathyroidism
  acromegaly
  sarcoidosis

Soft tissue involvement
  hyperlipidemia
  thyrotoxicosis
  sarcoidosis

Fig. 21.1 Some systemic diseases which may be complicated by rheumatological symptoms.

RHEUMATOLOGICAL PRESENTATION OF MALIGNANT DISEASE

Polyarthralgia/ Polyarthritis

  associated with carcinoma/ sarcoma

Local pain

  secondary deposit or myeloma produces –

  local pain
  vertebral collapse
  fracture
  arthritis of adjacent joint

Polymyalgia rheumatica/ Polymyositis/Dermatomyositis

  may precede development of clinically obvious malignancy

Fig. 21.2 Rheumatological presentation of malignant disease.

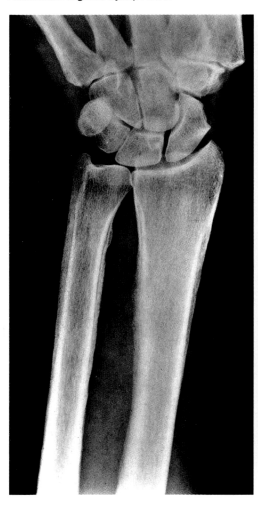

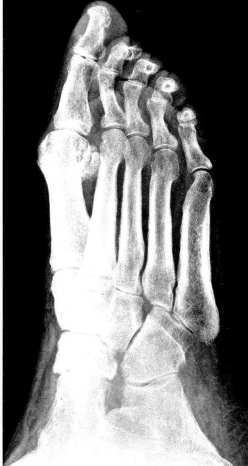

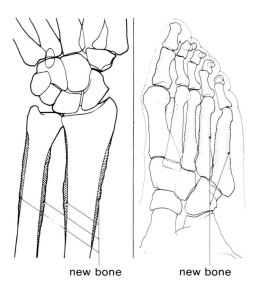

new bone   new bone

Fig. 21.4 Hypertrophic osteoarthropathy. Wrist radiograph showing periostitis at the distal ends of radius and ulna (left). The coarse layered appearance is most evident along the diaphyses. The relative sparing of the former epiphyses is characteristic. The foot radiograph shows periostitis in several metatarsal shafts (right).

manifestations of systemic disease may reflect the activity of the underlying condition, but often fluctuate independently. Some examples of diseases that may present with, or be complicated by, rheumatological symptoms are listed in figure 21.1.

NEOPLASTIC DISEASE

Malignant diseases affect bones and joints in many different ways (Fig. 21.2). Often the rheumatic presentation leaves no doubt as to the underlying diagnosis but sometimes a primary arthritic disorder is erroneously diagnosed, and a high degree of suspicion is required in order to make the correct diagnosis in every case.

Hypertrophic osteoarthropathy

This is characterized by finger clubbing and painful swelling of bones and joints, particularly forearms, wrists and ankles, with a mild recurrent, episodic synovitis (Fig. 21.3). The bones are often tender due to periostitis, which is the radiologically demonstrable lesion and has a coarse layered quality (Fig. 21.4). Radioisotope scanning will reveal periostitis before it is visible on plain radiographs (Fig. 21.5). The majority of cases are associated with a peripheral bronchial carcinoma but some non-neoplastic conditions including chronic lung sepsis, congenital cyanotic heart disease, cirrhosis and inflammatory bowel disease may cause it (Fig. 21.6).

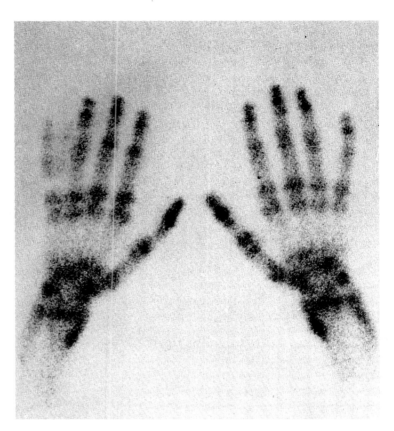

Fig. 21.5 Isotope bone scan demonstrating increased uptake in the periosteum in a patient with carcinoma of the bronchus. The plain radiographs were normal.

CAUSES OF HPOA
Bronchial carcinoma
Bronchiectasis
Aspergillosis
Cyanotic heart disease
Lymphoma
Hodgkins disease
Crohns disease
Ulcerative colitis
Primary biliary cirrhosis
Portal cirrhosis

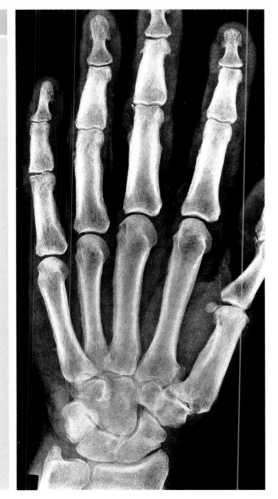

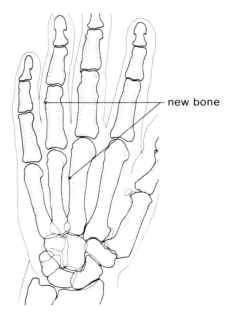

new bone

Fig. 21.6 Table of some causes of hypertrophic osteoarthropathy (HPOA) and a hand radiograph showing extensive periosteal new bone formation.

Carcinomatous arthritis

A number of malignancies may be associated with a polyarthralgia or polyarthritis, including carcinoma of the bronchus (Fig. 20.7), breast, prostate, bladder and pancreas. Pancreatic tumors may result in a dramatic, acute polyarthritis which is sometimes clinically indistinguishable from rheumatoid arthritis but may also be associated with skin lesions and fat atrophy. However, the arthritis of malignant disease is usually asymmetrical and involves larger joints producing an active synovitis with redness of the overlying skin; it may precede the presentation of the malignancy itself. Rarely, an atrial myxoma or sarcoma presents with arthralgia or arthritis (Fig. 20.8).

Malignant deposits

Local malignant deposits may also cause pain. The most common are secondary deposits in the spine or hip, and pain may result from the deposit itself or from secondary collapse or fracture of the bones (Figs. 21.9 & 21.10). An isotope bone scan may reveal more metastases than are detected on the plain radiograph (Fig. 21.11).

NEOPLASM
Bronchus
Breast
Prostrate
Bladder
Pancreas

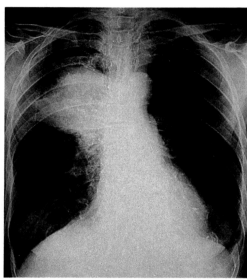

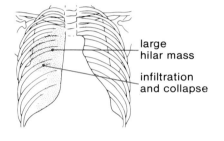

large hilar mass

infiltration and collapse

Fig. 21.7 Table of some neoplasms which may cause polyarthritis and a chest radiograph showing an oat cell carcinoma.

Atrial Myxoma (Right)
Valvular obstruction
Pulmonary emboli
Polyarthralgia
Raynaud's disease
Malaise and weight loss

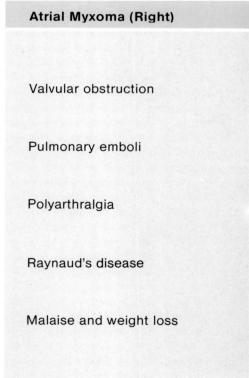

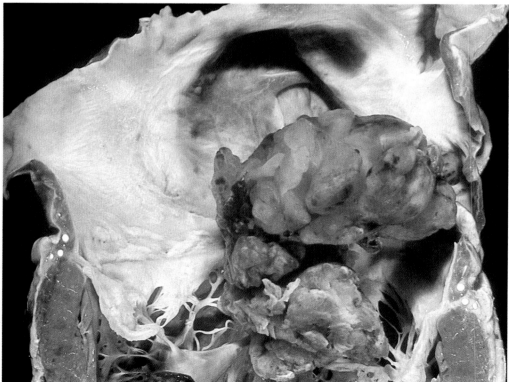

Fig. 21.8 Table of disorders due to atrial myxoma (left) and the post mortem appearance of a left atrial myxoma with a friable villous surface (right, courtesy of Professor A.E. Becker).

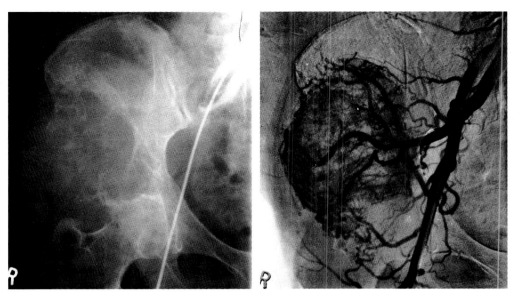
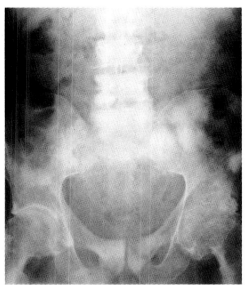

Fig. 21.9 Solitary metastasis from a carcinoma of the thyroid. The plain film demonstrates a huge destructive lesion in the anterior iliac crest (left). The iliac angiogram demonstrates the tumor to be highly vascular with a marked increase in the number and calibre of feeding vessels (right).

Fig. 21.10 Radiograph of the lumbar spine and pelvis in a patient presenting with back pain. There are multiple sclerotic deposits from a previously undiagnosed prostatic carcinoma.

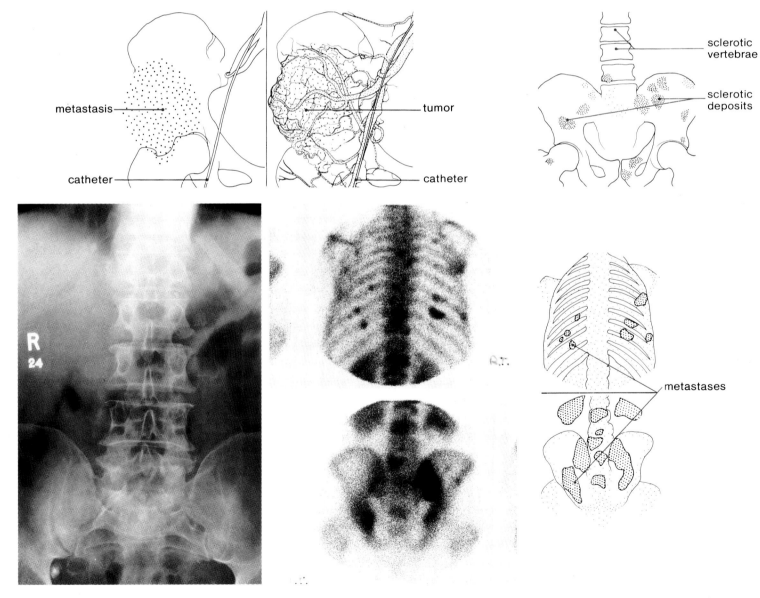

Fig. 21.11 A normal lumbar spine radiograph in a patient who had a bronchial carcinoma and complained of back pain (left). The isotope bone scans (right) reveal multiple metastases in the lumbar spine and pelvis. Note also metastases in thoracic vertebrae and ribs.

Myeloma deposits (Fig. 21.12) may produce the same effect although myelomatosis can also present with widespread arthralgia or diffuse back pain. A mono-arthritis may result from a deposit in bone adjacent to a joint (Fig. 21.13). Pain may also result from nerve entrapment as in the involvement of the brachial plexus by an apical bronchial carcinoma (Pancoast tumor) (Fig. 21.14).

Other musculoskeletal conditions

Other conditions such as polymyalgia rheumatica may be associated with malignant disease. A poor response to steroids, or other atypical findings may lead to the suspicion of the occult malignancy. Dermatomyositis, particularly in middle-aged men, may be associated with a tumor, and gout can result from myeloproliferative disorders (see below).

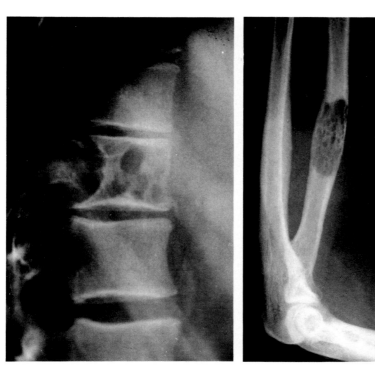

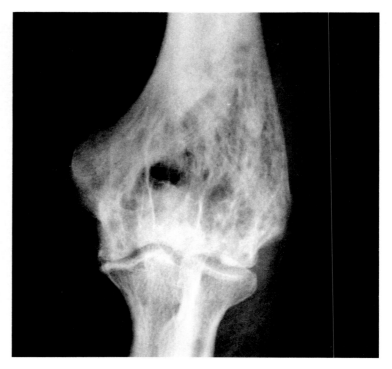

Fig. 21.12 Myeloproliferative disease. Multiple radio-lucencies due to myeloma in the body of T12 (left) and the deposit of myeloma in the mid-shaft of the radius in another patient (right).

Fig. 21.13 Radiograph showing irregular destruction of the lower end of the humerus in a patient who presented with an acute monoarthritis of the elbow. The primary tumour from which this metastasis arose was in the colon. Courtesy of Dr. D. Goldman.

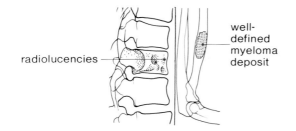

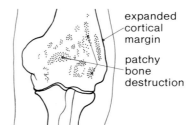

Fig. 21.14 Chest radiograph showing an apical bronchial carcinoma (Pancoast tumour). The patient presented with pain in the left arm. Courtesy of Dr. J. Webb.

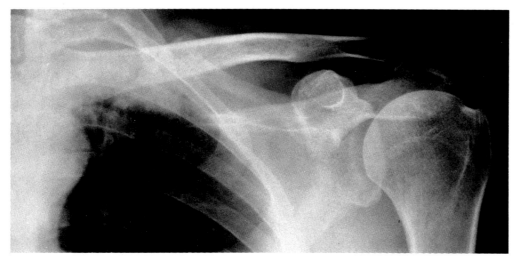

Infection

Various viral infections may provoke a non-specific arthralgia or polyarthritis (Fig. 21.15). Rubella arthralgia is the most common. Patients with bacterial endocarditis may occasionally develop arthritis and can also present with back pain.

HEMATOLOGICAL DISORDERS

A number of blood disorders are associated with arthritis or arthralgia of different types (Fig. 21.16).

Hemorrhagic diseases

The two commonest bleeding disorders are hemophilia A (classical hemophilia, Factor VIII deficiency) and hemophilia B (Christmas disease, Factor IX deficiency) (Fig. 21.17). The severity of the disease is related to the concentration of the deficient clotting factor, spontaneous bleeding being rare unless levels fall below 10% of normal.

Excess bleeding from wounds and bruising of the skin after minimal trauma is common. Soft tissue bleeding

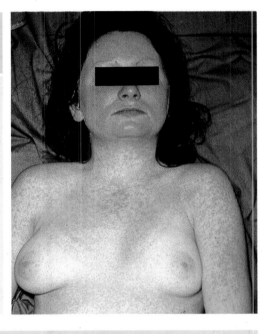

VIRUSES CAUSING POLYARTHRITIS/ POLYARTHRALGIA

Hepatitis B

Rubella

Rubella vaccine

Mumps

Infectious mononucleosis

Varicella

Fig. 21.15 A list of some viruses which may provoke a polyarthritis or polyarthralgia (left) and the characteristic rash of rubella (right, courtesy of Professor H. Lambert).

HEMATOLOGICAL DISORDERS AND RHEUMATIC DISEASE

Presentation	Cause	Mechanism
Hemarthrosis Muscle hemorrhage	Bleeding disorders (factors VIII and IX deficiency)	Bleeding
Hand-foot syndrome	Hemoglobinopathies eg. HbS, β−thalassemia	
Vertebral body 'step sign'		Microinfarction and marrow cavity expansion
Back pain		
Aseptic necrosis		
Polyarthralgia	Leukemia	Unknown
Gout	Leukemia PRV	Excess purine breakdown
	Other blood dyscrasias	Unknown

Fig. 21.16 Table of hematological disorders associated with rheumatic disease.

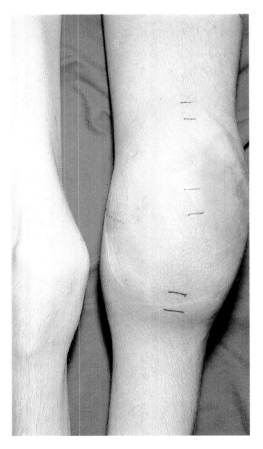

Fig. 21.17 An acute hemarthrosis in a patient with hemophilia. Note also the quadriceps wasting and bony deformity of the right knee due to previous hemarthrosis of the joint.

may occur spontaneously in severe cases but is usually related to trauma. Ligamentous strains, or the tearing of muscle fibers may result in large hematomas (Fig. 21.18), especially in children. The size of hematoma is greatly reduced by early replacement therapy but muscle contractures may result.

Hemarthroses are common and often the most disabling feature of hemophilia in adults. There may be a history of trauma but hemarthroses also appear spontaneously. In infants the ankle is commonly affected. In older children and adults the knees and elbows are the most frequently involved joints but ankles, shoulders and wrists are sometimes affected.

Acute hemarthrosis is treated by replacement therapy, and aspiration may be necessary. Temporary splinting may reduce the likelihood of recurrence or late contracture, but permanent joint damage develops after repeated bleeds in the majority of cases.

In infants and children hyperemia of the bone ends can cause epiphyseal enlargement, distortion and premature fusion. Subperiosteal hemorrhages may result in damage to the adjacent epiphysis (Fig. 21.19).

Other characteristic radiological appearances include the presence of growth lines in the diaphysis, which may mark the previous episodes of bleeding.

In adults the radiological features include trabecular widening and consequences of epiphyseal overgrowth, especially an increase in the size of the intercondylar notch in the knee and increased size and irregularity of the radial head at the elbow. Progressive joint damage leads to narrowing of the joint space, with irregular erosion and cyst formation in the subarticular bone (Fig. 21.20). Ankylosis may occasionally be the end result. Occasionally the hip is involved; avascular necrosis can occur and the outcome may eventually resemble that of Perthes' disease. Recurrent hemarthrosis may result in the deposition of hemosiderin in the capsule and the distended capsule may become radio-opaque. In addition, a large subperiosteal hematoma may result in adjacent bone destruction and the formation of a hemophilic pseudotumor (Fig. 21.21)

Hemoglobinopathies

Of the large number of abnormal hemoglobins that may be identified, Hemoglobin S, in which there is a single amino acid substitution in the β chain, is the commonest. Red cells containing such hemoglobin are susceptible to low oxygen tension when the distortion of hemoglobin molecules results in cell sickling (Fig. 21.22). The cells are abnormally fragile, lyse easily, and may sludge in capillaries. Patients who are homozygous for HbS develop episodes of sickling *in vivo*.

Diagnosis of the condition is usually made in childhood once levels of fetal hemoglobin have diminished significantly, usually after the first six months of life. Clinical manifestations include anemia and several systemic and rheumatological features.

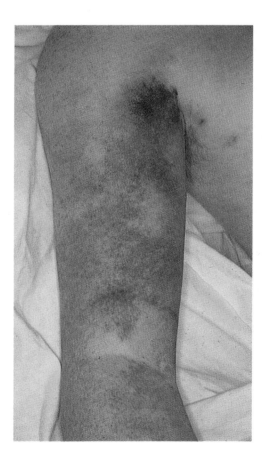

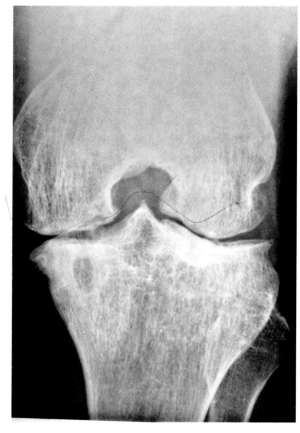

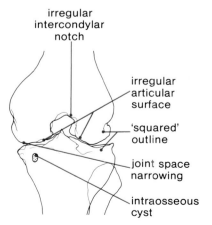

irregular
intercondylar
notch

irregular
articular
surface

'squared'
outline

joint space
narrowing

intraosseous
cyst

Fig. 21.18 Extensive subcutaneous hemorrhage with bleeding into the biceps muscle in a patient who caught his arm while walking through a door.

Fig. 21.19 Knee radiograph in hemophilia. This joint has suffered recurrent hemarthroses in childhood resulting in epiphyseal damage.

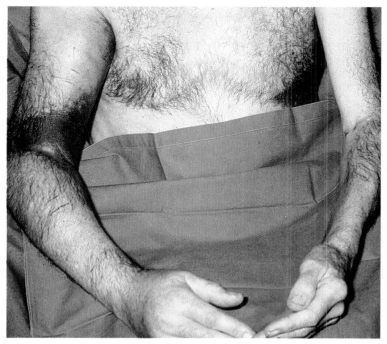
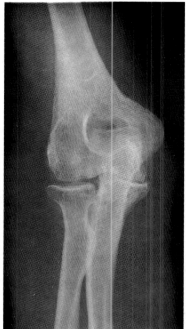
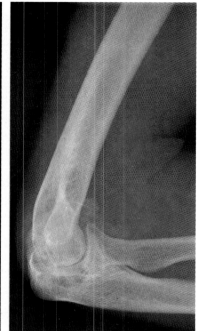

Fig. 21.20 A hemarthrosis of the elbow (left). The radiographs of this patient show irregularity of the radial head with joint space narrowing and irregular erosion and cyst formation (middle & right). The chronic deposition of hemosiderin in the synovium renders it radio-opaque.

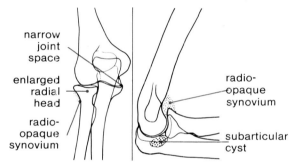

narrow joint space

enlarged radial head

radio-opaque synovium

radio-opaque synovium

subarticular cyst

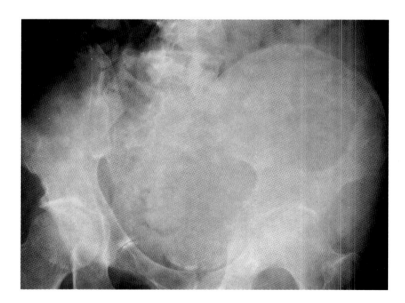

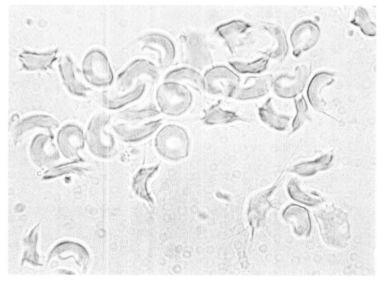

Fig. 21.21 Pelvic radiograph showing a hemophilic pseudotumor. Gross distortion in the pelvis is evident as a result of subperiosteal haemorrhage, which caused a pressure defect in the iliac blade.

Fig. 21.22 Sickle cell disease. Peripheral blood film in a patient homzygous for Hemoglobin S. Many of the red corpuscles are distorted, adopting a sickled shape. Courtesy of Professor J.W. Stewart.

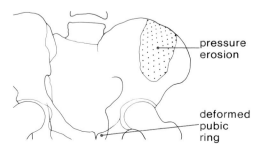

pressure erosion

deformed pubic ring

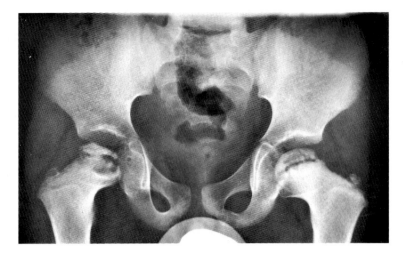

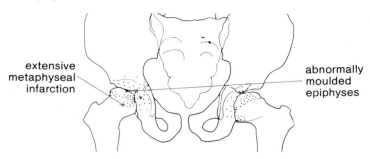

Fig. 21.23 Hip radiograph in sickle cell disease showing aseptic necrosis of the right femoral head with a large metaphyseal defect.

extensive metaphyseal infarction

abnormally moulded epiphyses

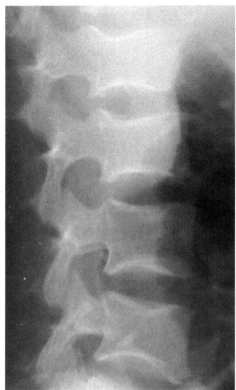

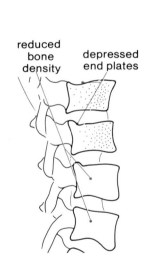

reduced bone density

depressed end plates

Fig. 21.24 Radiograph of the thoraco-lumbar spine in sickle cell disease showing widening of vertebral bodies. There are depressed end plates due to old infarcts and growth arrest.

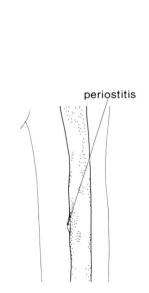

periostitis

Fig. 21.25 Radiograph of the femur in sickle cell disease showing periostitis. Courtesy of Dr. J. Sharp.

Fig. 21.26 Lateral skull radiograph in β-thalassemia showing a typical 'hair-on-end' appearance and alteration of bone trabeculation due to increased marrow volume.

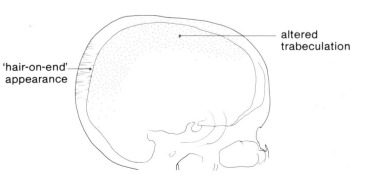

altered trabeculation

'hair-on-end' appearance

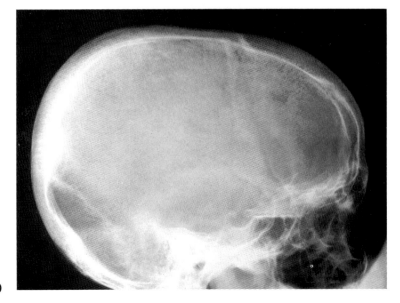

The rheumatological manifestations are caused by the increased volume of bone marrow and by tissue infarction due to cell sludging. Micro-infarction of the small bones of the carpus and tarsus results in episodes of painful swelling of the hands and feet with tenderness of the overlying skin known as the 'hand-foot syndrome'. Micro-infarction occurs in many bones and may result in aseptic necrosis and arthritis (Fig. 21.23). Marrow hyperplasia results in an increased size of marrow cavities with cortical thinning. Radiologically, there may be a coarse trabecular pattern. Vertebral bodies are widened and may develop a 'step' sign due to metaphyseal infarcts (Fig. 21.24), and periostitis may occur in long bones (Fig. 20.25).

CAUSES OF NEUROPATHIC JOINTS

Neurosyphilis	Leprosy
Syringomyelia	Diabetes
Paraplegia	Charcot–Marie–Tooth disease
Myelomeningocele	

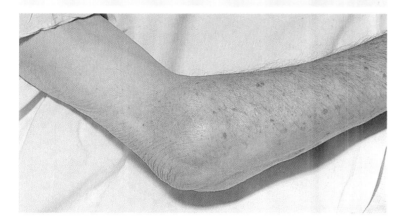

Fig. 21.27 Table of some of the diseases which result in neuropathic (Charcot) joints. The Charcot elbow joint shown here is due to syringomyelia. It is obviously swollen and is grossly unstable.

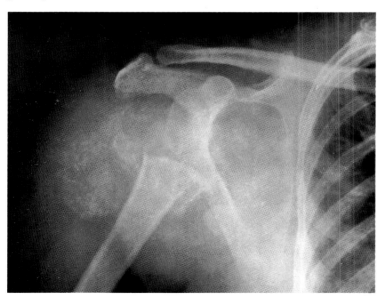

A patient with sickle cell disease is prone to 'sickle-cell crises' which are acute episodes of sickling resulting in small vessel occlusion and hemolysis. If there is a significant vaso-occlusive element then bone pain is a feature. Isotope scans may reveal perfusion abnormalities due to the ischemia, but plain radiographs are usually unchanged. Osteomyelitis, especially due to salmonella, is common in HbS patients.

Certain other hemoglobinopathies may cause musculoskeletal problems. In sickle cell-HbC disease, aseptic necrosis of large joints is a fairly common feature. In thalassemia, the increased marrow volume causes alterations in bone trabeculation seen particularly in the skull (Fig. 21.26) and occasionally spinal cord compression may occur as a result of distortion of vertebral bodies.

Other blood diseases

Gout can result from the increased cell turnover or myeloproliferative diseases. These include polycythemia rubra vera (PRV), leukemias, myelosclerosis and various hemolytic anemias. Treatment of leukemia and other malignant diseases with cytotoxic drugs may also provoke secondary gout. Myeloma may present to the rheumatologist particularly with back pain (see Fig. 21.12), and occasionally causes a polyarthralgia via hypercalcemia.

NEUROPATHIC JOINTS

Several diseases result in gross joint disorganization producing changes sometimes referred to as a Charcot joint (Fig. 21.27). The destruction apparent in the neuropathic joint is often attributed to a diminished sense of pain with impairment of position sense, thus allowing repeated trauma. Relatively painless instability with crepitus is usual.

The radiographic features are variable. There may be considerable sclerosis with new bone formation and loose debris (Fig. 21.28). In the atrophic variety there is attrition and loss of bony bulk. The destruction of involved joints is often a clue to etiology. Syringomyelia commonly affects the shoulders and upper limbs, and

Fig. 21.28 Radiograph of a Charcot shoulder joint showing the truncated shaft of the humerus and calcific debris and bony fragments in the grossly distended sub-deltoid bursa. This patient had syringomyelia.

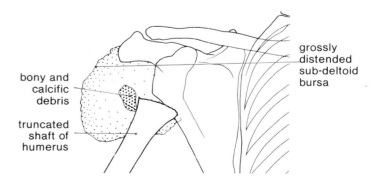

grossly distended sub-deltoid bursa

bony and calcific debris

truncated shaft of humerus

syphilis the knees. Diabetic neuropathy combined with infection and vascular problems can produce a peculiar type of neuropathic change in the feet (Fig. 21.29).

ENDOCRINE DISEASE

A number of endocrine diseases have rheumatological features (Fig. 21.30).

Acromegaly is associated with various arthritic symptoms. Low back pain is very common but movements are

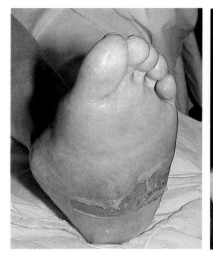 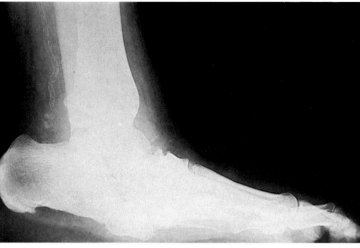 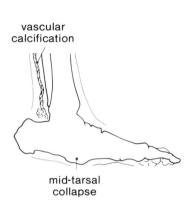

Fig. 21.29 Diabetic neuropathy and vasculopathy. There is gross and originally painless distortion of the foot anatomy (left). Pressure has resulted in an ulcer in the mid-foot which has become infected. The radiograph shows disruption of the intertarsal and tarsometatarsal great joints of the right foot and the interphalangeal joint of the great toe (right). The extensive disruption suggests a Charcot joint; the presence of arterial calcification makes diabetes mellitus a virtually certain diagnosis.

ENDOCRINE DISORDERS AND RHEUMATIC DISEASE

Acromegaly	arthritis entrapment neuropathy
Myxedema	polyarthlagia/arthritis entrapment neuropathy
Thyrotoxicosis	proximal myopathy thyroid acropachy
Diabetes mellitus	cheirarthropathy frozen shoulder neuropathic joints
Hemachromatosis	early osteoarthritis chondrocalcinosis disc calcification

Fig. 21.30 A table of some endocrine diseases and the rheumatological manifestations associated with them.

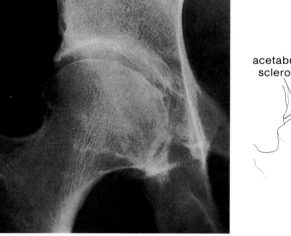 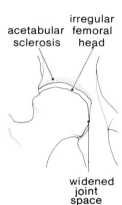

Fig. 21.31 Hip radiograph in a 38-year-old woman with acromegaly. There is joint irregularity and sclerosis due to the development of osteoarthritis.

Fig. 21.32 Shoulder radiograph in acromegalic arthritis showing exaggerted degenerative arthritis with large subarticular cysts and marked osteophyte formation.

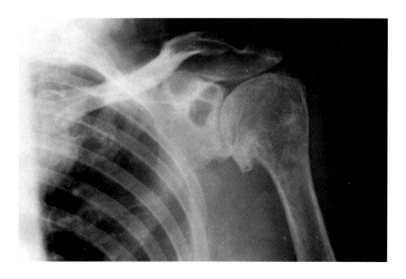 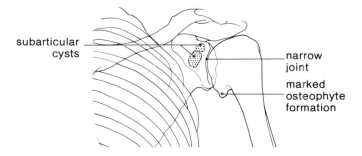

often maintained even when pain is severe. A peripheral arthropathy affects the larger joints; knees, shoulders and hips. Crepitus in affected joints is usual; the radiograph may show widened joint spaces due to thickening of cartilage but subsequent degenerative change may occur (Fig. 21.31). The finding of severe shoulder changes without any preceding history of inflammatory arthritis may suggest a diagnosis of acromegaly (Fig. 21.32). Bony overgrowth may result in a compression neuropathy such as carpal tunnel syndrome.

Diagnosis may be possible from the appearance of the patient (Figs. 21.33–21.35).

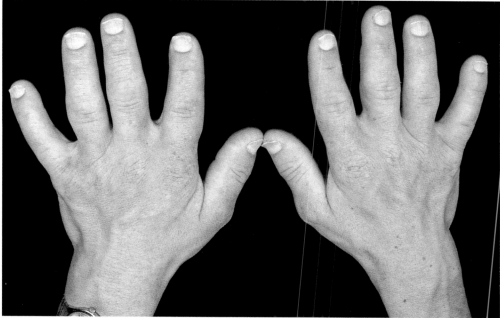

Fig. 21.33 The hands in acromegaly.

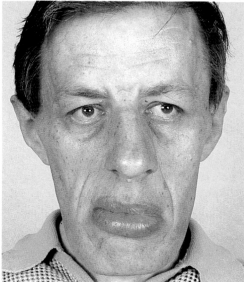
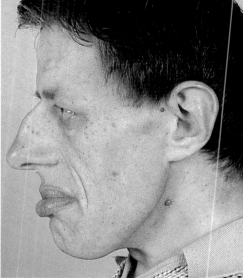

Fig. 21.34 The typical facial appearance of an acromegalic patient. There is overgrowth of the facial rather than skull vault bones producing the typical prognathous appearance.

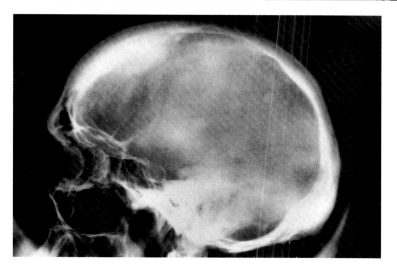

Fig. 21.35 Skull radiograph in acromegaly showing the usual features of a second vault, enlarged paranasal sinuses and an expanded pituitary fossa.

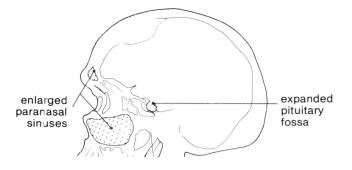

enlarged paranasal sinuses

expanded pituitary fossa

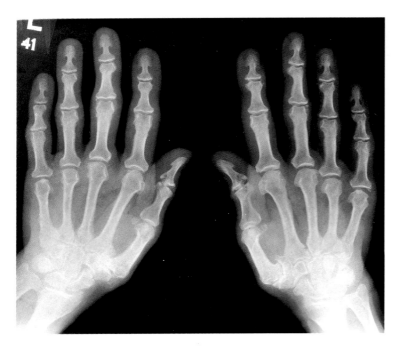

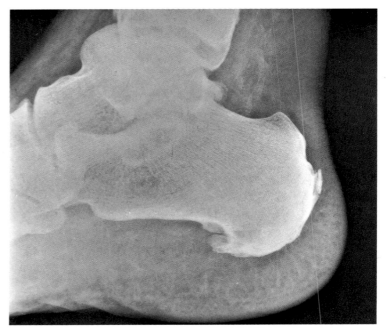

Fig. 21.36 Hand radiograph in acromegaly. Apart from generalized thickening of the soft tissues, joint space width is increased and broadening of the bone results in a 'squared-off' appearance at bone ends with marked enlargement of the terminal tufts.

Fig. 21.37 Lateral radiograph of the foot in a patient with acromegaly. The normal thickness of the heel pad is no more than 21.5mm in the female and 23mm in the male. In this patient the heel pad thickness was 25mm. This may be a useful confirmatory sign in diagnosis.

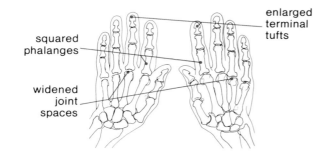

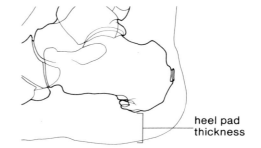

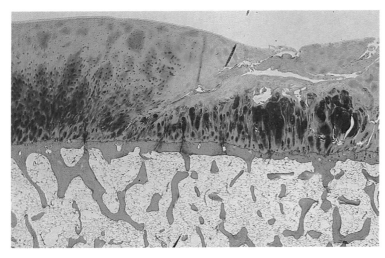

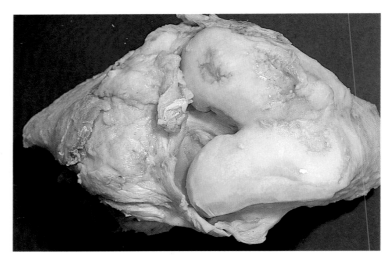

Fig. 21.38 Joint histology in acromegaly. There is heavy calcification in the deeper layers, with cartilage splitting and surface fibrillation. Many chondrocytes are seen on the left and relatively few on the right. H & E stain, x 180. Courtesy of Dr. E.G.L. Bywaters.

Fig. 21.39 Dissected post-mortem knee specimen in acromegaly showing a large condylar ulcer in the cartilage. Courtesy of Professor E.G.L. Bywaters.

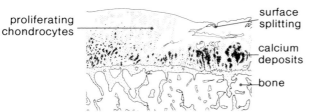

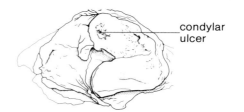

Hand radiographs show widened joint spaces and thickened phalanges with tufting of the terminal phalanges (Fig. 21.36). The heel pad is usually thickened (Fig. 21.37).

Joint histology reveals some synovitis with uneven and excessive proliferation of chondrocytes (Fig. 21.38). The surface cartilage may break down with the formation of well-demarcated ulcers which are a characteristic feature of acromegalic arthritis (Fig. 21.39).

Thyroid disease may present with rheumatological symptoms. Hypothyroidism is commonly associated with carpal tunnel syndrome, and musculoskeletal aches and pains are frequent. A true arthropathy may occur (Fig. 21.40). The synovial fluid is very viscous and may contain crystals (Fig. 21.41). Hyperthyroidism may cause a proximal myopathy. About 0.5% of patients develop thyroid acropachy which often appears after treatment by subtotal thyroidectomy. There is periosteal new bone formation involving the metacarpal and metatarsal bones alone. The forearm is never involved, thus distinguishing it from HPOA and the overlying skin may be thickened, hence the name (Fig. 21.42). Thyroid acropachy may be

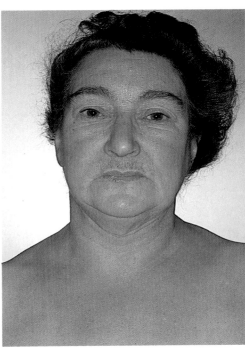
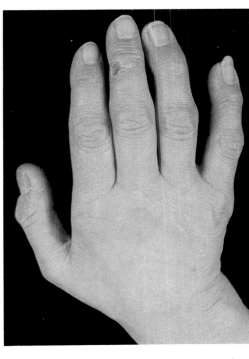
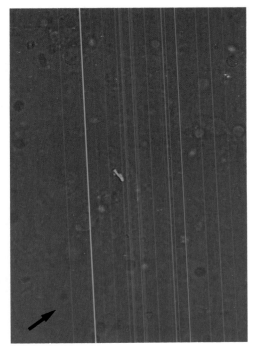

Fig. 21.40 Typical appearance of a patient with myxedema (left) and carpal tunnel syndrome (right). She has burnt her middle finger following the loss of sensation in the distribution of the median nerve.

Fig. 21.41 Smear of synovial fluid under polarized light microscopy showing pyrophosphate crystals in a patient with myxedema. With first order red compensator (arrow).

Fig. 21.42 Hand radiograph of a patient with thyrotoxicosis and thyroid acropachy. Periosteal new bone formation is seen on the mid-shaft of the thumb and index finger metacarpals.

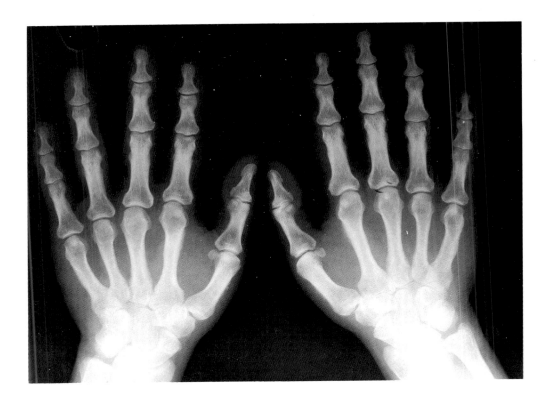

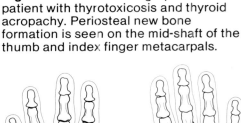

new bone

associated with pretibial myxedema (Fig. 21.43), both appear to be related to LATS (long-acting thyroid stimulator) production and occur in patients with exophthalmos.

Parathyroid disorders may present with joint symptoms either due to bone involvement or associated chondrocalcinosis (Fig. 21.44).

Diabetes mellitus may be associated with the development of neuropathic joints (see above). There is also an increased incidence of shoulder problems, including capsulitis and calcific periarthritis. Diabetic cheiroarthropathy (diabetic stiff hands) is an ill-understood condition characterized by skin thickening and limitation of movement (Fig. 21.45). It is common in Type I diabetes, but the pathogenesis is unclear.

DISORDERS OF LIPID METABOLISM

Hyperlipoproteinemia may cause xanthomata. These may appear as eruptive lesions in skin, and as local deposits in and around tendons (Figs. 21.46 & 21.47), or as lytic lesions in bone, which may produce local symptoms.

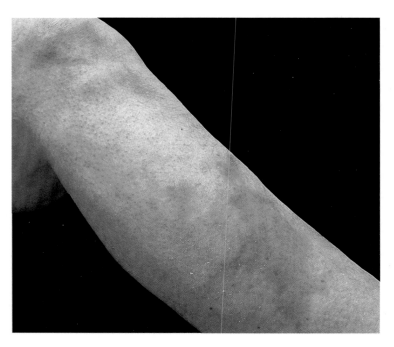

Fig. 21.43 Pretibial myxedema. The skin over the mid-tibial region is thickened and discolored.

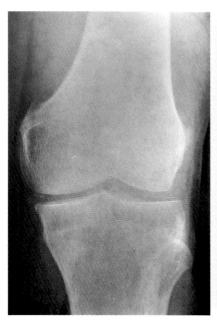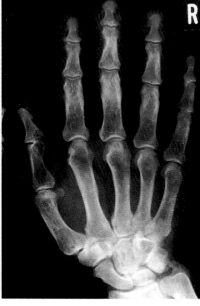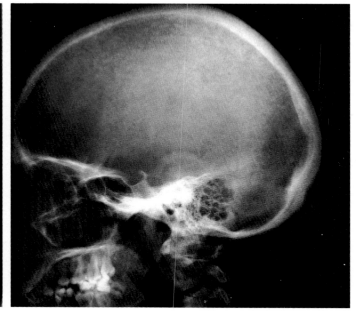

Fig. 21.44 Radiographs of a patient with severe untreated hyperparathyroidism showing cartilage calcification in the knee (left), characteristic phalangeal changes in the hand (middle) and the typical radiographic appearance of the skull – the numerous small translucencies with relatively dense areas between them produce the so-called salt and pepper appearance (right).

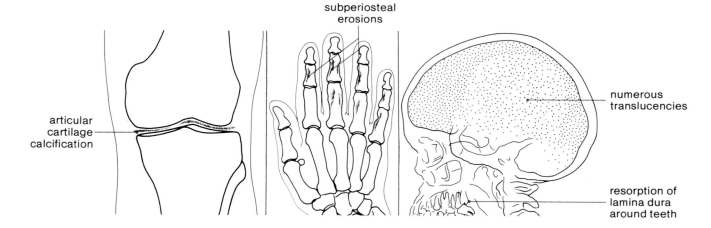

subperiosteal erosions

articular cartilage calcification

numerous translucencies

resorption of lamina dura around teeth

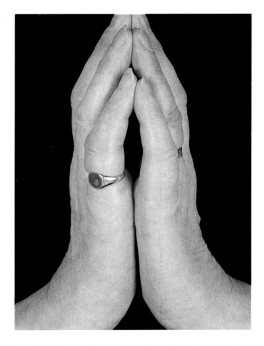

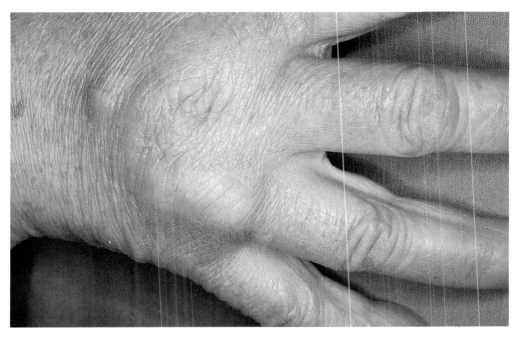

Fig. 21.45 Diabetic cheiroarthropathy. This patient is attempting to place her hands in the prayer position but is unable to straighten the fingers.

Fig. 21.46 Xanthomata involving the extensor tendon sheaths of the middle and ring fingers in a patient with Type 2 hyperlipoproteinemia. Such lesions may occasionally be confused with rheumatoid nodules.

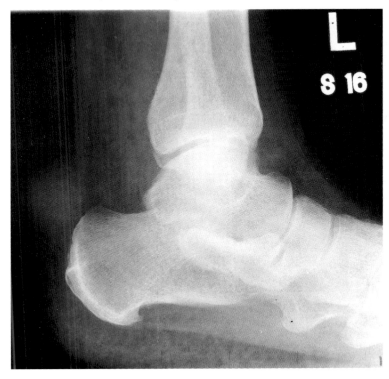

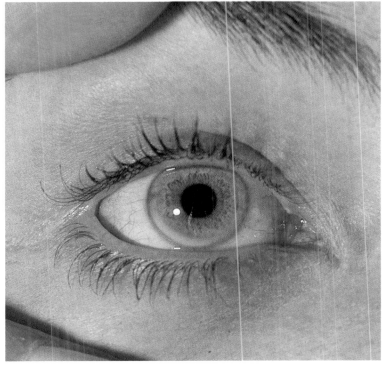

Fig. 21.47 Foot radiograph showing a xanthoma on the Achilles tendon just above its insertion into the os calcis (left)

and hyperlipidemia affecting the eye (right).

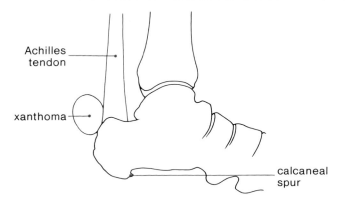

Achilles tendon

xanthoma

calcaneal spur

Type 2 hyperlipoproteinemia is also associated with a rare migratory polyarthritis.

Type 4 hyperlipidemia may also result in a polyarthritis. The joint effusions characteristically contain mono-nuclear cells. In addition, Types 3, 4 and 5 are all associated with hyperuricemia and acute attacks of gout may occur (Fig. 21.48).

MISCELLANEOUS CONDITIONS

Sarcoidosis is associated with two different patterns of arthritis. In 'acute' sarcoid with hilar lymphadenopathy (Fig. 21.49) and erythema nodosum (Fig. 21.50) there is not infrequently a polyarthritis or arthralgia which affects the medium and small sized joints especially the knees, ankles (Fig. 21.51) and wrists. It is usually sym-metrical, remitting without specific treatment and with-out any residual joint destruction.

The second pattern results from sarcoid infiltration in bone and joint; joint effusion is common and this form of arthritis is usually symmetrical. Bone involvement is associated with overlying tender cutaneous nodules (Figs. 21.52 & 21.53). Radiologically there are cystic

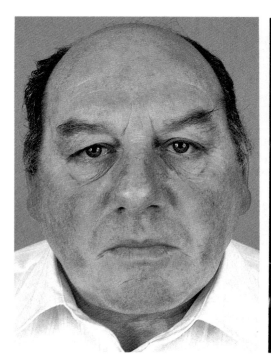
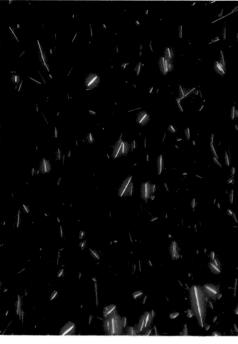

Fig. 21.48 Hyperlipidemia. This patient has Type IV hyperlipidemia. He developed an acute arthritis of the knee joint and birefingent crystals of monosodium urate monohydrate were found in the synovial fluid, using the polarized light microscope.

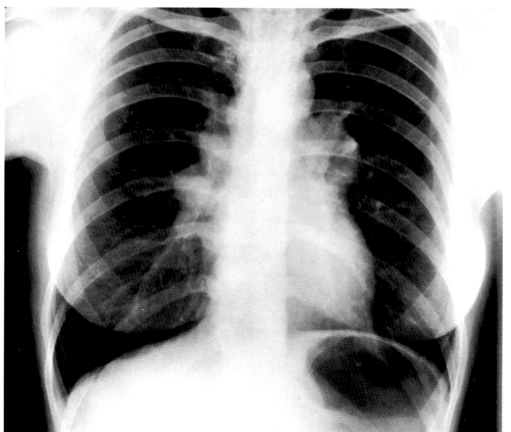

Fig. 21.49 Chest radiograph showing lymphadenopathy due to acute sarcoidosis in a patient who presented with a swollen painful ankle. Note the classical bilateral hilar and right tracheobronchial nodal distribution. The lungs are normal.

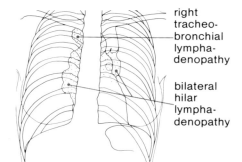

right tracheo-bronchial lympha-denopathy

bilateral hilar lympha-denopathy

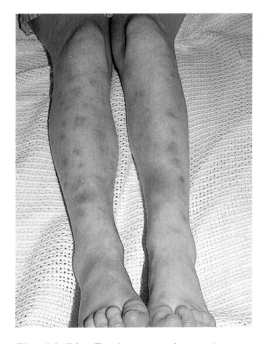

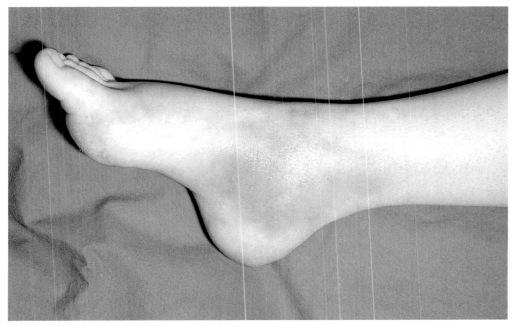

Fig. 21.50 Erythema nodosum in a patient with acute sarcoidosis.

Fig. 21.51 Ankle joint involvement in sarcoidosis.

Fig. 21.52 Chronic sarcoidosis. This patient has typical nasal changes usually referred to as perniotic lupus.

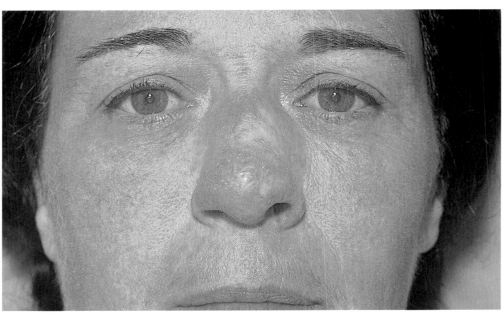

Fig. 21.53 A patient with chronic sarcoidosis showing deformity of several fingers due to granulomatous nodules.

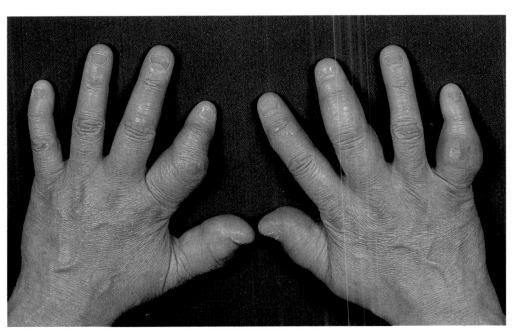

lesions, or an alteration of the normal trabecular pattern of bone which assumes a 'lace-like' quality (Fig. 21.54). Biopsy of involved synovium reveals the typical non-caseating granulomata (Fig. 20.55). This pattern of disease tends to be chronic or relapsing.

Other infiltrative disorders such as primary amyloidosis and Gaucher's disease may affect the bones and joints, and many other systemic disorders have rheumatological manifestations. Some other examples are illustrated in 'Miscellaneous Conditions'.

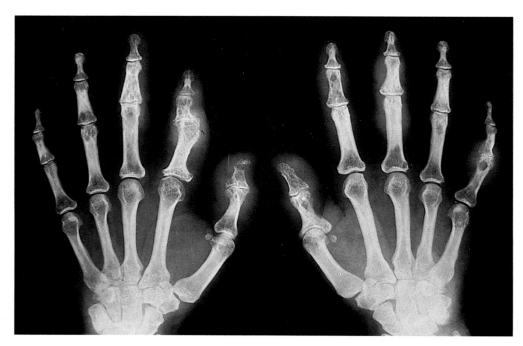

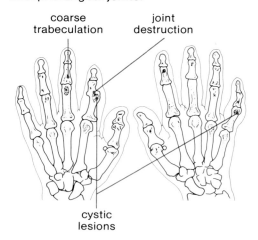

Fig. 21.54 Radiograph of the same patient as in figure 21.53. Typical cystic lesions are seen in several phalanges and there is adjacent joint destruction, in particular in the left index and right little fingers at the proximal interphalangeal joints.

coarse trabeculation

joint destruction

cystic lesions

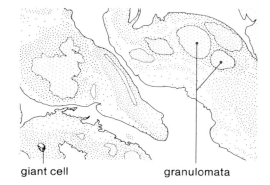

Fig. 21.55 Histology of a cutaneous nodule in sarcoid disease showing the typical non-caseating granulomata of sarcoidosis. H & E stain, x 400.

giant cell

granulomata

22

Bone and Collagen Diseases

with Dr. John A. Kanis

Metabolic bone disease impinges on many specialities. Patients may present to endocrinologists, orthopedic surgeons and nephrologists, as well as to rheumatologists, and the many manifestations of these diseases include articular signs and symptoms.

Generalized bone disease is a significant cause of morbidity and mortality. Of greatest clinical and socio-economic importance is osteoporosis, which clinically affects several million people. Very many people have Paget's disease but only some 5% of these are symptomatic. Other disorders of bone and connective tissue are less common but the management of osteomalacia, rickets and the bone disease of chronic renal failure still forms an important component of clinical practice.

Bone Structure and Turnover

Bone is a living tissue and after maturity undergoes a continual process of remodelling. Between 2 and 5% of the adult skeleton is renewed annually, this renewal being regulated by the numbers and activity of bone cells. In mature bone three main cell types occur (Fig. 22.1). The major constituent of bone matrix is Type I collagen, which is largely responsible for the tensile strength of bone. The mineral component of bone is predominantly calcium and phosphate in the form of hydroxyapatite. The skeleton consists of cortical (compact) and cancellous (trabecular) bone which may be affected by bone disease in different ways (Fig. 22.2). Examination of trabecular bone provides a sensitive index of disturbed bone remodeling.

Bone formation and resorption rates can be deduced from kinetic or histological studies (Fig. 22.3). In the latter case, administration of tetracycline – which is incorporated into bone at sites of active mineralization and fluoresces under UV light – can be used to determine the extent of the bone surface being mineralized; if two doses are given separated by a known interval the rate of calcification can be measured. A less direct but more readily measured index of bone formation is based on the estimation of plasma alkaline phosphatase, which is in part derived from osteoblasts. A simple biochemical estimate of bone matrix degradation is the measurement of urinary hydroxyproline. Different disorders may be characterized by different relationships between for-

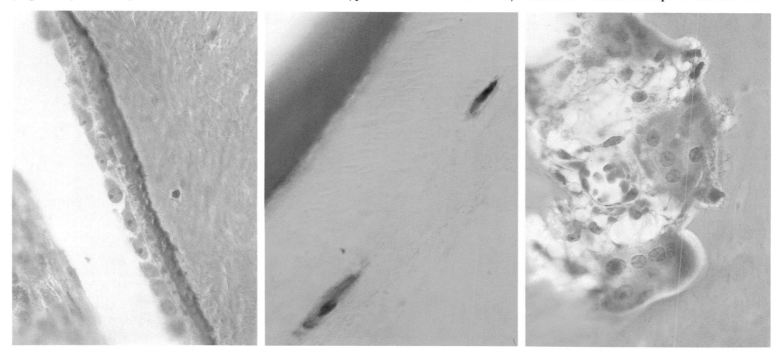

Fig. 22.1 Bone cell types. Using Goldner's stain mineralized bone appears green and osteoid red. Osteoid synthesis by *osteoblasts* (left); *osteocytes*, which control calcium homeostasis, buried in bone (middle), bone resorption by multinucleate *osteoclasts* (right).

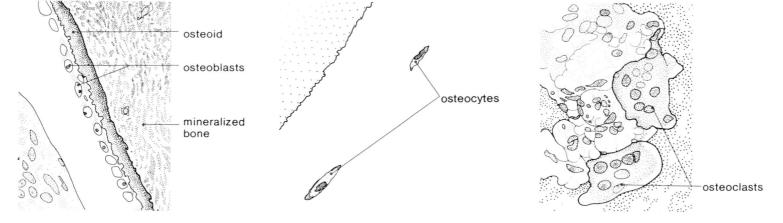

mation and resorption; thus in Paget's disease skeletal balance is often normal whereas in myelomatosis resorption is proportionately increased (Fig. 22.4). However, the relationship may also change with age so that in the elderly the rate of bone resorption exceeds formation and gives rise to a negative skeletal balance. However, it is difficult to achieve a sustained change in the relationship between formation and resorption with therapeutic agents.

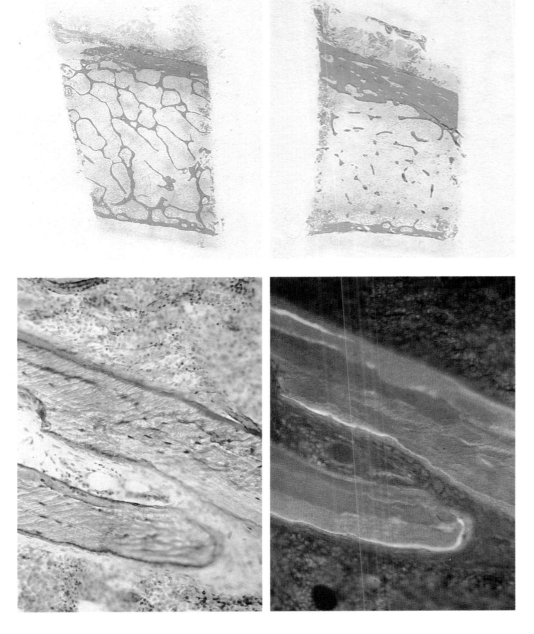

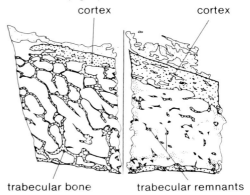

Fig. 22.2 Transiliac trephine biopsies in osteoporosis showing cortical loss with preservation of trabecular architecture (left) and cortical preservation with marked trabecular bone loss (right). Goldner's stain x 2.5

Fig. 22.3 Trabecular bone mineralization. Sites of active mineralization detected by the dark staining at the osteoid-mineral interface (toluidine blue, left) and tetracycline label incorporated at this site fluorescing under ultraviolet light (right). x 150.

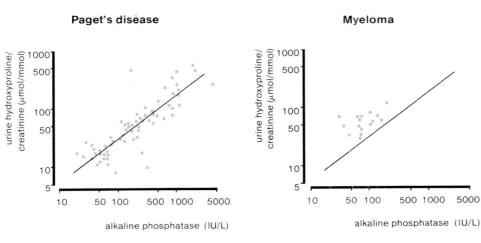

Fig. 22.4 Biochemistry of bone remodelling. Urinary hydroxyproline/creatinine ratio (measuring resorption) plotted against plasma alkaline phosphatase (measuring formation). In Paget's disease skeletal balance is maintained (left) whereas in myeloma resorption is proportionately increased (right).

Osteoporosis and Osteosclerosis

Osteoporosis is a diminution of bone mass without detectable change in the ratio of mineral to non-mineralized matrix and this distinguishes the condition from osteomalacia where the proportion of osteoid to calcified bone is increased (Fig. 22.5). Many disorders are associated with osteoporosis (Fig. 22.6) but the greatest problem in terms of the number of affected patients is due to osteoporosis associated with ageing, particularly ·in post-menopausal women.

A variety of techniques are available for measuring bone loss. With the exception of balance and kinetic studies they depend on indirect determinations of skeletal mass repeated at intervals; the rate of bone loss in osteoporosis may be small compared to the methodological errors (Fig. 22.7). Radiological reproducibility can be improved by using standardized radiographs and aluminium step wedges, but other techniques such as photon-absorptiometry or CT scanning are not widely available. Irrespective of the methods used it is clear that from the age of forty onwards there is a progressive loss of trabecular and cortical skeletal matrix (Fig. 22.8). Trabecular bone loss gives rise to vertebral fractures whereas significant cortical bone loss occurring in later life accounts for fracture of the femoral neck. While a diminution in bone mass may be one of the factors leading to skeletal failure (Fig. 22.9), a decrease in bone turnover and delayed repair of microfractures may also contribute (Fig. 22.10).

The cause of senile osteoporosis is unclear but it is probably multifactorial. These factors include the skeletal mass at maturity, nutritional factors, endocrine abnormalities (particularly the menopause) and immobilization (Fig. 22.11).

Osteosclerosis implies an increase in skeletal mass. This may be associated with decreased tensile strength of

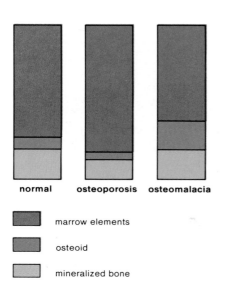

normal   osteoporosis   osteomalacia

■ marrow elements

■ osteoid

□ mineralized bone

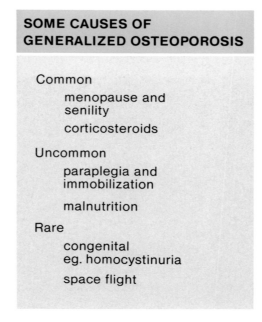

SOME CAUSES OF GENERALIZED OSTEOPOROSIS

Common
   menopause and senility
   corticosteroids

Uncommon
   paraplegia and immobilization
   malnutrition

Rare
   congenital eg. homocystinuria
   space flight

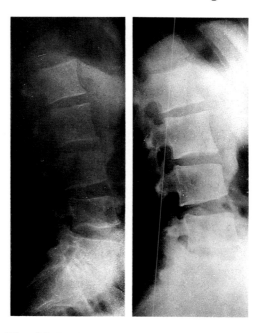

Fig. 22.5 Variations in the three elements of bone tissue in osteoporosis and osteomalacia. In osteoporosis there is a diminution in mineralized bone and osteoid, whereas in osteomalacia there is an increase in osteoid due to delay in mineralization.

Fig. 22.6 Some causes of generalized osteoporosis.

Fig. 22.7 Radiographs of the same patient taken three minutes apart using different techniques. These illustrate the difficulties in using radiographs to measure bone loss.

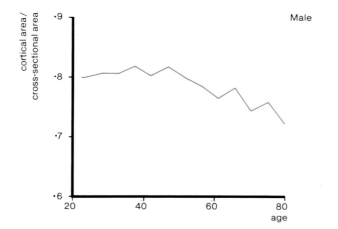

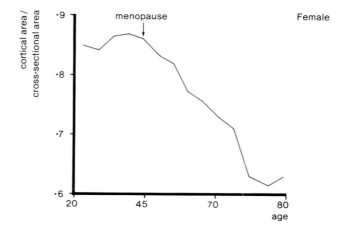

Fig. 22.8 Metacarpal morphometry showing the cortical area, expressed as a proportion of total cross-sectional area, as a function of age in men and women. Progressive loss after the age of forty is more pronounced in females. (After Nordin.)

bone so that fracture occurs. Important causes of generalized osteosclerosis include severe secondary hyperparathyroidism seen in chronic renal failure, fluor-osis, familial hypophosphatemic osteomalacia, carcinoma of the prostate and Albers-Schönberg or 'marble bone' disease.

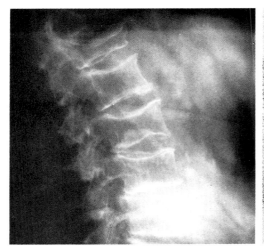 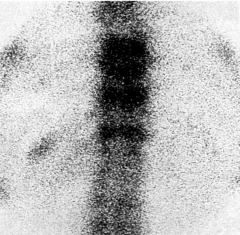 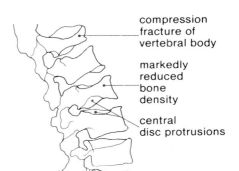

Fig. 22.9 Spinal osteoporosis. The lateral radiograph shows markedly reduced bone density (with apparent accentuation of the end-plates) and several compressions with loss of height and concavity or wedging (left). The isotope bone scan (right) shows the symmetrical, diffuse increased uptake typical of recent fractures.

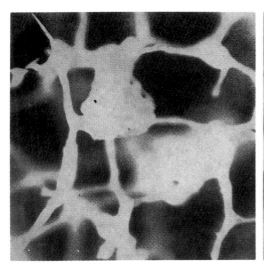 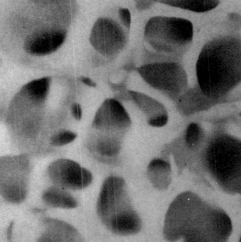 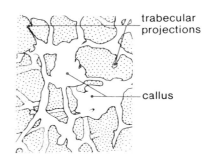

Fig. 22.10 Trabecular bone from an osteoporotic patient (left) and normal subject (right). Note the sparse and thin trabeculae in osteoporosis and also the presence of microfractures with callus formation. x 35.

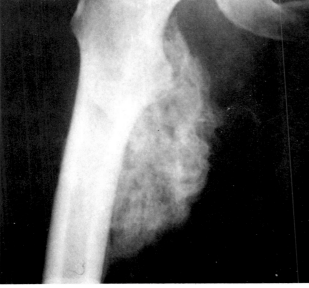 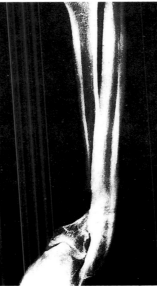 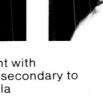 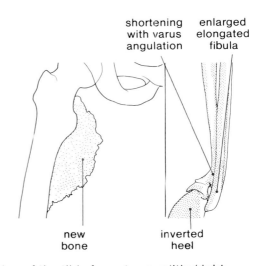

Fig. 22.11 Radiograph of the femur of a patient with paraplegia showing heterotopic bone formation secondary to rapid bone loss (left) and hypertrophy of the fibula subsequent to excision of the tibia for osteomyelitis (right, courtesy of Mr. J. Chalmers).

Paget's Disease

Osteitis deformans or Paget's disease of bone is characterized by enhanced formation and destruction of bone with an irregular distribution in the body. It affects approximately 4% of the population aged forty or over, but symptoms are rare, occurring in perhaps 5% of this age group. Abnormal osteoclastic proliferation, possibly due to a slow virus infection (Fig. 22.12), gives rise to rapid destruction of bone tissue which is then repaired. As the activity of the disease progresses, woven or non-lamellar bone is laid down and the normal architectural pattern is lost (Fig. 22.13). Although the overall formation and resorption of bone are closely matched, in any one area bone resorption may exceed formation and vice versa (Fig. 22.14). Thus, under steady state conditions both plasma alkaline phosphatase and urinary hydroxyproline are increased but there is no marked disturbance in plasma calcium unless the net bone balance is temporarily disturbed. This may occur during immobilization when the rate of resorption exceeds formation so that hypercalcemia and hypercalciuria develop. Most of the complications in Paget's disease arise because the diseased bone is structurally abnormal (Fig. 22.15). This gives rise to characteristic clinical and radiographic features (Figs. 22.16–22.21). Osteoarthritis often occurs in adjacent joints and it may be difficult to distinguish pain due to Paget's disease (usually unrelated to activity) from that of the joints (usually exacerbated by movement and weight-bearing).

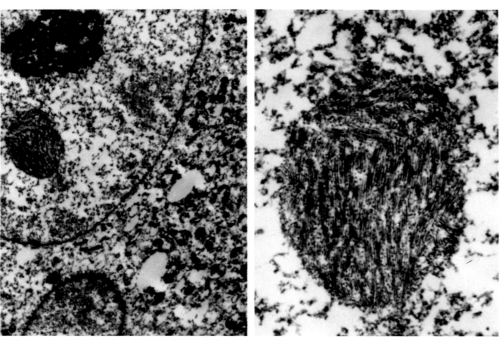

Fig. 22.12 Paget's disease. Electron micrograph showing inclusion bodies in the nucleus of an affected osteoclast (left, x 4500). Under high power they appear to share the morphological characteristics of the paramyxovirus group (right, x 14,000). Courtesy Dr. L. Harvey.

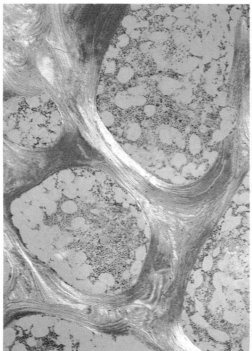
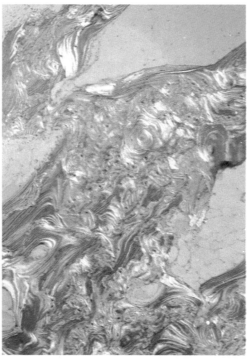

Fig. 22.13 Sections of trabecular bone showing the characteristics of normal lamellar bone (left) and woven bone (right) in Paget's disease. Note that lamellar bone is laid down in the direction of the long axis of the trabeculae. In Paget's disease, where bone turnover is greatly augmented, waves of osteoclast and osteoblast activity result in a mosaic disorganized appearance. Toluidine blue stain, x 650.

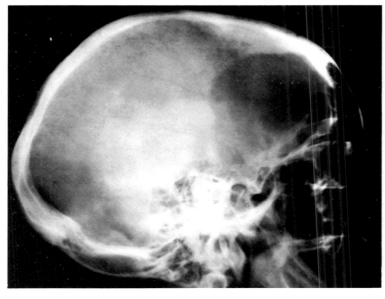
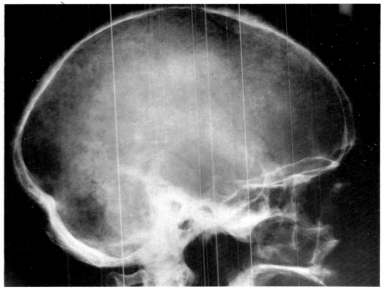

Fig. 22.14 Skull radiographs in Paget's disease. Wave of bone resorption ('osteoporosis circumscripta') in an early case appearing as a localized discrete area of radiolucency (left). Typical patchy osteosclerosis and osteolysis with platybasia and basilar invagination. The odontoid peg is above a notional line drawn from the foramen magnum to the hard palate (left).

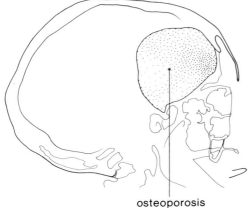

osteoporosis circumscripta

abnormal coarse trabecular pattern with sclerosis and lysis

tip of odontoid peg

Fig. 22.15 Complications of Paget's disease.

Fig. 22.16 Paget's disease of the lumbar spine showing an expanded vertebral body and involvement of the neural arches with marked sclerosis of the end-plates giving rise to a 'picture frame' appearance (left). In the absence of bony expansion it may be difficult to distinguish osteosclerosis due to Paget's disease from that due to prostatic carcinoma (right).

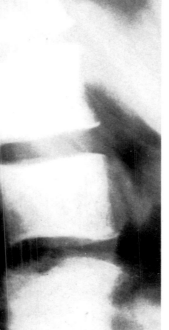
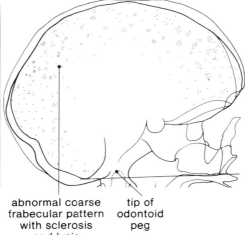

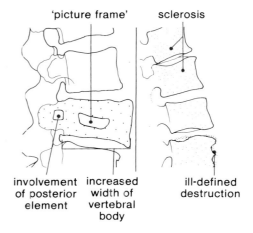

'picture frame'   sclerosis

involvement of posterior element

increased width of vertebral body

ill-defined destruction

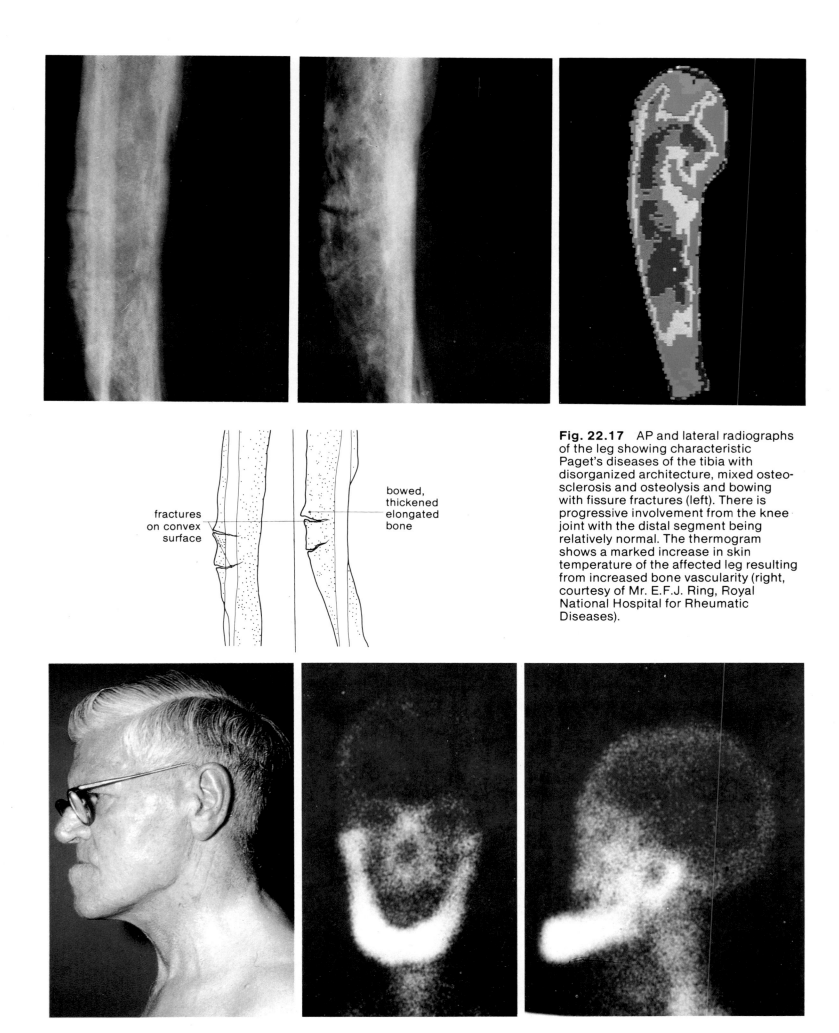

fractures
on convex
surface

bowed,
thickened
elongated
bone

Fig. 22.17 AP and lateral radiographs of the leg showing characteristic Paget's diseases of the tibia with disorganized architecture, mixed osteosclerosis and osteolysis and bowing with fissure fractures (left). There is progressive involvement from the knee joint with the distal segment being relatively normal. The thermogram shows a marked increase in skin temperature of the affected leg resulting from increased bone vascularity (right, courtesy of Mr. E.F.J. Ring, Royal National Hospital for Rheumatic Diseases).

Fig. 22.18 Paget's disease of the jaw. The technetium bone scans shows marked isotope uptake.

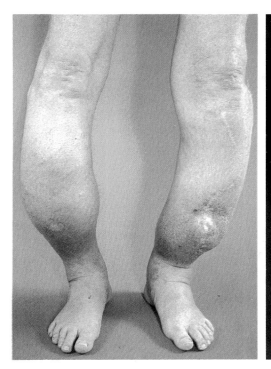 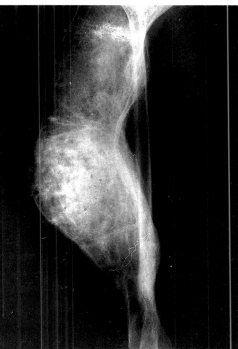

Fig. 22.19 Paget's disease of the tibia giving rise to severe deformity and ulceration of the overlying skin. Note the distal part of the tibia is at present unaffected.

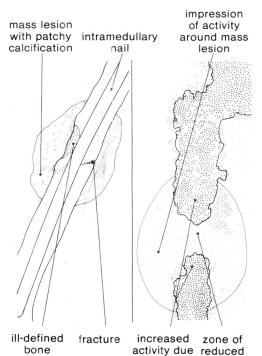

Fig. 22.20 A patient with Paget's disease involving the right thigh and leg resulting in a diffuse enlargement. He presented with rapidly increasing pain after a pathological fracture had been treated by pinning.

Fig. 22.21 Radiograph of the femur of the same patient as in figure 22.20, revealing the pathological fracture in the Pagetic bone and showing extension of calcification outside the cortical bone (left). This mass is ill-defined on the bone scan (right). The appearances are characteristic of osteogenic sarcoma.

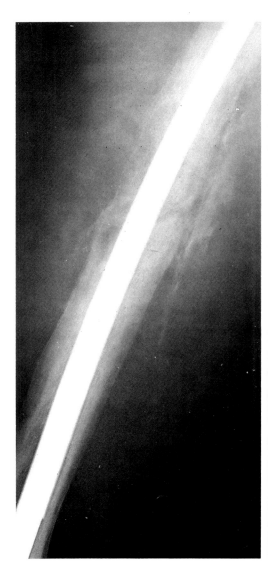 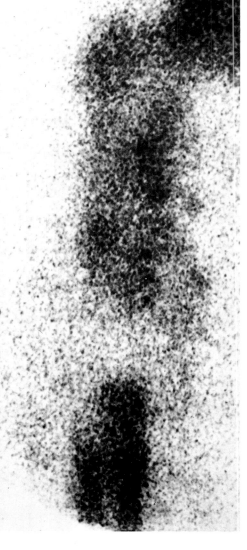

mass lesion with patchy calcification

intramedullary nail

impression of activity around mass lesion

ill-defined bone destruction due to sarcoma

fracture

increased activity due to Paget's disease

zone of reduced activity

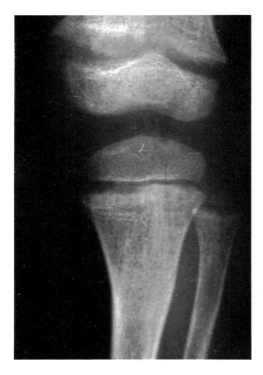

Fig. 22.22 Radiographic appearance of rickets in childhood. Note the widened epiphyseal seam and splayed metaphyses.

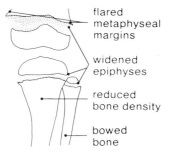

- flared metaphyseal margins
- widened epiphyses
- reduced bone density
- bowed bone

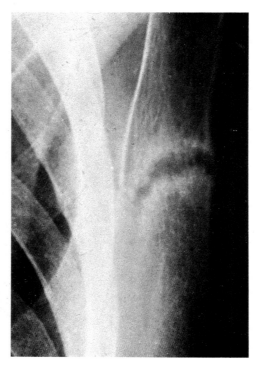

Fig. 22.23 Radiograph demonstrating a Looser's zone in the humerus.

- Looser's zone
- slightly expanded bone width
- sclerosis
- markedly reduced bone density and cortical thickness

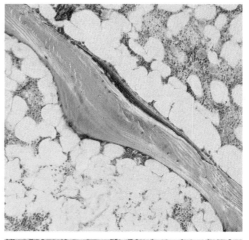

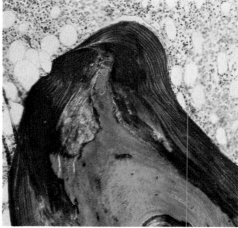

Fig. 22.24 Histology of normal (upper) and osteomalacic (lower) bone showing osteoid accumulation (stained red). More than twenty lamellae are seen – normally not more than four should be visible. Goldner's stain, polarized light, x 850.

CAUSES OF OSTEOMALACIA

Common
    abnormalities in vitamin D
    supply or metabolism

    vitamin D resistance

Uncommon
    renal tubular acidosis

    phosphate or calcium
    depletion
    eg. antacid abuse

Rare
    multiple renal tubular
    abnormalities
    eg. cystinosis

    drugs eg. fluoride and
    aluminium

Fig. 22.25 Causes of osteomalacia.

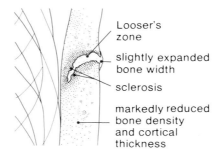

7-dehydrocholesterol   dietary intake

ultraviolet light

cholecalciferol D₃

liver hydroxylase

25 (OH) D₃

kidney 24 – hydroxylase   kidney 1α – hydroxylase

24,25 (OH)₂ D₃   **1,25 (OH)₂ D₃**

Fig. 22.26 The intermediary metabolism of vitamin D. Disorders may arise because of an inadequate supply of vitamin D, its impaired metabolism or target organ resistance.

DISORDERS RELATED TO IMPAIRED METABOLISM OF VITAMIN D

Privational deficiency
    eg. inadequate diet
        inadequate exposure to
        ultraviolet light

Malabsorption of vitamin D,
calcium and/or phosphate
    eg. pancreatic disease
        gastric surgery

Abnormal metabolism of
25–OHD

Defective production of
1, 25 (OH)₂ D₃
    eg. hypoparathyroidism
        renal impairment

Target organ resistance
    eg. celiac disease

Fig. 22.27 Disorders related to impaired metabolism of vitamin D.

22.10

Osteomalacia and Rickets

These are terms used to describe the delay between the production of organic bone matrix and its subsequent mineralization. Rickets is a disorder of childhood in which the disturbance of calcification is most marked at the epiphyseal growth plates. Vitamin D deficiency also delays cartilage cell maturation and this contributes to the increased thickness of the epiphyseal plates (Fig. 22.22). Looser's zones are diagnostic (Fig. 22.23) but osteomalacia commonly exists without radiographic abnormalities. The characteristic histological finding in osteomalacia is an increase in the osteoid (non-mineralized) matrix due to delay in mineralization (Fig. 22.24). Whereas normal mineralization depends on the presence of vitamin D not all forms of osteomalacia are due to disturbances in vitamin D metabolism (Fig. 22.25). Furthermore, osteomalacia is not necessarily the cause of excessive amounts of osteoid which are also seen in Paget's disease, hyperparathyroidism, fracture repair and thyrotoxicosis, where the rates of matrix formation are increased.

Vitamin D must undergo a series of further metabolic steps before becoming biologically active (Fig. 22.26) and bone disease may arise because of inadequate supply, or defective metabolism, of the vitamin. The usual cause of vitamin D deficiency in Europe is a combination of dietary and ultraviolet deprivation commonly seen in infancy and adolescence in large cities, particularly in the Asian communities. Vitamin D deficiency may also arise in intestinal malabsorption, particularly if this is associated with steatorrhoea. In all these disorders plasma values of 25-hydroxyvitamin D (25-OHD) are low and its measurement provides a useful index of the vitamin D status. An increasing number of disorders have been recognized to be due to disturbances in the production of 1,25 dihydroxy vitamin D (1,25 $(OH)_2D_3$) (Fig. 22.27). These disorders are collectively described as 'vitamin D resistant' since the doses of vitamin D necessary to achieve a therapeutic effect (10,000–200,000 IU) are greater than normal physiological requirements (20–1000 IU).

Clinical features of rickets in children include pain, deformity, fracture, myopathy and delayed growth, in addition to the characteristic radiological features. Appearances on bone scanning are variable (Fig. 22.28).

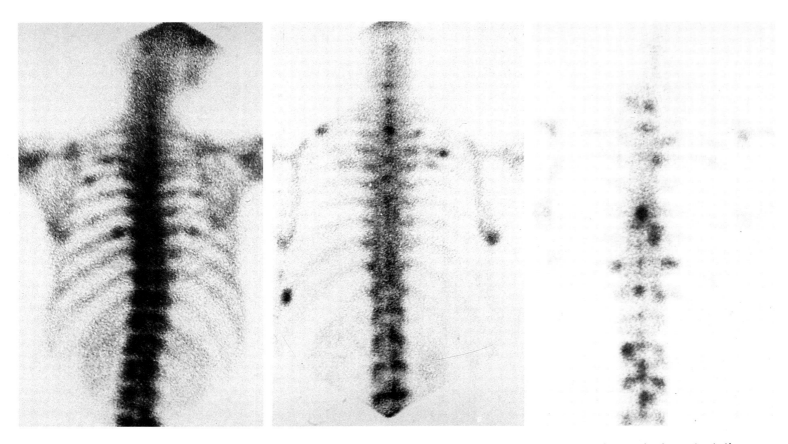

Fig. 22.28 Isotope scanning in osteomalacia. Generalized marked increase in uptake (left) and hot spots at fracture sites which are commonly bilateral and symmetrical (middle). This contrasts with the asymmetric uptake in metastatic disease (right).

Biochemical abnormalities (Fig. 22.29) include low plasma calcium due to impaired calcium absorption from the gut and impaired effectiveness of parathyroid hormone (PTH) in mobilizing calcium from bone. Many of the disorders associated with osteomalacia and rickets are characterized by low plasma phosphate due to mal-absorption and secondary hyperparathyroidism. There are several disorders of mineralization in which plasma phosphate may be low due to defective renal tubular reabsorption of phosphate, but levels of $1,25 (OH)_2D_3$ are normal. It may occur as an isolated defect, or in association with other renal tubular or systemic abnormalities. X-linked hypophosphatemia is an inherited disease with markedly variable phenotypic expression. Plasma calcium is characteristically normal but plasma phosphate is very low. Radiographic features may include increased cortical thickness and extra-osseous calcification, particularly in paraspinal ligaments (Fig. 22.30). Fluorosis or severe secondary hyperparathyroidism may also give rise to osteosclerosis associated with osteomalacia.

Renal Bone Disease
The skeletal disorders found in chronic renal failure are collectively termed renal osteodystrophy, and may occur singly or in various combinations. By the time patients with progressive chronic renal failure are about to start dialysis treatment the majority have histological abnormalities of bone, but skeletal symptoms are only present in a minority (less than 10%). However, the biochemical disturbances which give rise to bone disease commonly have other manifestations.

The major features of bone disease are osteitis fibrosa, thought to be due to increased secretion of PTH, and

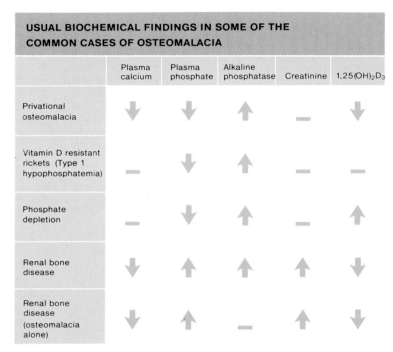

USUAL BIOCHEMICAL FINDINGS IN SOME OF THE COMMON CASES OF OSTEOMALACIA

	Plasma calcium	Plasma phosphate	Alkaline phosphatase	Creatinine	$1,25(OH)_2D_3$
Privational osteomalacia	↓	↓	↑	–	↓
Vitamin D resistant rickets (Type 1 hypophosphatemia)	–	↓	↑	–	–
Phosphate depletion	–	↓	↑	–	↑
Renal bone disease	↓	↑	↑	↑	↓
Renal bone disease (osteomalacia alone)	↓	↑	–	↑	↓

Fig. 22.29 Usual biochemical findings in osteomalacia.

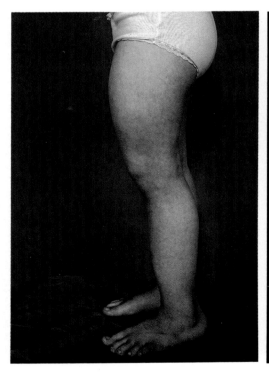

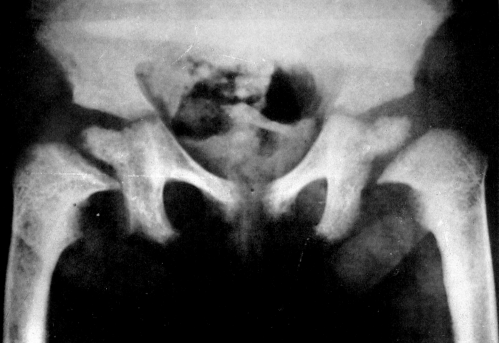

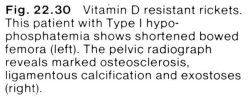

Fig. 22.30 Vitamin D resistant rickets. This patient with Type I hypophosphatemia shows shortened bowed femora (left). The pelvic radiograph reveals marked osteosclerosis, ligamentous calcification and exostoses (right).

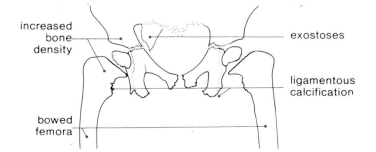

osteomalacia related to impaired renal production of 1,25 (OH)$_2$D$_3$ (Fig. 22.31). Changes in dialysis-treated patients are sometimes due to aluminium toxicity (see Fig. 22.47). Hyperparathyroid bone disease gives rise to subperiosteal bone erosion, periosteal new bone formation, fracture and, in adolescence, progressive skeletal deformity (Fig. 22.32). In adolescence severe hyperparathyroid bone disease may resemble rickets on radiography (Figs. 22.33–34).

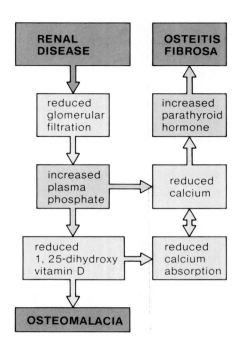

Fig. 22.31 Pathogenesis of renal bone disease.

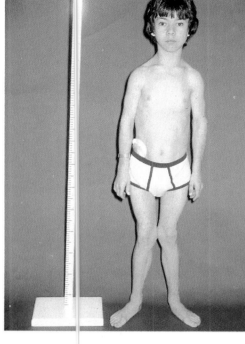

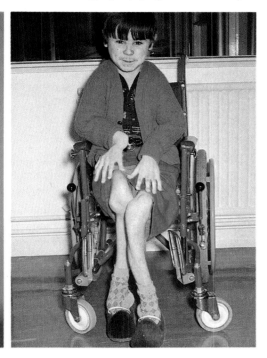

Fig. 22.32 Characteristic valgus knee deformities in osteomalacia due to renal failure (left) and metaphyseal resorption and deformity in hyperparathyroid bone disease (right).

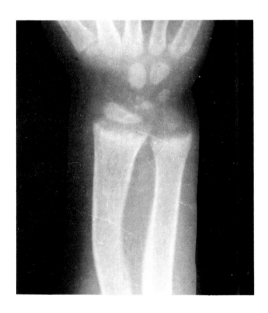

Fig. 22.33 Hand radiograph in renal osteomalacia showing widened epiphyseal margins and flared metaphyses.

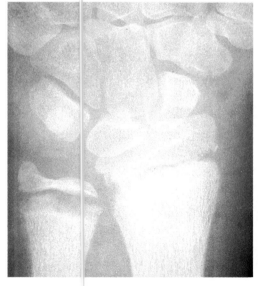

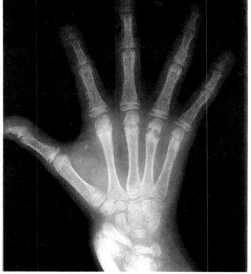

Fig. 22.34 Hand radiographs in hyperparathyroid bone disease. The apparent increase in size of the epiphyseal plate is due to metaphyseal resorption (left). The distal metaphyseal end is not splayed. When untreated, serious deformity may occur (right). Note also the terminal phalangeal resorption.

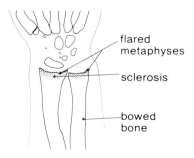

flared metaphyses

sclerosis

bowed bone

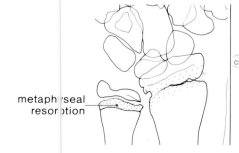

metaphyseal resorption

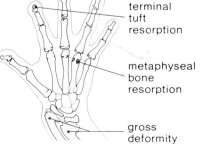

terminal tuft resorption

metaphyseal bone resorption

gross deformity

Progressive decrease in bone mass is common in patients on dialysis treatment, but osteoporosis is not invariable and patchy osteosclerosis of trabecular bone is also found (Fig. 22.35). Biochemical indicators of increased bone cell activity include raised plasma values of PTH, alkaline phosphatase and hydroxyproline. Osteomalacia is characterized by an increase in the amount of unmineralized bone matrix but it is important to distinguish increased amounts of osteoid due to augmented bone turnover from that due to a defect in its mineralization. In chronic renal failure osteomalacia and hyperparathyroidism commonly coexist. They can be distinguished by histological measurements on bone biopsy which estimate the rate of mineralization, for example by labelling with tetracycline (see Fig. 22.3).

The skeletal manifestations or renal bone disease include bone pain, bone tenderness, fractures, retardation of growth, joint disease and soft tissue calcification. Vascular calcification may interfere with access for dialysis. In renal units with a high incidence of osteomalacia reflecting a dialysis-induced cause (probably aluminium toxicity), indolent fractures occur.

Bone Disease and Hormones

The major calcium-regulating hormones are PTH, calcitonin and $1,25 (OH)_2D_3$. However, a variety of other hormones are known to influence skeletal metabolism and disturbances in their metabolism may give rise to bone disease.

Hyperparathyroidism

Primary hyperparathyroidism is a disorder due to auto-nomous hyperfunction of one or more parathyroid glands usually due to parathyroid adenoma (Fig. 22.36) and more rarely due to hyperplasia or carcinoma. In secondary hyperparathyroidism excess parathyroid hormone is produced because of the low ionized calcium concentration due to other causes, such as vitamin D deficiency. Additional disorders of parathyroid secretion include tertiary hyperparathyroidism, in which parathyroid tumors arise from prolonged secondary hyperparathyroidism, usually associated with chronic renal failure or intestinal malabsorption. Several features of primary hyperparathyroidism, especially hypercalcemia, may occur in association with malignant tumors.

The manifestations of primary hyperparathyroidism are mainly due to hypercalcemia. Approximately 50% of patients present with renal stone disease and primary hyperparathyroidism accounts for approximately 5% of patients with this problem. Radiographically evident bone disease is uncommon. Subperiosteal resorption of bone is characteristic of hyperparathyroid bone disease but is not usually as marked as in renal disease (Fig. 22.37, upper). In contrast, brown tumors, comprising fibrous tissue and osteoclasts (Fig. 22.37, lower), are rarely seen in renal bone disease and may give rise to pathological fracture. Associated disorders include multiple endocrine adenomata, gout, hypothyroidism, Paget's disease and diabetes mellitus; since the last four of these conditions are relatively common, the association may not always be causal. Chondrocalcinosis often develops, its frequency depending on the duration and severity of the hyperparathyroidism.

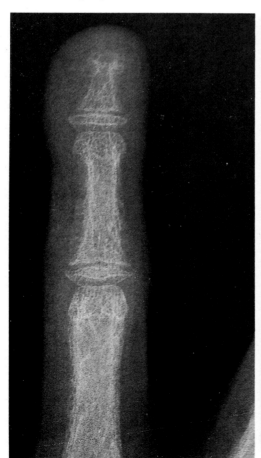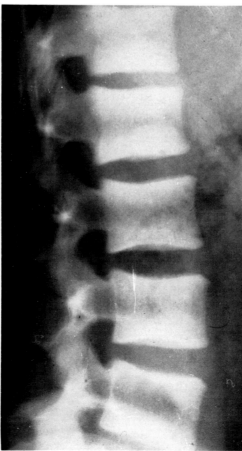

Fig. 22.35 Radiographic features of renal bone disease. A pathognomic feature of severe hyperparathyroidism is subperiosteal resorption of bone most marked in the radial border of the middle phalanx (left). Note also the marked intracortical erosion. In the spine osteosclerosis gives rise to alternate bands of osteosclerosis and osteoporosis to give the so-called 'rugger-jersey spine' appearance (right).

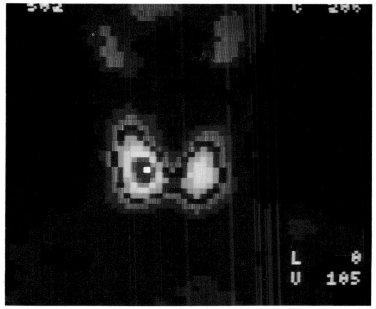

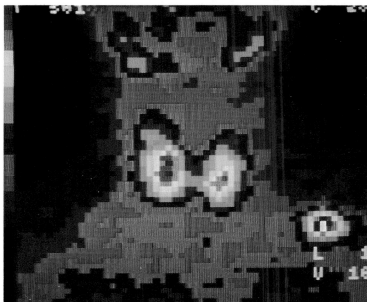

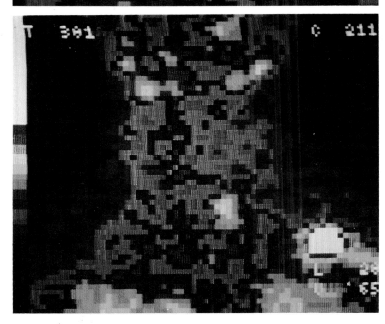

Fig. 22.36 Subtraction scan identification of a parathyroid adenoma. ^{99M}Tc scan with uptake in thyroid tissue (upper) and ^{251}Thallous chloride scan with uptake in vascular tissue (middle). Subtraction unmasks the vascular adenoma on the left side (lower). Courtesy of Dr. I. Blake and Mr. J. Williams.

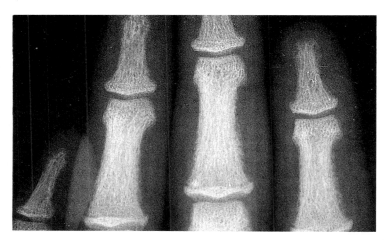

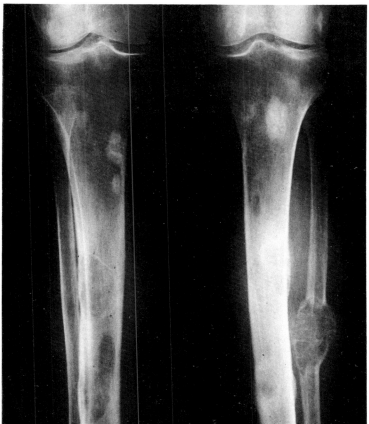

Fig. 22.37 Radiographic features of hyperparathyroidism. Subperiosteal resorption (upper) and lytic lesions due to brown tumors (lower, courtesy of Professor M. Kahn).

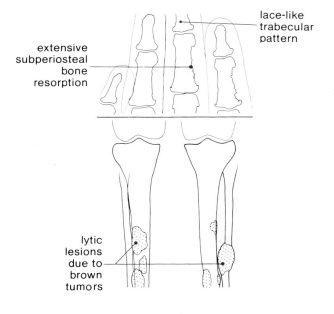

extensive subperiosteal bone resorption

lace-like trabecular pattern

lytic lesions due to brown tumors

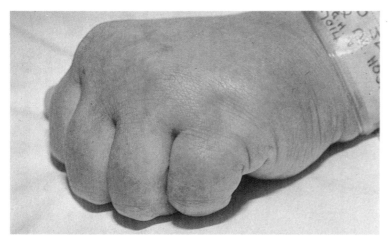

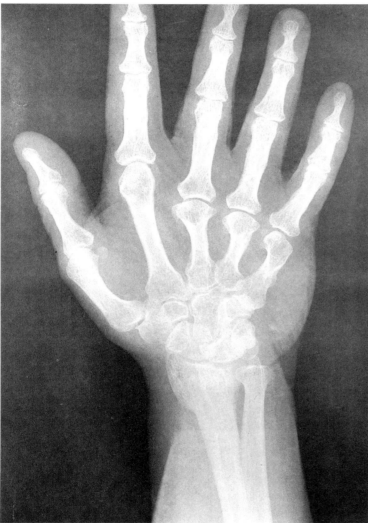

Hypoparathyroidism

PTH secretion is suppressed in hypercalcemia but the term hypoparathyroidism is usually reserved for those disorders with a defective secretion or action of PTH in the presence of hypocalcemia. These disorders are characterized by hypocalcemia and hyperphosphatemia and rarely give rise to clinically significant bone disease. Pseudohypoparathyroidism, which results from resistance of one or more target tissues to the action of PTH, may be associated with somatic and skeletal abnormalities (Figs. 22.38 & 22.39).

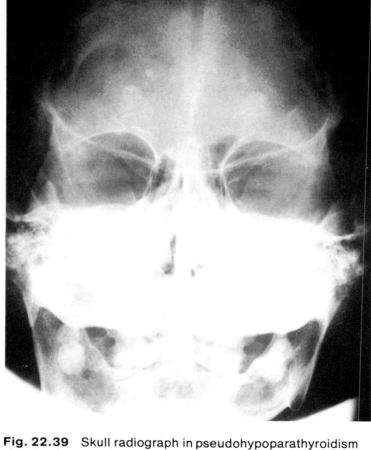

Fig. 22.38 Pseudohypoparathyroidism. A knuckle dimple in the clenched fist (upper, courtesy of Dr. D. Hosking) has resulted from the metacarpal shortening (lower, courtesy of Professor M. Kahn).

Fig. 22.39 Skull radiograph in pseudohypoparathyroidism showing intracranial calcification as a result of prolonged hypocalcemia. Courtesy of Dr. D. Hosking.

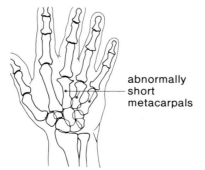

abnormally short metacarpals

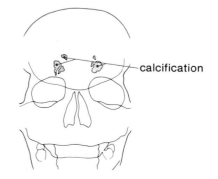

calcification

Other Hormones

Glucocorticoids regulate growth but their mode of action is complex and probably involves effects on many target tissues in addition to the effects on metabolism and on other hormones, including $1,25\,(OH)_2D_3$. In the adult, adrenal insufficiency is not associated with skeletal abnormalities but may cause hypercalcemia. Chronic glucocorticoid excess can induce osteoporosis (Figs 22.40–42).

Characteristic growth abnormalities are associated with deficiencies of either male or female sex hormones.

These appear to play a crucial role in epiphyseal closure and in the growth spurts seen before this event. They may also influence the amount of calcium present in the skeleton at the time of maturity. In adults the effects of estrogens are of particular interest because of the loss of bone that occurs in women after the menopause.

Drug-induced Bone Disease

Corticosteroids are responsible for the commonest form of iatrogenic bone disease, osteoporosis (see Figs. 22.40–42).

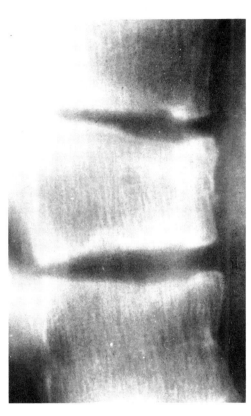
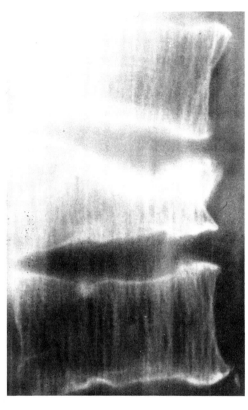
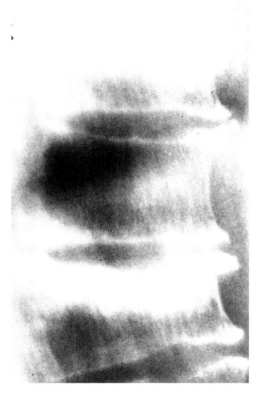

Fig. 22.40 Crush fracture due to trauma in a healthy patient. The vertebral bodies show a dense lattice of trabecular bone and no clear demarcation between end-plates and spongiosa. Courtesy of Professor B. Maldague.

Fig. 22.41 Crush fracture in idiopathic osteoporosis three weeks prior to this radiograph. There is preferential loss of horizontal trabeculae, hypertrophy of longitudinal trabeculae and an area of sclerosis and callus formation. Courtesy of Professor B. Maldague.

Fig. 22.42 Corticosteroid osteoporosis resulting in diffuse trabecular loss. Crush fractures of T6 and T8 have resulted in upper plate sclerosis which persists until withdrawal of corticosteroids. Courtesy of Professor B. Maldague.

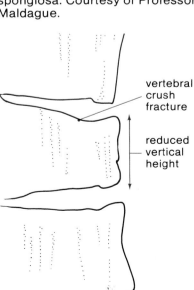
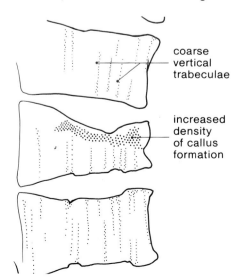
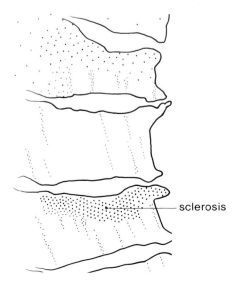

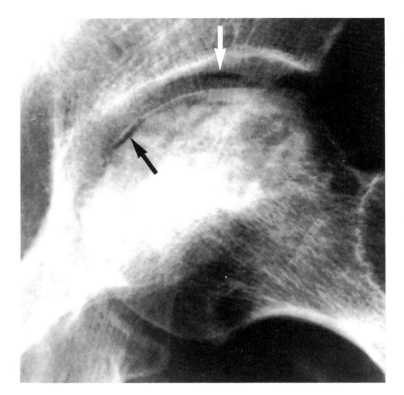

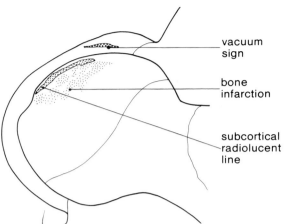

Fig. 22.43 Hip radiograph in aseptic necrosis showing early change with a radiolucent subcortical line (crescent sign). Distraction and abduction of the hip joint has produced the vacuum sign.

vacuum sign

bone infarction

subcortical radiolucent line

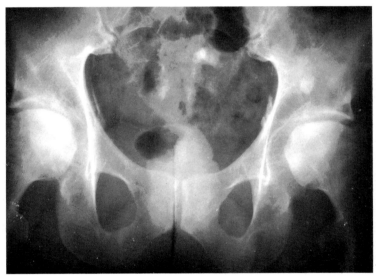

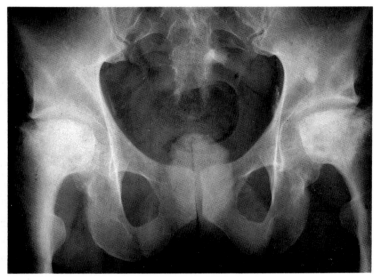

Fig. 22.44 Hip radiograph showing early aseptic necrosis. There is femoral head flattening and a cystic appearance with surrounding sclerosis. Courtesy of Professor M. Kahn.

Fig. 22.45 Hip radiograph showing advanced ischemic necrosis with severe destructive and resorptive changes. Courtesy of Professor M. Kahn.

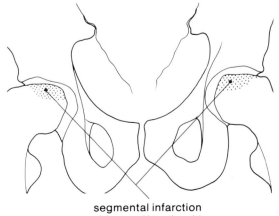

segmental infarction of femoral heads with flattening of dome

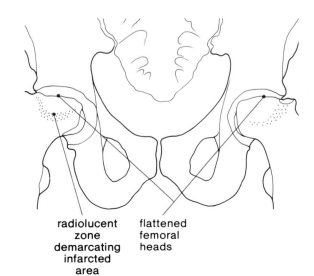

radiolucent zone demarcating infarcted area

flattened femoral heads

The pathophysiology is complex and related in part to secondary hyperparathyroidism, intestinal malabsorption of calcium and renal tubular defects. Vertebral collapse is common, but unlike senile osteoporosis it is associated with diffuse trabecular loss. In some cases marked pseudocallus formation occurs giving patchy areas of osteosclerosis. Corsticosteroids have also been implicated in the pathogenesis of aseptic necrosis (Figs. 22.43–45).

Several drugs induce osteomalacia. Anti-convulsants cause it, partly by inducing defective metabolism in 25-OHD, but also by inducing target organ resistance to the action of $1,25(OH)_2D_3$. High doses of the diphosphonate, etidronate, cause osteomalacia by direct action on bone (Fig. 22.46). Aluminium toxicity results in a form of osteomalacia refractory to treatment with vitamin D and typically associated with multiple fractures (Fig. 22.47).

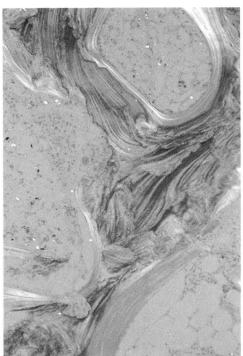
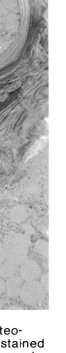
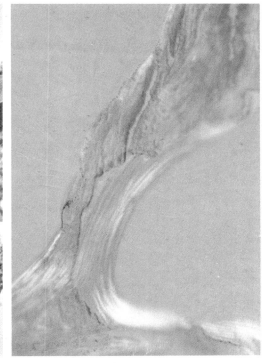

Fig. 22.46 Diphosphonate osteomalacia. The mineralized bone (stained blue) in this case of Paget's disease, is a mixture of lamellar and woven bone, while the surrounding osteoid (pale staining) is excessively thick and covers most of the trabecular surface. Toluidine blue stain, x 1000.

Fig. 22.47 Aluminium-induced osteomalacia. Excessively thick osteoid seams, stained red (left, Goldner's trichrome stain) and deposition of aluminium, stained red, at the osteoid/bone interface (right, aluminon stain, x 1000).

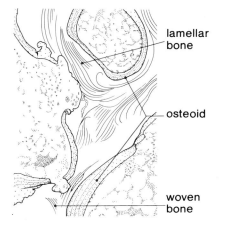
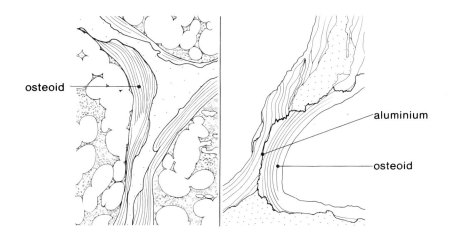

Vitamin D poisoning induces hypercalcemia. Complications of prolonged toxicity include nephrocalcinosis, renal failure and ectopic calcification (Fig. 22.48). On skeletal radiographs osteosclerosis and dense metaphyseal lines may be seen, but in severe cases diffuse osteoporosis is induced. Fluoride ingestion causes a more diffuse osteosclerosis (Fig. 22.49).

Abnormal Bone and Collagen Metabolism

Osteogenesis imperfecta, characterized by fragility of bone, may be associated with other disorders of connective tissues such as generalized joint laxity and capillary fragility. It exists in multiple forms (Fig. 22.50). The disorder arises from defective collagen formation.

Marfan's syndrome (Fig. 22.51) is characterized by increased length of the limbs, particularly the distal parts, dislocated lenses and generalized joint laxity with muscle hypotonia. The disorder is inherited as an autosomal dominant.

Ehlers-Danlos syndrome is an inherited systemic connective tissue disorder due to an increased fragility and friability of connective tissue which develops the capacity to stretch to an unusual length. Thus the major manifestations are hyperelasticity of the skin with easy bruising and the formation of atrophic scars. There is usually hyperextensibility of joints which is often striking (Fig. 22.52). Vascular collagen abnormalities may result in aortic or intracranial aneurysms.

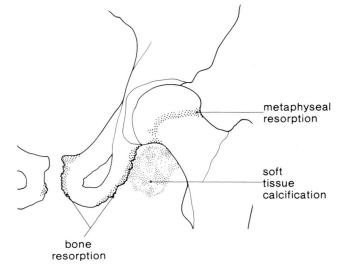

Fig. 22.48 Vitamin D toxicity in a patient with secondary hyperparathyroidism. Note the resorption of bone at the pubic symphysis and along the inferior pubic ramus. There is a discrete area of extra-skeletal calcification below the hip joint.

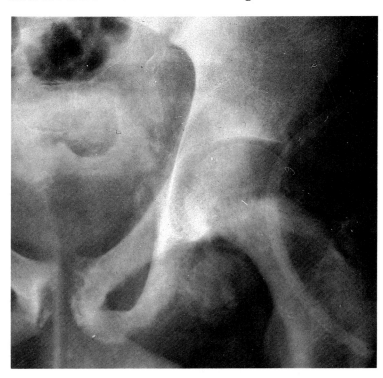

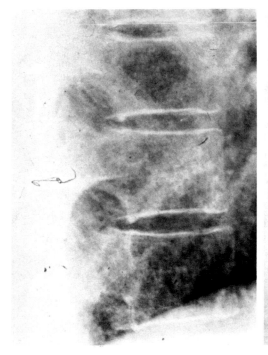
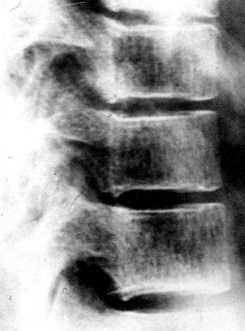
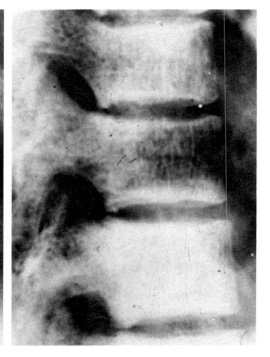

Fig. 22.49 Fluoride osteosclerosis. These sequential radiographs illustrate progressive osteosclerosis in a patient treated with sodium fluoride over a 5 year period. Courtesy of Dr. V. Parsons.

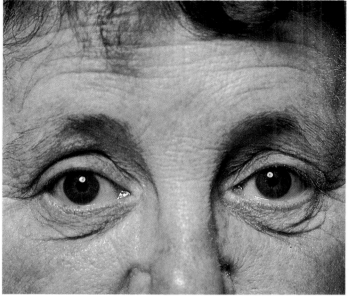

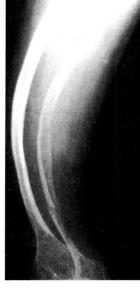

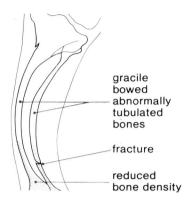

Fig. 22.50 The characteristic blue sclerae of osteogenesis imperfecta (left), more commonly seen in the milder autosomal dominant disease. The radiograph in osteogenesis imperfecta shows the slender bones with extreme cortical thinning (right). Callus formation following fracture is often exuberant.

gracile
bowed
abnormally
tubulated
bones

fracture

reduced
bone density

Fig. 22.51 Arachnodactyly in Marfan's syndrome.

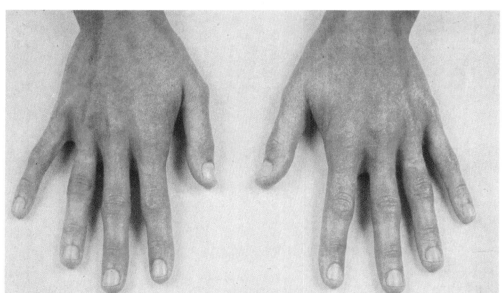

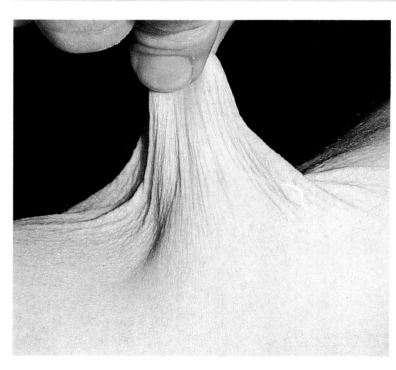

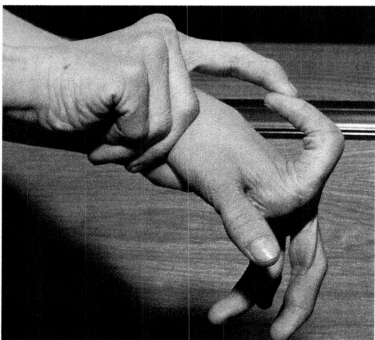

Fig. 22.52 Ehlers-Danlos syndrome. Excessive skin laxity (left, courtesy of Dr. H. Bird). The skin can be pulled away from the subcutaneous tissue and will snap back when released. An example of hypermobility is shown (right, courtesy of Professor M. Kahn).

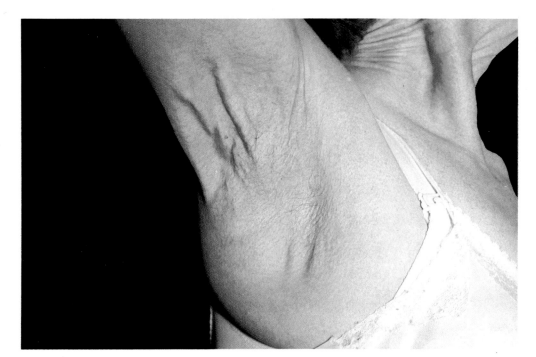

Fig. 22.53 Pseudoxanthoma elasticum. Note the yellow skin lesions in the axilla and loss of elasticity. The skin may calcify. Courtesy of Professor M. Kahn.

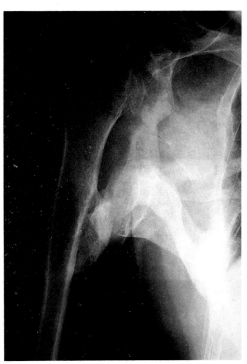

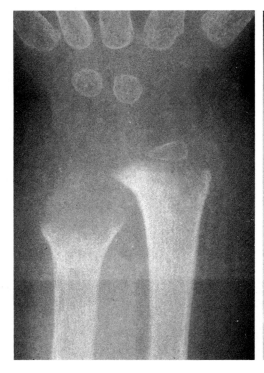

Fig. 22.54 Shoulder radiograph in myositis ossificans progressiva showing huge irregular bone masses. Gross new bone formation in the soft tissues bridges the shoulder joint, effectively causing an arthrodesis. Courtesy of Dr. R. Smith.

Fig. 22.55 Hypophosphatasia. Wrist radiograph in an infant showing the characteristic jagged radiolucent metaphyseal defect (left, courtesy of Dr. M. Whyte). Lateral radiograph of the spine in an adult showing narrowing of disc spaces and ligamentous calcification (right).

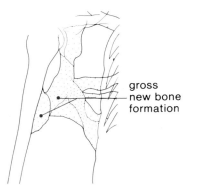

gross new bone formation

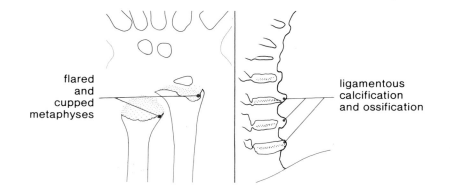

flared and cupped metaphyses

ligamentous calcification and ossification

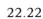

Pseudoxanthoma elasticum is an uncommon inherited disorder of connective tissue characterized by yellow skin lesions in flexural areas (Fig. 22.53). Chorioretinitis, arterial disease and visceral bleeding also occur.

Myositis ossificans progressiva is a rare developmental disorder characterized by progressive calcification followed by ossification of fasciae, aponeuroses and tendons (Fig. 22.54).

Inherited and Associated Bone Disease

The hypophosphatasias are recessively inherited disorders somewhat similar to rickets but characterized by a low serum alkaline phosphatase and, in infants, characteristic radiographic features (Fig. 22.55).

Osteopetrosis (Albers-Schönberg or 'marble bone' disease) is characterized by generalized osteosclerosis (Figs. 22.56 & 22.57).

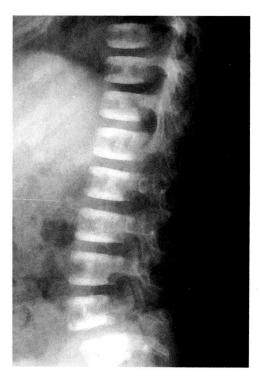

Fig. 22.56 Osteopetrosis. Spinal radiograph in the autosomal dominant form (Albers-Schönberg) showing a 'sandwich' appearance of the vertebrae with dense end-plate sclerosis.

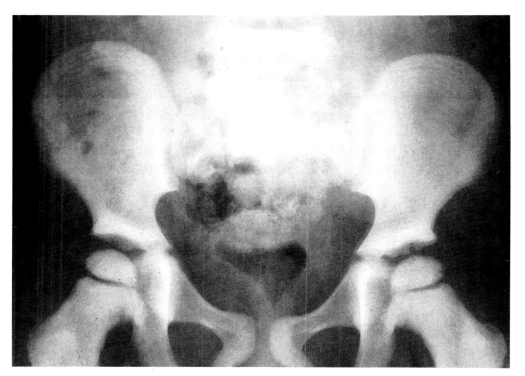

Fig. 22.57 Pelvic radiograph in osteopetrosis showing alternating zones of increased and decreased density parallel to the iliac crest. This 'bone within bone' appearance is due to intermittent disease activity and distinguishes osteopetrosis from other causes of sclerosis.

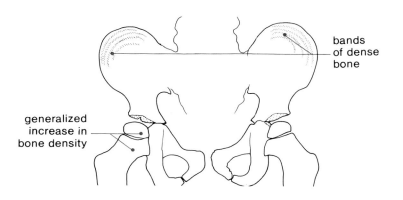

bands of dense bone

generalized increase in bone density

Metabolic bone disease associated with neoplasia includes periosteal new bone formation and generalized osteoporosis (Fig. 22.58), or osteosclerosis (Fig. 22.59) which may be diffuse and confused with Paget's disease.

Some solid tumours, particularly squamous cell carcinomas, may be associated with generalized skeletal rarefaction without evidence of skeletal metastases.

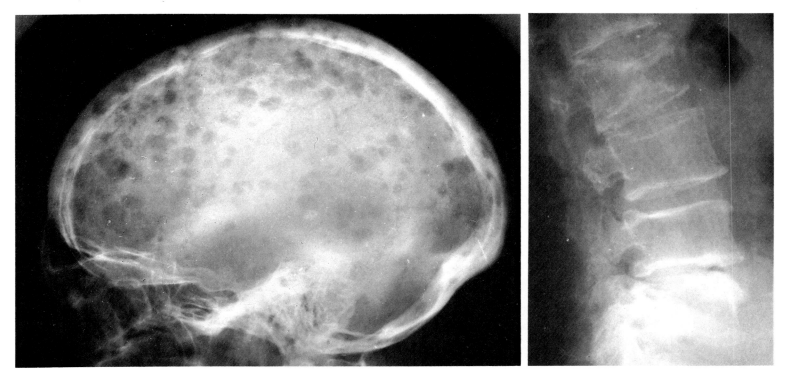

Fig. 22.58 Myeloma. Skull radiograph showing the characteristic punched-out lesions (left) and a spinal radiograph showing diffuse osteoporosis seen in about 5% of patients (right).

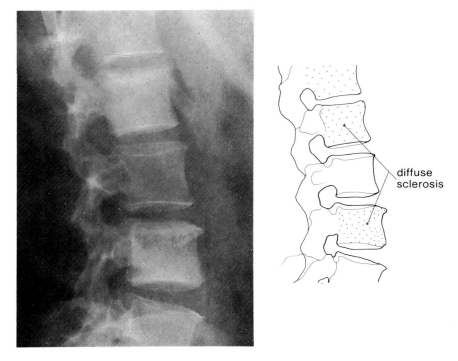

diffuse
sclerosis

Fig. 22.59 Spinal radiograph showing osteosclerosis due to Hodgkins disease. Prostatic metastases may produce an identical appearance.

23
Miscellaneous Conditions

Over two hundred separate rheumatic diseases have been described. Many of the common conditions have been included in this atlas and grouped according to a standard classification. Many cases presenting to the rheumatologist, however, cannot be conveniently described using this classification and some of these miscellaneous conditions will now be presented. This section does not provide a comprehensive account nor is it related to the incidence of these disorders. It provides an introduction to the wide spectrum of unusual conditions seen in rheumatological practice, many of which cause diagnostic confusion with common diseases.

Synovial Disorders
Case 1 Villonodular tenosynovitis

A 65-year-old lady presented with an uncomfortable swelling on the palmar surface of the middle finger of her right hand. This had slowly developed over the preceding six months. Examination revealed a swelling over the middle phalanx attached to the flexor tendon (Fig. 23.1). A radiograph showed a soft tissue mass and pressure lesion over the phalanx (Fig. 23.2). Surgical exploration was undertaken and the mass lesion removed from the tendon sheath (Fig. 23.3). Histology shows the typical features of villonodular synovitis (Fig. 23.4).

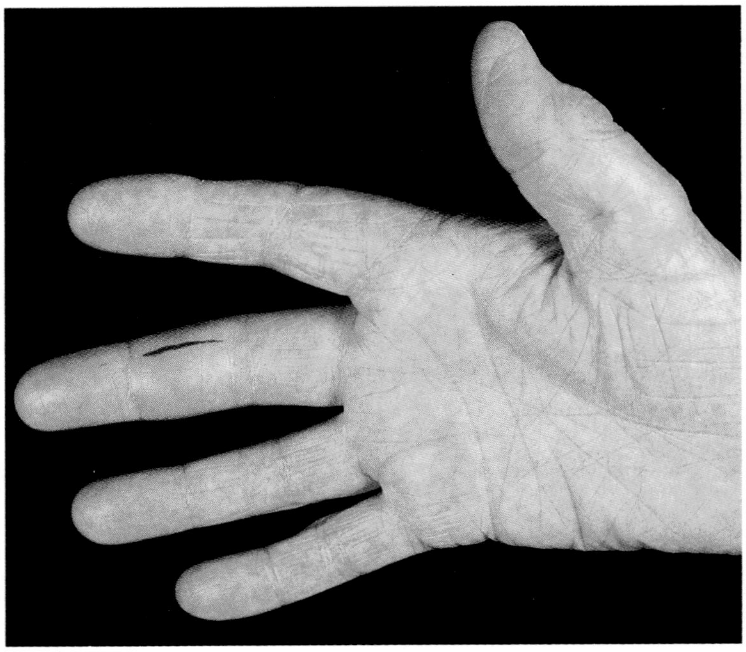

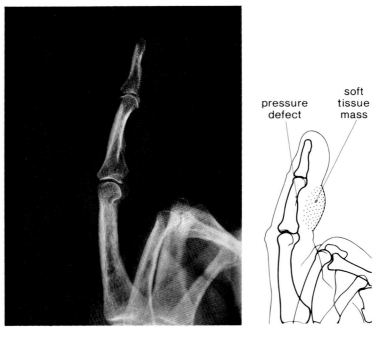

Fig. 23.1 Villonodular tenosynovitis. Swelling over the middle phalanx attached to the flexor tendon.

Fig. 23.2 Villonodular tenosynovitis. Plain radiograph showing a soft tissue mass and a pressure lesion over the phalanx.

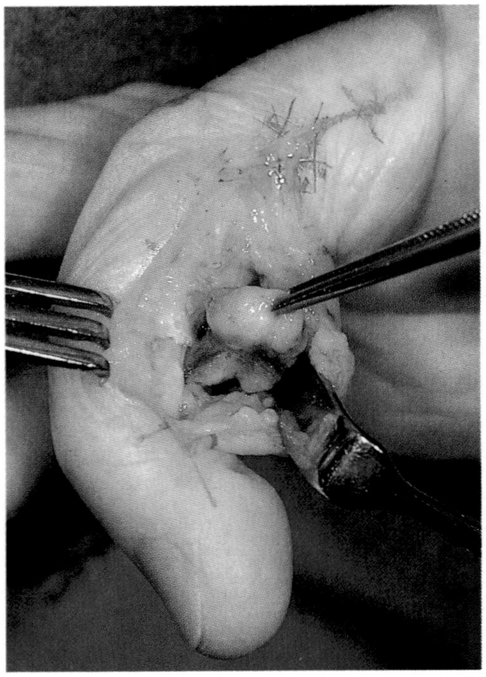

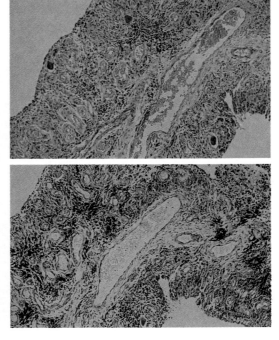

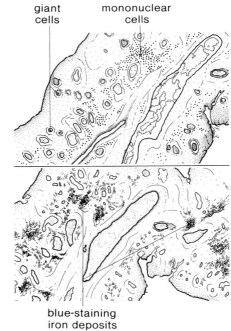

Fig. 23.3 Villonodular tenosynovitis. Surgical removal of a mass lesion from tendon sheath. Courtesy of Mr. I.J. Leslie.

Fig. 23.4 Villonodular tenosynovitis. Histology showing proliferative synovium containing large numbers of mononuclear cells and multinucleate giant cells (H & E stain, upper). The lower section has been stained with Perls to show the extensive accumulations of iron in the tissue. x 400.

Case 2 Synovial osteochondromatosis

A 34-year-old man presented with an 18-month history of gradually increasing pain and swelling of the right knee. The plain radiograph showed typical features of synovial osteochondromatosis (Fig. 23.5). A synovectomy was performed and masses of loose bodies and small chondromatous lesions attached to the synovium were removed (Fig. 23.6). Histological examination showed synovial metaplasia with the development of islands of cartilage, some of which were calcifying and ossifying within the synovium.

Case 3 Multicentric reticulohistiocytosis

A 57-year-old woman presented with painful hands. The history included early morning stiffness, mild constitutional symptoms and painful swellings of interphalangeal joints. A provisional diagnosis of rheumatoid arthritis had been made. On examination the interphalangeal joints were swollen and tender but in addition, small tumorous swellings were apparent around the nail beds in the hands and around the nose and mouth. Xanthomata were also present (Fig. 23.7). The radiograph of the hand showed destructive lesions

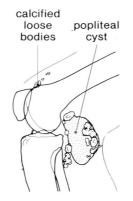

calcified loose bodies   popliteal cyst

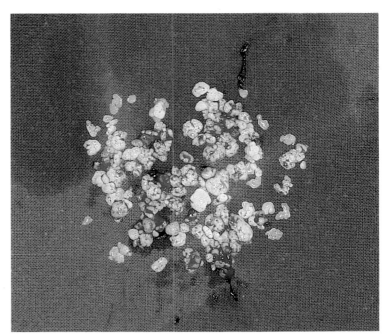

Fig. 23.5 Synovial osteochondromatosis. A lateral radiograph demonstrating multiple calcified loose bodies in the suprapatellar pouch and a popliteal cyst. The presence ·of trabeculae in some shows that they are partly ossified.

Fig. 23.6 Synovial osteochondromatosis. Masses of loose bodies and small chondromatous lesions which were attached to the synovium and removed during a synovectomy. Courtesy of Mr. J. Browett.

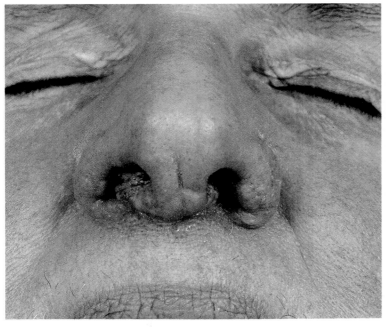

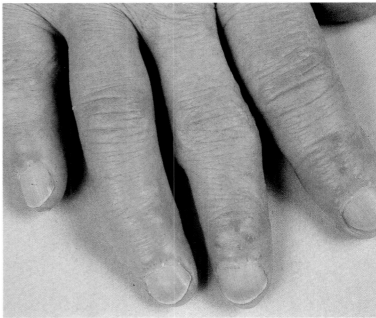

Fig. 23.7 Multicentric reticulohistiocytosis. Small tumorous swellings around the nose and xanthomata around the eyes (left). The typical nail bed tumors and interphalangeal joint arthropathy are also shown (right).

with widening of the joint space (Fig. 23.8). One of the tumorous swellings was biopsied confirming the diagnosis of multicentric reticulohistiocytosis.

Case 4 Plant thorn synovitis

A 13-year-old girl presented with a painful foot. Examination revealed tenderness isolated to the fourth metatarsophalangeal (MTPJ) joint of the right foot. A careful history uncovered the fact that this had first developed after she had gone cross-country running at school in bare feet. Plain radiographs showed soft tissue swelling and the subsequent development of a small erosive area in the painful joint (Fig. 23.9). The joint was explored and a synovectomy performed. Histological examination revealed the inclusion of fragments of plant thorn in the synovium confirming a diagnosis of plant thorn synovitis (Fig. 23.10). The symptoms and signs resolved post-operatively.

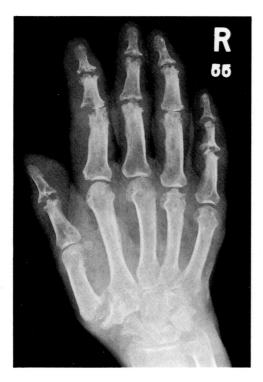

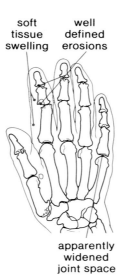

soft tissue swelling

well defined erosions

apparently widened joint space

Fig. 23.8 Multicentric reticulohistiocytosis. Hand radiograph showing well-defined erosions at many joints with normal bone density and normal, or apparently widened, joint spaces. Soft tissue swelling is present.

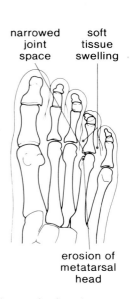

narrowed joint space

soft tissue swelling

erosion of metatarsal head

Fig. 23.9 Plant thorn synovitis. Plain radiograph showing narrowing of the joint space at the fourth MTPJ with ill-defined erosion of the metatarsal head. There is also periosteal new bone formation, separation of the 3rd and 5th metatarsal heads and soft tissue swelling.

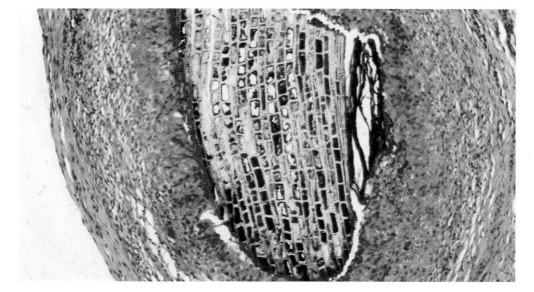

Fig. 23.10 Plant thorn synovitis. Synovial histology revealing the presence of a fragment of plant thorn.

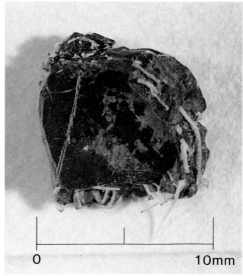

0   10mm

Fig. 23.11 Foreign body synovitis. A fragment of bakelite removed from the knee during surgical exploration.

Case 5 Foreign body synovitis

A 27-year-old girl was involved in a road traffic accident during which her knees struck the dashboard of the car causing an abrasion. This was washed, cleaned and sutured in a local casualty department. The patient continued to complain of persistent pain and intermittent swelling of the knee for several months. Radiographs were unremarkable. The joint was finally explored and a foreign body removed (Fig. 23.11). Analysis showed this to be a fragment of bakelite from the dashboard. Once the foreign body had been removed the patient's symptoms resolved completely.

Case 6 Cholesterol crystals

A 61-year-old man with chronic rheumatoid arthritis presented with a persistent swelling of the olecranon bursa (Fig. 23.12). The bursa was aspirated and a large amount of thick milky fluid was obtained (Fig. 23.13). Microscopy showed masses of cholesterol crystals (Fig. 23.14). Chronic effusions and bursae in both rheumatoid arthritis and osteoarthritis occasionally reveal this milky fluid full of cholesterol crystals which may contribute to the synovial and capsular reaction.

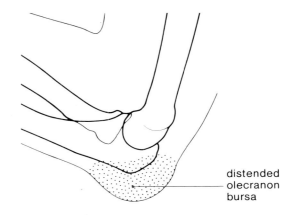

Fig. 23.12 Cholesterol-containing olecranon bursa. Radiograph showing an enormously distended olecranon bursa. The appearance is non-specific and could be due to rheumatoid disease, gouty tophi, or other disorders.

distended olecranon bursa

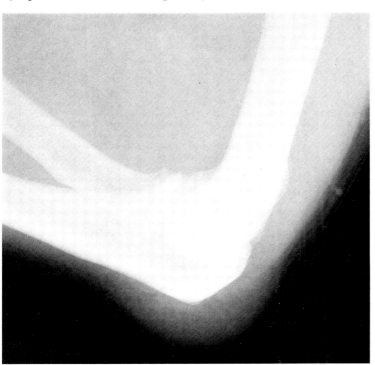

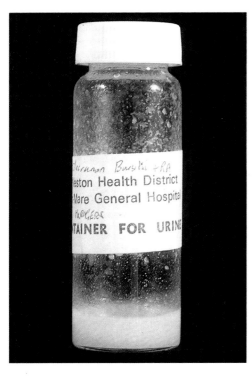

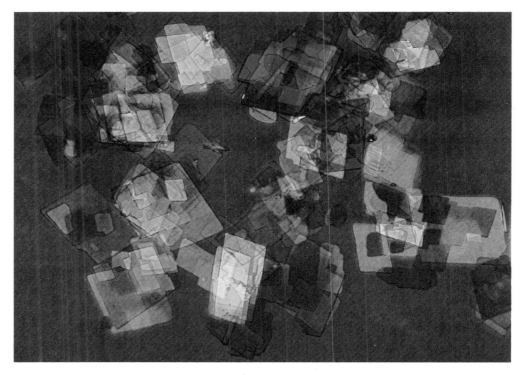

Fig. 23.13 Cholesterol crystals: synovial fluid aspirated from the bursa shown in Fig. 23.12. Note the 'milky' appearance of the fluid.

Fig. 23.14 Cholesterol crystals. Microscopical examination of the fluid aspirated from the bursa demonstrating the presence of cholesterol crystals. (Polarizing light microscope, first order red compensator, x 1600.)

Case 7 Hyperlipidemia

A 28-year-old lady presented with nodules on the hands and heels. Her father had similar swellings (Fig. 23.15). She also complained of transient attacks of arthralgia with small effusions developing in the knees. The family was hyperlipidemic, the lumps were xanthomata and diagnosis of hyperlipidemic arthritis was made.

Case 8 Palindromic rheumatism

A 42-year-old male Indian patient presented with a history of episodic small joint synovitis. He had seen many doctors but no abnormality was found. He was asked to attend during one of the acute episodes which generally lasted for three to four days only. On examination at that time tenosynovitis and metatarsalgia with marked redness of the overlying skin was apparent (Fig. 23.16). Twenty-four hours later this had resolved completely. A diagnosis of palindromic rheumatism was made. The patient was weakly seropositive and three years later developed classical rheumatoid arthritis.

Case 9 Adult onset Still's disease

A 33-year-old man presented with a history of arthralgia, fever, sore throat and general malaise. He was admitted to hospital for investigation. The temperature chart (Fig. 23.17) showed high fever in the evenings. Examination during the height of this fever revealed a mild rash. Investigations revealed a raised white cell count and ESR, and a raised IgG. Mild synovitis and pleuropericarditis developed. A diagnosis of adult onset Still's disease was made.

Case 10 Jaccoud's arthritis

A 47-year-old man with a past history of rheumatic fever was admitted for investigation of a cardiac lesion. A deformity of the hand was noted which included ulnar deviation and subluxation of the metacarpophalangeal joints (Fig. 23.18, left). The radiograph showed the deformity but no erosions or joint damage (Fig. 23.18, right). The history revealed that he had had significant joint disease during previous attacks of rheumatic fever in childhood and the diagnosis of Jaccoud's arthritis was made.

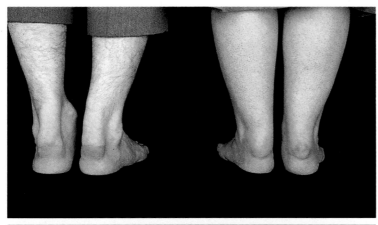

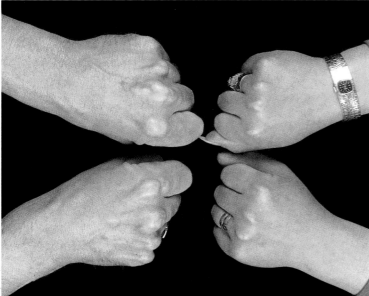

Fig. 23.15 Hyperlipidemic arthritis. Father and daughter with xanthomatous swellings on feet (upper) and hands (lower).

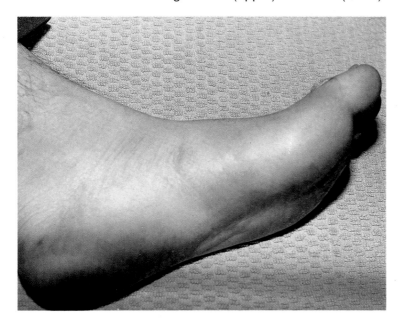

Fig. 23.16 Palindromic rheumatism. Tenosynovitis and metatarsalgia with marked redness of the overlying skin during an acute episode of small joint synovitis.

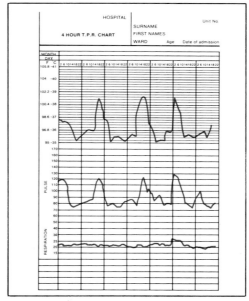

Fig. 23.17 Adult onset Still's disease: fever chart.

Case 11 Sarcoidosis

A 48-year-old man presented with a two-year-history of painful nodules in the hand. He was noted to have a nasal abnormality (Fig. 23.19). A radiograph showed cystic changes consistent with sarcoidosis (Fig. 23.20) and the diagnosis was confirmed by biopsy (Fig. 23.21).

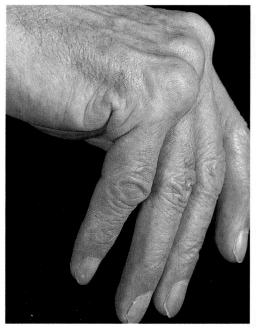

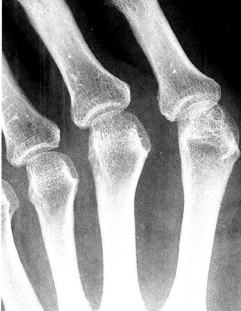

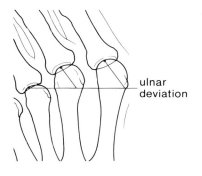

Fig. 23.18 Jaccoud's arthritis. Deformed hand showing ulnar deviation and sublaxation of the metacarpo-phalangeal joints (left). The hand radiograph (right) shows the deformity but no erosions or joint damage are present. Courtesy of Dr J.T. Scott.

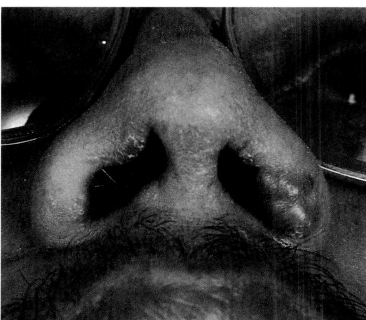

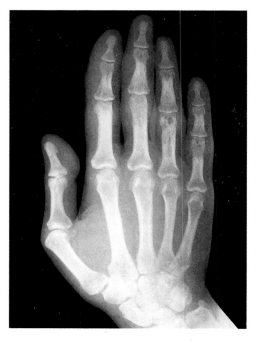

Fig. 23.19 Sarcoidosis: nasal tumors due to sarcoid granulomata. The patient also had lupus pernio.

Fig. 23.20 Sarcoidosis. Hand radiograph with widespread dactylitis characterized by lacy trabecular pattern. Large bone cysts and soft tissue swelling can also be seen.

Fig. 23.21 Sarcoidosis. Synovial histology showing granulomata with giant cell and epithelioid cell formation characteristic of sarcoidosis. H & E stain. Courtesy of Dr D.G.I. Scott.

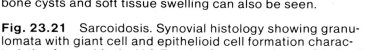

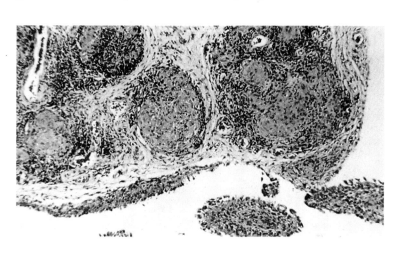

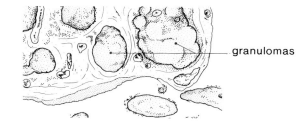

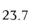

Bone and Cartilage Disorders
Case 12 Polychondritis

A 52-year-old man presented with recurrent episodes of painful red swelling of the ears (Fig. 23.22). He sub-sequently developed collapse of the bridge of the nose (Fig. 23.23). A diagnosis of polychondritis was made and antibodies to Type I collagen were found in the patient's serum. In spite of therapy with prednisolone he developed stridor and difficulty in breathing and chest radiographs showed collapse of the trachea due to polychondritis (Fig. 23.24).

Case 13 Spondylo-epiphyseal dysplasia

A 26-year-old girl of short stature presented with a history of pain and stiffness in the hips. Examination revealed skeletal deformity (Fig. 23.25). Radiographs showed typical features of epiphyseal dysplasia (Fig. 23.26). The pain and stiffness of the hips was due to development of premature osteoarthritis.

Case 14 Achondroplasia

A 28-year-old achondroplastic presented with pain, tingling and weakness in the legs related to exercise. The radiograph shows a spinal deformity of achondroplasia which has led to acquired spinal stenosis (Fig. 23.27).

Case 15 Traumatic osteochondritis

A 26-year-old man developed pain, swelling and stiffness of the right knee following a major injury incurred whilst playing rugby. The plain radiograph shows a fragment of bone in the suprapatellar fossa derived from the femoral condyle. A diagnosis of traumatic osteochondritis was made and the fragment of bone was removed (Fig. 23.28).

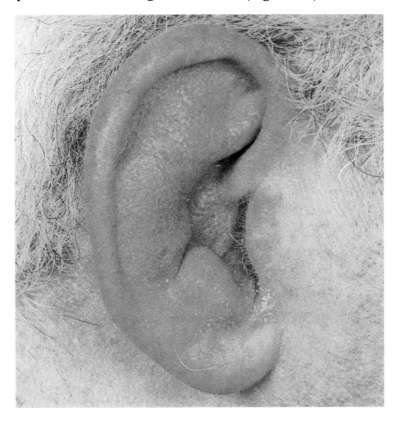

Fig. 23.22 Polychondritis: painful red swelling of the ears.

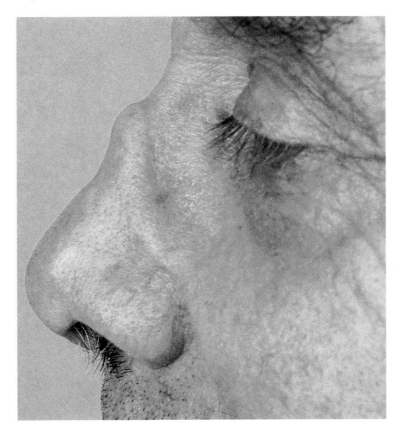

Fig. 23.23 Polychondritis: collapse of bridge of the nose.

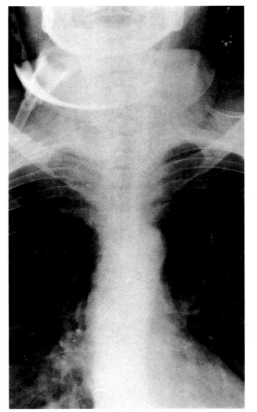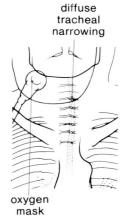

diffuse tracheal narrowing

oxygen mask

Fig. 23.24 Relapsing polychondritis. Chest radiograph showing diffuse tracheal narrowing. The laryngeal air shadows are completely obliterated.

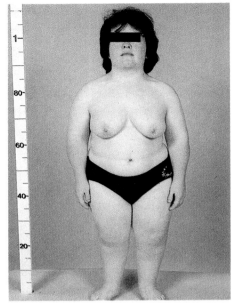
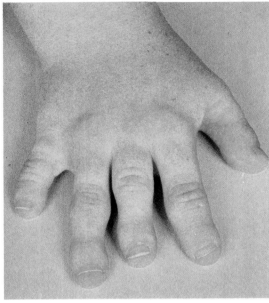

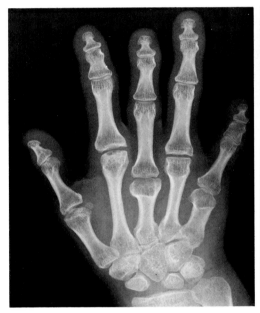
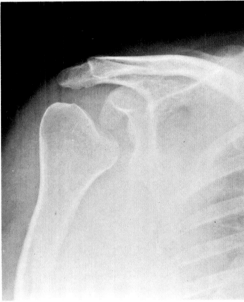

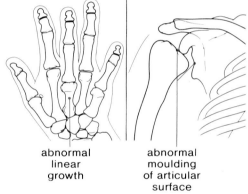

Fig. 23.25 Spondylo-epiphyseal dysplasia. The short stature is due to poor growth of the long bones.

Fig. 23.26 Spondylo-epiphyseal dysplasia. Hand radiograph showing abnormal linear growth, variable length of metacarpals (left), and shoulder radiograph showing abnormal moulding of articular surfaces (right).

abnormal
linear
growth

abnormal
moulding
of articular
surface

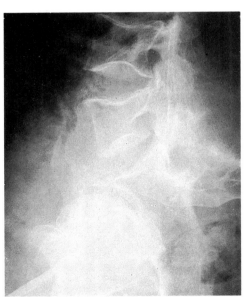
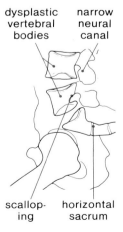

dysplastic
vertebral
bodies

narrow
neural
canal

scallop-
ing

horizontal
sacrum

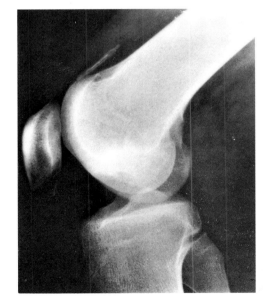

fragment
of avulsed
bone

site of origin of
bone fragment

Fig. 23.27 Achondroplasia. Lateral radiograph of the lumbo-sacral junction showing dysplastic vertebral bodies, markedly narrow neural canal with scalloping of the dorsal surface of the vertebral bodies and a horizontally positioned sacrum.

Fig. 23.28 Traumatic osteochrondritis. Knee radiograph showing a fragment of bone which has been avulsed and lies in the suprapatellar pouch. The site from which it has come can just be seen.

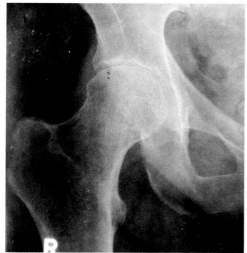

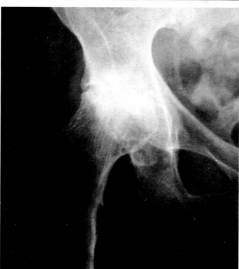

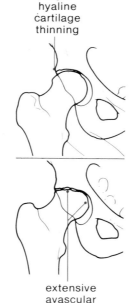

slight
hyaline
cartilage
thinning

extensive
avascular
necrosis
of femoral
head

Fig. 23.29 Avascular necrosis. The hip radiograph taken in 1981 (upper) reveals no abnormality apart from slight hyaline cartilage thinning. However the radiograph taken in 1985 (lower) demonstrates the existence of avascular necrosis of the femoral head.

Case 16 Avascular necrosis

A 46-year-old lady with rheumatoid arthritis treated with prednisolone for the last five years presented with a sudden increase of pain in the right hip. The radiograph showed evidence of avascular necrosis (Fig. 23.29, left) and this rapidly progressed to destruction of the hip joint (Fig. 23.29, right). Hip arthroplasty was performed and at operation the affected segment in the femoral head was clearly seen (Fig. 23.30).

Case 17 Ochronosis

A 64-year-old lady presented with painful knees and a painful back. There was a strong family history of arthritis and careful inquiry revealed that her sister had a similar disorder and that both patients' urine turned dark on standing. Clinical examination revealed patches of pigmentation in the eyes and nose (Fig. 23.31). A lateral radiograph of the spine showed the typical features of ochronotic arthropathy (Fig. 23.32).

Case 18 Diffuse idopathic skeletal hyperostosis (DISH, Forestier's disease)

An obese, hypertensive, 68-year-old man presented with stiffness and pain in the back accompanied by aching of the knees. Examination showed severe loss of movement throughout the spine and mild osteoarthritis of the knees. Radiographs confirmed the diagnosis of spinal and peripheral DISH (Figs. 23.33).

Case 19 Condensing osteitis of the clavicle

A 46-year-old lady presented with sudden onset of pain and swelling over the right sternoclavicular joint (Fig. 23.34). Radiographs showed the typical features of condensing osteitis of the clavicle (Fig. 23.35). The symptoms slowly subsided over the next few months, although the swelling persisted.

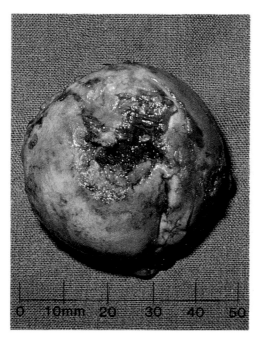

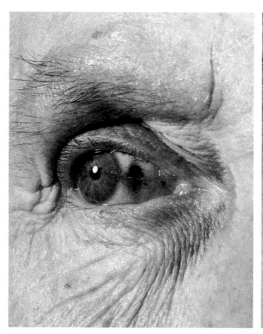

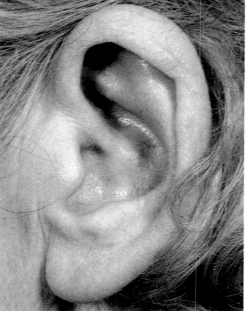

Fig. 23.30 Avascular necrosis. Affected segment in the femoral head removed during arthroplasty. Courtesy of Mr J. Browett.

Fig. 23.31 Ochronosis. Discoloration in the sclera of the eye and cartilage of the ear.

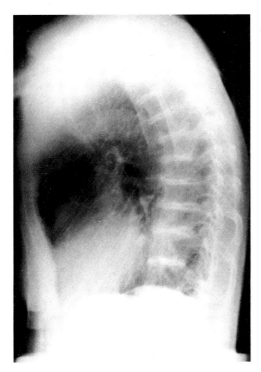
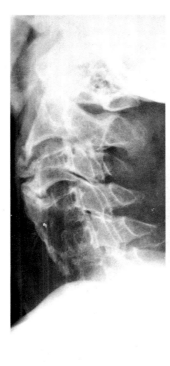
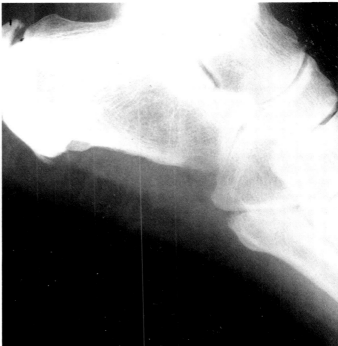

Fig. 23.32 Ochronosis. Lateral radiograph of the spine revealing typical features of disc space narrowing at all levels, subchondral sclerosis and disc calcification.

Fig. 23.33 Spinal and peripheral D.I.S.H. The spinal radiograph (left) demonstrates the presence anteriorly of a mass of consolidating new bone. There is, however, no new bone or osteophyte in the neural canal. The radiograph of the foot (right) shows the presence of new bone at tendon and ligament insertions without prior erosion.

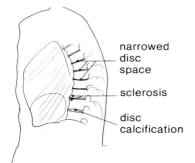

narrowed disc space

sclerosis

disc calcification

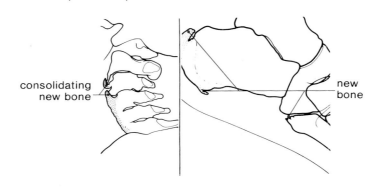

consolidating new bone

new bone

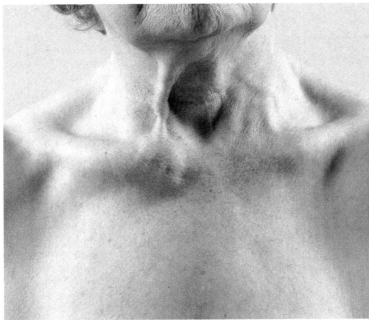
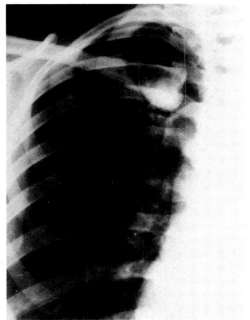
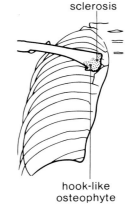

sclerosis

hook-like osteophyte

Fig. 23.34 Condensing osteitis of the clavicle. Swelling over the right sternoclavicular joint.

Fig. 23.35 Chest radiograph showing condensing osteitis of the clavicle. There is sclerosis adjacent to the distal part of the articular surface of the clavicle, which has a hook-like osteophyte.

23.11

Periarticular Disorders
Case 20 Knuckle pad syndrome (Garrod's fatty pads)

A 31-year-old lady was referred by her general practitioner to a rheumatology clinic because of mild discomfort of the proximal interphalangeal joints of the hands. Swellings over these joints had been noted

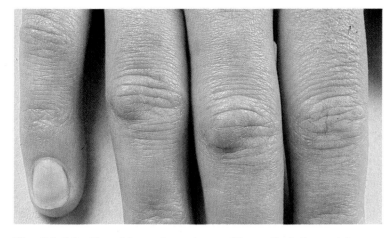

Fig. 23.36 Knuckle pad syndrome (Garrod's fatty pads). Typical swellings over the proximal phalangeal joints of the hands.

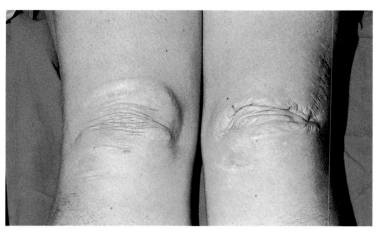

Fig. 23.37 Ehlers-Danlos Syndrome: skin abnormality at the knee. Courtesy of Dr H. Bird.

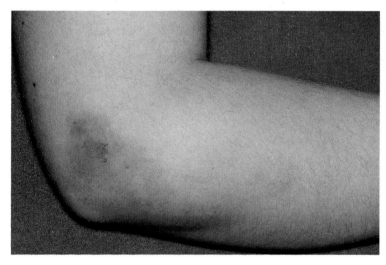

Fig. 23.38 Self-inflicted injury. Localized soft tissue swelling and fluctuant haematoma resulting from self-inflicted injury.

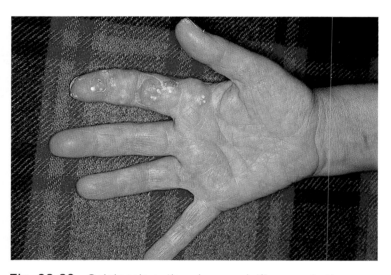

Fig. 23.39 Calcinosis cutis: a large calcific mass in the index finger.

Fig. 23.40 Calcinosis cutis. Hand radiograph showing substantial collections of subcutaneous calcification in the left index finger and smaller collections in other digits.

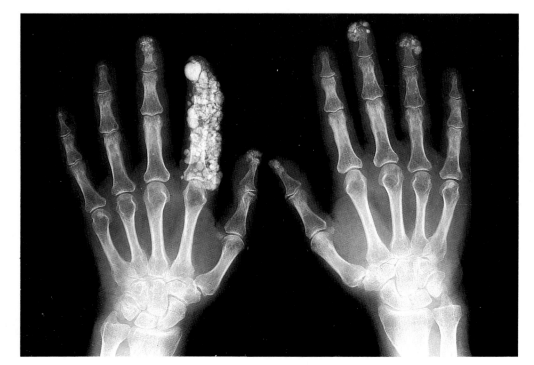

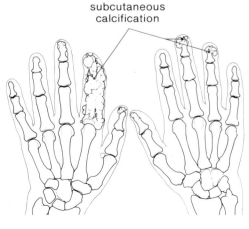

subcutaneous calcification

(Fig. 23.36). A diagnosis of rheumatoid arthritis had been made, causing the patient to become anxious about her future and decide to give up her job. Radiographs and blood tests were normal and a diagnosis of Garrod's fatty pads was made. The patient was reassured that she had no arthropathy and discharged from the clinic.

Case 21 Ehlers-Danlos syndrome
A 27-year-old lady with a known family history of Ehlers-Danlos syndrome presented with joint pain. Examination revealed marked hypermobility of the joints and tenderness over capsular insertions. The skin abnormalities of Ehlers-Danlos syndrome were apparent (Fig. 23.37). Radiographs and blood tests were unremarkable and the joint pain was diagnosed as being related to hypermobility.

Case 22 Self-inflicted injury
a 23-year-old lady presented with persistent tennis elbow related to an injury at work and which was

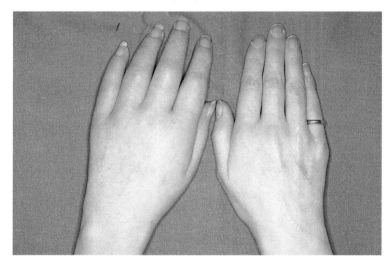

Fig. 23.41 Shoulder-hand syndrome: mottled edematous swelling on the left hand.

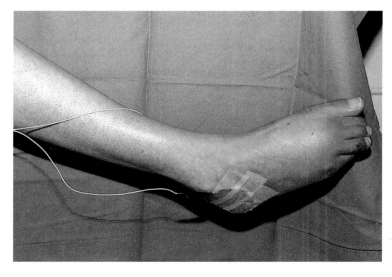

Fig. 23.42 Painful regional osteoporosis. Fixed inversion deformity of the foot accompanied by soft tissue swelling and discoloration. The electrodes are attached to a stimulator to provide pain relief.

unresponsive to treatment. A compensation case for the work injury was pending. Extensive localized soft tissue swelling and fluctuant hematoma was seen 7 months after injury (Fig. 23.38). There was no bruising elsewhere. A diagnosis of self-inflicted injury was made.

Case 23 Calcinosis cutis
A 61-year-old woman presented with pain and swelling of the index finger. This had developed gradually and occasionally ulcerated. Examination showed a large calcific mass in the finger (Fig. 23.39) and widespread calcinosis cutis was confirmed by the radiograph (Fig. 23.40). There was no evidence of connective tissue disease illustrating the unusual occurrence of solitary calcinosis cutis without scleroderma or any other causative disorder.

Other Disorders
Case 24 Algoneurodystrophy (synonym: Sudek's atrophy, shoulder-hand syndrome)
A 37-year-old lady presented with a painful shoulder and a painful swollen hand developing 3 weeks after a minor injury to the arm. Clinical examinations showed mottled edematous swelling of the hand (Fig. 23.41) and there was extreme pain on palpation of bones throughout the limb. The radiograph showed patchy osteoporosis and scintigraphy showed increased uptake of isotope confirming the diagnosis of algoneurodystrophy.

Case 25 Painful regional osteoporosis
A 32-year-old girl developed a painful discolored foot after surgery to correct a hallux valgus deformity. Clinical examination showed the soft tissue swelling with a fixed inversion deformity and skin discoloration (Fig. 23.42). Figure 23.42 also shows electrodes attached to a stimulator providing pain relief by transcutaneous electrical nerve stimulation. A radiograph shows typical patchy osteoporosis (Fig. 23.43).

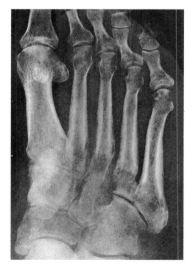
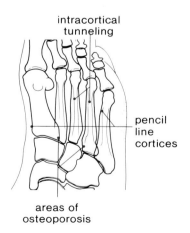

Fig. 23.43 Painful regional osteoporosis. Radiograph of the foot showing intense areas of osteoporosis at the tarsometatarsal and metatarsophalangeal joints. Features of acute disuse osteoporosis are present, with a predominantly subarticular distribution. Intracortical tunneling, pencil line cortices and slight soft tissue swelling can also be seen.

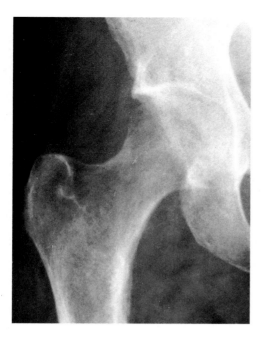

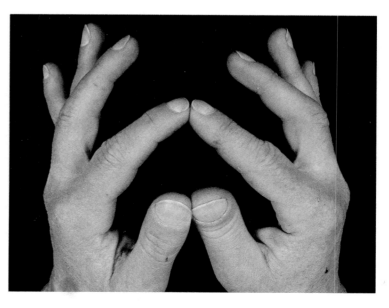

Fig. 23.44 Transient painful osteoporosis of the hip in pregnancy. The radiograph reveals marked osteoporosis of the hip and upper femur. Trabecular detail in the femoral head is 'washed out'. Other typical features which can be seen include the faint, thin line of the femoral head and evidence of rapid bone resoprtion with cortical splitting.

Fig. 23.45 Vinyl chloride disease: typical hand abnormality caused by resorption of the terminal phalanges. Courtesy of Dr C. Black.

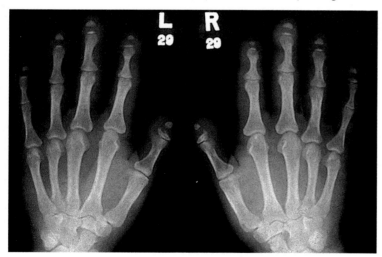

Fig. 23.46 Vinyl chloride disease. Hand radiograph showing destruction of the tufts and shafts of the terminal phalanges.

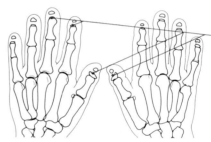

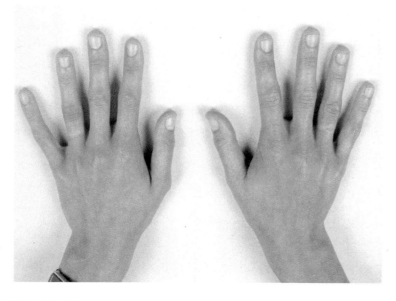

Fig. 23.47 Marfan's syndrome: arachnodactyly. Courtesy of Dr H. Bird.

Fig. 23.48 Thyroid acropachy: finger clubbing. The patient had exophthalmos and an arthropathy.

Case 26 Transient painful osteoporosis of the hip in pregnancy

A 31-year-old lady in the second trimester of pregnancy presented with acute onset of extreme pain in the left hip. She was unable to put her foot to the ground and was totally disabled by constant severe pain. Examination revealed little, although pain was exacerbated by all movements of the hip. After the patient had reached the third trimester no diagnosis had been made but the pain continued. Laboratory investigations revealed no abnormality. A single radiograph, taken with careful screening of the foetus, showed typical features of transient osteoporosis of the hip in pregnancy (Fig. 23.44). The condition resolved within a few weeks of delivery and the radiograph returned to normal.

Case 27 Vinyl chloride disease

A 54-year old man who had worked for many years in a factory known to expose employees to vinyl chloride presented with a hand abnormality shown (Fig. 23.45). The radiograph as well as the clinical findings were typical of vinyl chloride disease (Fig. 23.46).

Case 28 Marfan's syndrome

A patient presented with mild generalized joint pain. Laboratory investigations were unremarkable, but clinical examination revealed gross hypermobility of joints associated with the skeletal anomaly (Fig. 23.47). A diagnosis of Marfan's syndrome was made. Radiographs showed an abnormal metacarpal index.

Case 29 Thyroid acropachy

A 48-year-old man with a longstanding history of hyperthyroidism (Graves' disease) which had been treated, presented with painful wrists and fingers. The examination revealed exophthalmos and clubbing of the fingers and thumbs (Fig. 23.48). A radiograph showed the typical features of thyroid acropachy (Fig. 23.49).

Case 30 Primary Sjögren's syndrome

A 48-year-old lady presented with painful swollen parotid glands (Fig. 23.50). An initial diagnosis of mumps was made but the pain persisted without other features of this disease and the patient then developed arthralgia. On examination there was swelling of parotid and lacrimal glands. The patient had reduced tear secretion and a positive antinuclear factor. A diagnosis of primary Sjögren's syndrome was made.

Case 31 Scurvy

An elderly lady with longstanding rheumatoid arthritis complained of a sudden increase of pain in her shoulder associated with bruising of the upper arm (Fig. 23.51). The shoulder contained blood-stained synovial fluid. Investigations revealed her to be vitamin C deficient, dietary history revealing low intake as the cause. She had no other clinical signs of vitamin C deficiency.

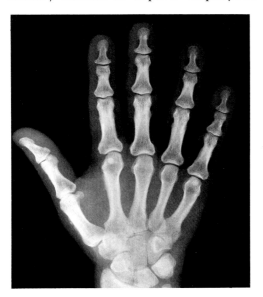

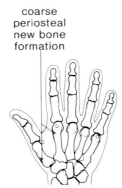

coarse periosteal new bone formation

Fig. 23.49 Thyroid acropachy. Hand radiograph showing typical coarse periosteal new bone formation along the radial aspects of the shafts of the thumb and index metacarpals.

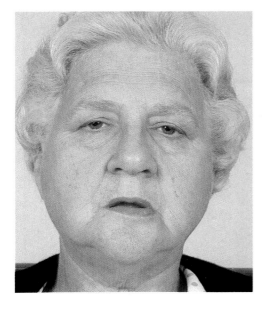

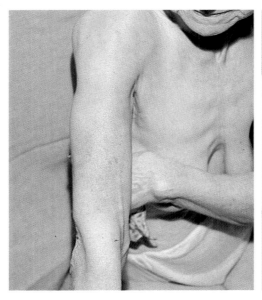

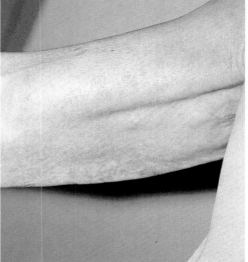

Fig. 23.50 Primary Sjögrens syndrome: swollen parotid and lacrimal glands.

Fig. 23.51 Scurvy: spontaneous bruising of upper arm. Courtesy of Dr I. Haslock.

23.15

Case 32 Apatite-associated destructive arthritis

A 76-year-old lady presented with increasing pain and disability in both shoulders and both knees. The joints were unstable and exhibited large cool effusions (Fig. 23.52). Radiographs showed atrophic destructive changes in the affected joints (Figs. 23.53 & 23.54). The synovial fluid was lightly blood-stained and contained large amounts of alizarin-red positive material. The same apatite-containing material was found in the biopsy (Fig. 23.55).

Case 33 Charcot joint

A 36-year-old man with known mild syringomyelia presented with mild discomfort and difficulty using his left shoulder and wrist. The wrist was swollen, deformed and limited in movement (Fig. 23.56), left). Radiographs showed the typical features of a neuropathic joint (Fig. 23.56, right).

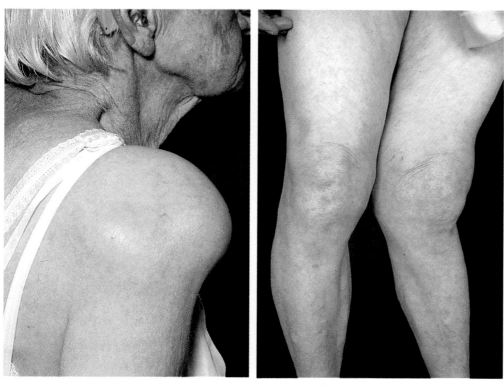

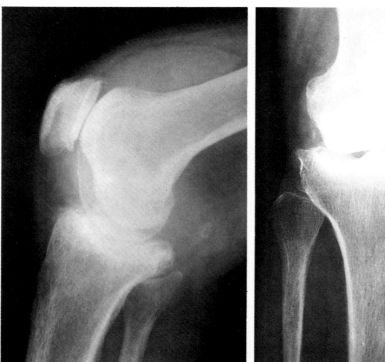

Fig. 23.52 Apatite-associated destructive arthritis: effusions of shoulder (left) and knees (right).

Fig. 23.53 Apatite-associated destructive arthritis. Knee radiograph showing a large joint effusion (left). Single compartment bone attrition has occured in the absence of reparative phenomena in the affected compartment. This can also be seen in the radiograph of a straightened knee, which shows valgus angulation (right).

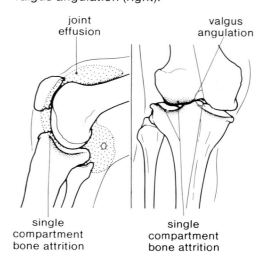

joint effusion

valgus angulation

single compartment bone attrition

single compartment bone attrition

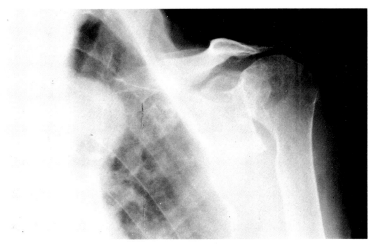

Fig. 23.54 Apatite-associated destructive arthritis. Shoulder radiograph showing typical changes which include marked bony attrition, cephalic migration of the humeral head and pressure defect on the humeral neck. The reparative or degenerative phenomenon is absent.

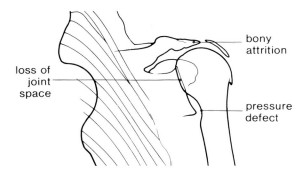

loss of joint space

bony attrition

pressure defect

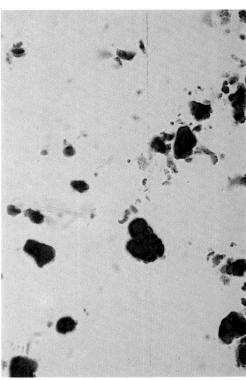

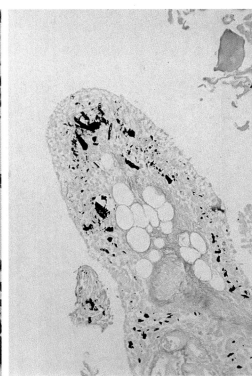

Fig. 23.55 Apatite-associated destructive arthritis. Alizarin-red stained slide of the synovial fluid showing masses of apatite spherulites (left, x 1000). A synovial section stained with Von Kossa shows extensive uptake of calcific material in the lining and subsynovial tissue (right, x 400).

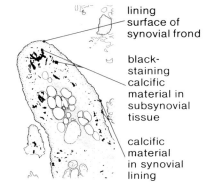

lining surface of synovial frond

black-staining calcific material in subsynovial tissue

calcific material in synovial lining

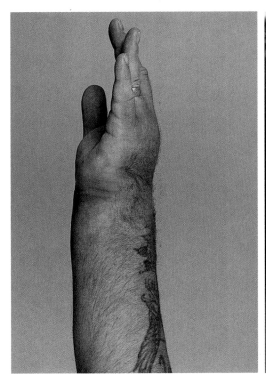

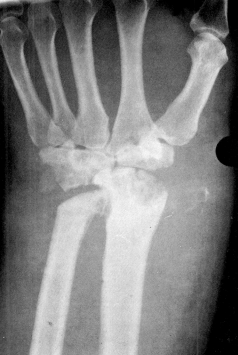

Fig. 23.56 Charcot joint. Swollen and deformed wrist (left) and a radiograph showing gross destruction of the proximal carpal row with attrition and simplification of bony margins (right). Residual fragments of bone and considerable soft tissue swelling can be seen.

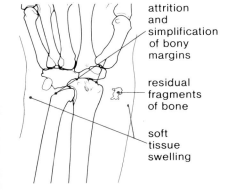

attrition and simplification of bony margins

residual fragments of bone

soft tissue swelling

23.17

Case 34 Nail-patella syndrome

A 47-year-old man presented with painful knees. Examination revealed absence of thumb nails and small patellae, and radiographs showed the typical features of the nail-patella syndrome (Fig. 23.57).

Case 35 Acne arthralgia

A patient with severe adolescent acne conglobata presented with a mild arthralgia of the hips and knees (Fig. 23.58). The ESR was slightly elevated, but other investigations were normal. The condition slowly resolved over the next few months, during which the acne also improved.

Case 36 'Long-leg arthropathy'

A 24-year-old lady presented with pain in the back and in the right knee. Examination showed a marked discrepancy of leg length (Fig. 23.59). The back pain was thought to be related to the scoliosis. The right knee was tender, and contained a moderate synovial effusion. A diagnosis of 'long-leg arthropathy' was made.

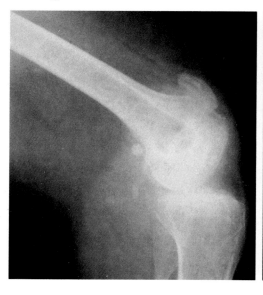
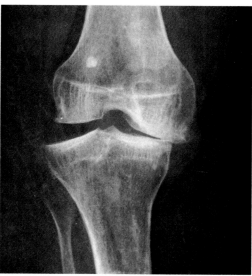
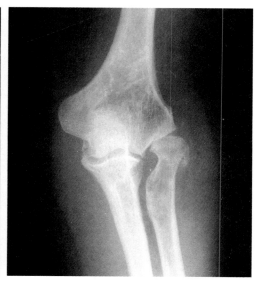

Fig. 23.57 Nail-patella syndrome. The knee radiographs (left and middle) demonstrate an abnormally high, small patella, dysplastic femoral condyles and osteo-arthritis of the medial compartment. The radiograph of the elbow shows hypoplasia of the capitellum with lateral sublaxation of the radial head (right). Degenerative arthritis is present at the radio-capitellar joint and there is secondary cubitus valgus.

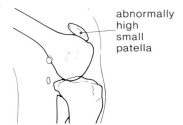
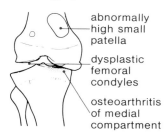
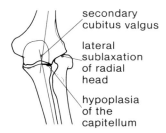

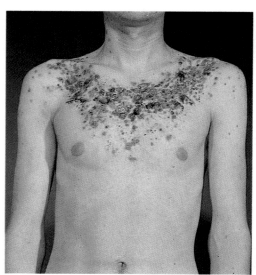
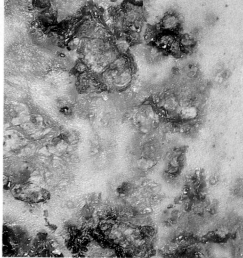
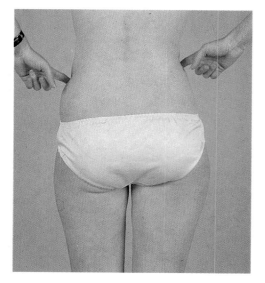

Fig. 23.58 Acne arthralgia: severe adolescent acne conglobata. Courtesy of Dr D.G.I. Scott.

Fig. 23.59 Long-leg arthropathy: examination revealing a difference in leg length.

Index